Notice

This book has been withdrawn from health library stock for one or more of the following reasons:

- There is a more recent edition of the title
- The book is more than 10 years old and more current material on the topic is available

You are therefore strongly advised to check any information contained within this book before using it to inform patient care

Clinical Orthopaedic Diagnosis

This book bagged "The Best Book Award" on National level, awarded by Bombay Orthopaedic Society

Clinical Orthopaedic Diagnosis

Second Edition

Sureshwar Pandey & Anil Kumar Pandey

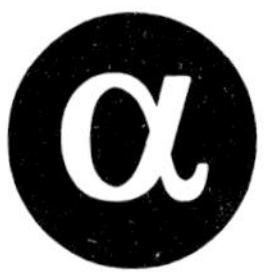

Alpha Science International Ltd.
Pangbourne England

Sureshwar Pandey MBBS(Hons) MS(Gen) FICS FIAMS MS(Orth) MACFAS FACS FNAMS
Professor Emeritus University of Ranchi

Anil Kumar Pandey MBBS CORM PhD(Orth) MAMS
Director and Consultant Surgeon Ramjanam Sulakshana Institute of Orthopaedics and Research, Ranchi

Alpha Science International Ltd.
P.O. Box 4067, Pangbourne RG8 8UT, UK

ISBN 1-84265-145-5

Printed in India

Printed at: Gopsons Papers Ltd, A-14, Sector 60, Noida

to
the fond memory of my beloved parents
Sulakshana Pandey
and
Ramjanam Pandey
who were, are, and will be
always with me to love,
teach and guide

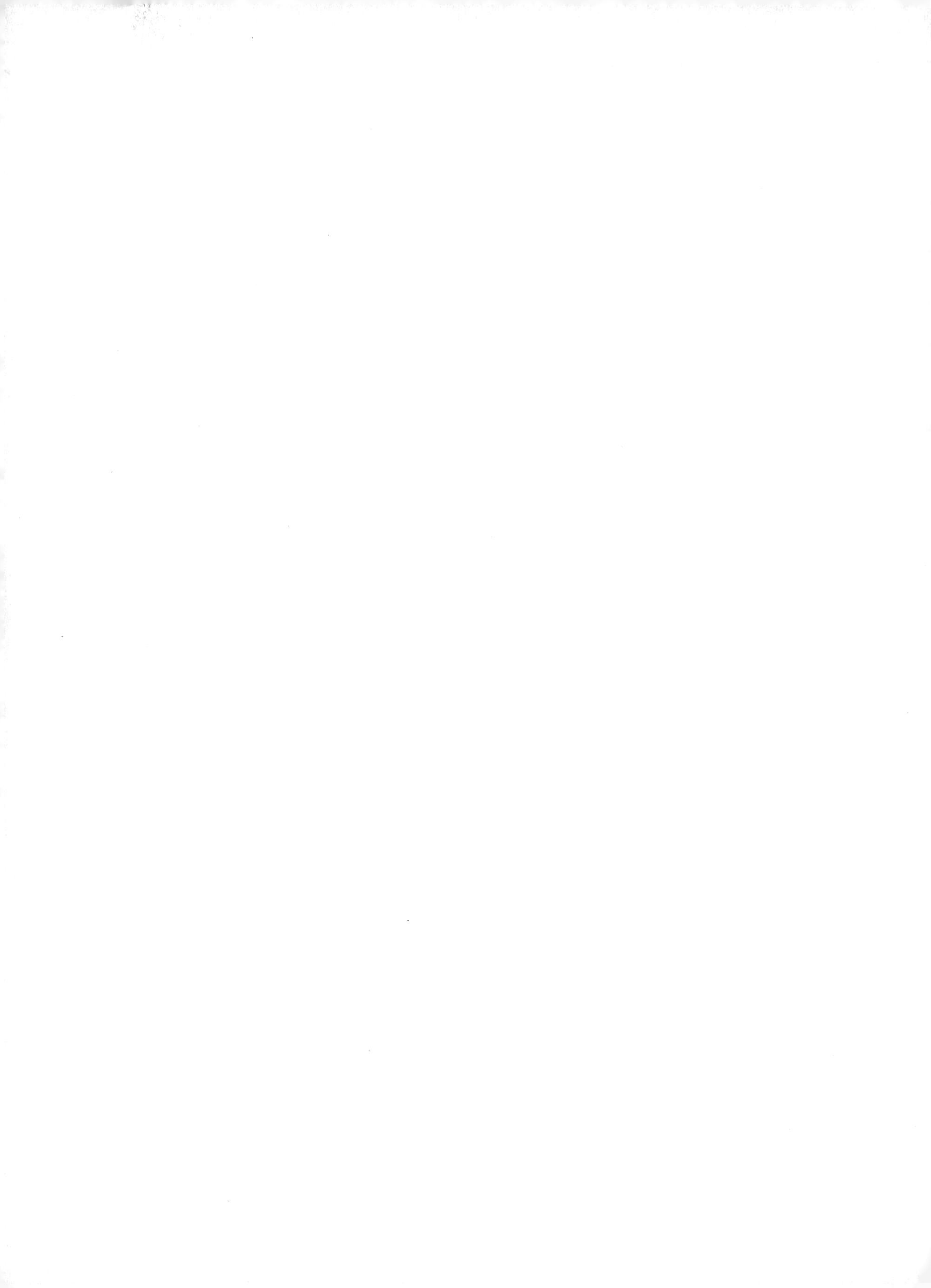

Foreword to the First Edition

Professor S Pandey has undertaken a very worthwhile project in writing a book on *Clinical Orthopaedic Diagnosis.* The importance of proper clinical examination needs no emphasis. All investigations are based on clues provided by proper and systematic clinical examination and a logical interpretation of the findings.

Unfortunately, there has been a lack of standard textbooks giving a detailed and systematic approach to a methodical clinical examination of orthopaedic patients, including correct interpretation of physical signs provided by such examination. Professor Pandey has produced a textbook which embodies all the methods utilised in a systematic clinical examination of the motor skeletal system.

By providing relevant line-drawings, which are very helpful in understanding clinical features and also providing charts that include a step by step interpretation of the clinical findings, he has made a proper clinical approach—logical and simple.

I feel confident that the approach he has adopted in eliciting and interpreting clinical features will be most useful not only to undergraduate and postgraduate students but even to practitioners so that they can look upon this book as a guide to reduce incidents of errors in examination.

I heartily congratulate Professor Pandey on this effort.

***Padmabhushan* Dr B Mukhopadhyay**
MBBS (Hons), MCh Ortho (L'Pool)
FRCS (Lond), FNAMS
Emeritus Professor, University of Patna
Saidpur Road, Patna 800004, India

Foreword to the Second Edition

The second edition of *Clinical Orthopaedic Diagnosis* is eagerly awaited by all those who had the opportunity to study the First Edition.

This is decidedly one of the most comprehensive presentation of a subject which has so far failed to receive the attention of practicing orthopaedic surgeons.

The book is oriented to help clinical diagnosis of all variety of orthopaedic cases—traumatic and non-traumatic. Its illustrations provide visual images and help in easy recognition of various conditions.

The second edition has been completely revised and additional chapters added to make it more comprehensive and up-to-date. I have no hesitation in recommending this book as one of the bedside volumes for all practicing orthopaedic surgeons and trainees. They can easily look up the contents of this book when faced with difficult problems of clinical diagnosis and the systematic manner in which investigations can be carried out in their proper schedule. This indeed is a useful addition to orthopaedic literature.

Padmabhushan **Dr B Mukhopadhyay**
MBBS (Hons), MCh Ortho (L'Pool)
FRCS (Lond), FNAMS
Emeritus Professor, University of Patna
Saidpur Road, Patna 800004, India

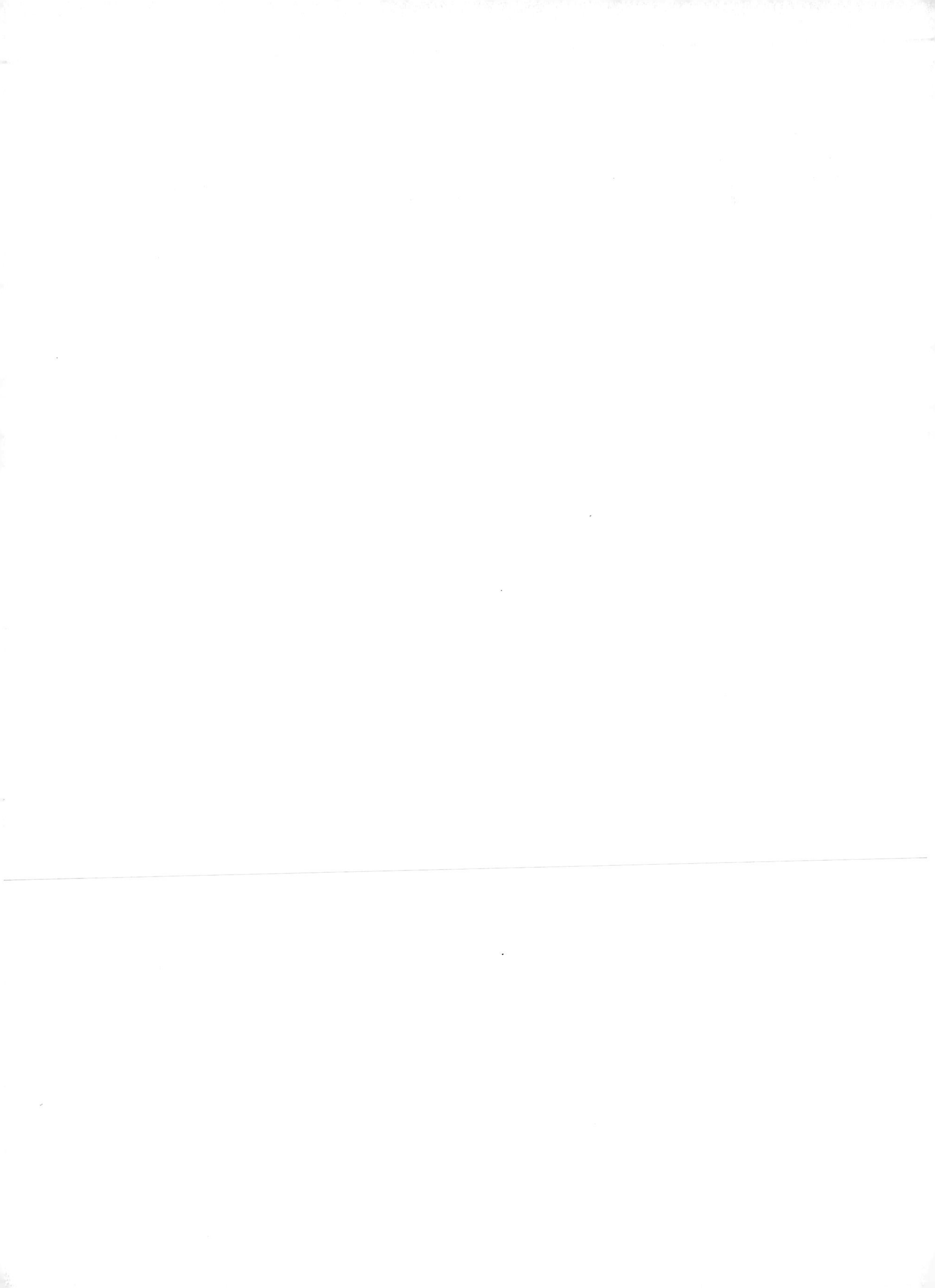

Preface to the Second Edition

"A lamp never lightens the other lamp unless it is burning itself"—this burning is mandatory in bringing out any further edition of any book—this has been literally done for this second edition.

The whole-hearted appreciation and acceptance of this book from every nook and corner, not only from India, but also from various countries of the world, stimulated us to bring out the second/international edition of this book.

The basic standard methodology cannot be changed, however, we have tried to update it judiciously as far as possible.

While examining the postgraduates (Diploma, MS, DNB, FRACS), I felt the necessity of adding few more chapters—and in that direction three chapters have been added in this edition: (1) Joints, (2) Syndromes related to Orthopaedics and Traumatology, and (3) Ulcers of Leg.

Considering the feedback from the students and teachers, the analysis and explanation of the symptoms and signs have been more elaborated.

Clinical photographs and the line-drawings form the backbone for such a book, which help in making the acquaintances with the clinical conditions easy and quick with lasting effects. Hence more clinical photographs have been added.

The comments in the Journal of Bone and Joint Surgery (Br) 1997 Vol 79B p 345, clearly reflects the depth and clinical dimensions of the book which has become very much in hot demand. The book has proved to be companion to not only the students, but the practitioners and teachers, who have preferred to keep it on the "out-patient clinic-desk".

Advances in technology, mirage of hardware, and dependency on the computer have been the driving forces in the practice of orthopaedics in the second half of the twentieth century. Unfortunately, the fertile, smart and sparkling brain of our young orthopaedists and traumatologists are slowly becoming the slave of computer, getting gradually distanced from the touch and feel of the patients, bubbling with the clinical features hard to be truly reflected on the computer screen. We are craving for the 3D pictures on the computer screen, but depriving our probing eyes and sensitive fingers to really see, feel and appreciate them in the body—no wonder *robots* are planning to replace us.

Unfortunately art and practice of medicine as a whole and orthopaedics in particular is increasingly changing into 'business' making the 'medicare' costly in spiral fashion. Most of the investigations (which are much costly today) can be cut down to the really needed ones by thorough examination of the patients.

If you will learn well, you will examine well, you will treat well, you will operate well, you will evaluate well—success will be yours and the ultimate all round gainful will be your patient who is "the centre of the medical universe around which all our works revolve and towards which all efforts trend"—JB Murphy (1857-1916).

We deeply acknowledge the encouragements of the students, trainees and teachers from all over the world, who have whole-heartedly accepted the FIRST edition and its two successive REPRINTS in such a short time.

We very humbly and deeply acknowledge the huge number of source books and the articles, which we have consulted to enlighten us at various steps in preparation of this book. We beg sincere apology for not mentioning their name due to paucity of time and space.

My (SP's) FAMILY—my loving wife, sons (Dr Anil, Arun, Akhil) and their wives (Dr Pushpa, Asha, Sandhya) continued to tolerate my eccentricities all through the period of preparing this Second/international Edition—I simply cannot repay their debt. My sweet grandchildren (Pallavi, Shivam, Vaishnavi, Shruti, Saumya and Satyam) continuously proved to be the real source of pleasure and encouragement in the tense and depressing moments. God bless them always...

"To study the phenomenon of disease without books is to sail an unchanted sea, while to study book without patients is not to go to sea at all..."—Sir William Osler (1849-1919).

Sureshwar Pandey
Anil Kumar Pandey

Preface to the First Edition

Orthopaedic practice demands repetitive and complex decision-making. All decisions are necessarily influenced by non-scientific considerations, such as limited facilities, patients' non-compliance, and financial constraints, as well as the current limitations of orthopaedic science. Despite these impediments we all strive towards accuracy in our decision-making. Accurate clinical diagnosis forms the basis of successful management of any ailment. No doubt, the development of a sound judgement is largely a matter of experience; yet one must remember the words of Sir Astley Cooper, "Nothing is known in our profession by guess, and I do not believe that from the first dawn of medical science to the present moment a single correct idea has ever emanated from conjecture..., there is no short road to knowledge." The great Indian surgeon Sushruta has also warned against diagnosing a disease merely on speculation. He gave explicit instructions regarding exploration of the history of the disease, thorough examination (inspection, palpation, auscultation, etc.) and analysis of the symptoms and signs, before coming to a conclusion.

The immense importance of systematic clinical examination cannot be overemphasised. No one can be familiar with the clinical signs and their interpretation in a short period or just by going through the text. A rigorous apprenticeship is mandatory to learn the clinical methodology step by step, lest a snap diagnosis based on a cursory examination may prove to be disastrous. Whatsoever may be the advances in the field of investigation procedures, these must remain the supplement to and not the substitute of thorough clinical examination.

With this backdrop, an attempt has been made to further enhance the importance of 'clinical methodology' in orthopaedics. The effort has been made to create an atmosphere of positive and practical approach towards diagnosing the clinical conditions on a sound basis, so that therapy becomes easy and less complex. No patient can be examined just for one system, rather it should be the total examination of the patient. However, for the osteoarticular and neuromuscular affections a more detailed examination than usual is necessary, such as assessment of movements, length disparities, neuromuscular status, etc.

A knowledge of clinical anatomy is quite essential for any orthopaedic student, trainee or even surgeon. To cover this, a brief description of the relevant clinical anatomy of the region dealt with was thought to be essential, and it has been given at the beginning of each chapter. Wherever it was necessary, a note on the basic physiology concerning that zone has been added. Quick and fairly clear conception of the subject can be had by going through a tabular form of description, which has been given whatever deemed to be essential. Reminder of the 'key diagnostic points' at the end of the chapters would help the clinicians come to a quick diagnosis, the trainees/residents to learn methods of elimination, and the students/examinees quickly revise the subject.

With due apology to the stalwarts, whose names could not be included due to my ignorance, an attempt has been made at the end of the book to recall the noted works of the pioneers of orthopaedics.

The manuscript has been revised through the scrutiny of more than seven batches of postgraduate and undergraduate students in orthopaedics and the project is the result of their inspiration, encouragement and criticism. However, a lot of improvements and modifications have to be done in future editions after reviewing the frank criticisms and remarks of the readers—the real watchdogs.

I am deeply obliged to my revered teacher, *Padmabhushan* Prof Emeritus B Mukhopadhyay, who lit the lamp of knowledge in my mind and soul. And also to my senior and contemporary colleagues all over the country and abroad, like Emeritus Prof N Tsuyama (Tokyo), Prof SM Tuli, Prof PT Rao, Prof DP Baksi, Prof NS Laud, Dr BB Joshi, Prof RR Ganguli, Prof RC Ram, Prof SV Sharma, Prof RP Singh, Prof KM Pathi, Prof NK Agarwal, Prof K Ono (Osaka), Prof T Koshino (Yokohama), Prof B Helal (London), Prof K Bose (Singapore), Prof JM Martorell (Barcelona), Dr R Bauze (Adelaide), and others who helped me to clear my confusion at several stages. I did derive benefit, pleasure, and profit from their stimulating exchange of ideas, which I very humbly and deeply acknowledge.

My colleagues, Prof RL Rajak, Prof B Alam, Prof HN Sinha, Prof AK Mishra, Prof KP Pandey, Dr PD Singh, Dr KN Jha, Dr SS Jha, Dr RC Mishra, Dr SN Sinha, and others with whom I have been privileged to work through the years and have helped by providing healthy criticism, I am indebted to all of them.

The tiresome work of proofreading has been ably assisted by my son Dr Anil, daughter-in-law Dr Pushpa and the fleet of my very dear postgraduate students, especially Drs SP Bhagat, Awadhesh Singh and Sanjeeva Kumar, whose help I cannot forget.

My family—my loving wife, sons (Dr Anil, Arun and Akhil) and their wives (Dr Pushpa, Asha and Sandhya) tolerated many of my eccentricities all through the period of preparation of this book. I cannot repay the debt. My grandchildren (Pallavi, Shivam, Vaishnavi, Shruti and Saumya) proved to be the real source of pleasure in tense moments. God bless them.

And finally, I sincerely acknowledge the help of Dr Ravi for preparing the line-drawings and Mr Ajit Kumar Shukla for typing the manuscript.

Sureshwar Pandey

Introductory Comments

This textbook authored by Prof S Pandey contains a large number of Orthopaedic diseases from children to adult ones. He spent really many years to collect all these materials to complete this marvellous book. From general common diseases to even quite special rare diseases and deformities, this book is dealing with orthopaedic disorders of many kinds. One can have very clear and concise picture of orthopaedic conditions described in this book.

The readers can easily understand and refer to the contents of this book presented in simple and lucid manner, especially the detailed instructional explanations on various diseases, tests, diagnosis strategies, etc. This book is ***sure to be suitable to be kept on the desk of the Outpatient Clinics to refer at every moment of questions.***

I really strongly recommend this book to undergraduate and postgraduate students and trainees who are interested in orthopaedics.

Tomohisa Koshino MD PhD
Professor and Director
Department of Orthopaedic Surgery
Yokohama City University School of Medicine and
President, University Hospital
Yokohama, 236-0004, Japan

Professor Pandey's 'Clinical Orthopaedic Diagnosis' arouses scepticism against fragmentation, so-called 'subspecialities of orthopaedics'. His suggestion for a "total orthopaedist" and comprehensive knowledge of the whole musculoskeletal system as the key point to make accurate decision in any situation deserves appreciation.

"The whole art of medicine is in observation, as the old motto goes, but to educate the eye to see, the ear to hear and the finger to feel takes time" (William Osler, 1906). We really hope this book would provide guidelines in favour of the saying, "teach him how to observe, give him plenty of facts to observe and make him proficient in his art through constant contact with diseases", and prove precious for those who want to know.

Congratulations for your great success in publishing such an excellent textbook—"Clinical Orthopaedic Diagnosis". I am very much impressed by the fact that it covers comprehensively such a wide area of Orthopaedic expertise yet implies concisely the wisdom of orthopaedics. You have presented so precious cases of wide variation...

I am very proud to have been working with such a wonderful orthopaedist and scholar.

Keiro Ono MD PhD
Ex-Professor and Chairman, Dept. of Orthopaedic Surgery
Osaka University Medical School, Osaka
Professor Emeritus, Osaka University Medical School
Director, Osaka Kosei-Nenkin Hospital, Osaka 553, Japan

I am indeed impressed with this book—"Clinical Orthopaedic Diagnosis" authored by Professor Sureshwar Pandey. It is a unique book on clinical methodology available today. It contains the wisdom of orthopaedics and traumatology as a whole, with an emphasis on the problems in tropical countries and developing world. Clinical methodology is quite clear supported by superb line-drawings and numerous clinical photographs.

The descriptions are simple and straightforward, but at the same time quite informative.

I am sure, those who are interested in orthopaedic surgery—students, practitioners or teachers—will find this book quite useful at all steps. ***It has great potential to be accepted all over the world.***

Chairuddin Rasjad MD PhD
Professor of Orthopaedic Surgery
Chairman, Department of Surgery
International Cooperation
Faculty of Medicine
Hasanuddin University
Ujung Pandang, Indonesia

Professor Sureshwar Pandey has accomplished a unique feat of collecting, analysing, and categorising the voluminous clinical material he managed to observe and treat during four decades of his active professional career. He has been a great enthusiast of proper clinical methods which are so essential for clinicians and society in general in the less privileged half of the world. A rational clinical assessment would help to employ the most appropriate and cost-effective newer modalities of investigations which are very expensive by any standards.

Most of the active orthopaedists in the Indian subcontinent deal with similar rich clinical material however it is to the credit of Prof. Pandey to put it in a fashion to be understood by any student and practitioner of orthopaedics.

Though extensive strides have been made in the diagnostic tools in the last two decades (almost threatening to replace the humane touch by robotics) however these serve best on the shoulders of the observations made by the clinical methods, Prof Pandey has re-emphasised for the newer generations. There is no substitute for clinical observations made by 'listening', 'looking', 'feeling', 'moving', 'measuring', 'percussing' and 'auscultating'. Clinical methods should be a way of Orthopaedics as is Yoga the way of life.

Though no compendium is complete and perfect however Prof Pandey deserves congratulations and gratitudes from all students of orthopaedics for his tremendous effort. I can assure Prof Pandey that he will cherish and continue to have a sense of accomplishment that he is leaving behind a monumental document for the posterity.

SM Tuli MS PhD FAMS
Former Director, Institute of Medical Sciences
Benaras Hindu University
Former Professor and Head, Dept. of Orthopaedics,
Benaras Hindu University and
University of Delhi

The Sureshwar Pandey's book "Clinical Orthopaedic Diagnosis" is a boon to the postgraduate students and practicing orthopaedic surgeons. It has also helped me in teaching the postgraduate students. His collection of clinical photographs is amazing. The language is so simple that Indian students can easily understand the clinical problems in orthopaedics. Postgraduate students in my institution are using it day in and day out and have expressed great satisfaction. Some have stated that they have passed MS (Ortho) and DNB (Ortho) because of this book. I am sure this new edition will be an exciting one.

Prof. GS Kulkarni MS MS(Ortho) FICS
Professor of Orthopaedics
Director, Postgraduate Institute of Swasthiyog Pratishthan, Miraj

I am glad to know that the second edition of "Clinical Orthopaedic Diagnosis" written by Prof Sureshwar Pandey will be published soon. The style of writing this book has got special characteristic features. Brief anatomical consideration at the beginning of the chapter, essential classification of diseases and trauma, detailed clinical tests of different diseases including those prevalent in the developing countries are the special aspects of this book. The excellent illustrations, tabular presentations of diagnostic features with keynotes at the end of each chapter will make the subject lucid to the undergraduate and postgraduate students and the practicing Orthopaedic Surgeons for their quick revision. The art of masterly presentation of clinical acumen of different diseases for their interpretation are important clues for its wide acceptance to the reader. The author deserves warm congratulation in his endeavour.

Dr. DP Baksi MS FRCS MS(Orth) PhD(Orth) FAMS
Ex-Professor and Head, Department of Orthopaedic Surgery
NRS Medical College, Calcutta
President, Indian Orthopaedic Association

It has been unique privilege for me to write my comments on the masterpiece work "Clinical Orthopaedic Diagnosis" by Prof Sureshwar Pandey. Prof Pandey, an eminent teacher in the field of Orthopaedics has utilised his wide knowledge of the subject to simplify the problems of Orthopaedic teaching, for which till now no other substitute was available. It is being, and will be always appreciated by the postgraduate and undergraduate students, orthopaedic surgeons, and none the less the teachers.

The text and the self-explanatory illustrations are superb and exemplary.

Prof P Tejeswar Rao MBBS (Hons) FRCS (Edin) FRCS (London) MCh Orth (L'Pool)
Ex-Professor and Head
Department of Orthopaedics, SCB Medical College, Cuttack
Ex-Director of Medical Education
Past President of Indian Orthopaedic Association
Medical Road, Ranihat, Cuttack, Orissa, India

I am indeed pleased to read your new book "Clinical Orthopaedic Diagnosis". I must confess that this is one of the concise, informative and complete principles on Clinical Orthopaedic and Diagnosis. The illustrations used in your book have clarity, the attempt to elicit clinical aids with precise analysis is noteworthy. I am certain, your book will be one of the best clinical aid for postgraduate students or young orthopaedic surgeons who can utilise it for clinical orthopaedic practice. I am certain, the book has potential of finding worldwide acceptance.

Prof NS Laud
Chief, Orthopaedic Surgery and Traumatology
LTM Medical College and Hospital, Mumbai
Past President, Indian Orthopaedic Association

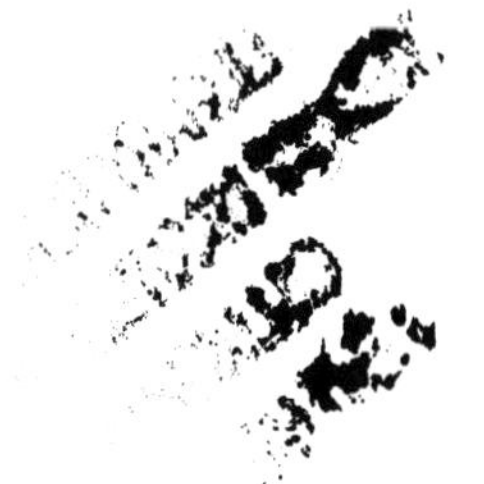

Contents

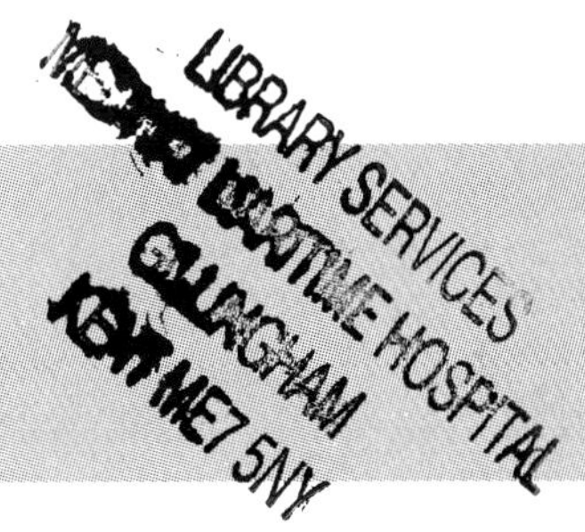

Plate 1

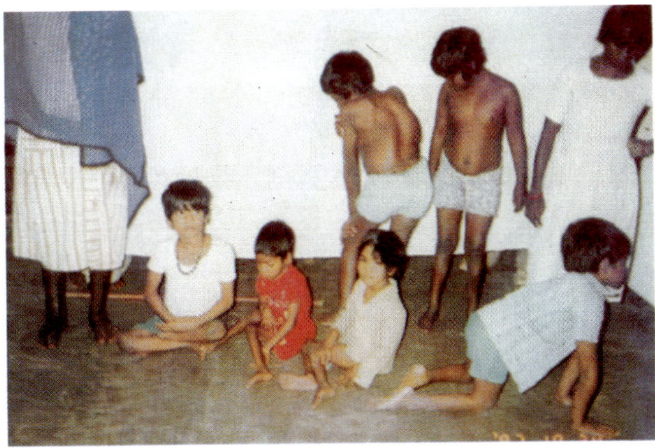

Fig. 1: Residual polio-paralysis in the different regions of the body of these children

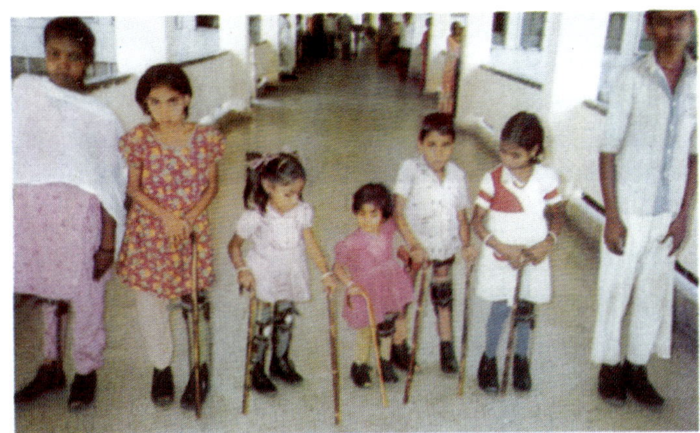

Fig. 2: A group of polio patients in the process of rehabilitation after surgical corrective and reconstructive procedures

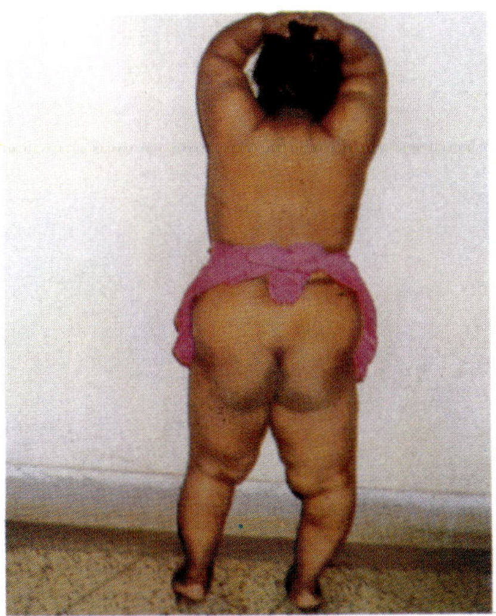

Fig. 3: Cushing syndrome

Plate 2

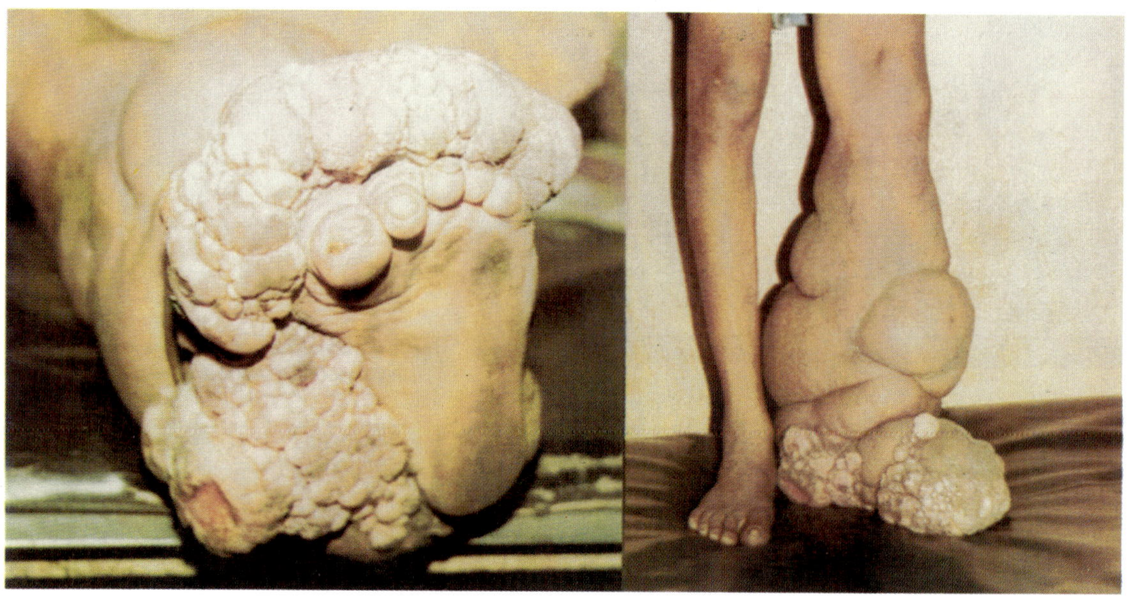

Figs 4 and 5: Huge elephantiasis of the leg and foot. Note that the toes and the sole are completely spared (tortoise foot)

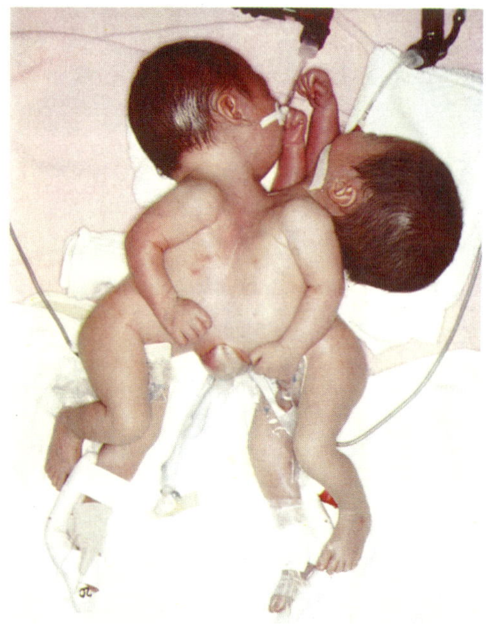

Fig. 6: Simmese twins

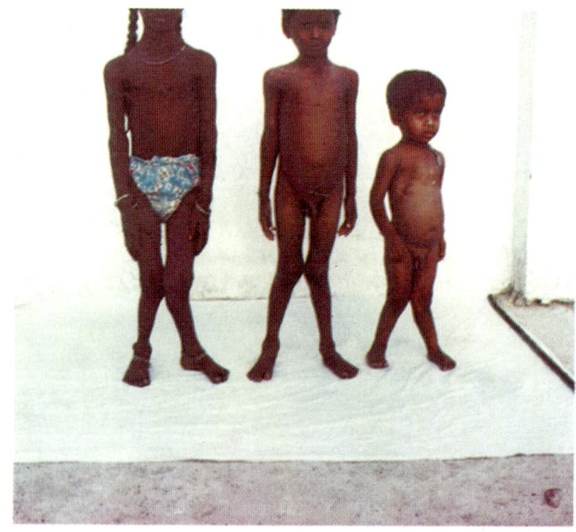

Fig. 7: Rachetic bilateral genu valgum in all three own brothers (2) and sister (1).

Plate 3

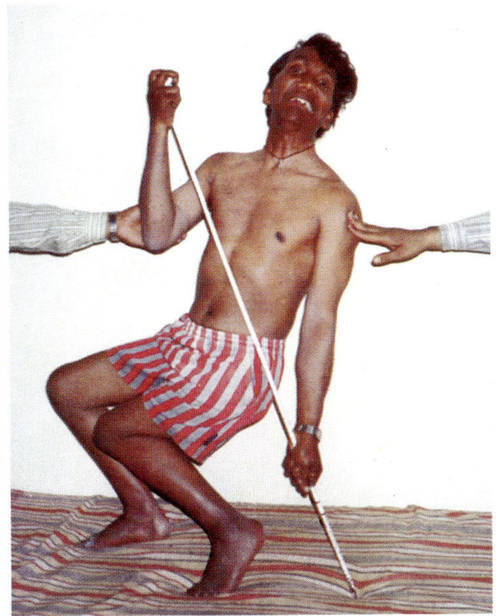

Fig. 8: Advanced patient of ankylosing spondylitis with fixed hips, knees, spine (including cervical spine), temporomandibular joints (he can not open his mouth for eating or chewing, and is more or less on liquid and semiliquid diets). He is bed-ridden for last 17 years. He can hardly stand like this with the support

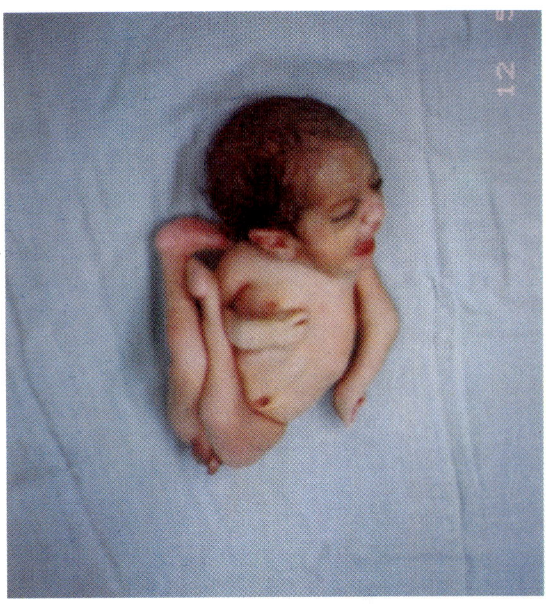

Fig. 9: Arthrogryposis multiplex congenita with deformities at hips, knees, ankles, feet, spine, shoulders, elbows, hands, heart, etc.

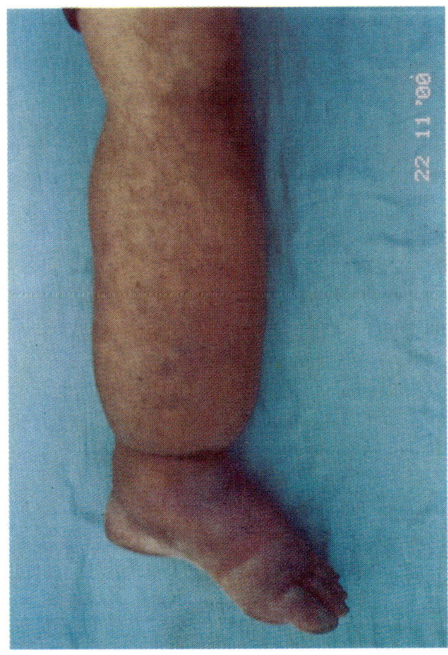

Fig. 10: Filarial elephantiasis — without fissuring, nodulations, ulcerations

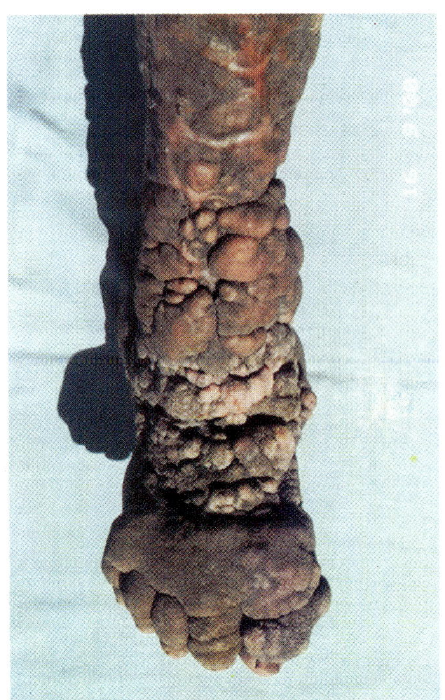

Fig. 11A

Plate 4

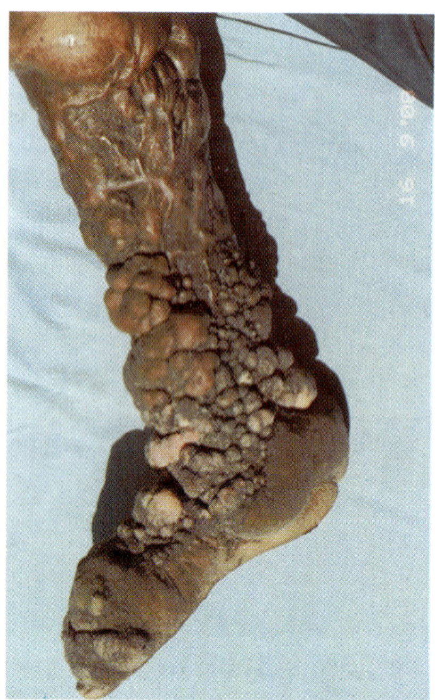

Figs 11A and B: Advanced filarial elephantiasis with numerous fissurings, nodulations, keratinizations, ulcerations etc. One attempt of surgical excision and skin grafting has been done with failure

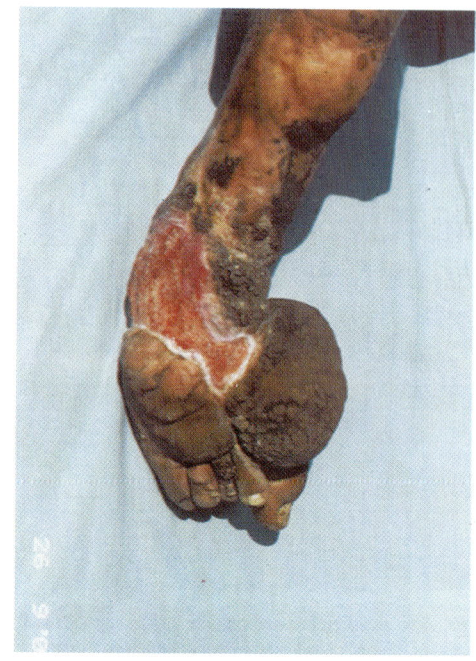

Fig. 12: Post-traumatic elephantiasis of leg and foot

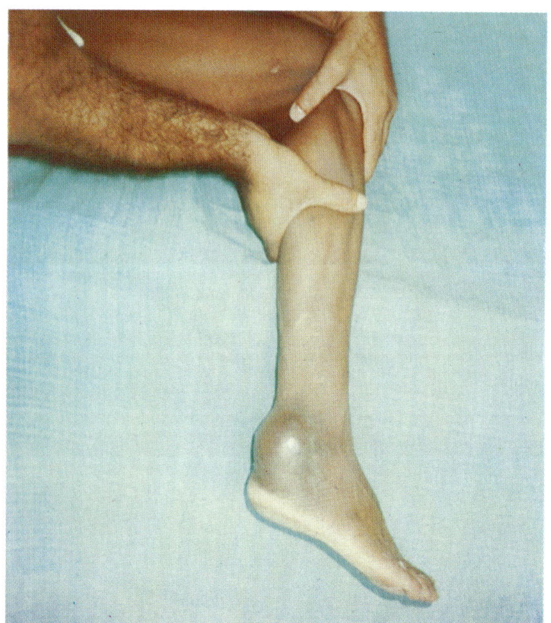

Fig. 13: Osteomyelitis of calcaneum with collection

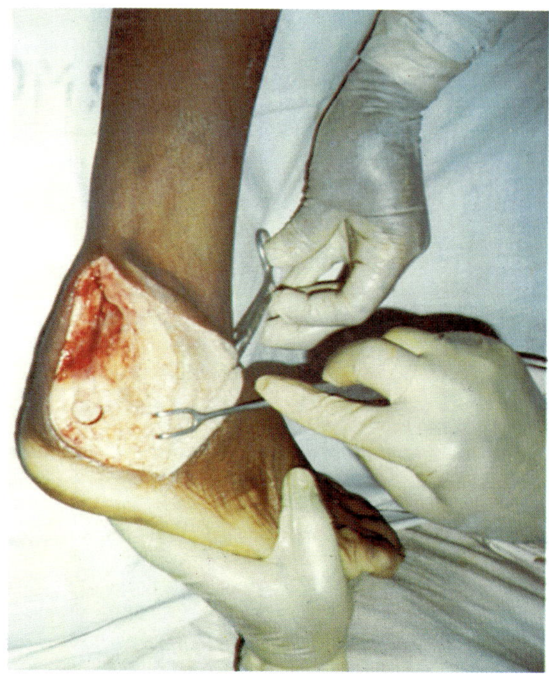

Fig. 14: Post-traumatic elephantiasis of leg and foot—showing the sequestrum sitting at the mouth of hole in osteomyelitic calcaneum

Plate 5

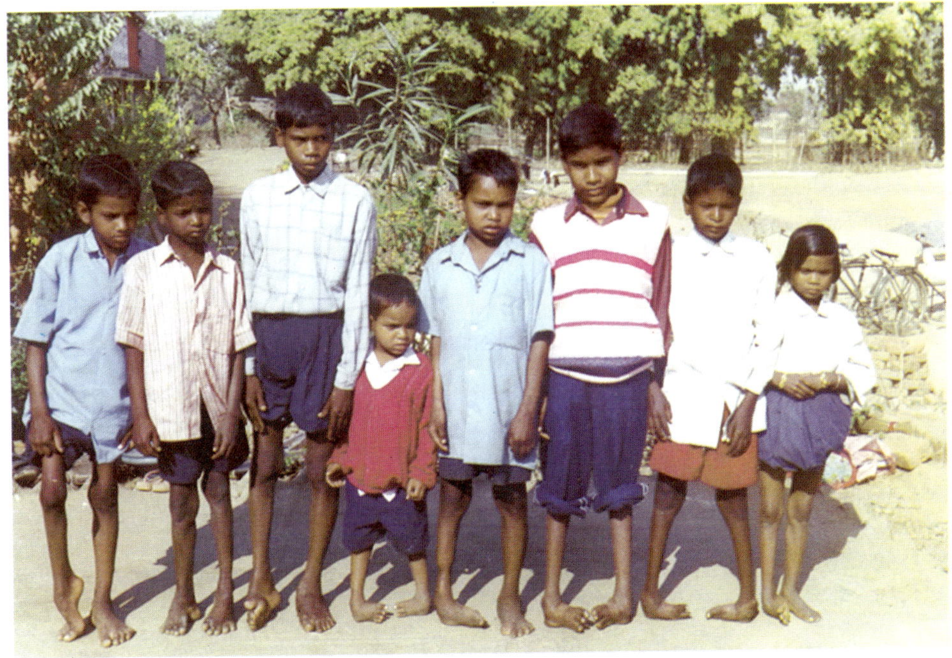

Fig. 15: A group of children with neglected clubfoot

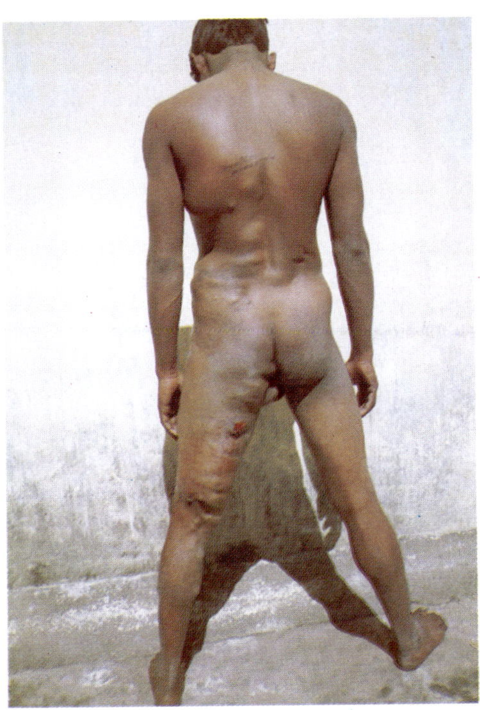

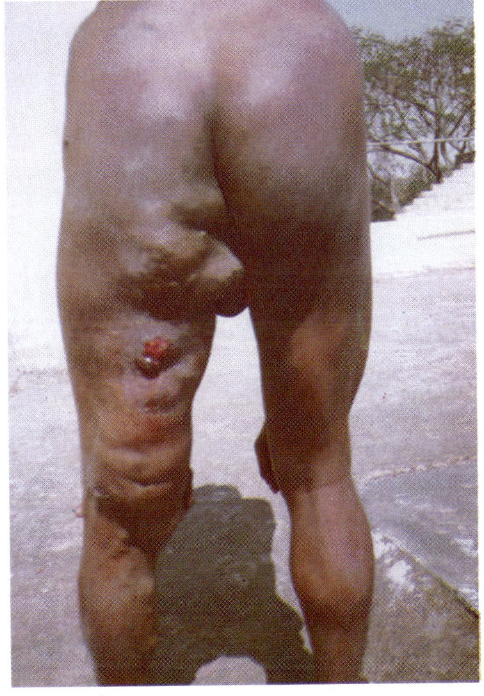

Figs 16 A and B: Extensive large vessel haemangioma

Plate 6

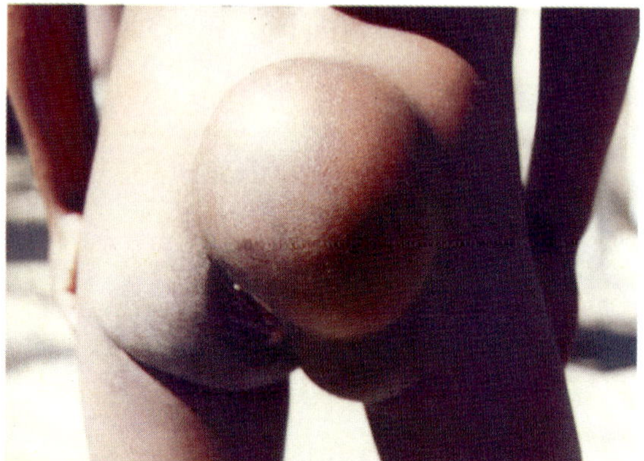

Fig. 17: Lipoma from sacrum

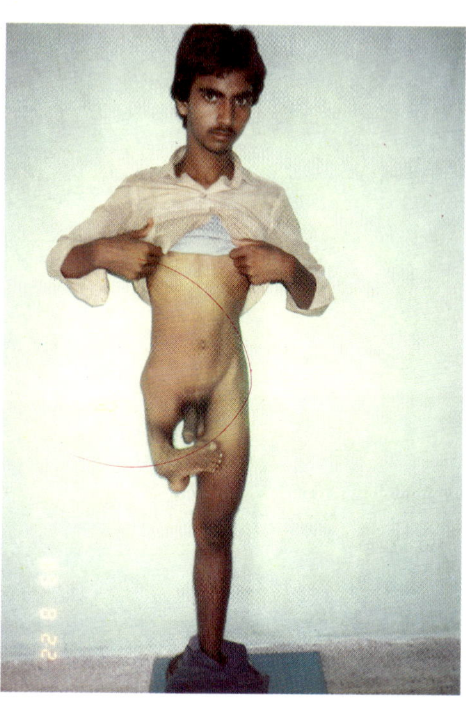

Fig. 18: Congenital absence of lower 3/4th of femur and almost of whole of leg bones on right side

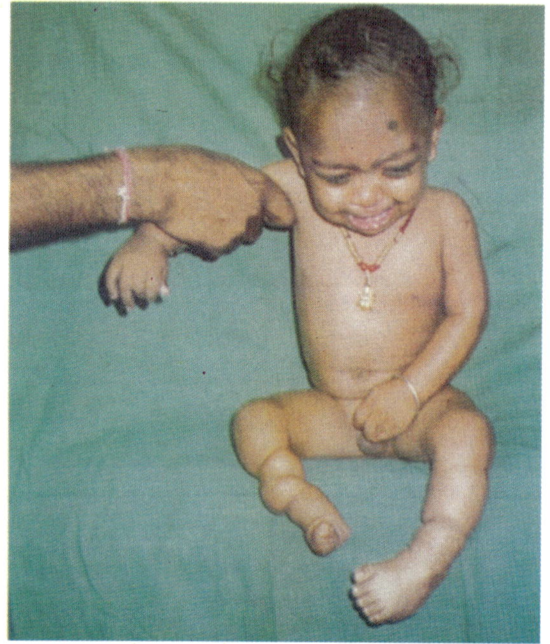

Fig. A1.3: Multiple congenital constriction rings in the legs with ill-developed right foot and associated clubfoot on left side

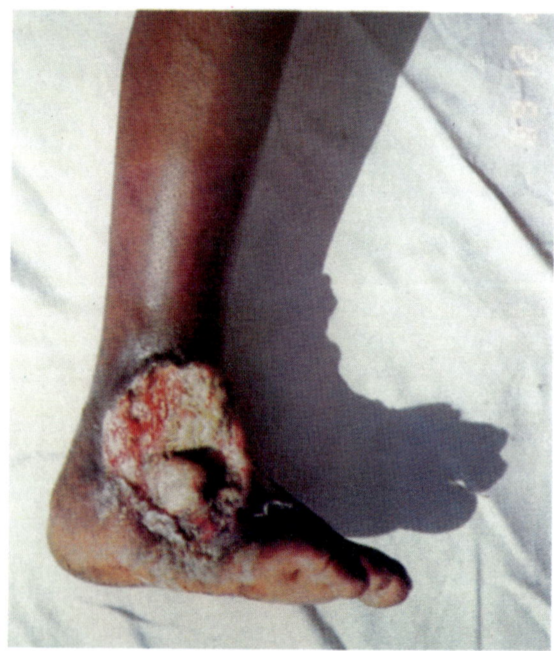

Fig. A2.12: Marjolin's ulcer developed over the post-traumatic scar

Plate 7

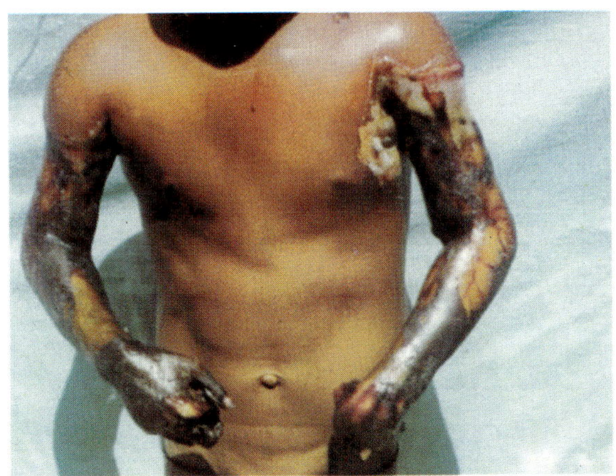

Fig. A2.13: Typical electrical burn of both upper limbs

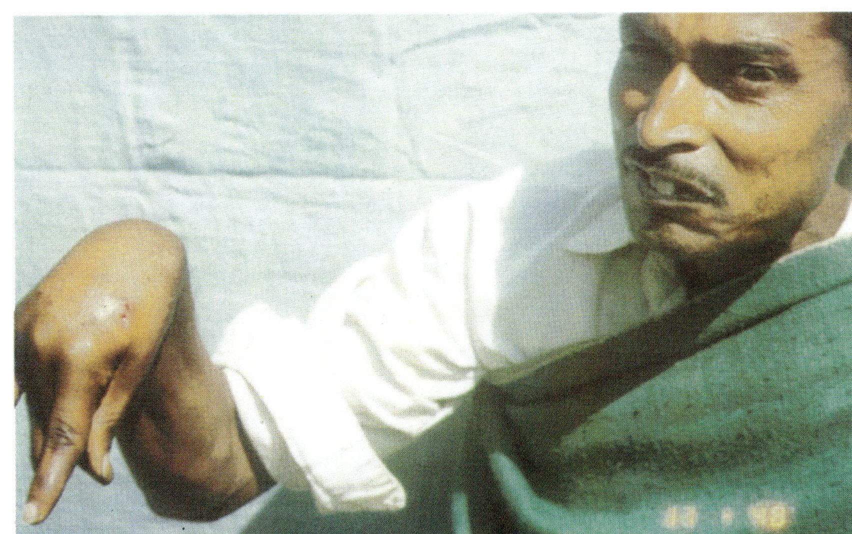

Fig. A2.14: Typical facial expression in tetanus (risus sardonicus). Note the tetanic spasm in the right hand and fingers. On the dorsum of the same hand there is the redish source prick wound

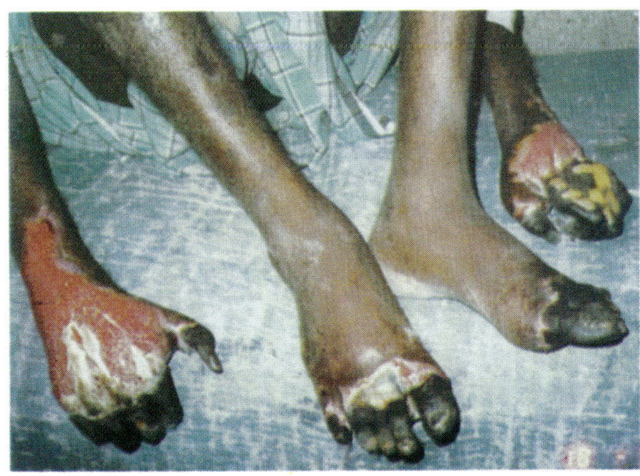

Fig. A2.15: Bilateral almost symmetrical gangrene of both hands and feet due to toxicity of an indegenous medicine

1 Introduction

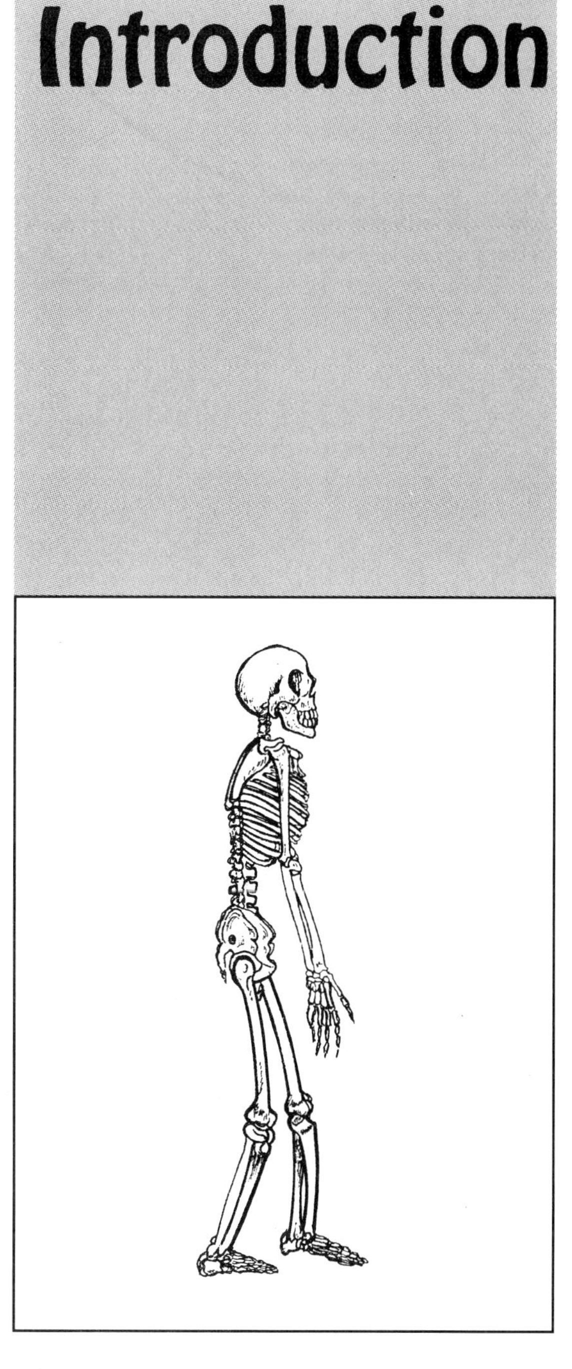

मिथ्या दृष्टा विकाराहि दुराख्याता स्तथैवच।
तथा दुष्परिमृष्टाष्च मोहयेयुष्चिकित्सकम्।।

Not taking a correct history and not doing a thorough examination by inspection and palpation can mislead the physician, in achieving the goal,

तस्मात् भिषक् कार्यं चिकीर्षुः प्राक कार्य समारम्भात्।
परीक्षया केवलं परीक्ष्यं परीक्षाय कर्म समारभेत कर्त्रुम्।।

Therefore a practitioner keen to carry out any procedure should first of all examine and thoroughly investigate the same before venturing on the actual treatment.

(SUSHRUTA c. 500 BC.)

Medicare represents the essence of life experiences, the pinnacle of education and the epitome of empathy and compassion. It is a mission to heal and to comfort, and to further dignify our fellow human beings.

HISTORY

The word 'orthopaedy' (derived from French word orthopédie and Greek word orthos+ paidion) came into existence, signifying an art of correcting deformities in children, by Nicolas Andry, a French Physician, in the year 1741 who designed orthopaedic oncography in his book entitled—'L' orthopaedic Ou L'art de prevenir et corriger dans les enfants, les difformite's du corps' in 1741. English translation of the title of Andry's book published in 1743, reads 'Orthopaedia: or the art of correcting and preventing deformities' in children ...... as may easily be put in practice by parents themselves, and all such as one employed in educating the children. The word 'orthopaedy' comprises of two Greek words—*orthos* (meaning straight) + *paidion* (meaning child). However, this speciality today, is none the less, "Orthogerontics". Frankly speaking, unless specified, all considerations in medical practice centres around the adults and middle age (40 to 60 years—mediatries) however with constant increase in the life expectancy, the orthopaedic and trauma problems of old age (more than 60 years of age—geriatrics) are non the less, rather more, demanding. Of course the orthopaedic problems of children (paediatrics) definitely deserve special considerations. Today orthopaedics has grown into a multifaceted discipline and is now one of the most comprehensive specialisation in the field of medical practice, leaving far behind the art and craft of traditional bone setters.

In order to support the curvatures of the spine, a supportive corset, made of punched iron sheet was first used by Ambroise Pare and Gersdorff (1530) had described an iron splint for stretching contractures, still it was not until after the First World War that the principles of rehabilitation were clearly included in the arena of orthopaedics.

In the western world, Hugh Owen Thomas (1834-1891) of Liverpool, propounded several fundamental principles of orthopaedics. These were later put on a sound footing by his nephew, Sir Robert Jones (1857-1933), who also concerned himself with different operative techniques in this speciality. Discoveries of anaesthesia (Crawford Long of Athens, Georgia, 1842); antisepsis (Joseph Lister 1867); fundamental research on bacteria by Louis Pasteur (1822-1895); and X-ray (Roentgen 1895) led to a phenomenally rapid evolution, of surgery as a whole, and orthopaedics in particular.

A probe into ancient Indian literature reveals that knowledge regarding the skeletal system has been mentioned in the three different systems of Atreya, Sushruta and Vagbhata. Even in the Vedic period, the craft of orthopaedic surgery was of an admirably high standard. In the oldest Aryan literature of the Rigveda, we find evidence of the use of suitable artificial limbs as substitutes for limbs accidently lost in war. (Rigveda, 15th, R, 1st Mandal, 176). In the above mentioned passage, the priest Agastya, requests the surgeon Ashwini to prepare an artificial limb for the queen Vishpla, which should be lighter than that of a bird's wing and made of steel.

Hua Tuo (141-203AD), in China performed many kinds of surgical operations, such as leparotomy, amputation of limb etc. He introduced general anaesthesia to China using the Chinese herb *ma-fei-san*, along with wine as the anaesthetic.

Today, orthopaedics has emerged as a distinct speciality in its own right, with even different sub-branches (Cold orthopaedics, Traumatology—Accident services, Sports medicine, Spine, Hand, Foot, Rehabilitation medicine and so on). Therefore the responsibility of an orthopaedic surgeon, in examining, investigating, diagnosing and managing the dysfunctions of the locomotor system (bones, joints, muscles and nerves), caused by congenital malformation, nutritional deficiencies, diseases, trauma, tumours and other known lesions, has also increased profoundly.

Accurate clinical diagnosis forms the basis for successful management of any ailment. No doubt, the development of a sound judgement is largely a matter of experience, yet one must remember the words of Sir Astley Cooper (1768-1848), "nothing is known in our profession by guess; and I do not believe, that from the first dawn of medical science to the present moment, a single correct idea has ever emanated from conjecture. It is right therefore, that those who are studying their profession should be aware that there is no short road to knowledge; that observations on the diseased, living, examinations of the dead, and experiments upon living animals, are the only sources of true knowledge; and that inductions from these are the sole basis of legitimate theory." The great Indian surgeon Sushruta (c. 600 B.C.) had also warned against diagnosing a disease merely on speculation. He gave explicit instructions regarding history taking, inspection, palpation, auscultation, etc. An indication of the details with which the symptoms and signs were analysed can be exemplified by the list of the types of pain which were enquired into—i.e. whether pain was of pricking, piercing, churning, bursting, pinching, uprooting, stiffening, benumbing, indurating, contracting, or of a spasmodic nature, etc. Pain, which came on or vanished without any apparent cause, or was varied and shifting in nature was supposed to be the effects of deranged 'Vayu'.

The immense importance of systematic clinical methodology in the practice of medical science can never be ignored. There is no short cut to familiarity with clinical signs and their interpretations. A 'snap' diagnosis based on a cursory examination may be disastrous for even an experienced clinician. On the other hand, an inexperienced apprentice examining his patient, methodically step by step, will certainly give a better account of himself.

The aim of the medical education should be familiarity with the scientific principles in an approach that will allow the physician to handle logically, correctly and safely even those diseases with which he/she may not have previous experience. The physicians of tomorrow should be educated rather than schooled. Medical science is nowadays characterized by more and more narrow specialisation burdened by new in-depth research works. Therefore, a threat emerges that the clinicians and subsequently the medical students loose their ability to see the sick persons in their totality. This phenomenon is one of the potential sources of dehumanisation of medicine.

The development of technical approach to the medical care has gradually led to the clinician to give less and less time to the patient. Earlier the clinician used to start the care taking with detail interrogations of the patient and/or relatives, which used to give an insight into the medical aspects of patient's past and present. Thorough physical examination was performed with great care before some tests were ordered. Though a little time consuming, such procedure promoted a holistic approach to the sick. Unfortunately there is a gradual reversal in that trend. Clinicians are cutting down their time spent in initial conversation and primary physical examination. The cult of numbers (uncritical acceptance of quantitative laboratory determinations) has almost replaced the cute clinical observation, the friendly attitude and psychic comfort of the former days.

Actually the computer addition is prevailing over many clinicians, medical teachers and also the medical students all over the globe. The abilities and competence of the computers are being overestimated. However, a computer, though most helpful and serviceable in medical education and practice, can not replace a thinking clinician and the practical examination. His associative reasoning can not be restricted to a software programme.

Today, in an era of rapid industrialisation and mechanisation, orthopaedics occupies an important place in the field of medical sciences. The examination and management of an osteo-articular problem, very much involves assessment of the patient as a whole. However, two factors, quite often missed, must get their place while examining an orthopaedic patient.

i. Proper documentation of case records, which has got immense value in this branch of reconstructive surgery.
ii. History taking and clinical examination should be rehabilitation oriented.

DOCUMENTATION

Accurate representation of the clinical findings, supplemented with sketches, graphs, photographs, X-rays, cine-films, writing tests, foot

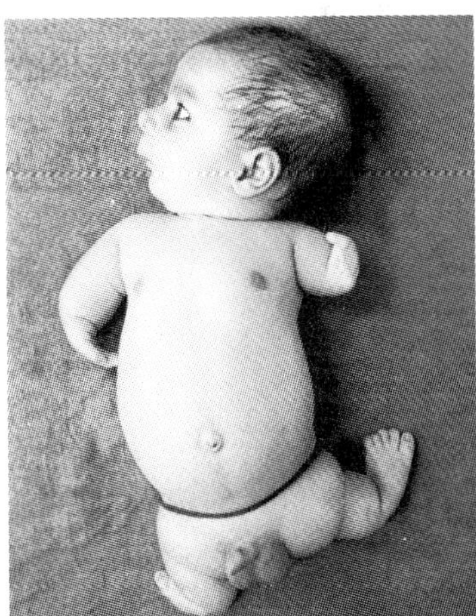

Fig. 1.1A: Congenital malformation of all the four limbs—rudimentary limbs

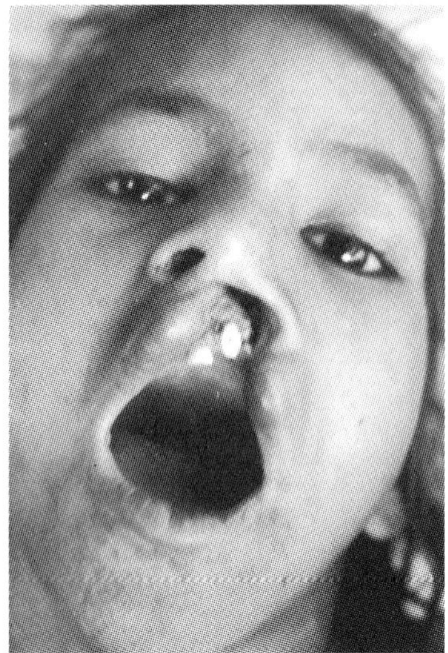

Fig. 1.1B: Congenital cleft lip and palate

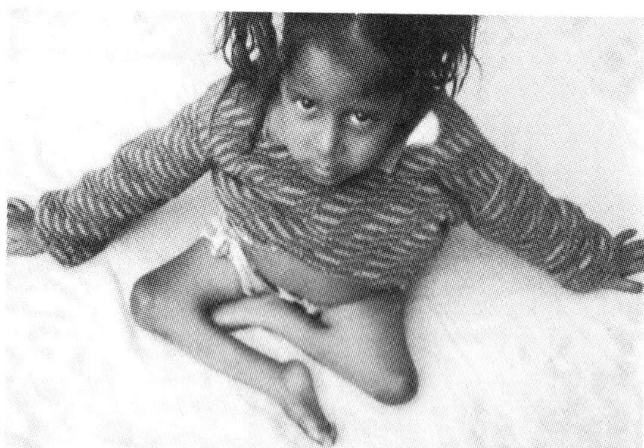

Fig. 1.2A: Congenital contracture of hip, knee, ankle and foot

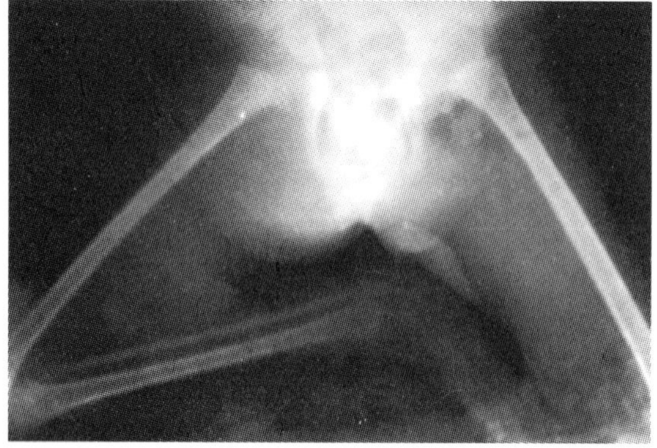

Fig. 1.2B: X-ray of same child (Fig. 1.2A)

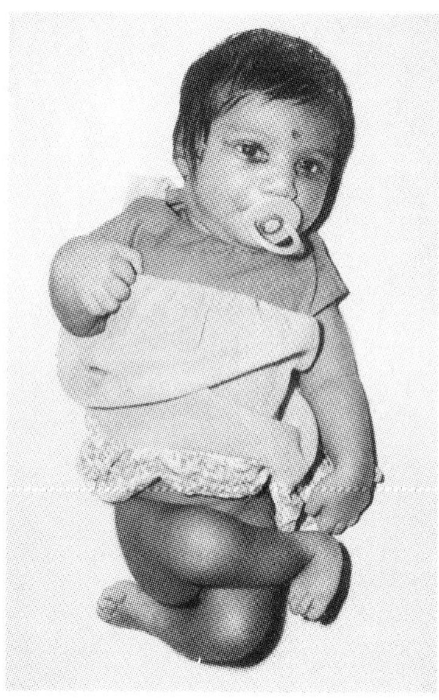

Fig. 1.3A: Arthrogryposis multiplex congenita. Note bilateral club hand, left club foot, bilateral flexion contracture of knee joint, wide perineum indicating bilateral CDH and congenital constriction band at right lower leg

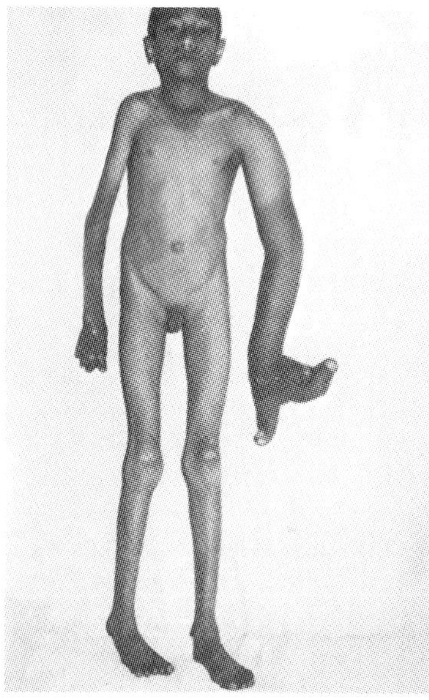

Fig. 1.3B: Congenital hyperplasia of left upper limb

prints, topographical representation and moulds go a long way in helping the clinician in diagnosing, planning of treatment, declaring the pro-

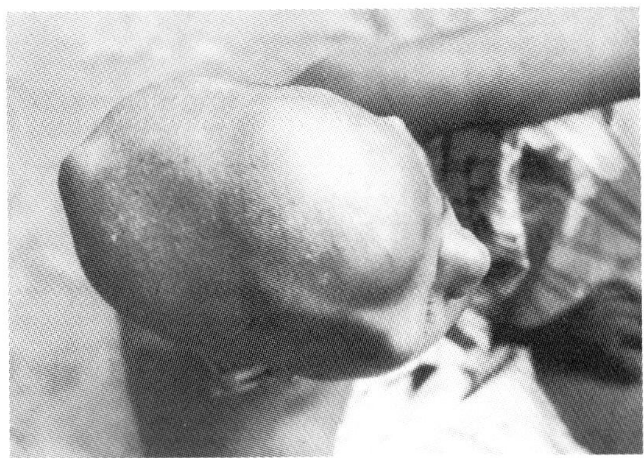

Fig. 1.4A: Pott's puffy tumour in a boy aged 16 years

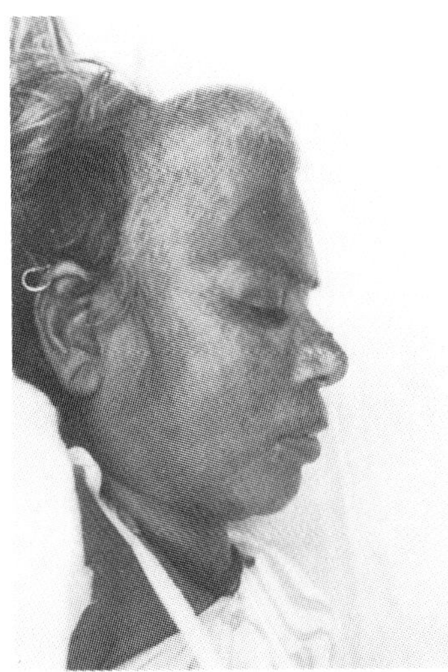

Fig. 1.4B: Pott's puffy tumour in a lady aged 46 years

gnosis and assessing the results of follow up.

An orthopaedic problem in a patient may arise from any of the following:

1. Congenital, infective and developmental malformations (Figs 1.1–1.9).
2. Affections of bones.
3. Affections of joints (Figs 1.10 and 1.11)
4. Affections of soft tissues around and controlling the joints e.g.—skin (burn contracture), subcutaneous tissue (*Dupuytren's* contracture), muscles, tendons (Figs 1.12 and 1.13).

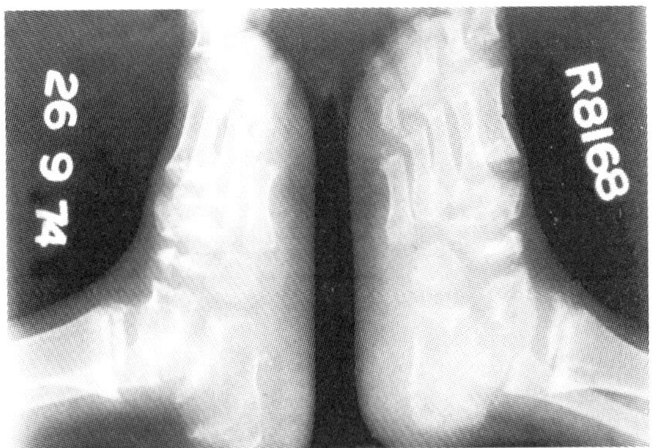

Fig. 1.5: Typical X-ray of multiple epiphysitis

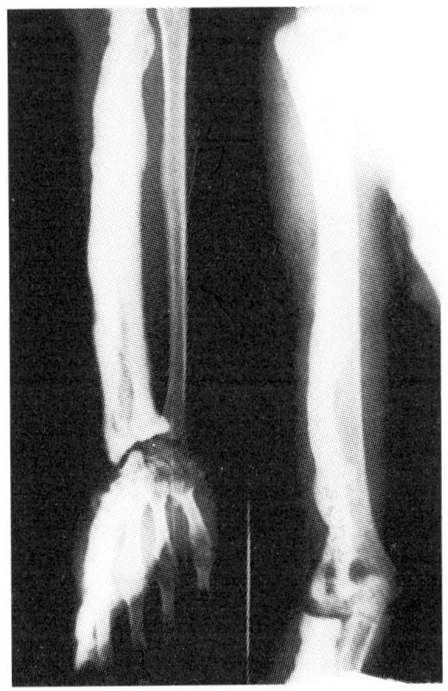

Fig. 1.6: Melorheostosis (candle bone disease). Note that affections are mainly of radius, lateral half of humerus and hand. The peculiar streaked sclerosis of bone resembling candle driplings. It is oftenly associated with congenital neurofibromatosis

5. Affections of nervous system (Fig. 1.14).
6. Vascular affection of limbs (Buerger's phenomenon; Volkmann's ischaemic contracture, etc.).
7. Postural abnormalities (Fig. 1.15) e.g., (1) Pisa syndrome—a dystonic syndrome characterised by lateral flexion of the trunk associated with slight rotation due to high dose of chlorpromazine, given for neuro-

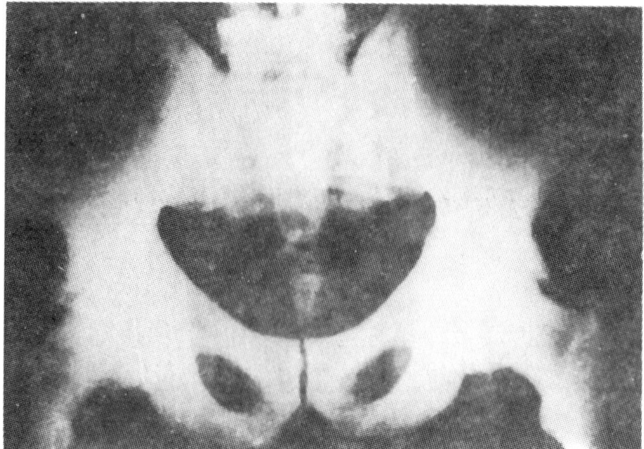

Fig. 1.7: Marble bone disease (osteopetrosis)

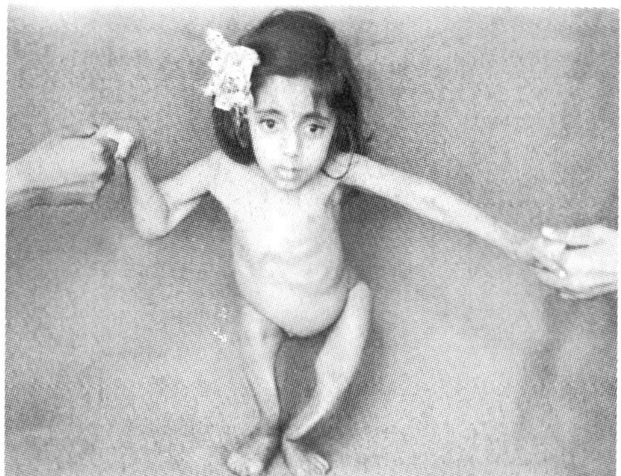

Fig. 1.8A: A girl with osteogenesis imperfecta with multiple deformities following multiple fractures

epileptics. There may be associated tardive dyskinesia; (2) Tortipelvis (L. tortus= twisted+pelvis= basin) meaning thereby muscular spasms in children distorting the spine and hip.

EXAMINATION OF THE PATIENT

Medical knowledge alone is not enough to meet the patient's expectations from us. Fellow feeling, friendly intentions, moral support, relief from fear, human attitude towards the patient, as well as physician's efficiency, all these are essential.

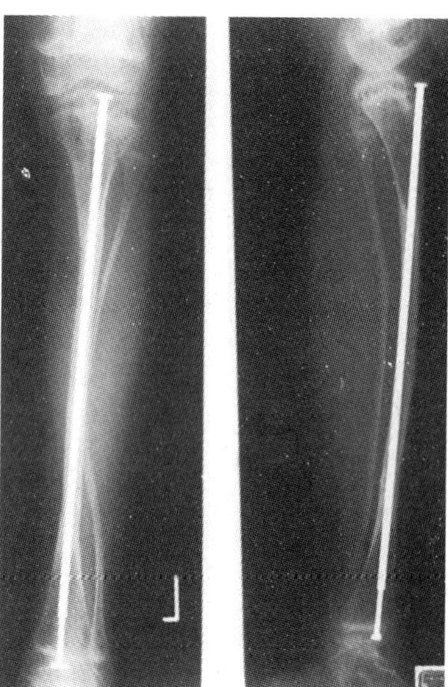

Fig. 1.8B

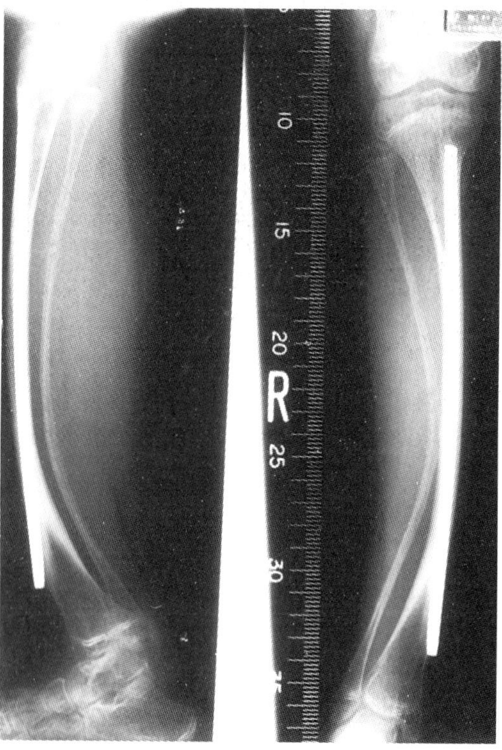

Figs 1.8B and 1.8C: In osteogenesis imperfecta the fractures can be avoided by using telescoping rods

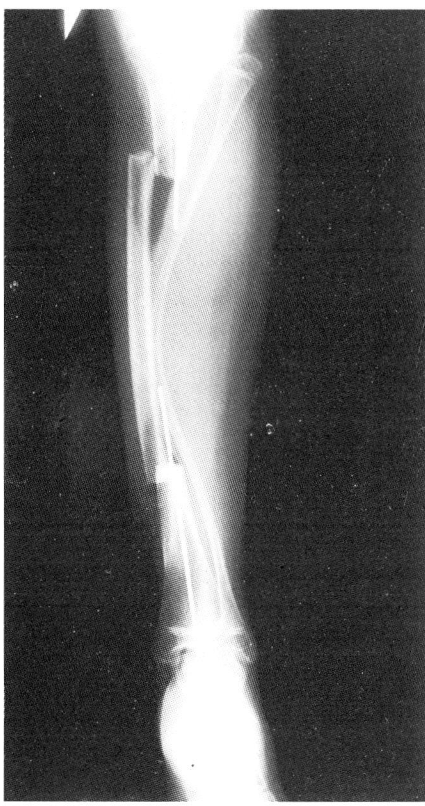

Fig. 1.8D: Prophylectic telescopic rodding of the long bone to prevent pathological fractures in osteogenesis imperfecta

1. Armamentarium Necessary for Examining an Orthopaedic Patient

1. A measuring tape.
2. Goniometer (large and small).
3. A tendon rubber hammer.
4. A pocket torch.
5. A pin with protected point.
6. Skin marker pencil.
7. A stethoscope.
8. A diagnostic set (tongue depressor, auroscope, ophthalmoscope).
9. A plain white paper and impression ink for taking prints.
10. Camera (more important than even a stethoscope for a reconstructive surgeon).
11. For neurological cases—cotton wool, tuning fork, test tubes.

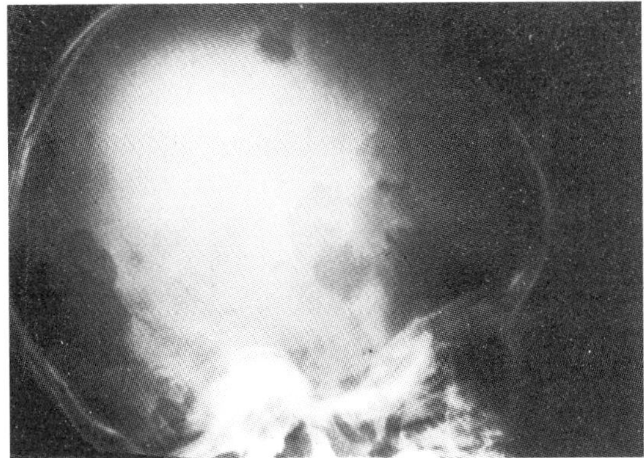

Figs 1.9A

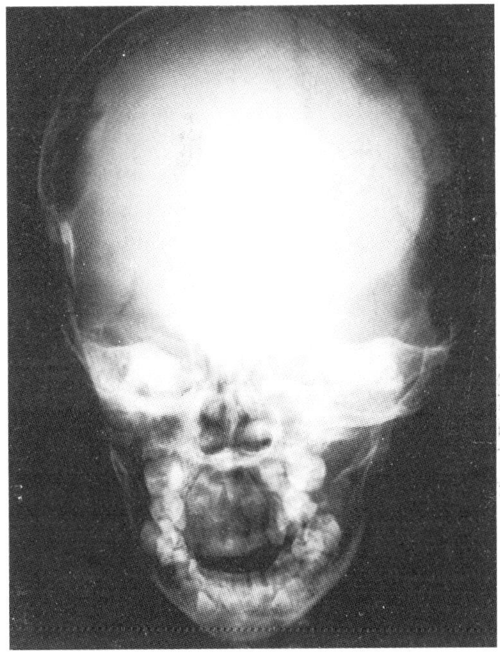

Figs 1.9A and B: Hand-Schüller-Christian disease (a typical histiocytoses) with classic geographic skull: (A) Lateral view of skull, (B) Anteroposterior view of face and skull

2. Certain Factors Essential for Examining an Orthopaedic Case

1. Hear the patient with patience, even if he is confused, disoriented and annoying.
2. Reassuring the patient and gentle handing of the affected parts.
3. Good bedside manners.

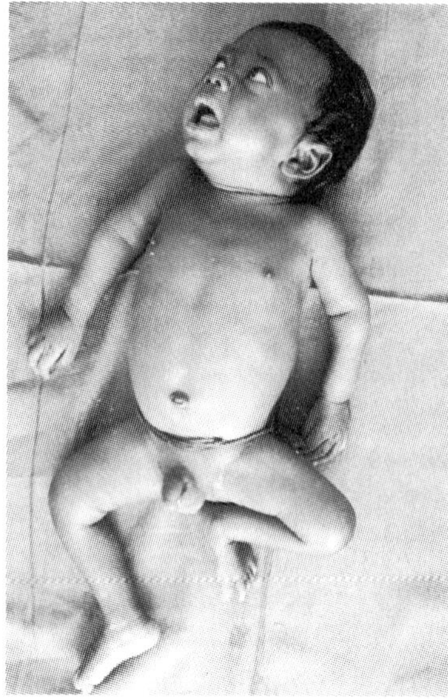

Fig. 1.10: Congenital syphilis with multiple joint affections and pseudoparesis

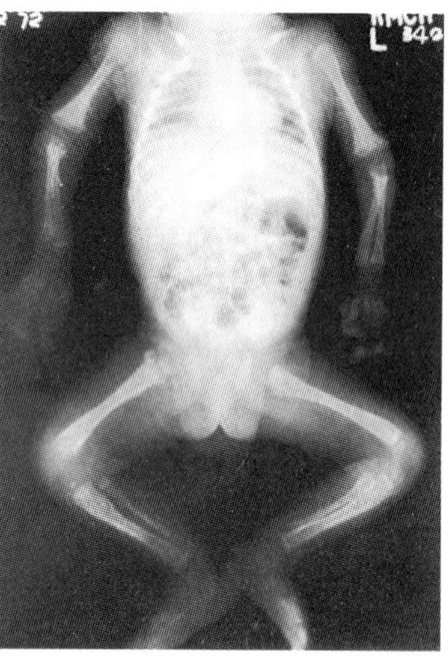

Fig. 1.11: X-ray of the same child showing multiple metaphysitis with collection in the joints, bilaterally (in knees, hips and shoulders)

4. Sympathetic appreciation of the patient's problems.
5. Doctor should be well-dressed, composed, and not in hurry.

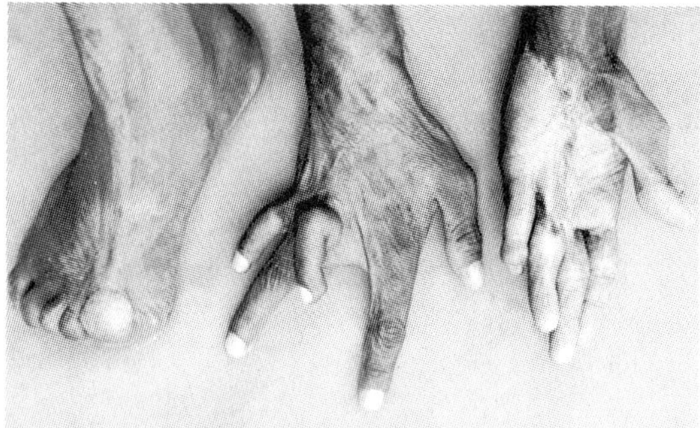

Fig. 1.12: Burn contracture producing multiple problematic deformities of foot and hand

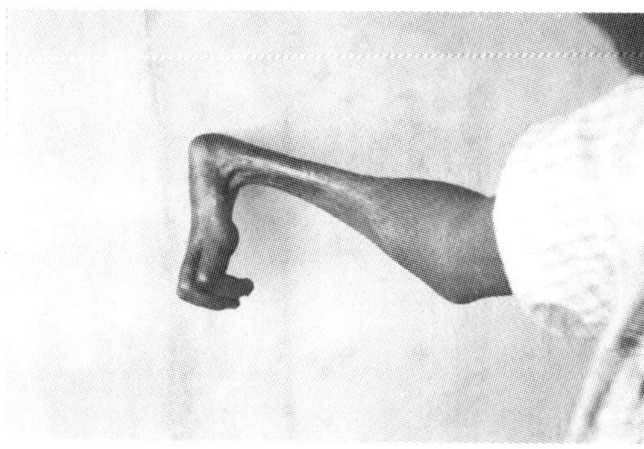

Fig. 1.13: Grotesque deformity of wrist and hand—very severe Volkmann's ischaemic contracture

6. As far as possible communicate with the patient in his/her language to get the clear story and facts.
7. All physical complaints should be taken up seriously.
8. Remember that the patient is almost always right while narrating the problems.
9. Remember that the snap-diagnosis can be mostly wrong.
10. Diagnosis of Functional Neurotic Disease (FND) should always be at the last, after excluding all possible diagnosis.
11. An insight into the patient's future rehabilitation programme.
12. Need for examining the patient as a whole, and not a particular limb or system.
13. The patient must be placed in comfortable position.

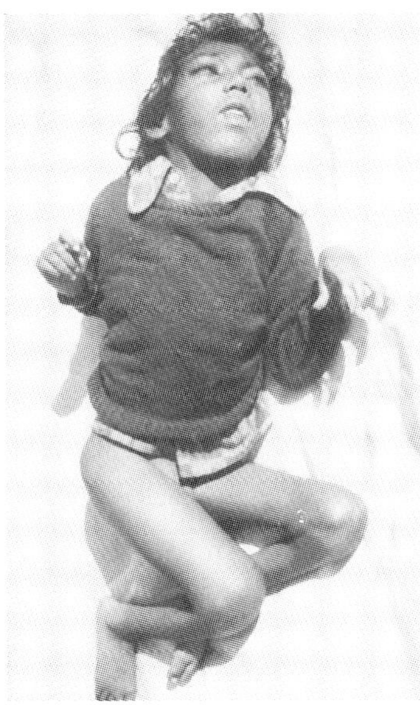

Fig. 1.14: A cerebral palsy child (spastic) with mental retardation

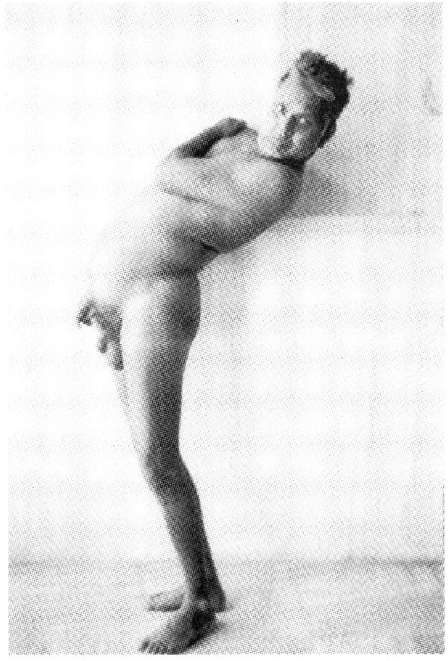

Fig. 1.15: A typical spinal deformity due to Pisa Syndrome

14. Usually patients feel comfortable, confident and free, when one of their own man remains there while being examined.
15. The patient is to be fully exposed, at least the corresponding part or limb.
16. Do not hurt the patient during examination.

The first impression, that a keen clinician gets of his patient while he is entering the examination room, forms the basis for his onward assessment.

Common Orthopaedic Complaints

1. Pain.
2. Disability in using the limb.
3. Inability in using the limb.
4. Deformity.
5. Stiffness of the joints.
6. Swelling/abscess.
7. Discharging wounds/sinus.
8. Limb length disparity.
9. Altered power and sensations.
10. Cramps in the calf.
11. Allied complains e.g. hyperhydrosis, tremors, muscular fasciculations.

History Taking

History of complaints forms the key step for making the diagnosis. History taking is an art of collection of datas over which you are planning your examination. The importance of relevant, detailed history taking can never be overemphasised.

Do not forget that your responsibility does not cease on getting a disease cured or a fracture united, rather management is incomplete without total rehabilitation of the patient. Therefore, history taking and examination must be rehabilitation oriented.

At first, note the full name, age, sex, race, religion, occupation and complete postal address of the patient. Carefully listen his/her story about the problem in his/her own language and words.

Enquire about the complaints in order of their appearance and note their duration. Each symptom should be thoroughly analysed. 'Suck each symptom dry, like a dog sucks a bone'.

Chief Orthopaedic Complaints Center Around the Following

Pain is one of the four elementary sensations. It is the master symptom in medicine. Pain may be defined as "an unpleasant sensory and emotional experience associated with actual or potential tissue damage (except in psychological pain)".

Depending on the site of origin and nature, pain may classified as:

1. *Nociceptive pain*—Pain produced by activation of normal nerve by noxious stimuli (mechanical, thermal, chemical). Site of origin of pain may be: (a) somatic, e.g. skin, muscles, bone, joints, (b) visceral—Pain in tubular structure (especially in abdominal viscera) is colic in nature, usually severe, deep pain; palpation may not reproduce pain.

Pain in solid structure is continuous in nature, usually dull, superficially felt; and palpation always reproduces it.

2. *Neurogenic pain*—Origin of pain is in nerve itself, e.g. herpetic neuralgia , diabetic neuralgia (neuritis), post-infarction pain, causalgia.

Causalgia is a clinical syndrome associated with a lesion of a peripheral nerve containing sensory fibres, first described by S W Mitchell *et al* (1864). It is manifested by pain in the extremity coming spontaneously or with any stimuli, with or without change in the patient's mental state. Pain is usually of intense burning character, and may be intermittent or persistant diffused in the area of cutaneous supply of the involved nerve.

Perhaps the only manifestation of (complains) pain in the neonate or young children is "weeping" (which may be due to hunger or fear even). Infants must not be taken as the young adults, and they should be examined with deep scrutiny.

For correct diagnosis of pain it is better to follow 'PQRST' approach:

P = Palliative factor (what makes it less; Provocative factor (what makes it more)
Q = Quality of pain (type of pain)
R = Radiation of pain
S = Severity of pain
T = Timing of pain (is it all the time or intermittent, etc)

3. *Psychological pain*—with no organic cause various factors are responsible for origin and perpetuation of pain.

4. *Total pain*, in which all the above three factors are responsible, e.g. pain in cancer.

5. *Phantom limb pain*—It was originally described by Ambroise Pare in the seventeenth century. It may be defined as an unpleasant sensation often painful with or without burning sensation distal to the site of a nerve injury (phantom sensation), and may result in marked physical and psychological morbidity.

Certain Sitewise Reference of Pain

- From cervical region to shoulder, arm and even up to fingertips (brachalgia or cervicobrachial neuralgia)
- From supraclavicualr region to arm, forearm, fingers
- From shoulder to arm, forearm, hand and fingers
- From wrist to thumb, index finger (mainly from front of wrist)
- From upper mid dorsal spine to side of chest (girdle pain)
- From lower dorsal spine to abdominal wall
- From lumbar region to loin, groin, upper medial aspect of thigh
- From lower lumbar region to lumbosacral region to—along sciatic roots—sciatica
- From sacro-iliac joint to back of thigh and knee
- From hip to anteromedial aspect of thigh and knee
- From thigh to knee according to the aspect of thigh involved
- From knee to shin of tibia.

1. *Concerning pain*: Note its site, depth of severity (ignorable—trivial; not ignorable as it interferes in activities—moderate; constant even in rest—severe; tossing and incapacitating—very severe), mode of onset, character, diurnal variation, path and site of radiation, relation with activities and rest, relieving/aggravating factors. Reference of pain can be due to same source of sensory supply or cortical confusion between embryologically related areas.

2. *Deformity*: Mode of onset, progressive or static, any attempt at earlier correction, disabilities due to deformity.

3. *Disability* or *Inability:* in using the limb, with clear description.

4. *Limitation of Movement*: How it started, whether progressive or static; any massage done and, how it hampers the activities.

5. *Swelling*: Site, how it started, associated with pain or painless, size, increasing gradually or rapidly, any decrease in the size if ever, any similar or other type of swelling elsewhere.

6. *Discharging wound*: How it started, type, colour and nature of discharge, intermittent or continuous, painful or painless, any history of indigenous applications or cauterization and any history of bony spicules in the discharge.

7. *Constitutional features*: Like fever, anorexia, constipation, headache, urinary trouble, eye trouble, night sweating.

8. *Cramps*: Cramps and cramp-like complaint in both calves are not uncommon. There can be several causes, which may be specific or nonspecific. *Claudication* (the word derived from Latin 'Claudicatio'= to limp. The Roman emperor Claudius (10 BC to AD 54)— walked with limp probably due to polio should be differentiated from the cramps. Claudication may be due to neurological (e.g. spinal stenotic syndrome) or vascular causes (e.g. Buerger's phenomenon), and they can be confused with each other. In rare cases both causes may co-exist presenting with superimposed features. The neurogenic and vascular claudications can be differentiated as in Table 1.1.

In claudication (vascular e.g. Buerger's phenomenon; neurogenic e.g. spinal stenotic syndrome), the patient feels gradually ensuing catch in both calf muscles after some walking. The walking distance, before the symptoms start appearing, gradually decreases. The claudication of spinal origin usually disappears after sitting or bending forward in chair, while that of vascular origin requires rest from walking for relief.

In cramps, the patient feels a sudden painful catch in the calf muscles with or without the contracted muscles forming a hard ball (systremma), which almost disappears within a few seconds, either following local massage or rest or itself, leaving behind a dull aching pain lasting for few hours to a day or two. Constipation, overexertion and walking without habit can precipitate cramps in the calf. Calcium deficiency, and advanced pregnancy can also induce these cramps. However, symptoms like cramps can also be seen in vague ankylosing spondylitis, thyrotoxicosis, poly-insersinitis, metabolic diseases e.g. hyponatraemia (as in heat stroke) and hypomagnesaemia, myopathies, aesthenia and depressive syndromes in adults. Chronic leg compartment syndrome and stress fractures should be differentiated from intermittent claudication.

9. Any other complaints, even unrelated to orthopaedics, should be noted chronologically. Usually there are more than one presenting complaints, which may appear one after another or simultaneously. Note the sequence of their appearance.

Hyperhydrosis (Excessive Sweating)

Normally sweating occurs when ambient temperature is greater than 32.5°C and during exercises.

Table 1.1: Difference between neurogenic and vascular claudication

Neurogenic claudication	*Vascular claudication*
• Claudication is in the calf muscles due to pressure on or affection of cauda equina (spinal nerve roots). Patient after exerting/walking for sometime develops neurogenic pain and paresthesia along the lower limb (mainly the calves, but may be in buttocks as well).	• Claudication in the calf muscles due to narrowing of the vascular tree (earlier spasmodic, but gradually organic narrowing due to athromatous deposits and fibrosis). Pain may be also in thigh.
• Spinal canal stenosis is commonest cause.	• Buerger's disease is the commonest cause.
• Persons beyond 40 yrs. of age are usually affected.	• Young and middle age groups are usually affected.
• Males are more affected.	• Mostly in males.
• Patient complains of pain usually, in both calves/legs; catch and tightness in muscles; difficulty in walking; paresthesia.	• Patient complains of gradually increasing pain and fatigue and burning sensation, usually to start with in one leg, but later on in both after some walking.
• Burning is not associated with pain.	• Burning is usually an accompanying symptom.
• Pain is aggravated by extension of back.	• Pain is aggravated by continuation of walking.
• There is no particular time or walking-distance for initiation of the claudication. Rather distance of walking before precipitating of symptoms may remain same.	• Claudication always starts after walking some distance, which gradually decreases (the length of distance) with the advancement of pathology.
• Claudication pain is relieved only by bending forward or sitting, not only by resting in standing. Rather as soon as patient stands from sitting posture, the pain is initiated.	• Claudication pain gets relieved after rest for sometime. Pain is not relieved after stooping.
• Going uphill reduces the pain.	• On going uphill pain is not reduced, rather it may increase.
• Cycling reduces the pain.	• Cycling does not reduce the pain, rather it may increase.
• Peripheral vascular pulsation normal (according to the age).	• Peripheral vascular pulsation (dorsalis pedis pulsation upwards) is decreased, or even may not be felt.
• There may be neurological deficit features (muscular weakness, wasting, sensory or visceral affection).	• No neurological deficit.
• Usually there is no trophic changes	• Trophic changes do develop.
• Gangrene does not develop.	• Gangrene develops in advanced cases.
• X-ray, CT Scan, MRI helps in confirming the diagnosis.	• Doppler flowmetry is helpful to assess the status of the peripheral circulation.
• Management mainly consists of surgical decompression of the spinal stenosis. Non-operative management like limitation of activities, spinal exercises, neurotropic vitamins, orthotics have limited role.	• In early stages management mainly consists of antiplatelet, antiathrogenic, vasodilator drugs (medical sympathetomy). If no response—surgical sympathetomy. For gangrene—amputation.

Causes of Generalised Sweating

1. During shock, vaso-vagal attack, anxiety, excruciating pain, motion sickness.
2. In systemic diseases, e.g. rickets, infantile scurvy, hyperthyroidism, pink disease, tuberculosis (night sweating).
3. Drugs, e.g. alcohol, salicylates, pilocarpine.
4. Occasionally during menstruation.

Localised Hyperhydrosis

Localised hyperhydrosis occurs due to:

1. Injury to spinal cord or nerve
2. Brain tumours
3. Post-encephalitic Parkinsonism.

Few Common Sites of Hyperhydrosis

Site	*Cause*
• Palms and Soles	• May be normal Psychoneurosis Rheumatoid arthritis
• Sweating at tip of nose	• Granulosis rubra nasi
• Generalised with small vesicles on the skin and trunk	• Miliaria or sudamiel
• Lesions in crops on any part of body with perspiration.	• Miliaria papulosa or rubra (prickly heat),

Tremor (L-tremor, Tremere, Shake, Tremble; Greek—tremein, tremble)

Tremor may be defined as involuntary shaking of the body or limbs (regular or irregular; fine or coarse) with an oscillatory character.

Tremor may be grouped under following headings:

a. Physiological, e.g. due to fear, weakness, anxiety, alcoholism, or fever, nervousness.

   The tremor of anxiety is usually fine and rapid but it may be coarse and irregular.

b. Benign essential tremor: It occurs as a familial disorder as the coarse distant tremor, usually exaggerated in awkward postures, e.g. when the patient holds his outstretched fingers pointing to each other in front of his nose. Though it is usually relieved to some extent during movement, but it is present both at rest and movements.

c. Senile tremors are similar to benign essential tremor.

d. Parkinsonian tremor: In Parkinsonism, tremor is usually the initial presentation for which patients seek advice. It first involves the fingers and spreads to proximal portion of arm, and gradually it may extend to the tongue, lips and legs. The tremor is rapid, rhythmic, and alternating tremor, mainly in flexion/extension, but often with rhythmic rotatory component between finger and thumb (**pill-rolling tremor**). It is often associated with features of extrapyramidal disease such as hypokinesia, cogwheel rigidity, postural abnormality, gait disorder (festinant gait—short and shuffling steps), and expressionless quite voice.

e. Cerebellar tremor: It usually occurs in elderly persons, in whom the tremor occurs only during movements (intention tremor). Such tremors increase when the limb approaches a target and gets relieved when the affected limb is supported and relaxed.

f. In thyrotoxicosis, tremor is always rapid.

g. Hysterical tremor usually involves a limb or whole body and is characteristically worsened by examiner's attempt to control it.

h. Tremors of hand may be even congenital.

i. Tremors may also occur in multiple sclerosis, uraemia, hepatic failure, mercurial poisoning, etc.

Muscular Fasciculations

These are spontaneous contractions of groups of muscle fibres. They originate from abnormal generator sites in the peripheral nervous system. They vary in distribution and frequency and most commonly occurs in motor neurone disease (anterior horn cell disease), however may also occur in fatigued normal subjects.

History of Present Illness

Let the patient narrate the story of his ailments in his own words from the beginning to the present condition. Pick up the salient points. Dilate on each point with relevant leading questions. Any history of injury or febrile attacks must be explored through leading questions. Treatment received for the present complaints should be noted in detail.

Broadly orthopaedic problems fall in two major groups—injury related or noninjury related.

(A) *In Case of Injury*—Enquire about its mode and nature, and if associated with any abnormal sounds, the amount of impact, the portion of body hurt, immediate effects of injury, delayed effects of injury, could he/she stand and walk or was carried (then mode of carriage), did the injury affect mobility/activities.

High velocity injuries are getting more and more common and usually produce multiple injuries with or without injury to vital organs. Hence enquire with leading questions about the general effects of polytrauma (e.g. shock, haemorrhage, etc) and about level of consciousness at the time of trauma and later on.

MODES OF INJURY

i. Direct hit (Contact injury).
ii. Indirect injuries.
    —Rotational strains (e.g. fracture neck femur).
    —Violent muscle pulls (e.g. fracture of patella).
    —Compression injuries (e.g. compression fracture of vertebra).

In Case of Fall—height of fall, surface on which fallen, level of consciousness after falling, if he could stand up or walk or even take weight on the affected side or not following the injury, immediate posture after injury, any manipulation at the site of injury by himself or any one else.

AFTER THE INJURY

—Mode of transportation to home or hospital.
—Attempts by bone setters or quacks and/or any other treatment given.

(B) *Fever*: Onset, any associated rigor, range of temperature, continuous or intermittent, if only at particular time, e.g. in the evening, sweating, response to treatment, accompanying symptoms.

Enquire about appetite, polyuria, loss of weight.

History of Past Illness

Any earlier injury; history of earlier infections, specially tuberculosis, syphilis, leprosy, pyogenic; average duration of bleeding after any cut; any particular treatment received. History about TORCH profile (To= toxoplasmosis, R= rubella, C= cytomegalovirus, H= herpes virus), which can be detected with ELISA test.

Personal History

Occupation, any tobacco/drug habit, personal hygiene, hobby, sensitivity or allergy to any drug or object.

In case of females—marital status, number of children, any gynaecological complaints.

Family History

Any familial incidence related to the recent complaints, tuberculous infection in family, any hereditary disorder (Figs 1.16 to 1.17B).

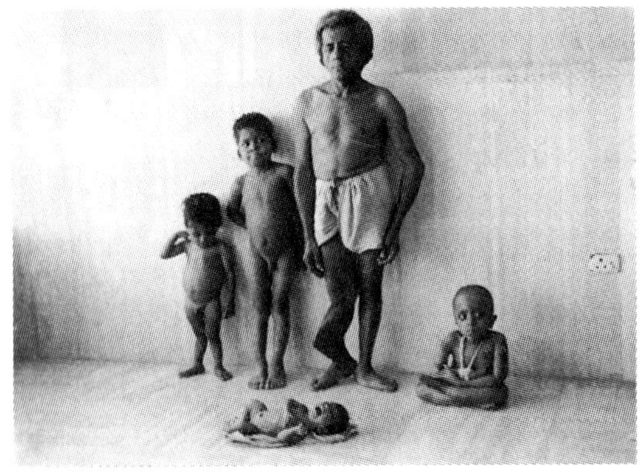

Fig. 1.16: A family of five, all having deformities of the limbs due to osteogenesis imperfecta—hereditary familial disorder

History and Record Chart

Name	Age Sex Marital status and family. Photographic records with dates	Race	Religion	Occupation	Registration No. Complete postal address: Telephone: Fax: E-mail:
Complaints	—Pain —Deformity —Disability —Disparity of limb length —Swelling —Any other.				

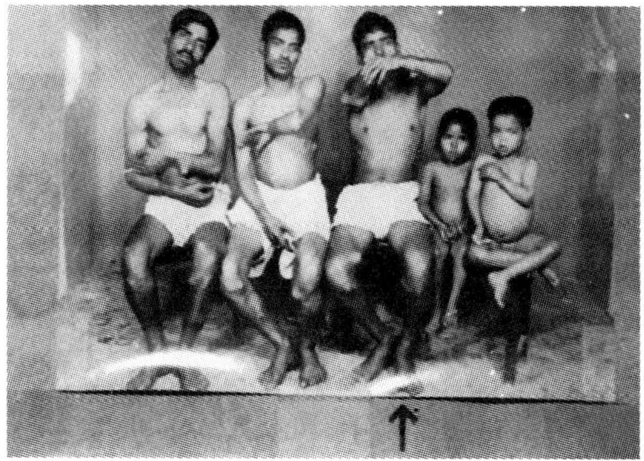

Fig. 1.17A : Group photograph of available family members showing multiple exostosis, familial incidence had been followed upto four generations. Third brother in this group consulted for his foot lesion (exostosis in 1st web)

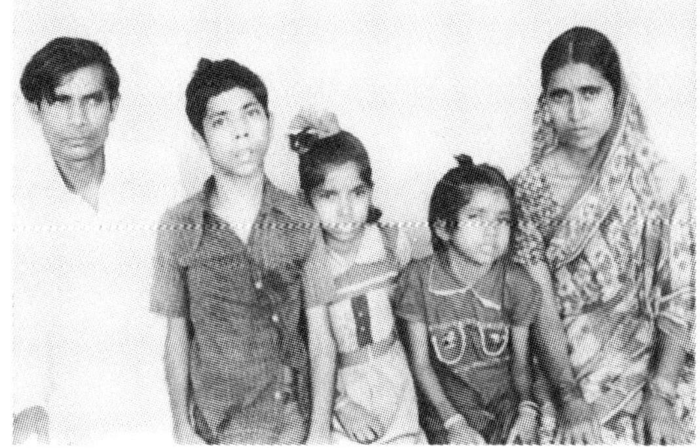

Fig. 1.17C: A family of five—all suffering from myopathy

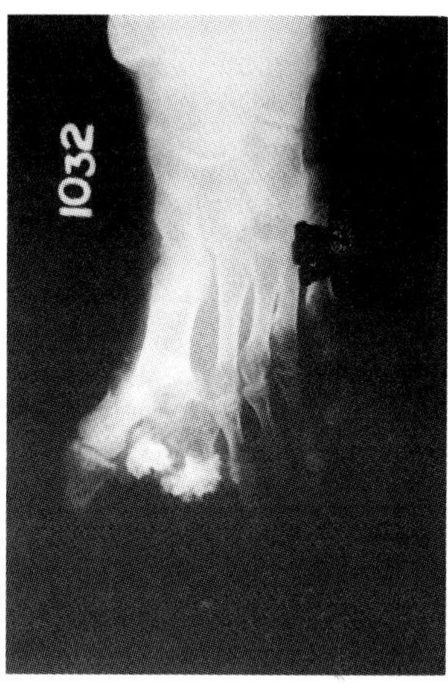

Fig. 1.17B: X-ray of the foot of the third brother in the family of Fig. 1.17A. Note the disabling exostosis from the first metatarsal head region

Social History

—Economic background, status of living.
—Topographical surroundings.
—Barriers in and around home.
—Education in the family.

History of present illness: Analysis of relevant points. The onset of the symptoms can provide clue to the origin of the disease, e.g. Congenital (present since birth); Developmental (defect in developmental period of childhood and adolescence); Infective/Inflammatory (associated with constitutional features); Metabolic (nutritional and/or economic deficit); Endocrinal (evidences of harmonal imbalance); Traumatic (history of injury); Neoplastic (painless or painful, gradually or rapidly, increasing swelling or ulcer—benign or malignant); Degenerative (in older age groups, or chronic or old pathologies); Idiopathic (causes not known).

History of past illness: Trauma, tuberculosis, syphilis, gonorrhoea, bleeding diasthesis.

Personal history: Addiction, immunization, allergy or sensitivity to drugs, education, hobby.

In case of females: Any gynaecological disorder, number of children.

Family history and social status: Social status, hereditary disorder, economic status, infectious disease.

EXAMINATION

- General examination
- Regional examination
- Local examination.

General Examination

i. Look, intelligence, built, any special posture, cyanosis, oedema, pulse, temperature, blood pressure, jaundice, lymph glands, nail conditions (the appearance of nails can serve as a barometer of a patient's general health).

ii. Attitude—While entering the examination room, note the first impression and posture (general, regional, local).

iii. Attitude of standing
—with full weight
—with partial weight
—with support.

If patient can stand, also perform Trendelenburg's test.

iv. *Gait*
A. Limp or lurch
B. Specific gait (also see page 179 & 180):
- waddling
- high stepping
- hemiplegic (spastic)
- ataxic
- scissor
- festinant
- lathyriatic
- stamping
- knock knee, etc.

Systemic Examination

1. Skull and face—Contour, swelling, decubitus ulcer, and any stigmata (of syphilis, rickets, etc.).
2. Neck—Lymph nodes, venous engorgement, any swelling.
3. Cardiovascular system—Pulse, blood pressure, heart.
4. Respiratory system—Thoracic cage, rib contour, chest expansion, abnormal shape of chest (flat, barrel, pigeon), rib hump, rachitic rosary,
   Harrison's sulcus, scorbutic rosary).
5. Abdomen—liver, spleen, kidney, any lump, iliac fossae, any abnormal finding.
6. Central nervous system: Higher mental functions
   - Cranial nerves
   - Motor system: power, bulk, tone, reflexes, coordination, involuntary movements
   - Sensory system.
7. Genitourinary system.
8. Endocrinal functions.

Regional Examination

The examination of the part complained of only, does not complete the examination, because sometimes the symptoms felt in one part have their origin in another. For example, pain in the leg is often caused by a lesion in the spine, pain in the knee may have its origin in the hip, a pain or tingling and numbness in hand may have its origin in the cervical spine. Hence, the necessity of regional examination.

- For lower limb examine lumbar region to tip of toes.
- For upper limb examine cervical region to tips of fingers.
- For trunk examine as a whole (and the supply region if cord is involved).
- Also examine the regional lymph nodes.

Local Examination

Inspection (look for)

i. Posture of the patient and position of part/limb—attitude.

Table 1.2: Ulcers (discontinuity of epithelial surface)

Non-specific ulcer	*Specific ulcer*	*Malignant ulcer*
• Varicose ulcer (ulcer developing on underlying varicose veins)	• Tuberculous (undermined edge)	• Carcinomatous (everted edge)
• Trophic ulcer [trophe (Greek)=nutrition] (ulcers developing due to impairment of nutrition which depends upon properly intact vascular and nerve supply) e.g.—Ischaemic ulcer, —Diabetic ulcer, —Ulcers developing in spina bifida, tabes dorsalis, leprosy, peripheral nerve injury—due to anaesthetic skin, and are called neuropathic/perforating ulcer.	• Pyogenic (sloping edge) • Syphilitic (usually punctated) • Actinomycotic (multiple ulcer with sulphur granules)	• Rodent ulcer (basal cell carcinoma usually occurring on upper face. • Marjolin ulcer (carcinoma developing on scar).
• Tropical ulcer		

ii. Inspect from different sides.
iii. Normal anatomical points
  —bony
  —soft tissue.
iv. Skin:
  • colour
  • texture
  • erythematous changes
  • puckering
  • cafe-au-lait spots
  • tattoo marks
  • 'pachh'/vaccination scar
  • superficial cuts or scars (linear scar with/without suture mark—usually operative scar; irregular scar—injury; broad, adherent puckered scar—old suppuration)
  • warts or callosities
v. Muscle condition:
  • swelling
  • wasting
  • spasm
  • contracture
  • fasciculations.
vi. Vascular:
  • venous prominence
  • pulsation
  • varicosities.
vii. Abnormal findings: e.g. swelling, sinus, ulcer.

In case of ulcer (s), note the followings: site, size, shape, surface, floor, base, margin (edge), relation to deeper tissues, surrounding tissues, discharge on the surface [(specially ICHOR (a thin watery discharge from an ulcer or unhealthy wound) which usually denotes chronicity and deeper involvement], pigmentation, regional lymph nodes.

Broadly the ulcers are classified as (i) Non-specific, (ii) specific, (iii) malignant (Table 1.2).

Examination of Any Sinus

A sinus (Latin= a hollow; a bay or gulf) is a blind track opening onto the skin or mucous membrane [cf. Fistula (Latin= a pipe or tube) is a tunnel connecting two epithelial or endothelial surfaces]. Note:

— number, site, relation with deeper tissues, relation with skin, margin, discharge—intermittent/continuous colour and type of discharge, relation with pain, possible source, any bony spicule, nature of scar (if healed).

— sinus tract—feel, traceability to parent site, fixed to bone or mobile. Probing should be avoided.

Causes of Persistance of Sinus

Persistance of infection; presence of dead tissue within, e.g. bony sequestrum; presence of any foreign body, e.g. bullet, metallic foreign body, pieces of cloth, etc; persistance of cavity within the bone; epithelialisation/endothelialisation of sinus track; puckering of soft tissues around the tract; intractable infection, e.g. fungal infection; malignant changes in the tract; diabetese; general debility, prolonged use of corticoids; persistent discharge, e.g. of urine, cerebrospinal fluid, faeces, etc. after irradiation.

Palpation

(A) *Superficial (touch)*: Skin condition; temperature; sensation; superficial tenderness; anatomical points—bony, soft tissue; induration (oedema)—regional/local; arterial pulsation; crepitus (may be due to entrapped gas, e.g. in surgical emphysema, gas gangrene (Fig. 2.14); fracture; tenosynovitis).

(B) *Deep Palpation (feel)*: Deep tenderness: It should be avoided in presence of any inflammation (clinically diagnosed by noting the cluster of symptoms and signs of colour (heat due to vasodilatation), dolor (pain), rubor (redness due to vasodilatation), tumour (swelling mainly due to oedema, exudate) and functio-laesa (less or loss of function). It can be tested by direct pressure, indirect twist, and deep thrust. Tenderness of a bone, joint or soft tissue can be classified into four grades according to the reaction (facial and verbal) of the patient during examination for tenderness.

Grade I — The patient says that part is painful on pressure.
Grade II — The patient winces.
Grade III — The patient winces and withdraws the affected part.
Grade IV — The patient will not allow the part to be touched.

Deep Palpation of the Bone

Bone should be palpated for surface, alignment, deep tenderness, abnormal prominence, disturbed relationship of the normal bony landmarks, any crepitus (fracture).

Palpate the girth of bone for THICKENING (there is increase in almost all surfaces which are usually irregular, anatomical configuration is distorted. Bone is thickened usually due to deposit from outside, e.g. in chronic osteomyelitis); BROADENING (breadth of the bone increases, surfaces of the bone almost regular, anatomical configurations are usually identifiable. Broadening occurs from within, e.g. in rickets); EXPANSION OF BONE (bony surfaces are expanded, surfaces are usually nodular or bluntly irregular, all dimension of bone in the affected zone are increased).

Deep Palpation of a Joint

Palpate for:

i. Synovial thickening—soft/boggy/doughy feel—any tenderness.
ii. Joint line—a slit all around in between the articular ends—feel for any tenderness, any abnormal mass.
iii. Fluid in the joint—yielding/cystic/fluctuant/tense feel.
iv. Articular ends—for any tenderness, roughness, crepitus.
v. Adjoining bones—for any thickening, expansion, crepitus, irregularity, tenderness.
vi. Abarticular (at a distance from or not involving a joint) structures and tissues.

Palpation of Fossae (if any)

Palpation of muscles: Girth, feel, tone and pliability of muscles.

Examination of any swelling should be in detail: skin over the swelling, site, size, margin, extent, surface, any veinous prominence, hyperaesthesia on the surface, shape, vascularity, tenderness, consistency (cystic, very soft, soft, doughy, firm, hard, stony hard), fixity, deeper relations, mobility, fluctuation test, transillumination test (if cystic).

Springing

To elicit pain at the site of lesion by intermittently compressing the distant part of the parallel bones, e.g. in fracture of the neck of radius pain can be elicited by compressing the lower forearm.

Transmitted movement: In case of fractures, feel for transmitted movements across the fracture site.

Percussion (tap)

Specially over the bone in suspected crack fracture; over the spinous processes to elicit tenderness in spine.

Auscultation (hear)

— If needed, e.g. for systolic bruit (haemangioma).
— May be of value in localising crepitations, snaps, mild friction rubs in joints.

Measurements

A. Linear measurements
B. Circumferential measurements
} to the tip of medial malleolus.

A. *Linear Measurements*
(a) Apparent measurement
(b) True measurement

a. *Apparent measurement*
— make the limbs parallel to each other and to the trunk.
— handle the unaffected limb to make the limbs parallel.
— measure from any fixed central point to the most distal sharp bony point of the long limb bone.

Therefore, in the lower limb, measure from:
— manubrium sterni
or xiphisternum
or umbilicus.
— in the upper limb—from vertebra prominence (C_7) to radial styloid.

b. *True measurement*
— Reveal the concealed deformity by handling the affected limb.
— Limbs to be kept in identical position.
— Measurement is ipsilateral and then comparison with the other side is done.

Lower limb
i. Total length—from anterior superior iliac spine to medial malleolus.
ii. Segmental length.
— Anterior superior iliac spine to mid-medial knee joint line (thigh length).
— Mid-medial knee joint line to tip of medial malleolus (leg length).
— The components of thigh length are measured as follows:
• Infratrochanteric—tip of greater trochanter to knee joint line.
• Supratrochanteric—indirect measurement—e.g. through Bryant's triangle.

Upper limb
i. Total length—from acromial angle to radial styloid process tip.
ii. Segmental length
— from acromial angle to lateral epicondylar tip (arm length).
— from lateral epicondylar tip to radial styloid process tip (forearm length).

(B) *Circumferential Measurements*
i. At affected point—for any swelling.
ii. At fixed distances, proximal and distal, from the affected part
—for muscular wasting
—for muscular hypertrophy
iii. for disorganised joint.

Across Measurements (for cross check-up of measurements)

In identical position of the limbs:
—From left anterior superior iliac spine to right medial malleolus tip.
— From right anterior superior iliac spine to left medial malleolus tip.

Movements

(Ask to perform—*Active*; performed by others—*Passive*).

Always compare with the opposite joint. In general, the range of movements at any joint, is

Table 1.3: Types of joint stiffness

Extra-articular	*Intra-articular*
• Obvious evidences of extra-articular tightness or adhesion like scars subcutaneous fixity, musculo-tendinous contracture, sinus tract in vicinity.	• No obvious scar, adhesion, sinus or contracted tissues.
• Joint line is usually nontender, except when any inflammatory process lies over the joint line.	• Joint line tender.
• Painless range of free movements active and/or passive.	• Possible movements are usually painful, especially at the extremes.
• On X-ray joint space sharply defined and clearly visible; articular ends nearly normal.	• Joint margins fluffy, joint space reduced. Articulating bony ends usually osteoporosed with or without evidences of underlying pathology.
• Dealing with the contracted extra-articular tissues, releases the stiffness.	• Dealing with the extra-articular tissues does not release the stiffness.
• Manipulation under general anaesthesia is not helpful in mobilising the joint.	• Manipulation, may mobilise the joint. Arthroplasties of different types are usually required for mobilising the joint.

more in females than males. First look for *ankylosis* or *stiffness of the joint.*

Ankylosis (no apparent movement in a joint)

Types of Ankylosis

i. Bony (True)
   —No movement even on using force.
   —No pain.
   —Bony trabeculation across the joint in X-ray.
ii. Fibrous (False)
   —Slight yield on using force.
   —Pain on using force.
   —Joint line visible in X-ray.

Stiffness in the joint: (i.e. joint in which complete movements cannot be obtained—either active or passive): Limitation of movements can be:

a. In all directions—due to arthritis
b. Not in all directions—due to synovitis and/or spasm of muscles.
c. Fixed movement in one or more direction —due to fixed deformity.

Limitations of movements are painful in active arthritis (due to stretching of or pressure on the inflammed capsule and/or rubbing of exposed subchondral bone) and painless in healed ones (due to short fibres fibrous bondage).

TYPES OF JOINT STIFFNESS (Table 1.3)

i. Extra-articular, e.g. due to burn contracture, myositis ossificans, post-infective contracture of periarticular tissues, congenital contracture, e.g. quadriceps contracture, arthrogryposis multiplex congenita, etc.
ii. Intra-articular, e.g. due to septic arthritis, tuberculous arthritis, intra-articular fractures, etc.

If there is no ankylosis, assess the movements in various planes:

A. Sagittal plane—flexion/extension
B. Coronal plane—abduction/adduction
C. Rotational plane—external/internal; supination/pronation.

For each movement:

—Fix the zero position.
—Mark lag of movement (usually extensor lag).
—Assess angle of fixity of any movement (e.g. fixed flexion deformity).
—Range of active movement.
—Range of passive movement.

— Range of utility or activity = Free active movement.
— Range of possibility = Free active movement + Free passive movement.
— Any pain during the movement—If painful focus is in the vicinity of the joint (not in the joint), patient will still be reluctant to initiate active movement. Taking the patient in confidence, passive movement can be demonstrated to variable range, in such cases.
— Limitation of terminal range.
— Achievement of 'critical arc'.
— Achievement of ADL (activities of daily living).
— Any abnormal movement (e.g. hypermobility in neuropathic joint, e.g. *Charcot's joint*).
— Any abnormal sound during the movement (heard/felt).
— Assess the power of controlling muscles.

Active movement of a joint—Movement produced by patient himself, without any assistance.

Passive movement—Movement produced at a joint either by patient's other limb and/or examiner.

Fixed deformity: It is a fixed position of a joint from where the limb cannot be brought back to neutral position, but further movement in the same axis (direction) may be possible.

Normally active and passive ranges are equal. Passive range is more than active in:
— Paralysed joint.
— Lax/Torn
  - Capsule
  - Ligament
  - Tendon
  - Muscle
— Subchondral/condylar fracture.

Test for any laxity or tear of the aforesaid components.

Critical Arc

For any joint, the minimum range of active movement, which is necessary for the important functions of the joint.

ADL

The bare minimum necessary for daily living, like—eating, clothing, cleaning the private parts and minimum necessary mobility.

Power of Controlling Muscles (Table 1.4)

The assessment should be accurate from prognostic point of view. According to Medical Research Council (MRC) scale, muscle power is grouped under five grades. We feel that each grade is further divisible into 4 quadrants; depending upon lag of completion of full range, the deficit can be assessed as e.g., '2- - -', '2- -', '2-', '2'.

Table 1.4: Grading of muscle power

MRC scale		*Suggested sub/grouping*
'0'—	Not even flicker of contraction	'0'.
'1'—	Flicker of contraction	'1'.
'2'—	Contraction of muscles with no assistance and gravity eliminated, but moving the joint to full range.	Depending upon lag of completion of full range 2- - -, 2- -, 2-, 2.
'3'—	Contraction of muscles against gravity but with no resistance, moving the joint to full range.	Depending upon lag of completion of full range 3- - -, 3- -, 3-, 3.
'4'—	Contraction of muscles against gravity and with moderate resistance, moving the joint to full range.	Depending upon lag of completion of full range 4- - -, 4- -, 4-, 4.
'5'—	Normal	Depending upon lag of completion of full range 5- - -, 5- -, 5-, 5. (While '5' is normal, the rest are subnormal in that order).

Special tests: (Pertaining to individual joints) Diagnostic tests must have the following qualities: sensitivity, specificity, reproducibility, predictability, accuracy, minimum hurting to the patient.

Heel Walking/Toe Walking

If the patient can walk, quick inferences can be drawn by making him walk on heels and toes alternately.

If he can walk swiftly in both positions without any complaints—probably there is no serious affection in the lower limbs including its neuromuscular control.

Erect posture along with integrity of the hip, knee, ankle and foot are essential for painless, quick, heel/toe walking.

Any limb-length disparity will obviously affect these walking and any inequality will be apparent.

If patient cannot walk swiftly, there are two broad probabilities:

(A) *If There is Inability/Difficulty in Walking on Heels, it may be due to:*

i. *Weakness* of muscles and/or abnormal joint condition:
 - Weakness of dorsiflexors of ankle; stiffness of the ankle joint.
 - Probable weakness in quadriceps femoris and erector spinae
 - unstable hip.

ii. *Pain*—This may be felt due to any of the following pathologies:
 - Pain in back of thigh, knee and leg—due to sciatic stretch.
 - Pain in sacroiliac region, in hip region—(affection of the joint line e.g. trauma, tuberculosis).
 - Back of the knee, e.g. in cases of trauma— posterior cruciate lesion (?), condylar fracture/crush of tibia (upper end).
 - Pain at ankle—In any traumatic, inflammatory, degenerative or neoplastic condition.
 - Pain at heel—Any cause of painful heel syndrome (see chapter on Foot).

(B) *If There is Inability/Difficulty in Walking on Toes, it may be due to:*

i. *Weakness* of muscles and/or abnormal joint condition:
 - Weakness of plantar flexors; stiffness of ankle (except where in equinus); genu recurvatum; unstable hip.

ii. *Pain*—Pain in the forefoot—trauma, metatarsalgia, inflammatory lesion.

 Usually pain in ankle is not complained of in early affections because the gravity line falls forwards.
 - If pain is in knee region—in case of trauma—probably anterior cruciate involvement, involvement of anterior horn of semilunar cartilage, affection of the quadriceps apparatus.

Peripheral circulation: Impaired peripheral arterial circulation may produce symptoms in a limb, especially in lower limb. So a thorough examination should be done to assess the state of circulation, which is done by examination of the colour and temperature of skin, the texture of skin and nails and by palpating for arterial pulsation, which must always be compared with opposite side.

Peripheral Nerves

(e.g. lateral popliteal nerve, ulnar nerve, etc.).

- tenderness
- thickening
- beading
- irritability
- detailed muscle power and sensory charting.

Investigations: For confirming the clinical suspicion, certain investigations are needed. One must not have a 'shortgun approach' in ordering the investigation (all around investigations), rather it must be an 'arrow head' targeted approach to order the really just needed investigations.

A. General investigations.

B. Special investigations.

C. Electrical investigations.
D. Radiological and allied investigations.

A. General Investigations

— Routine haemogram.
— Erythrocyte sedimentation rate (ESR).
— Routine urine examination.
— Stool examination.
— Grouping and cross-matching of blood. (Also for AIDS and hepatitis B).

B. Special Investigations

i. Serum biochemistry, e.g. sugar, urea, calcium, phosphorus, alkaline and acid phosphatase, fluorine, creatinine.
ii. Serology—Washerman's reaction (WR)—presently not necessarily recommended, Kahn, VDRL, Rheumatoid factor (Rose Wallar test).
iii. Aspiration of any collection and its examination—physical, chemical, cytological, serological, culture and sensitivity, inoculation test.
iv. Foot print, Ichnogram (imprint of the soles of the feet taken in standing position), hand print.
v. Arthroscopy (Diagnostic/therapeutic—knee, shoulder, ankle, elbow, and even IP joints).
Arthroscopy: Nowadays, arthroscopy is being widely used to diagnose and variably deal the pathology (mainly traumatic) affecting the interior of the joints. It is particularly useful for the knee.
vi. Biopsy:
—FNAC (Fine needle aspiration cytology)
—Needle biopsy
—Aspiration biopsy
—Core biopsy
—Endoscopic/arthroscopic biopsy
—CT aided biopsy
—Open biopsy
—Excisional biopsy.

C. Electrical Investigations

— Electrocardiography (ECG)
— Electroencephalography (EEG)
— Electromyography (EMG)
— Strength duration curve
— Nerve conduction test
— Electrophoresis.

D. Radiological and Allied Investigations

i. *Plain radiography; xeroradiography: Xero = dry*, thus xeroradiography does not involve the wet process of developing and fixing the film (using the photoconductive behaviour of a selenium plate and by photoelectric process, the conventional X-ray exposure is recorded as positive image)
—Routine projections
• Antero-posterior/postero-anterior view
• Lateral view
• Oblique view
—Special projections
• Axial view
• Stress radiography.

ii. *Contrast radiography*
• Air contrast radiography.
• Radio-opaque dye contrast radiography [water soluble (metrazimide), oil soluble].
• Myelography.
• Radiculography.
• Discography.
• Arthrography.
• Sinography.
• Venography: After applying a fine tourniquet just above the malleoli a nonionic contrast medium is injected to outline the veins.
• Plathysmography assesses changes in volume of a limb or digit over the cardiac cycle.
• Arteriography: In arteriography a radio-opaque solution is injected into the arterial tree, generally by a retrograde percutaneous method involving the femoral (occasionally brachial or axillary artery).
• Cystography is done by injecting the contrast medium through a catheter

introduced into the bladder. The micturating cystogram is done to look for the presence of vesicoureteric reflex.

- Lymphangiography is used to demonstrate the nature of lymphatic abnormalities and to diagnose lymphoedema. Pedal lymphangiogram is done by injecting blue dye subcutaneously between the toes to outline the lymphatic vessels.
- Duplex imaging—A duplex scanner uses B mode ultrasound to provide an image of vessels.
- Doppler flowmetry—to assess the status of the peripheral circulation, a continuous wave ultrasound signal is beamed at an artery and the reflected beam is picked up by a receiver.
- Laser doppler flowmetry—for direct measurement of the circulatory disorders in chronic compartment syndrome (CCS).
- Doppler ultrasonography—A doppler flow probe is used to exclude arterial disease, and to determine the patency of a vein. A bidirectional flow probe is used to detect venous reflex.
- Bone densitometers—to assess the bone mineral density (BMD)—the single best method to diagnose osteoporosis and to assess the future risk of osteoporotic fractures. Of many types of densitometers, two commonly used are:
  1. Ultrasound densitometer—nonionising, safe and cheap, but not that precise.
  2. Dual energy X-ray absorptiometry (DEXA): it is accurate, precise and reproducible 'Gold standard results', but is costly.

iii. Tomography (stratigraphy; planigraphy; Tomos=cut or section): X-ray taken after being focussed at a desired depth blurring all the structures above or below, and anterior or posterior of the area of interest.

iv. Stereoscopic—bi-dimensional picture studies.

v. Cine-radiography.

vi. Scintography (Radio-active isotope studies or radio-nuclide studies). A three phase study aiming to show the vascular, soft tissue and bone uptake is performed using TC-99 m MDP. It is sensitive for detecting osseous abnormalities, but should be correlated with plain radiograph or other techniques, since it is nonspecific.

vii. Ultrasonic scanning, and high resolution ultrasonography.

viii. Computer assisted X-ray tomography.

ix. Computerised tomography and intrathecal low osmolarity contrast media studies.

x. Nuclear Magnetic Resonance Imaging (NMRI) or Magnetic Resonance Imaging (MRI)—In order to avoid using the word nuclear, which induces fear, the changed terminology is MRI.

xi. Spinal cord monitoring—Recording of somatosensory evoked potentials (SEP).

xii. Meterecom (a 3-D skeletal analyser)—A precise, computer-based, non-invasive, 3-dimensional digitizer designed to access bony landmarks, at any point on the body for various patient's positions.

xiii. Roentgen-Stereophotogrammetric Analysis (RSA) allows the accurate three-dimensional measurement of relative implant movement and in certain circumstances, measurement of wear. The accuracy of RSA can be upto the detection of 0.1 to 0.8 mm for translation movement and 1 to 2° for rotation at the 99% significance level.

xiv. MSI (Roser Boldlex 1995): The combination of technique of MRI and Magneto Encephalographic Recording (MEG) is being known as Magnetic Source Imaging (MSI). This indicates a functional description rather than only anatomical detail.

Clinical Diagnosis

Basically clinical diagnosis is based on sound knowledge of anatomy, physiology, and pathology; a specific history and detail clinical examination. In the process of making a diagnosis at the end of careful listening and analysing the history, guess the diagnosis; after thorough clinical examination make a provisional clinical diagnosis, which should be nearly confirmed by the relevant investigations. But the final confirmed diagnosis should be made only after histopathological examination (medicolegal aspect).

Thorough clinical examination leads to more or less accurate clinical diagnosis. However, in certain situations, this may not be possible. In such conditions, provisional diagnosis with immediate differential diagnosis should be mentioned. The most probable provisional diagnosis should be reached by the process of elimination, starting from the common to rare conditions.

In expressing the diagnosis of the disease, it is essential to make it a complete expression under the following headings:

i. Duration
ii. Anatomical site affected
iii. Causative pathology with its stage of advancement,
iv. Any obvious complication
v. Any particular treatment given
vi. Affection of the patient's routine life, specially the activities of daily living (ADL). e.g.:
   A. 5 months old, untreated, advanced tuberculous arthritis of right hip joint with discharging sinus, and patient not able to perform ADL.
   or B. 7 weeks old conservatively managed traumatic ununited fracture of neck of left femur with 2 cms. of supratrochanteric shortening and patient not able to perform ADL.

BIBLIOGRAPHY

1. Pare A: The works of that famous Chirurgion Ambroise Parey—translated by T Johnson. London, R Cotes and W Du-gard, 1649.
2. Roger Boldlex: *A century of Medical Imaging*, Paraplegia, **33**: 685-686, 1995.

2 Examination of Long Bones

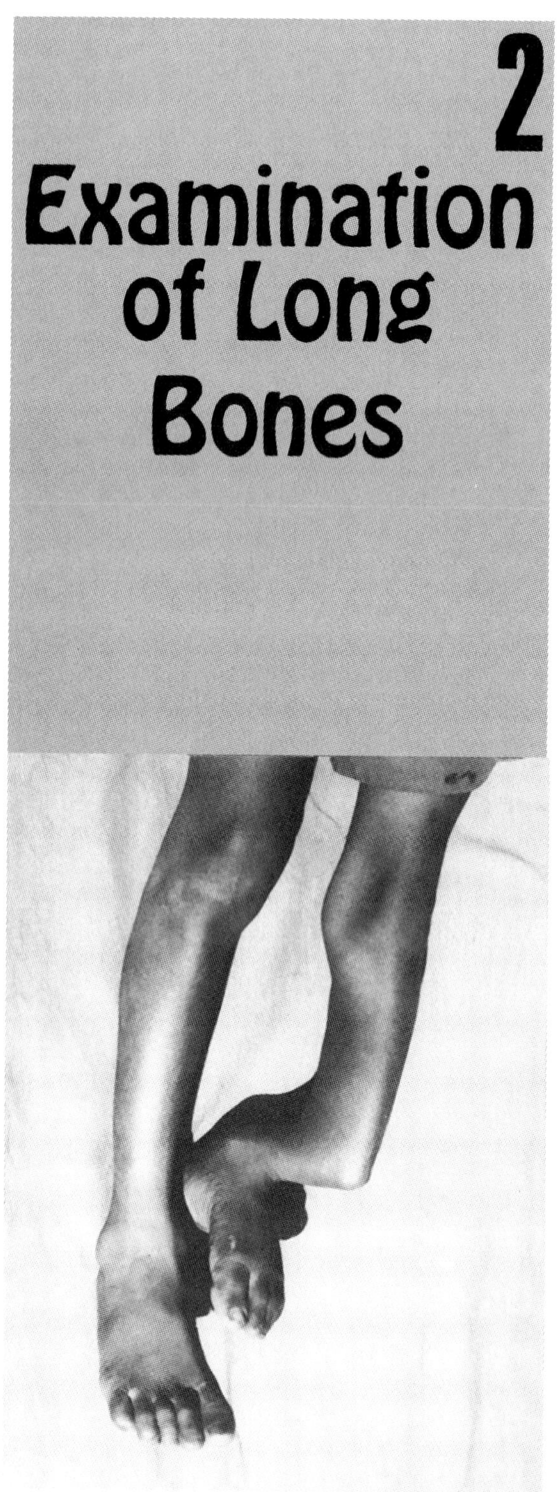

INTRODUCTION

Except when it is acutely affected, e.g. fracture or acute inflammatory lesions, the affections of the shaft remain unheeded for varying periods. The movements of the adjoining joints are not affected in the majority of shaft affections. Therefore, the patient has comparatively less disability. Of course, in all shaft affections, the examination of the adjoining joints is essential. The shaft of the short long bones, e.g. metacarpals, metatarsals and phalanges will be examined as discussed in the chapter of Hand and Foot.

ANATOMICAL CONSIDERATION

The long bone, before fusion of its growing epiphyses can be descriptively divided into:

1. *Diaphysis*: The central portion of shaft upto the metaphysis at both ends.

2. *Metaphysis:* (The flared transitional zone between the diaphysis and epiphysis). Metaphysis are the ends of diaphysis proximal to the epiphyseal growth plates on each side. It is difficult to draw an exact line of demarcation between diaphysis and metaphysis. The structure of the bone is much more compact in diaphysis than in the metaphyseal region. At the metaphysis, the cortical layer of bone is very thin. However, the metaphyseal region contains mostly highly vascular cancellous or spongy new bone.

3. *Epiphyseal growth plate:* Epiphyseal growth cartilage or plate lies transversely between metaphysis and epiphysis, and is responsible for longitudinal growth of the bone.

4. *Epiphysis*: The ends of the long bones are the epiphysis (between growth plate and articular cartilage). In infancy, most of the bulk of the epiphysis is cartilaginous, having a central area of ossification. With the advancement of age, the bony bulk of the epiphysis increases.

5. *Articular cartilage*: The epiphysis is capped with a layer of hyaline cartilage at its extreme ends. This smooth gliding shiny surface is bathed all the time with the synovial fluid for facilitating the movements of the joints.

A typical long bone is cylindrical with expanded ends. The periosteum, a tough thin connective tissue layer, is more and more closely adherent as we go from the centre to the ends. It covers the entire bone except the articular cartilage, and attachments of tendons, ligaments and joint capsule. However, in infants and children, the periosteum is thick, more vascular and cellular and is on the whole comparatively loosely attached. With increasing age it becomes thinner, less vascular, less cellular and more firmly attached.

Periosteal blood vessels lie on the outer face of periosteum anastomosing with the adjacent muscular blood vessels.

Nerve supply of the periosteum is mainly vasomotor and run along the periosteal blood vessels.

The periosteum is a fibrocellular structure having two layers—outer fibrous (dense collagen fibrous tissue and fibroblast like cells) and inner cambium (vascular) layer. In the inner cambium layer osteoblasts, having very potent osteogenic activities, are interspersed here and there. They are responsible for the circumferential growth of the long bones.

BLOOD SUPPLY OF LONG BONES (Fig. 2.1)

Taking all together the volume of blood supply of the long bones account for 5 to 10% of the cardiac output.

The long bones have three main sources of blood supply:

1. Nutrient system
2. Periosteal system
3. Metaphyseal system

1. *Nutrient system*: The nutrient artery usually perforates the shaft of a long bone in its middle third. After piercing the cortical layer at a definite place for each bone, it divides into ascending and descending branches. These branches travel along the Haversian canal, forming anastomosis at different levels all around and ultimately form anastomotic rings in the metaphyseal area.

2. *Periosteal system*: The periosteum receives blood supply from the adjoining soft tissues especially the muscles, which send tiny perforating branches almost to their attachment to the bones. These small branches ultimately anastomose with the branches of the nutrient system and are responsible for supplying about outer two-thirds of the bony wall.

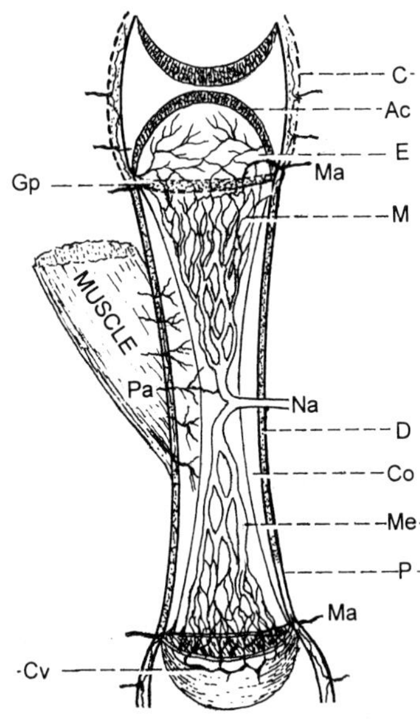

Fig. 2.1: Different parts of long bone and its blood supply. C = capsule; AC = articular cartilage; GP = growth plate; Ma = metaphysical artery; M = metaphysis; Na = nutrient artery; D = diaphysis; Co = cortex; Me = medulla; P = periosteum; Pa = periosteal artery; Cv = circulus vasculosus

3. *Metaphyseal system:* Direct branches from the articular blood vessels or the adjoining muscular blood vessels form an anastomotic leashing, almost all around the metaphyseal surface. From this circular arterial system, multiple perforating branches enter the metaphysis. They heavily interlace among each other as well as with the ends of the nutrient system.

Short bones are supplied by numerous periosteal blood vessels. A rib is supplied by a nutrient artery and periosteal vessels.

Veins

Variable sinusoidal networks are formed in the regions of epiphysis, metaphysis and diaphysis.

These in turn drain into venous channel leaving the bone through all its surfaces which are not covered by articular cartilage. Valveless nutrient veins accompany the nutrient arteries.

Lymphatics

Lymphatic vessels are found accompanying the periosteal vascular plexuses but their presence within the bone substance has never been convincingly demonstrated.

Nerves

They are distributed freely within the layer of the periosteum. Finely myelinated and non-myelinated nerve fibres accompany the nutrient vessels into the interior of the bone and even into the perivascular spaces of the *Haversian* canals. Articular ends of the long bone are very rich in nerve supply.

Most of the part of the shaft of a long bone is protected by several layers of soft tissues—i.e. muscular, fascial, fibrofatty, subcutaneous and cutaneous layers. However, all the layers may not be complete all around all over in all bones, e.g. in tibia. Therefore, examination of the shaft of a long bone mandatorily implies the examination of soft tissues, neurovascular bundles and the bony axis. The long bone supports the central core axis of the limbs, and it also provides surface for attachment of different muscles.

The marrow of long bones are mostly red, specially at the ends, therefore, the haemopoietic activity is also subserved by the long bones. The long bone also acts like a long lever for effective functional mobility at the adjoining joint fulcrum.

METHODOLOGY

History Taking (As in the chapter on Introduction)

General Examination

General, systemic and cursory regional examination must precede the local examination of the shaft (As in the chapter on Introduction).

LOCAL EXAMINATION

1. Inspection
2. Palpation
3. Percussion
4. Squeezing
5. Measurement
6. Auscultation

Examination of the shaft is not complete till the adjoining joints are thoroughly examined.

1. Inspection Prerequisites

i. The part to be examined or even the entire limb must be adequately exposed for examination.
ii. The corresponding part of the opposite limb must be examined for comparison.
iii. Both limbs must be kept in identical position (position the unaffected limb in the same posture, in which the affected limb has been kept comfortably by the patient).

Look For

A. The position, shape, thickening or thinning of the part.
B. Skin surface regarding its look, texture, colour, creases, vascularity, presence of scar, sinus, obvious pulsation through skin. Any abnormal swelling must be examined as per the examination of the swelling anywhere in body (shape, surface, mobility, consistency, relationship to deeper structures and surrounding structures, fixity, etc.).
C. Look at the long bone from diaphysis to epiphyseal end and compare its symmetry with the opposite side. There may be angulation or bowing [congenital (Figs 2.2A to 2.4) traumatic, syphilitic—sabre tibia, degenerative collapse, Paget's desease, etc.]. Look at metaphyseal area for any broadening (if bilateral—usually rickets, if unilateral—usually traumatic or neoplastic).
D. Epiphyseal area may be thickened or there may be swelling.
E. With a suspicion of rickets or syphilis always look for their stigmata.

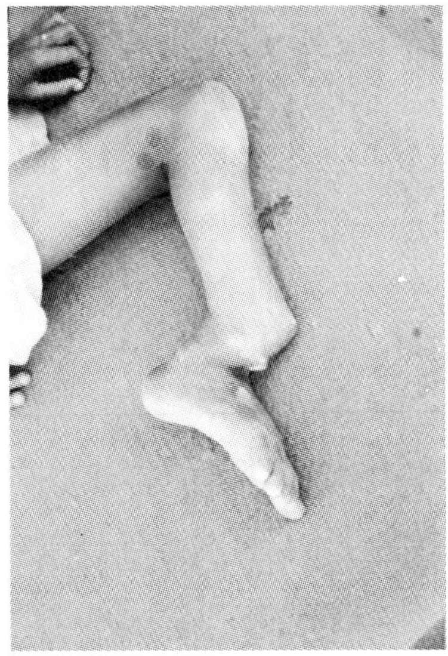

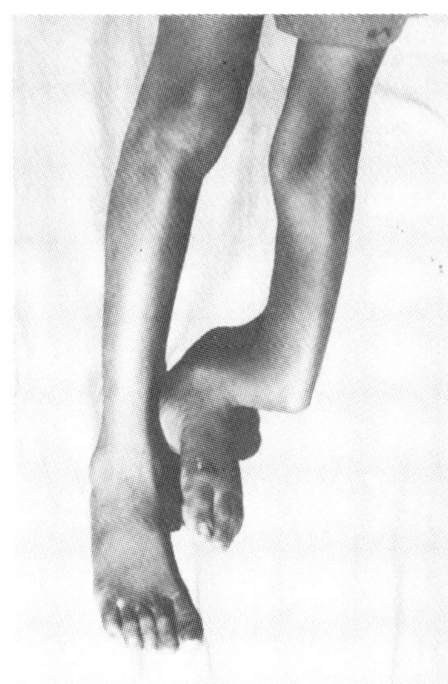

Figs 2.2A and B: Congenital pseudoarthrosis (often associated with neurofibromatosis) of tibia with gross angulation is most frequently encountered, but this pseudoarthrosis may occur in any long bone (e.g. forearm bones—usually only ulna or raidus; femur)

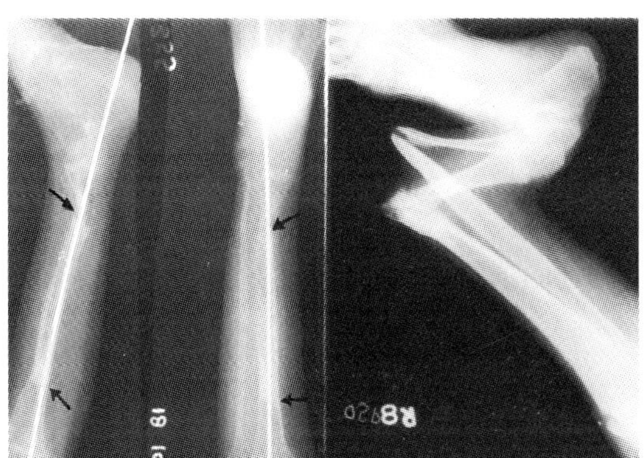

Fig. 2.3: X-ray picture of congenital pseudoarthrosis of lower third of leg bones (common site) — Pre and post correction radiographs

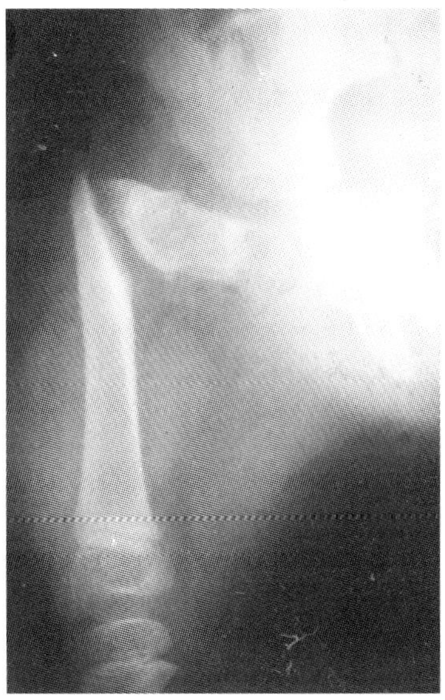

Fig. 2.4: Congenital pseudoarthrosis of femur (unusual site)

Stigmata of Rickets

- Delayed closure of fontanellae, cranio tabes, frontal bossing.
- Delayed eruption of teeth, decaying of teeth.
- Pigeon chest, rachitic rosary, Harrison's sulcus.
- Protuberant abdomen, hepatomegaly.
- Broadening in wrist region.
- Coxa-vara, anterolateral bowing of femur, genu valgum or varum, anterolateral bowing of lower third of tibia with flattening of tibia and secondary adaptive changes in the foot (for genu valgum, varum or bowing) (Figs 2.5A to 2.5D).
- Rachitic dwarfism (especially in renal rickets).

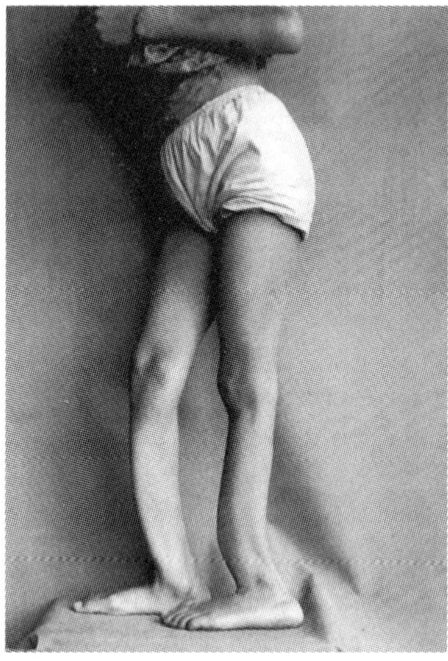

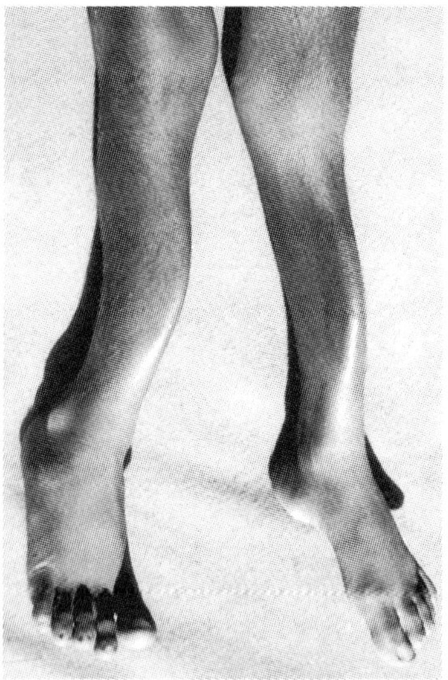

Figs 2.5A and B: Rachitic bilateral bow leg. Note the bowing in the lower third with side to side flattening of tibia

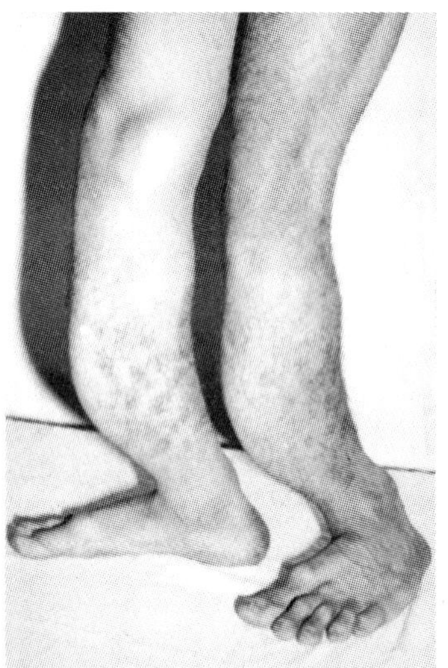

Fig. 2.5C: Sabre tibiae

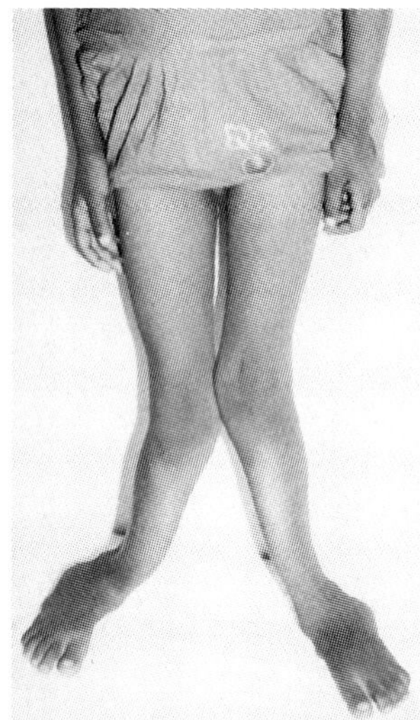

Fig. 2.5D: Rachitic bilateral genu valgum with anterior bowing in the lower third junctional zone

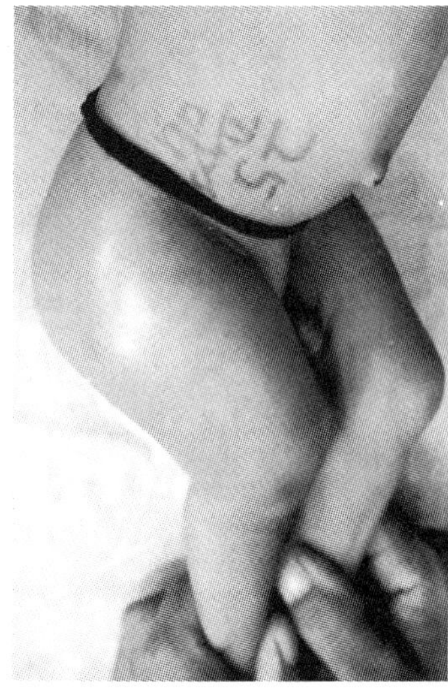

Fig. 2.5E: Acute haematogenous osteomyelitis

Stigmata of Syphilis
- Alopecia
- Frontal bossing
- Depressed nasal bridge, perforation of nasal septum. (cf. flattening of nose-tip in leprosy)
- Hutchinson's teeth
- Keratitis
- Auditory nerve deafness
- Snuffles.

| Hutchinson's triad.
≠

- Enlarged lymph nodes—occipital and epitrochlear.
- High arching palate, perforation of palate, mucous patches.
- Gumma of testis.
- Condylomatas (anal region, mouth) (Fig.9.1).
- Sabre tibia (Fig. 2.5C).
- Clutton's joint (symptomless symmetrical synovitis with boggy fluid distension usually in childhood due to congenital syphilis).
- Charcot's joint (Fig. 12.53).

2. Palpation

Confirm the findings of inspection.

A. *Superficial Palpation (touch)*

Temperature, hyperaesthesia, hypoaesthesia, anaesthesia, texture of skin (smooth, rough, etc.), superficial crepitation, superficial tenderness to be noted.

B. *Deep Palpation (feel)*

Feel the muscles, deeper soft tissues and normal bony shaft after displacing longitudinal muscle fibres to the sides wherever possible. Note any abnormality like crepitus, abnormal swelling, fixity of the soft tissues, irregularity of the bone, etc. Crepitus may be an important finding while examining the shaft of a long bone (confirms fracture, if with history of injury; confirms pathological fracture in expansile lesion of the bone, e.g. giant cell tumour). However, it should not be attempted only for the sake of confirming fracture in clinical examination. After all, crepitus results from rattling of the bony fringes at the fractured ends. This crackling is going to break the thin fragile fringes and thereby reduce the possibility of locking of the fragments following reduction. If it is done for diagnosing an expansile lesion (giant cell tumour),the thin expanded fragile cortical shell sustains microfractures, thereby allowing leakage of the underlying contents and dissemination of the pathological tissues hitherto confined within the bony cortical shell. In the course of gentle examination or gentle handling of the limbs, if crepitus or abnormal mobility are felt, they will be a welcome finding. However, one must not attempt to demonstrate these clinical signs in acute lesions.

If the general curvature of the shaft is not identical with the opposite side this should be clearly noted. Note the site of abnormal contour, the direction of bulge, and the change in curvature. Palpate surface of curvatures as far as practicable as if examining a bony lump. Whenever possible, any abnormal vascular finding should be noted (pulsation, thrill, compressibility, pulsatile swelling, ballooning and varicosities). Palpate the soft tissues, layer by layer all along. Any abnormal tender spot should be thoroughly scrutinized. At times, nodular or oblong firm soft tissue swellings are felt at varying depths which are usually tender on direct pressure (neurofibroma). In case of neoplasm, its status, as regards benign or malignant, should be decided clinically as described in the chapter on Bone Tumours.

3. Percussion

Percussion of a long bone usually subserves more or less the function of squeezing. However, tenderness in the shin of tibia is well demonstrated by this method.

4. Squeezing

Periosteal tear and haematoma, a very minor crack fracture or a deep seated painful bony lesion may not be accurately diagnosed by the routine method of examination. In such cases, squeezing of the palpable portion of the shaft of the bone may provide a clue. By squeezing, pressure stress is generated on the surface of the bone which travels along the long axis of the bone. The moment the wave encounters the discontinued area, the subperiosteal nerve endings are triggered by the vibratory waves and the patient complains of pain at the site.

5. Measurement

Linear measurement of the shaft includes total and segmental length measurement of the limb (as described in the concerned chapter).

The circumferential measurement of the shaft must be done at the symmetrical levels of the shaft (e.g. mid shaft levels) for muscular wasting or increase in girth. Besides, the girth at the level of any abnormal swelling must be compared to that of the unaffected limb.

6. Auscultation

This clinical ritual sometimes is much informative, e.g. hearing for a systolic bruit in a highly vascular swelling of the long bones.

7. Investigation

i. Beside the routine haemogram and urine analysis, X-rays are very important. This should be taken preferably in three planes, i.e. anteroposterior, lateral and oblique. If possible, X-ray of the corresponding part of the shaft of other limb must be included in same plate for comparison. This helps in detecting the minor changes in the texture, girth and curvature of the bones. In the X-ray—the entire shaft must be exposed specially where inflammatory and neoplastic lesions are suspected. The skip lesions in the same shaft have been noted in several cases.
ii. Orthotomography—It is done to detect any suspicious lesion, which cannot be detected by ordinary X-rays, e.g. osteoid osteoma.
iii. Radioisotope-scanning.
iv. Computerised axial tomography.
v. Magnetic Resonance Imaging (MRI).
vi. For confirmation of any lesion histopathological examination may be necessary. Of course before this, other investigations including radioscanning must be completed. Histopathological examination can be done by either aspiration biopsy or open biopsy. The latter is more authentic.

KEY DIAGNOSTIC POINTS OF COMMON AFFECTIONS OF LONG BONES

A. Osteomyelitis (Table 2.1)

Broadly 'osteomyelitis' is inflammation of bone, but it comprises of two words—osteitis (inflammation of bone) + myelitis (inflammation of marrow). Inflammation may be defined as the reaction of vascularised living tissue to local tissue injury or insult by different stimuli. Osteomyelitis can be acute, subacute, and chronic depending upon the period of infection, the virulence of dose of infective organism and the immune system, age, general nature and condition of the host.

1. *Acute Haematogenous Osteomyelitis* (Fig. 2.5E) (= infection of bone and marrow by circulating organisms in the blood from a distant source in the body)

- Usually occurs in childhood.
- Vague history of insignificant trauma, followed by pain.
- Constitutional features—high temperature (around 39°C) persisting for few days, patient looks ill and toxic.
- Affected part (metaphyseal region) swollen, warm, distended, erythematous; pitting oedema (indicates deep pus collection, e.g. sub-periosteal abscess).
- Clinical features base on pathophysiological evolution of acute haematogenous osteomyelitis as summarised in three stages (Treuta 1968): Stage I—a boil in the bone manifesting as constant severe pain, swelling, local tenderness; Stage II—features of established inflammation with increase in above clinical features; Stage III—sub-periosteal abscess stage (clinical features as noted above).
- Neighbouring joint mildly swollen, however fair range of passive movement can be demonstrated. But patient does not want to move his limb due to pain.
- Regional lymph nodes enlarged, soft and tender.
- When asked for, he can point to the site of maximum pain, which is also very tender, i.e. this is the point of focus in the metaphysis.
- Bacterial pyomyositis (infection of skeletal muscle by staphylococci or other organisms) is common in tropics, which can be easily confused with, especially in adults.

Table 2.1: Characteristics of osteomyelitis in different age groups

Infancy	*Childhood*	*Adult*
• 1 year (0-1 Year)	— Maxm. incidence (1-17 Years).	— 17 onwards.
• Usually secondary to umbilical infection	— Haematogenous from any septic focus.	— Open fractures, — Haematogenous.
• Constitutional features less marked.	— More marked.	— Moderately marked.
• Site—Usually intra-articular metaphysis and epiphysis.	— Metaphyseal.	— Usually diaphyseal
• Local temperature—very little/ insignificant/or even not raised.	— Always raised.	— Mild to moderately raised.
• Pus not under pressure.	— Pus under tension.	— Less pus (located in medullary, cavity).
• Veil like periosteum is easily perforated by pus.	— Sub-periosteal pus collection persists for sometime elevating periosteum for longer and wider distance before bursting.	— Adherent periosteum does not allow wider spread of pus.
• Diffuse local oedema manifest quite early—even whole limb may be swollen.	— Pitting oedema more or less localised to area of affection.	— Pitting oedema localised to area of affection.
• Joint affection frequent because infection can easily penetrate along the communicating blood vessels through epiphyseal growth plate.	— Joint affection less frequent except at sites where metaphysis is intracapsular.	— Joint affection in late cases due to muscular adhesions.
• *Sequestrum* formation much less	— Very common.	— Smaller/thin sequestra, except in open fractures (where bigger sequestrum).
Complications		
• Dissolution of intra-articular cartilage.	— Extensive diaphyseal affection.	— Flares
• Unstable joint	— Pathological fracture. — Persistant sinus	— Pathological fractures — Persistant sinus
• Marked shortening	— Limb length disparity—lenghening more common.	— Shortening and/or deformities due to malunited pathological fractures
• Angular deformities more common.	— If joint involvement—epiphyseal separation.	
• Chronic conversion much less	— Chronic conversion much common.	— Chronicity more common Malignancy—epithelioma in sinus — Sarcoma in bone — Amyloidosis
• Organisms: Staphylococci H. influenza Streptococci Pneumococci	— Staphylococci Streptococci Pneumococci Salmonella and others. In sickle cell anaemia, salmonella group more common.	— Staphylococci, pseudomonas, bacillus proteus, and others. In heroin addicts pseudomonas aeruginosa is predominant organism, besides staphylococcus aureus and gram-negative bacilli.

Investigations

Total differential count of WBC—polymorphonuclear leucocytosis.

—Blood ESR raised.

X-ray: May be non-contributory till 10-12 days.

—Within 48 hours	• Loss of normal delineation between the subcutaneous and muscular shadows (*Glenn* 1948). • Linear transverse lines extending from muscle outwards.
—10 to 12 days	• Localised rarefaction at the site of origin of the disease (earlier in infancy). • Early subperiosteal new bone formation.
—12 to 20 days	• Soft tissues present almost homogeneous look. • Surrounding bone also rarefied due to increased vascularity. • Increasing subperiosteal reactionary longitudinal bone laying.

—Blood culture may be positive

—Culture of the aspirate and/or scraped tissue indicates the causative organism (also true for subacute and chronic osteomyelitis).

—Special investigation

—Radioisotope studies for hot spots.

—CAT scanning and MRI.

2. *Subacute Osteomyelitis*

- The second half of the 20th century saw truly, the remarkable advances in the therapy of bacterial infections, still it is not uncommon to see the cases of subacute or chronic osteomyelitis.
- For convenience acute osteomyelitis presenting beyond 3 weeks may be known as subacute one, however, pathology may start *de-novo* as subacute presentation.
- Constitutional features present but less marked.
- Patient can move the affected part slightly.
- Part swollen (but not so much as in acute osteomyelitis).
- Local temperature raised, local tenderness and appearance of bony thickening.
- Neighbouring joint is less swollen but with terminal painful limitation of the movements (due to the fact that the controlling muscles which were oedematous at the beginning now start developing adhesions).
- Regional lymph nodes enlarged but less tender.

X-ray:

- Soft tissue shadow starts getting smaller.
- Localised rarefaction irregularly spreads in the medullary cavity and/or towards cortex.
- Periosteal longitudinal bone laying well marked.
- In extensive diaphyseal affections there may be indication of early pathological fracture.

3. *Chronic Osteomyelitis*

—Prolonged history.

—No constitutional features except when there is flare.

—Discharging or healed sinuses, usually fixed to the bone.

—History of discharge of small bony spicules.

—May be deformities (usually angulation) (Figs 2.6 and 2.7); neighbouring joint usually stiff or having limited movement; affected bone thickened for variable lengths; may be tender.

—May be limb length disparity (usually affected bone is longer) (Figs 2.8, 2.9, 2.9A, 2.9B) [cf. other common causes of limb disparity, e.g. congenital (Figs 2.10A to 2.10C), haemangiomatous (Figs 2.10F and 2.10G), lymphangiomatus (Figs 2.10H and I), and dyschondroplasia (Figs 2.10J to 2.10L)].

—Regional lymph glands insignificant.

X-ray: Soft tissue shadow usually shrunken (due to wasting and adhesions).

—May be sequestrum (a dead piece of bone separated from the living in the process of necrosis, by granulation tissue and/or pus). (Fig. 2.11)

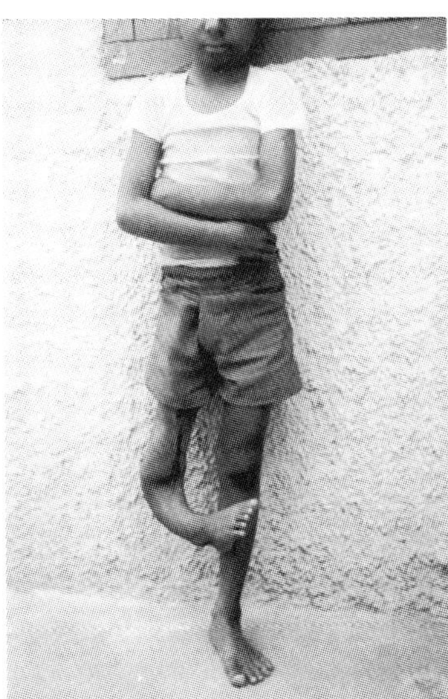

Fig. 2.6: Gross angulation and shortening due to destruction and bone loss following chronic osteomyelitis

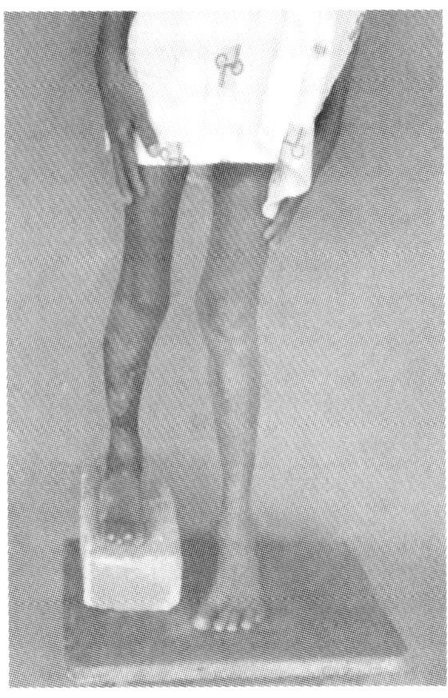

Fig. 2.6A: Same patient after fibular muscle pedicle graft

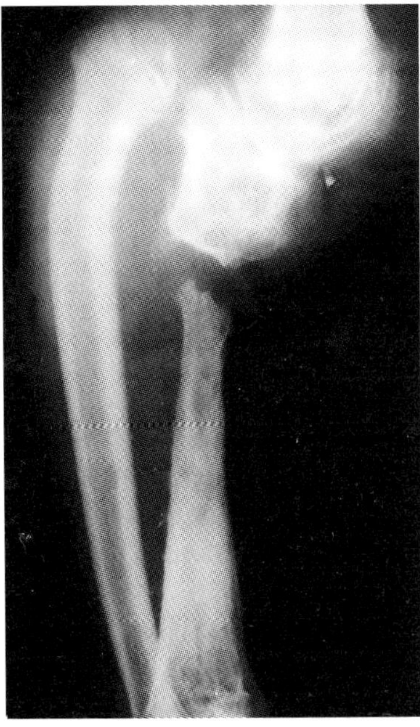

Fig. 2.7: Gross deformity and shortening following sequestrated out a diaphyseal segment in pyogenic chronic osteomyelitis

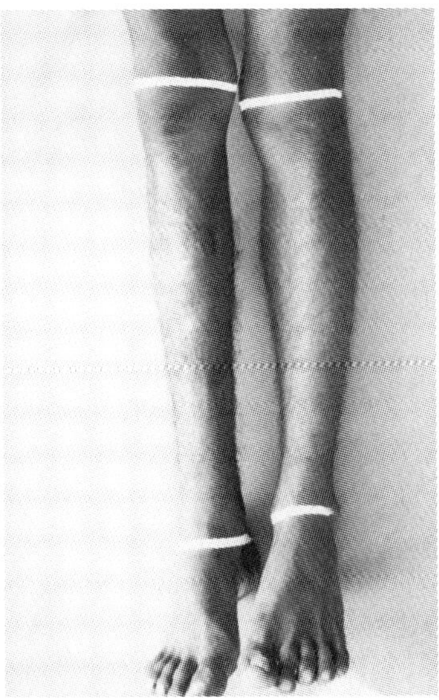

Fig. 2.8: Lengthening of leg due to chronic osteomyelitis of right upper third of tibia

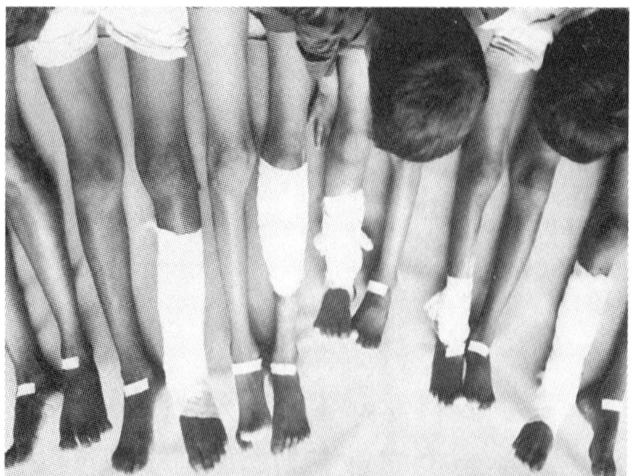

Fig. 2.9: Group photograph of patients having limb-length disparity (usually lengthening) which is quite common following chronic osteomyelitis

— Sinus track denoted by irregular translucent passage reaching upto the bone (due to entrapped air).
— Surrounding new bone formation—involucrum.
— Evidence of healed pathological fracture, malunion, may be non-union.
— Relics of damaged cartilaginous growth plate.

4. *Brodies Abscess*
— Usually in the upper end of the tibia, upper end of the femur, lower end of the tibia, lower end of the femur, upper end of the humerus.
— Usually in late teens or in young adults; present with chronic dull pain in the metaphyseal zone, specially after work or exertion; slight to moderate pitting oedema.
—Underlying bone is tender.
— Neighbouring joint usually not affected.

X-ray: Localised area of irregular rarefaction surrounded by sclerosed zone.

B. Fractures (Tables 2.2 to 2.5)

Fracture of Long Bones

Examination of closed fracture markedly differs from that of an open one. Open fractures are almost always diagnosed by the patient/ relatives themselves. What is required is, after relevant X-ray, war footed management of these open fractures with the sole aim of converting

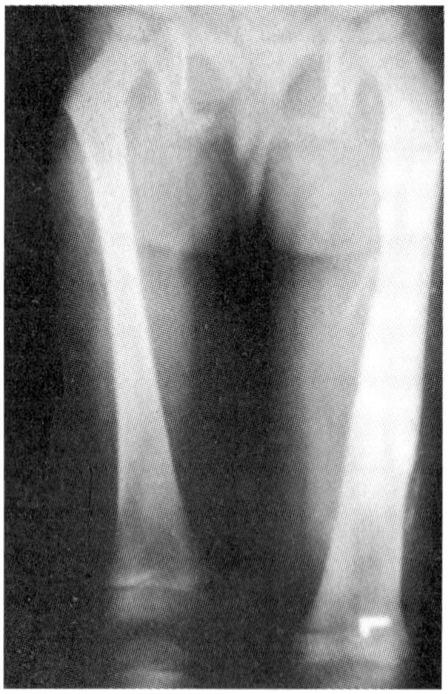

Fig. 2.9A: Lengthening of left femur due to chronic osteomyelitis (diaphyseal affection)

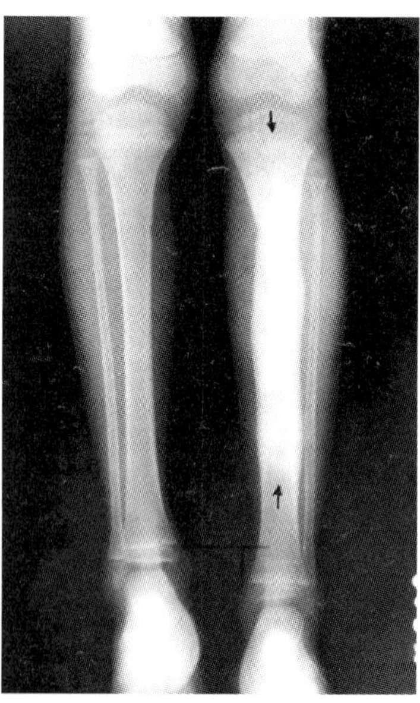

Fig. 2.9B: Lengthening of left tibia due to (metaphyseal) chronic osteomyelitis

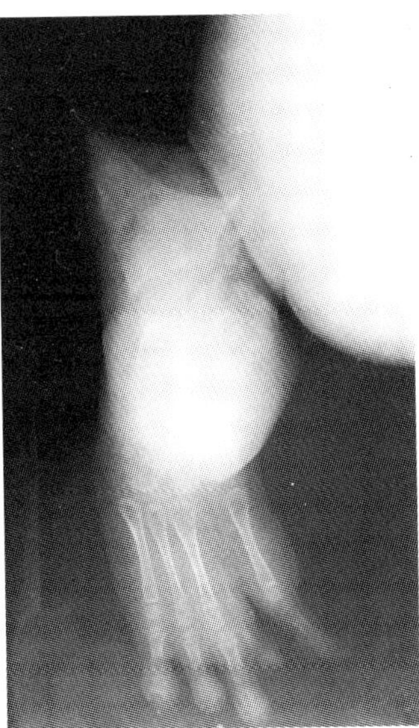

Fig. 2.10A: Congenital abscence of right thigh, knee, leg, ankle and hind-foot, which have been represented by a mass placed in horizontal continuity of the spider like forefoot

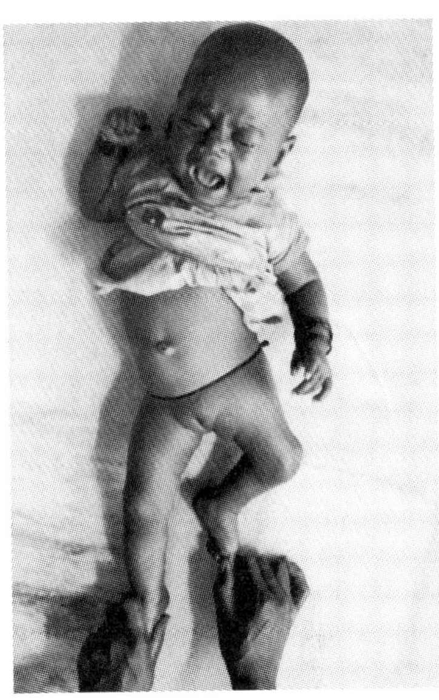

Fig. 2.10B: Congenital short femur and leg bones with gross dysplasia of hip and flexion deformity of knee

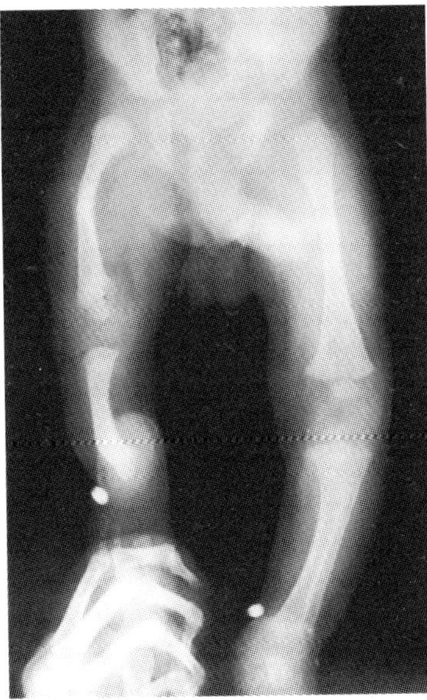

Fig. 2.10C: Congenital shortening and bowing of ipsilateral femur and tibia and abscence of fibula

them to closed type. Fractures around the joints and intra-articular fractures present more or less with joint problems.

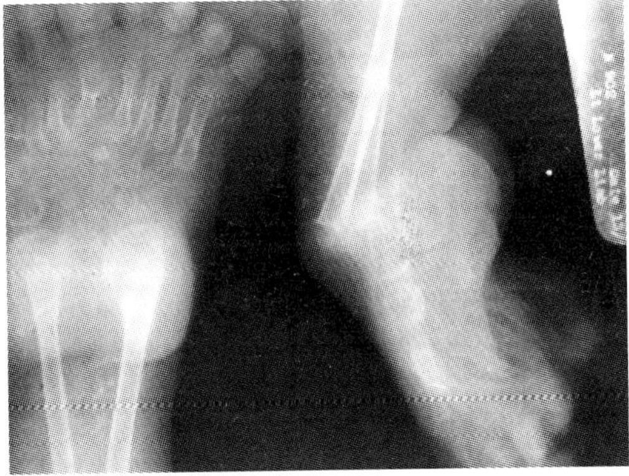

Fig. 2.10D: Congenitally disorganised leg bones, ankle and foot

Green Stick Fracture

It is an incomplete fracture in which only one cortex is broken with the fractured ends telescoped within each other, while the opposite cortex usually bends in the same direction, as occurs in an attempt of breaking a green bamboo stick. Infants and children are brought with bowed affected part, which is swollen and tender

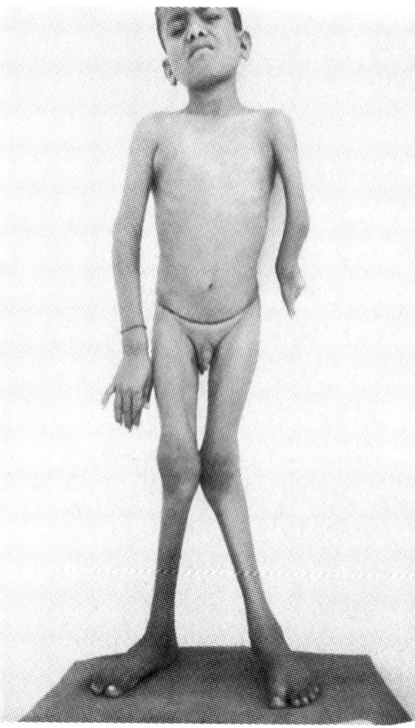

Fig. 2.10E: Congenital shortening of arm, forearm, and hand with ankylosed joints (elbow, wrist, fingers and thumb) and marked genu valgum with comparatively long legs

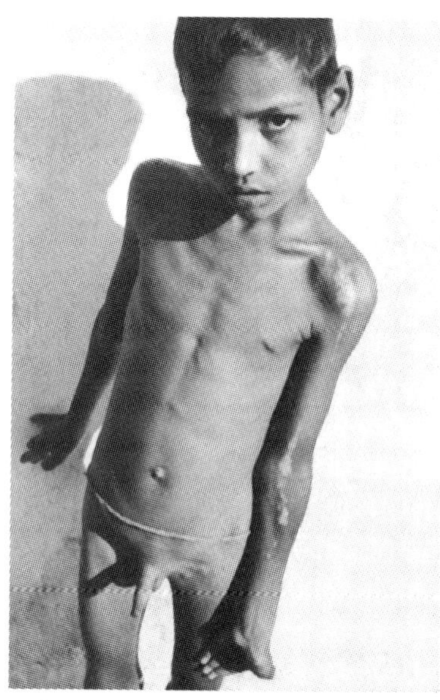

Fig. 2.10F: Haemangiomatous lengthening of the left upper limb. Note the capillary patches almost in continuity in front of shoulder, arm, elbow, wrist and thumb

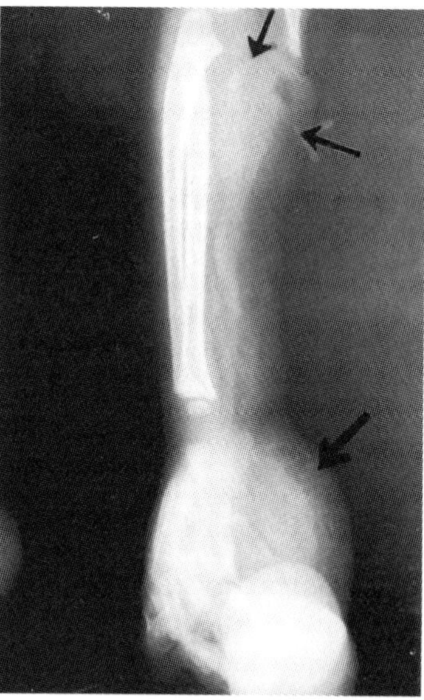

Fig. 2.10G: X-ray of forearm and hand of same boy (Fig. 2.10F). Note the swelling and the calcified mass shadow in haemangiomatous zone in front of forearm and hand

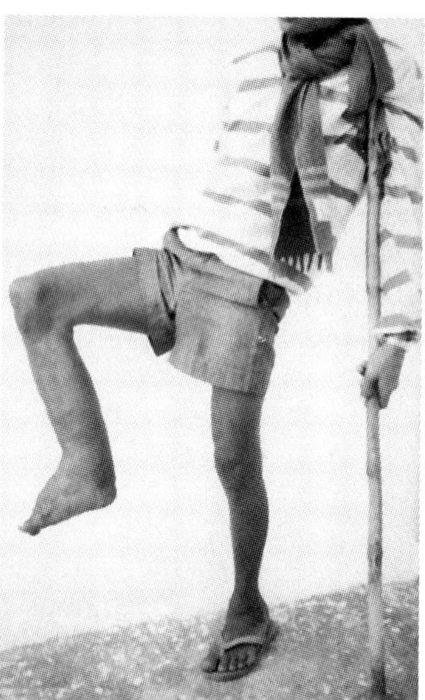

Fig. 2.10H: Congenital lymphoedema leading to enlargement of right lower limb (both length and breadthwise)

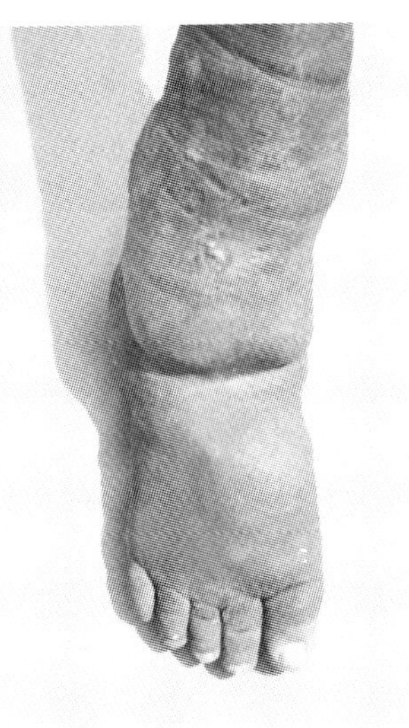

Fig. 2.10I: Filarial lymphoedema and elephantiasis with grooves and eczematous ulcers

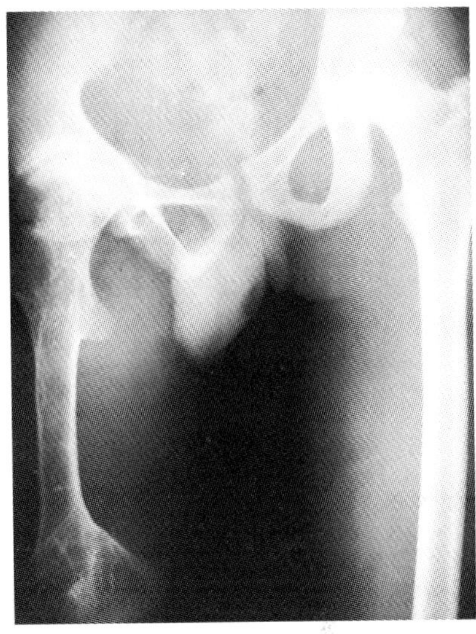

Fig. 2.10J: Dyschondroplasia. Note metaphyseal enlargement, thickened shaft, shortening of bone and mottled epiphysis

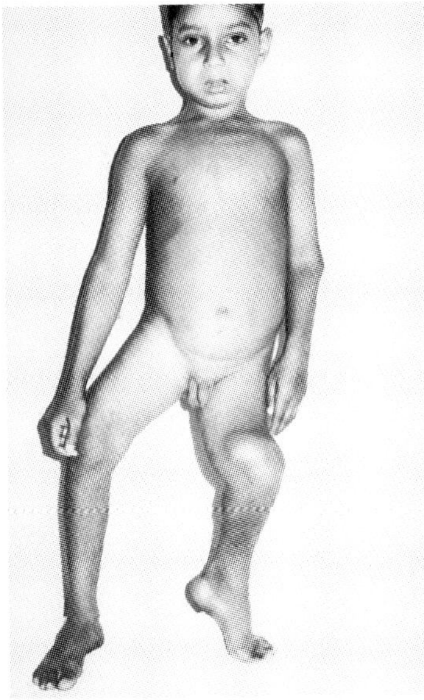

Fig. 2.10K: Dyschondroplastic femora and tibiae

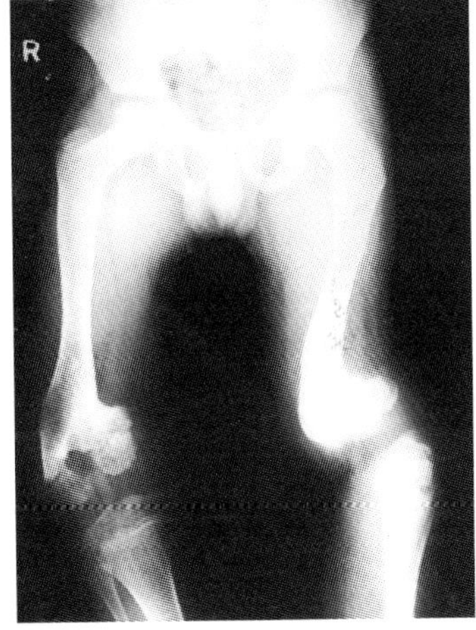

Fig. 2.10L: X-ray of the same boy (Fig. 2.10K)

at the fracture site, however, limb can be used to a fairly good extent. Since the fracture is always incomplete and impacted, there is no abnormal movement at the fracture site.

Features of a Fracture

- History of optimum indirect or direct violence.
- Immediate or delayed appearance of ecchymosis.
- Immediate feeling of pain; may be some rattling noise during the fracture; difficulty or inability in using that limb; gradually

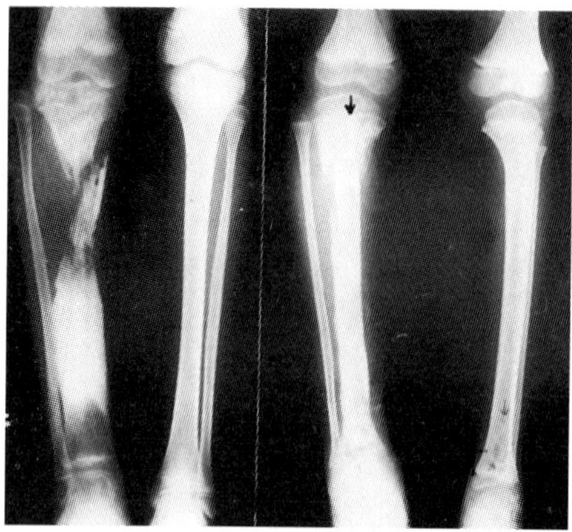

Fig. 2.11A: On the left half—extensive osteomyelitis of right tibia with pathological fractures and sequestrating out necrosed segment. It is bound to end up in a shorter leg. On the right half—shortening of right tibia due to chronic osteomyelitis with affection of growth epiphysis

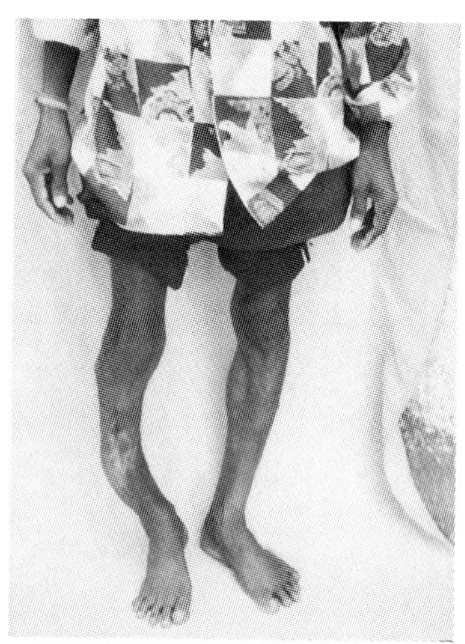

Fig. 2.11B: Malunited pathological fracture in osteomyelitis with marked bowing and shortening of leg

increasing swelling; deformities according to displacements, angulation and rotations.

— Localised persistent bony tenderness; squeezing of proximal and distal end of fractured bone leads to pain at the site. To elicit tenderness, press through healthy tissue (pressure on contused soft tissue may be misleading).

— Crepitus: If one gets crepitus during casual examination it should be noted, but do not attempt to demonstrate it.

— Irregular bony ends (with or without gap) may be felt.

— Abnormal mobility at the suspected fracture site; however in impacted fractures (e.g. *Colles* fracture, fracture upper end of humerus, Garden type I fracture of neck of femur), where one fracture end is partially or completely telescoped within another end, there will be no mobility at the fracture site and patient can invariably use the limb of course with variable pain.

— May even present with early complications of fractures, e.g. wrist drop in fracture shaft humerus; skin necrosis in dislocation of the ankle; effect of partial cessation of blood supply—early features of ischaemic changes (as written in Elbow chapter).

Juxta-Articular and Intra-Articular Fractures

— They may be associated with ligamentous injury of the joint (especially the intraarticular ones).

— Presentation mainly concerns with adjoining or affected joints.

— The affected bony ends may be widened and tender.

— Joint movements are painfully restricted.

— The concerned joint is swollen and tender.

— Deformities are due to angulation and subchondral collapse of bones.

— In the knee joint stress tests must be done to recognise, the possible internal derangements of the knee joint.

— In battered baby syndrome, the fractures are usually juxta articular with or without intra-articular communication (Fig. 2.13).

Pathological Fractures (Figs 2.11A and 2.11B)

— History of minor trauma (suboptimal for that age and bone).

— May be history of earlier local pathological lesion with persistent or occasional pain at the site, with or without swelling.

Table 2.2: Classification of fractures (Considering broad etiological factors)

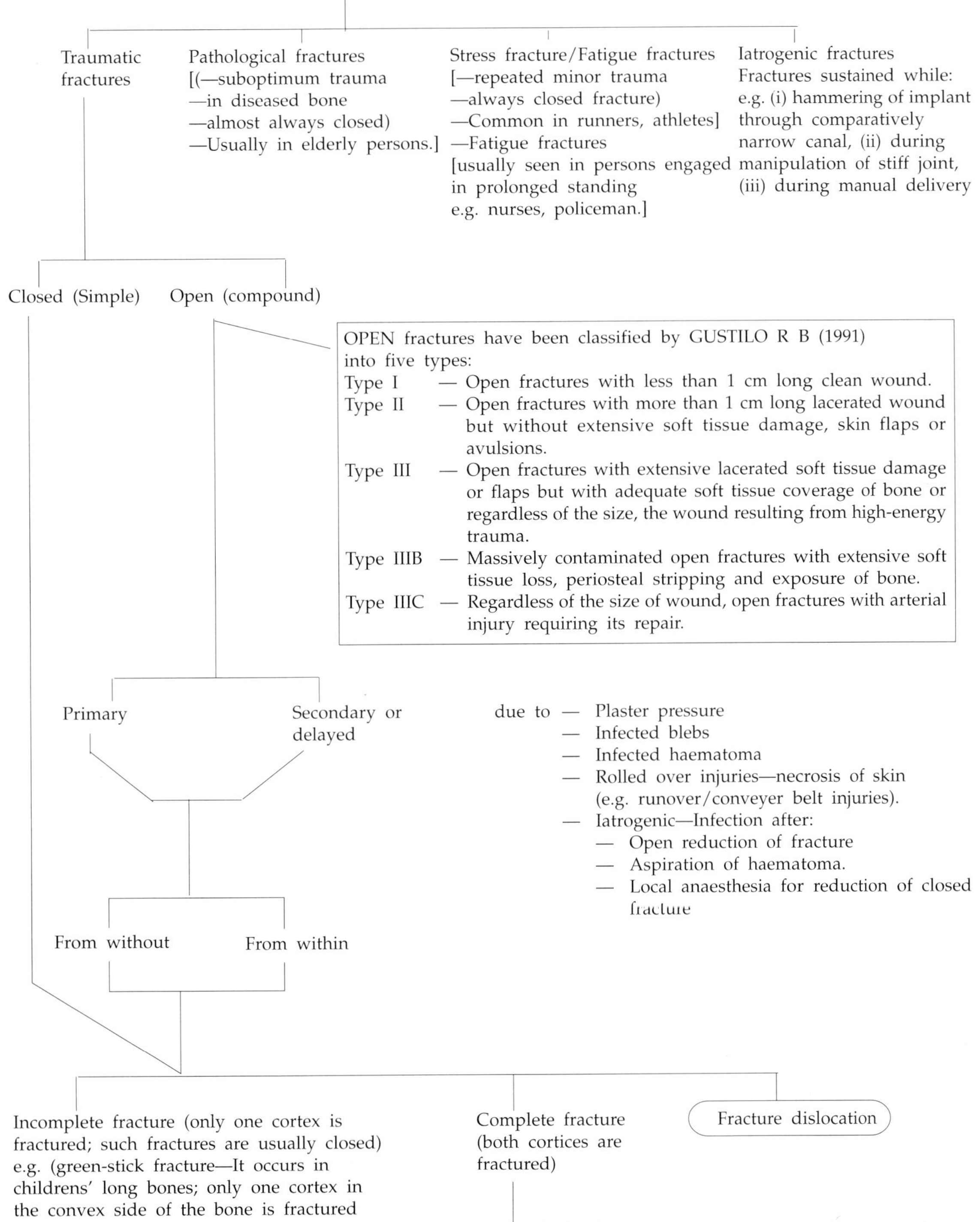

Contd.

Table 2.2: Contd.

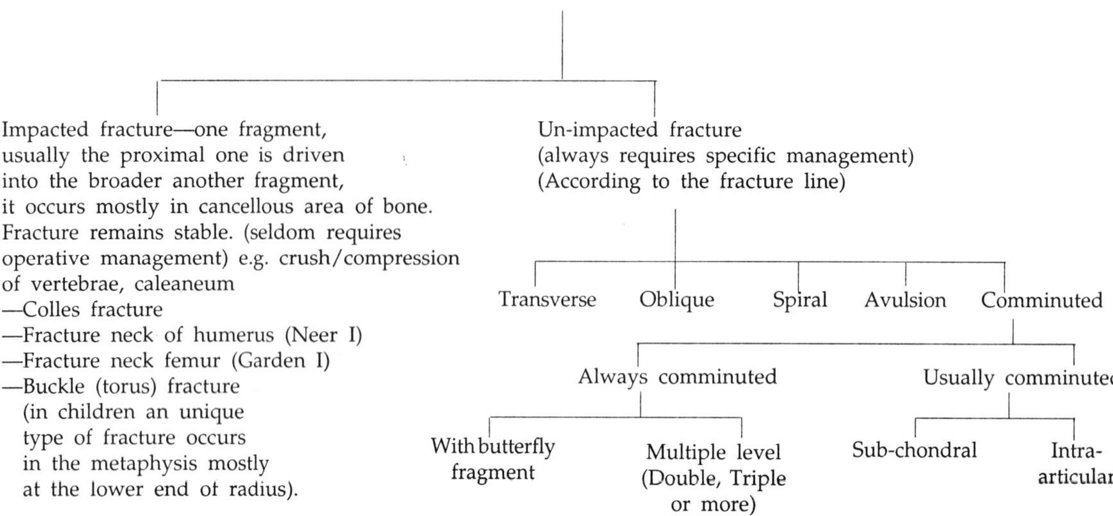

Displacements of Fractures: (Distal fragment is always to be considered for describing displacements in relation to the proximal fragment	(i) Shifts—Upward (overlap), downward (distraction) (ii) Tilts/Angulation—(consider convex side) mainly the valgus, varus, anterior or posterior angulation, (iii) Rotation/twist—external/internal Translation: —sidewards (lateral and medial) —forwards/backwards.

Table 2.3: Working time table for different stages of uncomplicated fracture healing—in weeks
(Based on Perkins G.)

	Ensheathing callus (gluing)	Clinical union	Consolidation	Radiological union
Child, Upper limb, long bone, Spiral fracture	5-6 days (¾th week)	1-1½	3	6
For each of the following, multiply by 2 • Adult • Lower limb long bone fracture • Transverse fracture.				

— Enquire for general debilitating conditions like diabetes mellitus, tabes dorsalis, alcoholism, malnutrition and prolonged hypoproteinaemia, prolonged morbidity, osteomalacia.
— Paget's disease, malignancy.
— Osteogenesis imperfecta (Figs. 1.8 and 2.13).
— Osteoporosis—a systemic bone disease, progressing with the population longevity, and characterised by low bone mass and micro architectural detereoration of bone tissue with a consequent increase in bone fragility and susceptability to fracture; gradual dorso-lumbar, lumbar kyphosis and loss in height.

Complications of Fractures

Whenever a fracture is diagnosed one must look for its possible complications.

Table 2.4: Salient features of different stages of fracture healing

	Ensheathing callus	*Clinical union*	*Consolidation*	*Radiological union*
Symptoms	— Pain +++ — Swelling +++ — Cannot bear any stress — Two ends at fracture move separately.	— Pain + — Swelling ++ — Can bear gravitational stress but not angulatory one. — Two ends at fracture move as one.	— No pain — Swelling + — Can bear upto angulation stress. — Two ends at fracture moves as one.	— No pain on any stress. — Swelling ±
Signs	— Warm — Firm fusiform swelling— due to organising haematoma and soft tissue swelling over and around the fractured ends. — Tenderness +++ — Surface at fracture site smooth except at the spiky ends.	— Slight warm — Fracture ends not felt. — Surface regular. — Firm or hard swelling. — Tenderness + — Fracture ends not felt. — Surface regular.	— Local temperature normal — Swelling less and hard — No tenderness — Surface regular	— Hard, more or less uniform non-tender slightly fusiform swelling
X-ray	— Fracture line clearly visible. — Hazy soft tissue swelling.	— Fracture line visible. —Callus • Exo callus. • Endo callus. • Interstitial callus.	— Fracture line may be visible. — Callus • Exo callus. • Endo callus. • Interstitial callus	— Fracture line not visible. — Callus • Exo callus – • Endo callus ± • Interstitial callus converted to trabecular bone — Medullary continuity ±

Table 2.5: Complicated status of fracture

	Delayed union	*Ununited fracture (Rarely it can include delayed union, but left to as such it usually proceeds to non-union)*	*Non-union*	
			Fibrous union	*Pseudoarthrosis*
1	2	3	4	5
1. Pain	+	+	None/slight	None
2. Swelling	+	±	+	No
3. Local temperature	±	±	Normal	Normal
4. Movement at fracture site.	May yield on stress	Present	Slight movement on stress (Patient may not be aware of).	Painless hypermobility (patient complains of it).
5. Angulation	May bear	Cannot bear any stress.	Slight yield on angulation stress.	No need to test—being hypermobile e.g. "double elbow" (Fig. 5.5A),
6. Tenderness at fracture end.	Tender	Tender	Not tender	Not tender.
7. Surrounding muscles.	Wasting +	Wasting + (or slightly).	Wasting ±	Marked wasting.
8. Functional affection.	Varying	Fully affected	Not much.	Markedly affected.
9. Optimum period	Optimum period for stages of clinical union and consolidation delayed.	Optimum period crossed (but not to the limit of non-union) for clinical union still there is stress-mobility at fracture site.	24 to 36 weeks (on average).	24 to 36 weeks or more (on average).
10. Bondage of fracture ends.	Organising callus (but delayed).	Fibrous tissue.	Dense fibrous tissue.	A cavity forms in fibrous tissue lined by pseudosynovial tissue.
11. X-ray	Callus not sufficient Fracture line visible.	Callus none or irrelevant Fracture line clearly visible Ends rarefied Medullary canal open.	Callus: —atrophic type—no callus —Oligotrophic-slight, irrelevant callus —hypertrophic—elephantoid callus at the fracture ends. Fracture ends may not be sclerosed Medullary cavity may not be closed.	Callus none; fracture ends rounded and sclerosed (as if there was no fracture). Medullary canal closed.
12. Suggestion	Prolonged immobilisation; Osteo-induction; Phemister's graft.	Osteo-induction Open reduction— • internal fixation. • bone graft • replacement arthroplasty	Osteo-induction Phemister's graft. May require open reduction and internal or external fixation	Open reduction, freshning of sclerosed ends. Internal fixation/external fixation e.g. Ilizarov's method Bone grafting ±.

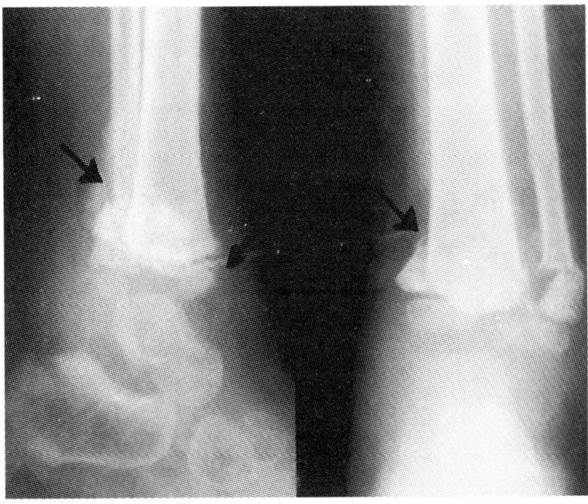

Fig. 2.12: Multiple injuries of twisting strain produced in same ankle—battered baby.

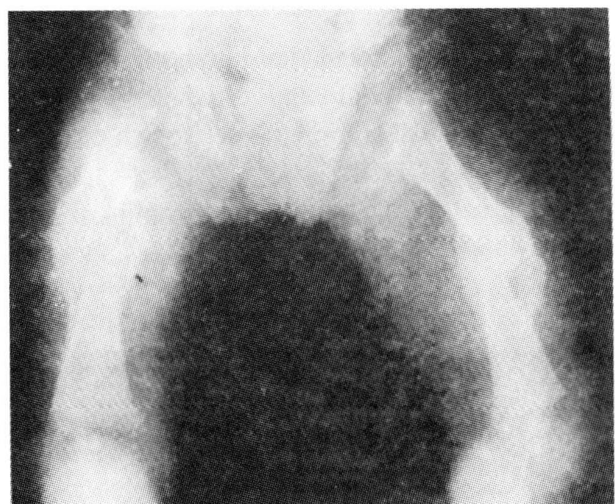

Fig. 2.13: Osteogenesis imperfecta with multiple fractures of femoral shaft

(i) *Early Complications* (0-2 weeks)

— *General*: Haemorrhage, shock, acute respiratory distress syndrome (ARDS), fat embolism, crush syndrome, thromboembolism, fracture fever; infection, tetanus, *gas gangrene* (Fig. 2.14) in open fractures.
— *Local:* Compounding (primary) at the site.
— Affections of peripheral nerves. (In spinal injuries—damage of spinal cord).
— Affections of main blood vessels (partial—leading to ischaemia; complete—leading to gangrene).
— Torn/ruptured tendon.
— Blister formation.
— Acute Volkmann's ischaemia.

(ii) *Intermediate Complications* (2-12 weeks)

— *General*: Deep vein thrombosis, pulmonary embolism; tetanus; *decubitus complications* (renal failure, pressure sore, chest infection).
— *Local compartmental syndrome:* Setting in of the features of ischaemic changes in hands or foot; development of different deformities and stiffness of adjoining joints.
— Secondary compounding of the fracture.
— *Myositis ossificans*: Basically, it is a subperiosteal calcification though it has been thought to occur in muscles. Usually, injuries around elbow and hips, are associated with myositis ossificans or heterotopic ossification. Other established risk factors for heterotopic ossification include head injury (CNS injury), severe burn, personal factors such as gender, age, and probably genetics.
In early stage: Area of impending myositis (usually cubital fossae, antero-inferomedial aspect of groin, around the shoulder, etc.) feels indurated and resistant, warm and slightly tender, with limitation of movements at the affected joint.
X-ray: Fluffy to irregularly calcified radio-opaque area with no definite margin and no trabecular pattern of bone (usually seen after 3 weeks).
In late cases: Area neither tender nor warm, localised plaque like bony mass may be felt after six weeks. Though movements improve but are still limited.
X-ray: Localised, regular, condensed radio-opaque shadow with sclerosed, circumscribed margin and usually not related to site.
— *Nerve affection*: e.g. *lateral popliteal nerve palsy* (due to pressure by splint or bed).
— *Plaster disease:* (Stiffness of joints, wasting of muscles, skin changes, pressure point sores).

(iii) *Late Complications* (after 12 weeks)

— *General Complications*: Accidental neurosis; depressive psychosis; tetanus.

— *Local Complications*:

- Malunion
- Delayed union
- Nonunion
- Sudeck's osteoneurodystrophy
- Avascular necrosis of bone
- Post-traumatic degenerative arthrosis
- Friction tendinitis
- Tendon rupture
- Growth disturbances
- Delayed nerve complication (e.g. carpal tunnel syndrome, tardy ulnar palsy)
- Stiffness of the joint, which may even be ankylosed.

Interposition of soft tissue is a potent cause of delayed and nonunion. It should be suspected when:

- There is no sensation of crepitus while manipulating the fracture.
- When there is wide gap in between the fragments.
- There is no or hardly any callus formation (in X-ray).

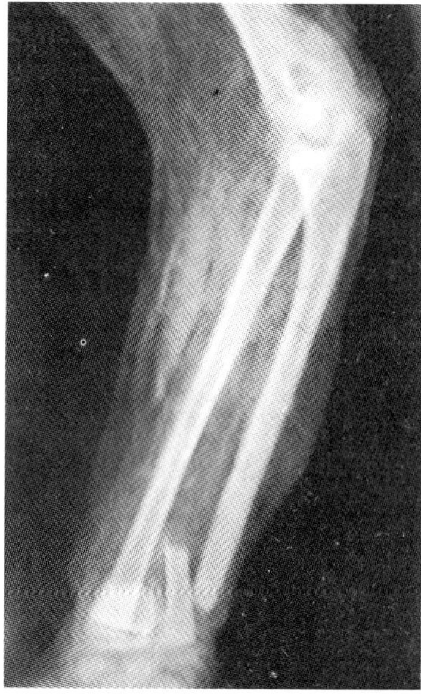

Fig. 2.14: Extensive linear gas along muscles and soft tissue planes in gas gangrene

Osteoporosis

It is a multifactorial systemic bone disorder resulting in increased bone fragility due to low bone mass and micro architectural detereoration of bone tissue. It is one of the most important and commonest medical disorders affecting the post-menopausal women. Low bone mass is the main determinant of osteoporosis and determination of bone mineral density (BMD) is the single best method for diagnosing osteoporosis and to asses future risk of osteoporotic fractures.

Ladies (usually more than 50 years old), complain of vague pain in the bones, more in the flat bones, more in the night, and features of fracture with even trivial injuries.

The WHO defined osteoporosis in adult women using T-scores as follow:

- Normal—A value of BMD within 1.0 standard deviation (SD) of the young adult reference mean.
- Osteopenia—A value of BMD more than 1.0 SD but less than 2.5 SD below the young adult reference mean.
- Osteoporosis—A value of BMD that is 2.5 SD or more below the young adult mean.
- Severe osteoporosis—A value of BMD that is 2.5 SD or more below the young adult reference mean in the presence of one or more fragility (osteoporotic) fracture (e.g typical osteoporotic fractures like compression of spine, colles fracture, femoral neck fractures).

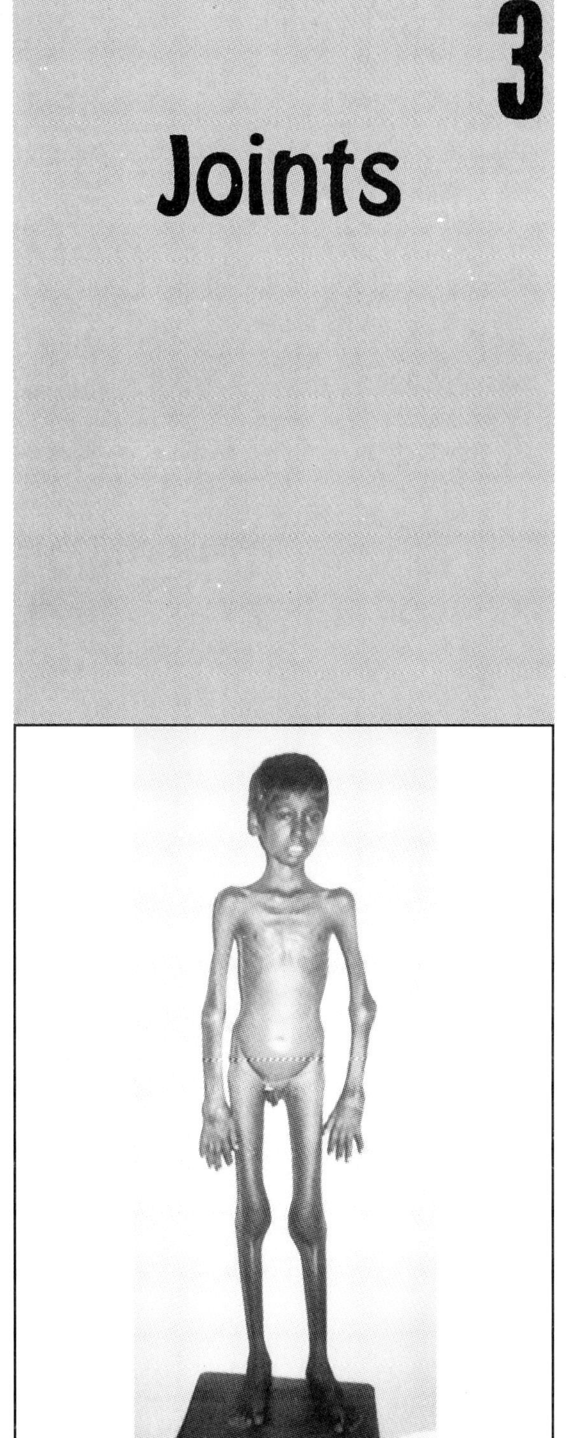

3 Joints

The junctions between the skeletal components, where slight to free, movements occur may be defined as the *'joints'* or articulations or arthrosis or juncturae.

The joints (ARTHRON) in between the skeletal structures are essential for mobility. So the jointed exoskeleton of crustaceous and insects accounts for the name of their phylum—the ARTHROPODAE.

Basically the *joints can be placed into two broad groups:*

A. *Synovial* or freely mobile joints (juncturae synoviales or diarthroses)
B. *Nonsynovial joints,* which can be (a) Fibrous or Fixed joints (juncturae fibrosae or synarthroses). (b) Cartilaginous or slightly movable joints (juncturae cartilaginae or amphiarthroses).

VARIANTS OF NONSYNOVIAL JOINTS

a. *Sutures* e.g. in between skull bone components.
b. *Synchondroses*: Temporary cartilaginous junctions between the diaphyses and epiphyses in the growing age group.
c. *Scindyleses*: In this articulation a rigid bone fits into a groove on a neighbouring element e.g. junction between the vomer and the rostrum of the sphenoid bone.
d. *Gomphosis:* (peg and socket joint)—It is a specialised form of fibrous articulation in which the teeth are fixed in the mandible and maxillae.
e. *Syndesmosis:* In this articulation two bony surfaces are bound together by an interosseous ligament, where little movement is possible, e.g. in sacroiliac joint.
f. *Symphysis:* It is a fibrocartilaginous articulation of nonsynovial type, in which there is an intervening fibrocartilaginous disc or connecting pad. A limited range of movement is possible, e.g. symphysis pubis.

SYNOVIAL JOINTS

In a synovial joint the concerned bones are linked together by a *fibrous capsule,* which mostly encloses the joint completely (except the hip joint) and *intra or extra capsular accessory ligaments*. The *articulating surfaces* of the bones are covered with a thin layer of *hyaline cartilage* (rarely fibrocartilage), which accounts for a very low coefficient of friction (0.002 or less). The capsule is lined by *synovial membrane* (developed from embryonic mesenchyme), which also covers almost all the intra-articular structures except the articulating surfaces which remain in contact and compression. This membrane secrets synovial fluid and also removes materials from the joint cavity, e.g. cystalloid, soluble dyes, etc. The synovial fluid acts like a lubricant and also provides nutrition to the articular cartilage. The *SYNOVIAL FLUID* (synovia) is a clear or pale yellow highly viscous (fluid remains intact when slowly pulled between thumb and the index finger) glairy fluid of slightly alkaline pH (at rest). It shows viscous, elastic, and plastic components.

It contains some protein (about 0.9 mgm/ 100 ml) with mucin; glucose (within 60% or more of serum glucose); cells (about 60 per ml) consisting of monocytes (predominantly), lymphocytes, macrophages, free synovial cells and occasionally polymorphonuclear leucocytes. The *synovial joints* can be:

1. *Simple*—have only two articulating—male and female—surfaces.
2. *Compound*—have more than one pair of articulating surfaces, e.g. elbow joint.
3. *Complex*—where an articular disc or meniscus of fibrocartilage is present, e.g. knee joint.

According to the approximate shape of the synovial joints they have been classified as follows:

1. *Plane joints*, in which apposing articular surfaces are fairly flat. Movements at this type of joint are sliding and translational, e.g. intercarpal joints, intermetatarsal joints.
2. *Hinge joints* (ginglymi) are uniaxial joints, having to-and-fro movements in one plane, e.g. elbow joint.
3. *Pivot* (trochoid) joint is uniaxial joint, in which rotational movements occur around a longitudinal axis running through the centre of the central bony pivot. The pivot may rotate within the ring, e.g. in proximal radioulnar joint, the radial head rotates within the annular ligament; or the ring may rotate around the pivot, e.g. the ring formed by anterior arch of atlas and its transverse ligament rotates around the dens of axis vertebra.
4. *Condylar joint* is basically an uniaxial joint but some additional rotational movements also occur, e.g. temporomandibular joints in which two convex knuckle shaped male surfaces (condyles) articulate upon two concave female surfaces.
5. *Ellipsoid joints* are biaxial joints, in which oval convex male surfaces articulate with an elliptical concave female surface, e.g. radiocarpal joints, metacarpophalangeal joints.
6. *Saddle (Sellar)* joints are biaxial joints with their apposing surfaces concavoconvex, e.g. carpometacarpal joint of thumb; ankle joint; calcaneo-cuboid joint.
7. *Ball and socket joints* are multiaxial joints in which a globular head of one bone articulates with the cup like concave surface of other, e.g. hip joint, shoulder joint.

ARTHRITIS

Literally arthritis means= the inflammation of the joint.

Pathologically it includes inflammation at different levels:

Capsulitis = inflammation of capsule

Synovitis = inflammation of synovium

Chondritis = inflammation of articular cartilage

Subchondral osteitis = inflammation of subchondral bone.

Clinically *Synovitis* and *true arthritis* should be differentiated on their merits (Table 3.1).

Table 3.1: Difference between synovitis and true arthritis

Synovitis	*True arthritis*
• *Inflammation of synovial tissue* Synovitis, if remains untreated or inadequately treated, leads to arthritis.	• *Inflammation* (with or without destruction) of *articular cartilage.* Arthritis always *includes synovitis.*
• Clinical presentation: Pain, swelling, with or without variable flexion (spasmodic), cautious movements.	• Pain, variable swelling, spasmodic or fixed flexion and/or other deformities, limitation of movements.
• *Good range of movements* are possible after taking the patient in confidence. *Only terminal movements in one or more directions may be painfully limited* due to mechanical intracapsular pressure over the inflammed synovial tissue.	• *Movements are limited in almost all directions.* Pain starts almost from very beginning or quite early when the movements are attempted.
• More common in children especially in tuberculous and pyogenic synovitis. However rheumatoid, villonodular, traumatic, and degenerative synovitis usually occur more in adults.	• In any age group (according to the causative factor.
• X-ray findings: *Joint space is usually increased* due to synovial proliferation and secretion; There is no destruction of the articular cartilage, nor subchondral cystic destruction.	• In X-ray the *joint space is* variably *reduced* depending upon the extent of destruction of the articular cartilage; subchondral and articular destructions are obvious. There may be collapse of the articular surface.
• After proper treatment complete recovery is possible.	• Complete recovery is never possible and some form of legacy is bound to persist.

PRESENTATION OF ARTHRITIS

According to acuteness of presentation, virulence of the organisms, and registance of the patients, *arthritis may be grouped under three headings:*

A. *Acute arthritis*—
  a. specific, e.g. pyogenic (bacterial)
  b. nonspecific, e.g. allergic, haemophilic

B. *Subacute arthritis*—
  a. specific
    —pyogenic —tuberculous (?)
    —gonococcal —syphilis
    —filarial
  b. nonspecific
    —allergic
    —villonodular synovitis
    —post-diarrhoeal
    —haemophilic

C. *Chronic arthritis*—
  a. specific (infective)
    —tuberculous —pyogenic (Figs 3.1 to 3.3)
    —syphilis —Hansen's disease.
    —actinomycosis
  b. crystal arthritis
    —gout
    —pseudogout
  c. collagen arthropathy—rheumatoid arthritis and its variants.
  d. villonodular synovitis
  e. osteoarthritis
  f. haemophilic arthritis

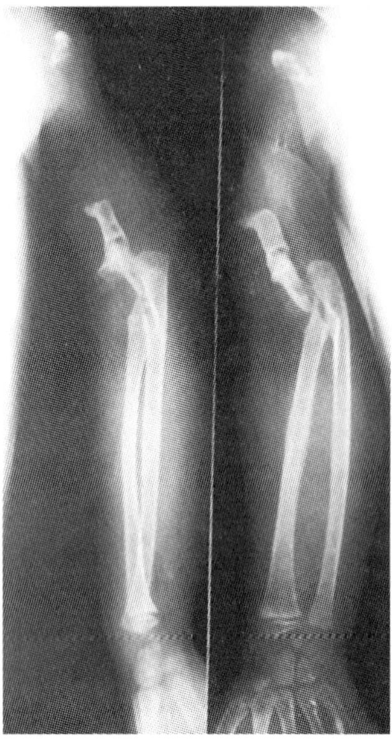

Fig. 3.1: Pyogenic arthritis of shoulder and elbow with extensive osteomyelitis of humerus which has sequestrated out

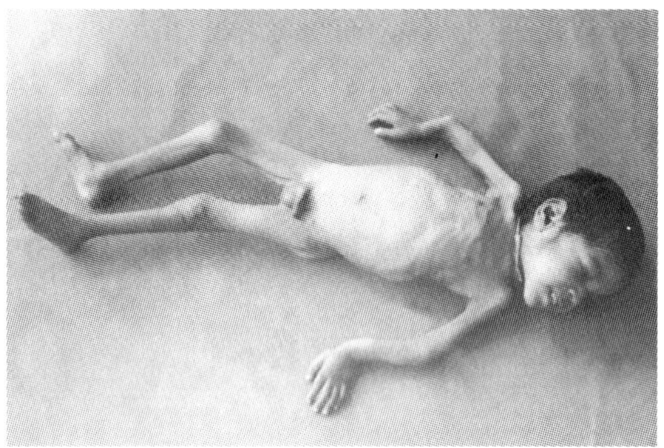

Fig. 3.3: Multifocal pyogenic arthritis in a marasmic child

g. neuropathic arthropathy usually results from:
   i. neuromuscular disorders, e.g. syringomyelia
   ii. chronic infection, e.g. syphilis, Hansen's disease
   iii. chronic alcoholism
   iv. diabetese
   v. vanishing bone disease (Gorham disease) may also manifest as neuropathic arthropathy.

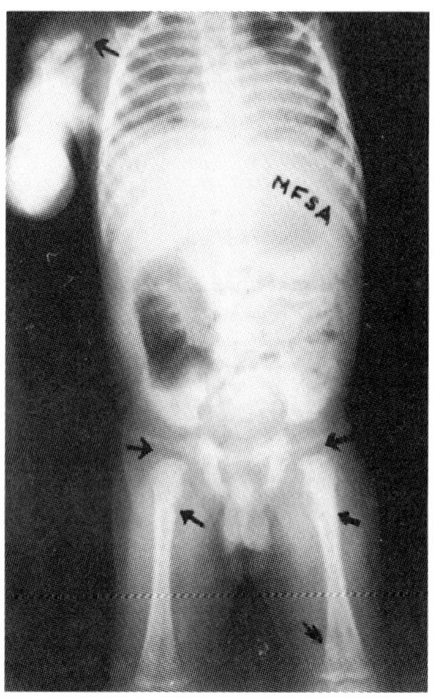

Fig. 3.2: Multifocal pyogenic arthritis (both hips and right shoulder). Note the associated congenital malformations of right upper limb

According to the number of joints involved the arthritis can be prefixed as:

A. Monoarticular (arthritis)
B. Polyarticular (polyarthritis)

INFLAMMATORY ARTHROPATHIES are:

- Rheumatoid arthritis
- Rheumatic fever
- Juvenile rheumatoid arthritis
- Collagen vascular:
  —systemic lupus erythematosus (SLE)
  —scleroderma
  —polymysitis (dermatomysitis)
  —mixed connective tissue disease
  —polyarteritis nodosa
- Psoariatic arthritis
- Reiter's syndrome
- Polymyalgia rheumatica
- Gonococcal arthritis
- Crystal arthritis—Gout; Pseudogout
- Miscellaneous
  — Tuberculous
  — Peripheral arthritis of inflammatory bowel disease

— SABE (subacute bacterial endocarditis
— Viral arthritis
— Amyloid arthropathy

SALIENT FEATURES OF INFLAMMATORY POLYARTHRITIC CONDITIONS

A. RHEUMATOID ARTHRITIS

- *Ladies* in thirties are mainly affected
- Several joints (three or more than three) are affected—mainly the small joints of hands and feet (but distal interphalangeal joints are not affected). Usually symmetrical joints are affected
- *Morning stiffness* of the joints (especially the fingers and wrists)
- Pain stays for hours, more in the morning; increases with activities and massage
- May be low grade fever
- Secondary weakness in the limbs
- Some muscle wasting (but less than tuberculosis)
- *Swelling in and around the joint*; locally warm; joint tenderness; synovial thickening; deformities according to the joint affected and the neglect
- Involvement of the tendons
- Rheumatic nodules
- May be associated systemic diseases
- Cardiovascular system affected in about 15% of cases.

X-ray findings:
— In *early stage* periarticular soft tissue swelling
— Later on periarticular osteoporosis
— Joints erosions occur within first 2 years, though cartilage damage manifest at a much earlier stage
— Pencilling of cortex

With progress of disease:
— Reduction of joint space, but the bony margins are sharply delineable
— Destruction of articular cartilage, then of subchondral bone (much less than tuberculosis)
— Subluxation of joint due to ligamentous laxity and destruction

Aspiration of joint: Fluid is serous and cloudy; On clinical viscosity test, the fluid breaks into droplets easily and becomes watery.

Joint fluid contains 2000 to 50,000 cells/mm with 40-80% polymorphs.

Total hemolytic complement (C/H50) is not depressed.

Outline of Management

— Drugs: Aspirin (methyl salicylate); NSAIDs; Gold or D-penicillamine; methotrexate; sulfasalazine; chloroquine; steroids—intra/periarticular and/or systemic.
— Rest to the inflammed part in functional position
— Guarded physiotherapy; hydrotherapy; heat therapy; mud therapy.
— Supportive/corrective orthotics
— Surgery:
  - synovectomy with or without joint debridement (after 6 months of drug therapy and when the synovium is affected)
  - Joint replacement—partial or total
  - Arthrodesis
— Rehabilitation.

B. COLLAGEN VASCULAR CONDITIONS

1. *Systemic Lupus Erythematosis*
   - More common in female;
   - Systemic joint involvements
   - Mucosal lesions
   - Rashes
   - Systemic reaction
   - Brain or visceral organ involved
   - Hair loss
   - Leucopenia
   - Serological test for syphilis falsely positive
   - X-ray noncontributory, no erosion.

Lab findings:
- Aspiration—noninflammatory joint fluid with good viscosity and mucin clot; Total WBC count 1000-2000 WBC/mm, cells are mostly small lymphocytes
- Serum C/H50 mostly depressed

- Antinuclear antibody titre elevated
- Anti-native-human DAN antibody titre increased.

2. *Scleroderma*
   - Tight tough skin
   - Raynod's phenomenon
   - Resorption of digits
   - Constipation
   - Lung, heart, kidney involvement
   - Symmetrical kidney contractures
   - Little/no synovial thickening
   - Positive ANA with speckled or nuclear pattern
   - X-ray—calcinosis circumscripta.

3. *Polymyositis* (dermatomyositis)
   - Proximal muscle weakness—mainly the pelvic and pectoral girdle muscles.
   - Muscular tenderness
   - Skin changes
   - Typical nail and knuckle pad erythema
   - Symmetrical joint involvement
   - Elevated CPK (creatine phosphokinase)
   - EMG shows combined evidence of myopathic and denervation pattern.

4. *Mixed Connective Tissue Disease*
   - Swollen hands
   - Raynaud's phenomenon
   - Tight skin
   - Symmetrical joint and tendon involvements
   - X-ray—may be joint erosion
   - Positive ANA speckled pattern
   - Antiribonucleoprotein antibody increased
   - Good response to corticoid therapy.

5. *Polyarteritis Nodosa*
   - Symmetrical involvement
   - Diverse clinical picture of systemic disease
   - Diagnosis is usually histologically.

C. RHEUMATIC FEVER

- Children and young adults (0-35 years) are affected
- Persistent sore throat
- Group A streptococci responsible
- Migratory arthritis
- Rashes
- Heart/pericardial involvement
- Elevated antiseptolysin O titres
- Joint involvements respond dramatically to aspirin

D. JUVENILE RHEUMATOID ARTHRITIS (Figs 3.4A and B)

- Symmetric joint involvement
- Rashes
- Fever
- RA Factor—negative
- X-ray—periostitis, erosion in late cases
- Recur in adults.

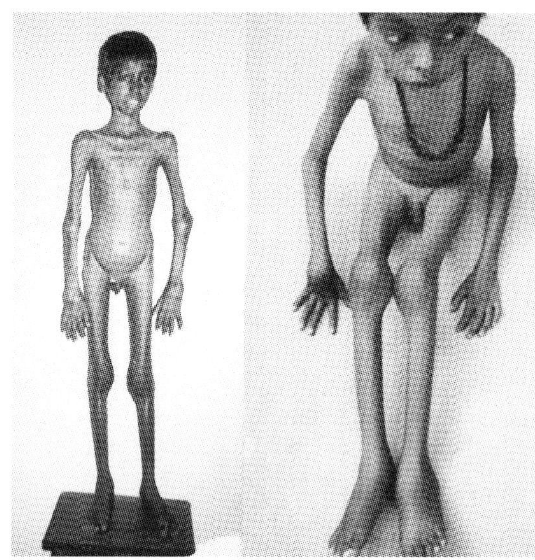

Figs 3.4A and B: Juvenile rheumatoid arthritis

E. PSORIATIC ARTHRITIS

- Asymmetric boggy joint and tendon swelling
- May be skin or nail changes prior or post to arthritis
- Distal interphalangeal joints predominantly involved
- X-ray—periostitis and erosion
- RA Factor—negative
- Aspirated joint fluid—inflammatory changes with polymorph preponderance
- C/H50 mostly not depressed.

F. REITER S SYNDROME

- Males much more affected
- Associated urethritis, iritis, conjunctivitis
- Keratosis blennorhagia
- Asymmetric joints affection mostly in lower extremity
- Balanitis circinata
- Painful ulcers in mucous membrane
- Loss of weight; generalised weakness
- C/H50 increased in serum and joint fluid with 3-5 Reiter's cells (phagocytosed polymorphs)
- Joint fluid show 5000-30,000 leucocytes/mm^3
- Prepondering macrophages in joint fluid.

G. GONOCOCCAL ARTHRITIS

- Migratory arthritis/tenosynovitis (settles fully in one or more joints)
- Either sex affected
- Primary focus in urethra, female genitourinary tract, rectum or oropharynx
- Skin lesion—vesicles mostly in genitalia
- On smear examination gramnegative diplococci isolated
- Positive culture from primary site, blood, joint fluid BUT NOT from vesicular fluid.

H. POLYMYELGIA RHEUMATICA

- Elderly age group affected (more than 50 years)
- Symmetric pelvis or pectoral girdle affection, but no loss of strength
- Morning stiffness of long duration
- Easy fatigue is prominantly manifested
- Loss of weight
- Joints involved: shoulder, sternoclavicular, knees, etc.
- ESR—markedly elevated
- Alpha 2 and gamma globulin elevated
- Anaemia
- Serum CPK (Creatine phosphokinase)—normal
- Prednisolone even in low dose (10-20 mgm) relieves well.

I. CRYSTAL ARTHRITIS

A. Gout

- Mostly hereditary disease (occurs in family)
- Usually males in forties or more are affected
- Onset usually acute, coming in very early morning
- Joints affected: Pain in big toe (metatarsophalangeal joint, ankle, elbow, knee, shoulder, hand joints
- Joints are swollen, warm, tender, and look inflammed; movements are painfully limited
- Tophi may be present in chronic cases
- In late cases deformities may develop
- Serum uric acid is raised
- Blood ESR is raised
- X-ray: soft tissue swelling; subchondral variable irregular sized cystic appearances; chalky white deposits of urates; joint space reduced; destruction of adjoining bones; deformities develop
- Decreased urinary 17-ketosteroids—reduction below 3 mg/24 hours is a constant finding in gout
- SYNOVIAL FLUID contains WBC (10 to 60,000/mm^3 with predominating polymorph. It contains monosodium urate monohydrate crystals seen by compensated polarized light microscope (or sometime by ordinary light microscopy) as negatively birefringent needle shaped rods.

Outline of Management

Rest —General for few days
—Local support, e.g. elevation on pillow. (physical strain, trauma, surgery, mental stress, over eating may precipitate or exaggerate the acute attacks)

Drugs

In acute cases

- Colchicin (0.6 mgm tablet even upto 6 to 8 tablets on the first day depending on severity; thence one tablet twice daily for few months

- Indomethacin-50 mgm QID to 25 mgm TID

In chronic cases:

- Colchicine 0.6 mg BID for 9 to 12 months
- Xanthine oxidase inhibitor, e.g. alpurinol 100-200 mgm daily
- Uricosuric agents (if uric acid remains increased), e.g. probenecid 0.5 to 2 gm/day.

B. *Pseudogout*

Same elderly age group as gout;
Onset less acute than gout
Knees are more commonly affected. Other joints affected are metacarpophalangeal, wrist, elbow, shoulder, hip, knee

- Mental stress, over physical activities, surgery may precipitate the acute attack
- May be flexion contracture
- X-ray: Chondrocalcinosis (calcium deposit in cartilage, ligaments, meniscus, joint capsule) is common (cf. chondrocalcinosis is also common in hyperparathyroidism, hemosiderosis, hemochromatosis, hypophosphatasia, hypomagnesemia, hypothyroidism, neuropathic joints, gout, in elderlies).
- Other changes may be like those is gouty arthritis.

SYNOVIAL FLUID contains calcium pyrophosphate dihydrate crystals, which are weekly positively birefringent but have a different extinction angle compared to the urate crystals.

The WBC count in this synovial fluid is 5 to 60,000/mm^3 with polymorphs predominating.

Outline of Management

- Colchicin may give quick relief
- Indomethacin as in gout
- Intra-articular corticoids after aspirating the fluid, if any

J. MISCELLANEOUS JOINT INFLAMMATION

Peripheral arthritis of inflammatory bowel disease, tuberculosis, SABE (subacute bacterial endocarditis), viral arthritis

ACUTE SEPTIC ARTHRITIS

- Acute onset with high fever (with or without rigor and fluctuations)
- Vague or insignificant history of injury
- Clinical evidences of local severe inflammatory changes including hyperaesthesia, and painful limitation of movements.
- X-ray:
  - enlarged soft tissue shadow;
  - joint space may be increased (due to collection in the joint)
  - there may be fuzzy appearance across the joint
- Blood examination: high leukocytosis with polymorphs predominence; Blood ESR—raised
- Blood culture may be positive for the infective organism
- Joint aspiration: purulent joint fluid with yellow, yellow-whitish flakes; turbid fluid; on clinical viscosity test—very watery; total count of WBC—increased usually more than 15,000 with predominating polymorphs; synovial glucose very low (less than 60% of the concurrent serum glucose); synovial culture usually reveal the causative organism.

Outline of Management

- General rest; hydration; nourishment
- Rest to the part
- Repeated aspirations, joint lavage, intra-articular antibiotics
- Systemic broadrange antibiotics @ to culture and chemosensitivity
- Arthrotomy—drainage, lavage, removal of necrosed materials, installation of antibiotics.

TUBERCULOUS SYNOVITIS/ARTHRITIS (Fig. 3.5)

- Subacute onset to chronic onset
- May be vague history of trauma
- May be history of primary focus in the body, e.g. lung, gland, abdominal viscera
- History of chronic immunodeficiency
- History of chronic drugs
- Alcoholics

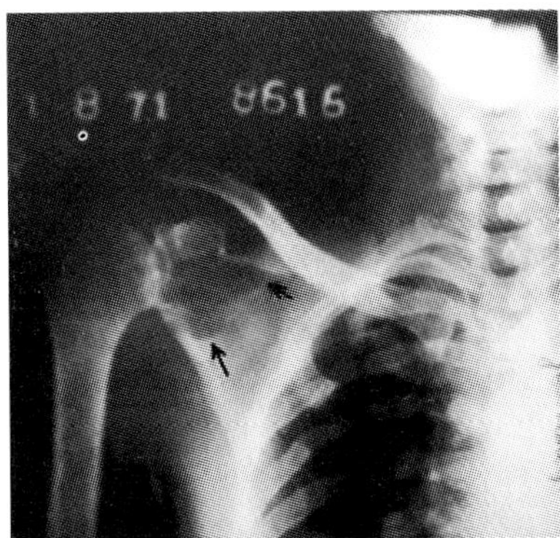

Fig. 3.5: Tuberculous caeca of right shoulder with a destructive cystic lesions in adjoining scapula and humeral head

- Complains of pain, swelling, deformities, limitations of movements, stiffness of the joint, cold abscess, sinuses
- Warm tender swollen joint,
- Movements restricted (due to muscular spasm, destruction of the articular cartilage, still later on ankylosis
- Cold abscess in the dependant part of the joint (usually), or at distant places due to tracking of the pus along the path of the least resistance
- Sinuses—typical of tuberculous nature (usually)—multiple, undermined margins; pigmented surroundings; serous, serosanguinous or sanguinous discharge)
- Aspiration of the swollen joint: serous or serosanguinous fluid which may contain yellowish-white flakes; predominant polymorph lecocytosis
- Blood ESR raised; differential leucocytes count is increased
- Culture may show acid-fast bacillus (about 65%)
- X-ray: Initially joint space may be increased due to collection of fluid; generalised osteoporosis of the adjoining bones; reduction of joint space due to destruction of the articular surface; subchondral destruction—irregular cystic spaces; tuberculous sequestra; collapse; cold abscess, if present, casts soft tissue shadow.

Outline of Management

- General rest
- Local rest (by plaster/splint support; traction)
- Chemotherapy (antituberculous)
- Orthosis in the convalescing stage (non-weight bearing for the lower limb)
- If cold abscess—repeated aspiration through nondependant zone and installing of streptomycin; if not satisfactory response—excision of the cold abscess along with or without excision of the source and the tract.

SURGERY for the tuberculous joint: when nonoperative management is not satisfactory OR in complicated cases:

- Arthrotomy, lavage, and synovectomy
- Excision of the diseased tissue
- Arthrodesis in second stage (i.e. after exicison in first stage) OR in one stage itself as excision arthrodesis
- Arthroplasty: excisional arthroplasty, e.g. in hip joint, elbow and shoulder joints
  Replacement arthroplasty only when the treated joint has remained healed for at least three years.

OSTEOARTHRITIS (Degenerative arthritis; Nonnodal nonerosive degenerative joint disease)

- Primary osteoarthritis is always in elderly people
- Secondary osteoarthritis can occur in earlier age as well (e.g. post-traumatic; healed infections of the joint; old Perthes disease or otherwise osteonecrosis of the bone involved in the joint, etc.
- Pain mainly after rest and fairly relieved after mild to moderate activities (severe activities usually increase the pain)
- Variable asymmetric joints may be involved at a time
- Distal interphalangeal joints are affected (cf. rheumatoid arthritis where these joints are not affected)
- May be disuse atrophy of the muscles
- Local temperature not raised except when there is flare with collections in the joint
- Coarse crepitations in the joint

Chart 3.1: Evaluation of a hot swollen joint

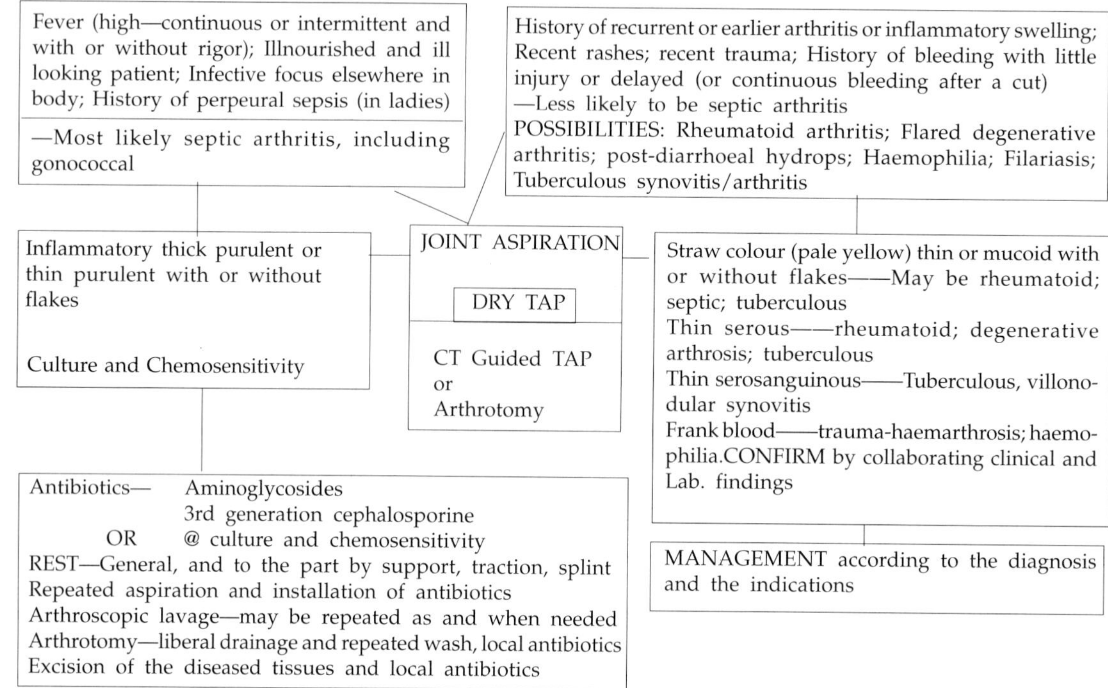

- Effusion in the joint (usually when there is flare)
- Range of the movements are reduced especially in the terminal range (more in flexion)
- Deformities of the joints—mainly it is angular deformity, especially in direct weight bearing joints, e.g. in knee and ankle
- Contractures may develop.
- X-ray:
  - joint space gradually narrows down
  - subchondral sclerosis,
  - subcortical cysts
  - marginal osteophytes (and eburnations).
  - Collapse of joint
- On aspiration of the joint (when there is effusion):
  - fluid is usually clear and straw colour/serous
  - Clinical viscosity test—fluid remains intact when slowly rubbed (pulled) between thumb and the index finger, i.e. viscosity is high or good as in normal cases.
  - Glucose content is normal,
  - Cell count is 2000/mm^3 (cf. normal is 200/mm^3) with more of monocytes

Outline of Management

- Drugs—NSAID (Nonsteroidal-anti-inflammatory drugs)
- Aligning the weight transmission in lower limbs by the alteration of the shoe heel; providing inserts; bracing
- Limited supports (to maintain the functions simultaneously)
- Postural adjustments, e.g. sitting, standing, sleeping postures; chair adjustments
- Intraarticular steroids and allied injections
- SURGERY:
  - Arthroscopic lavage; arthroscopic/open joint lavage and clearing
  - Osteotomy (e.g. high tibial osteotomy for knee and McMurray's osteotomy for the hip)
  - Joint replacement (e.g. total hip and knee replacements)

Table 3.2: Causes of ankylosis

	Extra-articular	*Intra-articular*	
		Soft tissue	*Bony*
Skin	• Contracture • Congenital • Post burn	• Capsular contractures • Synovitis • Intra-articular ligamentous affections	• Intra-articular fracture • Infective conditions e.g. pyogenic, tuberculosis • Collagen arthropathy • Degenerative changes • Neoplasm
Subcutaneous tissue	• Dupuytren's contracture • Fibrosis		
Muscles	• Fibrosis • Myositis • Neoplasm		
Tendon	• Fibrosis • Neoplasm, e.g. Xanthoma • Bursitis		
Vessels	• Aneurysm e.g. in popliteal fossa		
Bone	• Inflammatory condition of bones in the vicinity. • Neoplasm in the vicinity.		

- Arthrodesis of the joint (more suitable in manual workers and labourers)

VIRAL ARTHRITIS (Fig. 3.6)

History of preceeding or concomitant systemic viral illness

- Mixed clinical picture of viral and septic infections

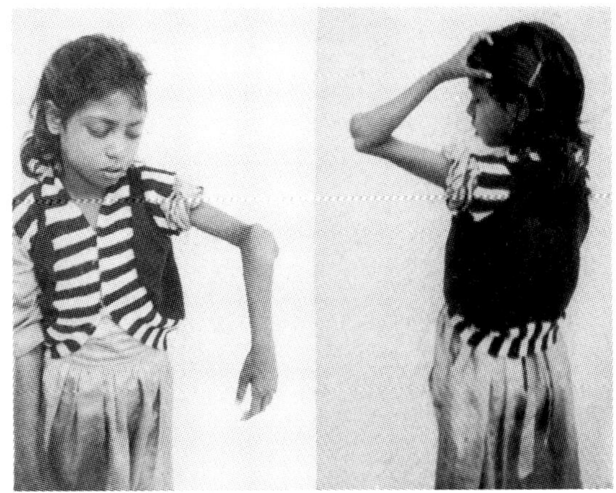

Figs 3.6A and B: Post vareolar arthritis of left elbow

- Aspirated joint fluid can show inflammatory changes with polymorphs preponderance.
- Culture of virus from the joint fluid.

POST VARIOLAR ARTHRITIS manifests as disorganised variably stiff joints (usually bilateral; elbow is a common site). Though small pox has been eradicated, but its legacies would be seen for few more decades, especially in tropical and allied countries.

5. DYSENTERIC ARTHROPATHY

- Sterile seronegative synovitis/arthritis as a complication of intestinal infection with *Shigella* or *Salmonella* or cases of *Yersinia*.
- Clinical manifestations of asymmetric polyarthritis or arthralgia, following weeks of definite diarrhoeal illness, abdominal pain.
- Knee, ankle, and wrist are commonly affected
- Diagnosis is by stool examination and agglutination tests.
- Usually it clears in weeks or months with management of intestinal infections.

6. PONCET'S DISEASE OR TUBERCULAR RHEUMATISM

- Poncet (1897) described cases of polyarthritis occurring in patients suffering from tuberculosis.

Table 3.3: Types of ankylosis

	True or bony	False or fibrous
	— No yield even on stress	— Yield on stress
	— No pain even on stress	— Pain on stress
	— Marked atrophy of the surrounding soft tissues especially muscles	— Comparatively less atrophy of the surrounding soft tissues
	— Causes of ankylosis usually intra-articular	— Mixed causes (intra-or/extra-articular)
Radiological findings	—Trabeculations across the joint	— No trabeculations across the joint
	—No joint line left	— Joint line always present
Management	—Detailed assessment specially related to functional loss	— Detailed assessment
	—If adjustments possible, rehabilitation in original or changed job	— Planned physiotherapy — Analgesic — Reassurance
	—If treatment required	— Management of primary cause
	—Operation: • Excisional arthroplasty • Total joint replacement • Planned arthrodesis	Operation: • Total joint replacement • Excisional arthroplasty • Planned arthrodesis

- Polyarthralgia may be associated with tuberculosis (usually extraarticular tuberculosis), however this association may be controversial
- The joint aspirate is watery or straw-coloured fluid whose (mostly) culture is negative
- Symptoms may subside with NSAIDs and physiotherapy, however antitubercular drugs may be given for six months.

Ankylosis: Ankylosis of a joint means fixity of the joint, in any position depending upon the pathology and posture (cf. arthrodesis is a planned operative fusion of a joint in possible functional position).

Aims of Examining an Ankylosed Joint (Tables 3.2 and 3.3)

—To know the possible cause.
—To know the type of ankylosis.
—To evaluate the capability of the joint in presence of the ankylosis or incapacitating effects of the ankylosis.
—To plan the treatment.
—Stretchability of the ankylosed joint:
- Yield of skin.
- Yield of subcutaneous tissue.
- Yield of blood vessels and
- Yield of tendons.

—To predict the prognosis.
—To assess the effects of ankylosis on the adjoining joints and posture.

4 Shoulder Joint

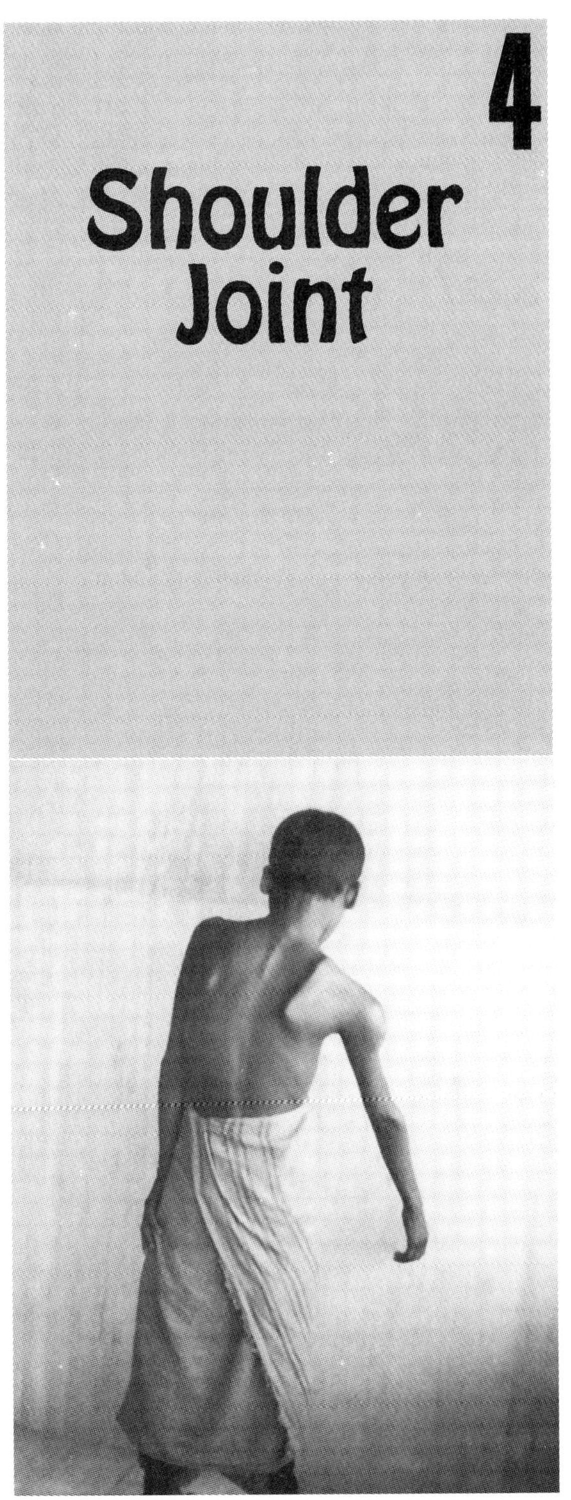

INTRODUCTION

In the process of evolution from quadrupeds to bipeds, the forelimbs developed into upper limbs. In quadrupeds they serve the purpose of weight bearing and attack. In bipeds their responsibilities are mainly concentrated on subserving fine functions, holding an object, attack and defence. The main axis of the upper limb also changed with some rotational element at the root joints, i.e. at forequarter girdle. Therefore, the long axis of the upper limb in human beings is neither set parallel nor at right angles, but oblique to the trunk.

ANATOMICAL CONSIDERATION

The upper limb more or less hangs from the body. The only skeletal connection from the trunk to the upper limb is the strut of the clavicle. It, therefore, assumes the responsibility of a shock absorber, preventing a thrust from the upper limb from being transmitted to the trunk. For a clinician, the word 'shoulder' should include the shoulder girdle as a whole, since an affection anywhere in the shoulder girdle has to affect the shoulder functions.

The movement at shoulder is the sum total of movements at different joints of the shoulder girdle (i.e. gleno-humeral articulation, scapulo-thoracic gliding, acromioclavicular and sterno-clavicular joints). In most of the affections of cervical spine, the shoulder region may be involved. Rather, at times, the complaints lie only in the shoulder for a pathology in the cervical spine. Therefore, it is imperative to examine fully the cervical and cervicodorsal regions for shoulder complaints. The rotator cuff consists of musculotendinous attachments to the greater tuberosity (teres minor, supraspinatus and infraspinatus), lesser tuberosity (subscapularis) and adjoining capsule of the shoulder joint. The dynamic interplay of the rotator cuff and deltoid muscle is essential for smooth functioning of shoulder. The rotator cuff acts as horizontal stabilisers and steerer holding the humeral head in the glenoid during the abduction of shoulder.

The glenohumeral joint is superiorly protected by osseous-ligamentous arches formed by the coracoid process, coracoacromial ligaments, and the under surface of the acromial process. The subacromial bursa lying between the capsule and the arches virtually protect the humeral head from impingement against the acromial process and is liable to undergo degenerative inflammation quite often.

The non-specific inflammation and adhesions affecting the capsule, the rotator cuff, subacromial bursa and the surrounding ligaments, manifest more or less in the same way, ultimately resulting in frozen shoulder. The coracohumeral ligament, mainly meant for acting as checkrein against extreme external rotation of humeral head, gets variably contracted in rotator cuff syndrome/frozen shoulder thus earlier limiting the external rotation.

The clavicle subserves its strut action through strong coracoclavicular ligaments (trapezoid and conoid parts) which helps in suspending and stabilising the arm in its allocation. Hence any rupture of this ligament, associated with injury of acromioclavicular ligament causes subluxation/dislocation of the joint.

Long head of biceps originates from supraglenoid tubercle, invaginating through the synovium and passes in the bicipital groove, strapping the head of the humerus firmly in the glenoid cavity in all its movements. This makes this tendon vulnerable to degenerative inflammation, attrition and even varying ruptures.

The shoulder is notorious for undergoing stiffness, not only following its own pathology, but also following the pathology situated centripetally or centrifugally, e.g. in cervical spondylosis or shoulder hand syndrome (Steinbrocher *et al* 1943).

METHODOLOGY

History Taking

The usual complaints concerning shoulder are: (i) Limitation of movements, (ii) Pain in the region of shoulder joint, (iii) Inability to lift the limb, (iv) Swelling in the region of shoulder joint, and (v) Wound or sinus in the region of shoulder joint.

Injuries of shoulder joints are usually the result of indirect violence. Of course, falling on the shoulder point can also produce various injuries. The actual mode of sustaining the injury should be noted, e.g. (i) fall on outstretched hand or point of shoulder or on point of elbow, (ii) direct hit from any direction at shoulder, (iii) hyperabduction strain of the shoulder.

Pain

Besides enquiring about the nature, site, relation with activities, diurnal variation of pain, always ask about its radiation, especially from or to the cervical region, arm, forearm, or hand. Note the actual direction and point of radiation. Pain in the shoulder region may be referred from the affections of the viscera, e.g. on right side, from subdiaphragmatic, supradiaphragmatic and diaphragmatic pathology (specially gall bladder affection). Cardiogenic pain may radiate through the left shoulder and along the inner aspect of left upper limb.

General and Systemic Examinations

As in chapter on "Introduction".

Regional Examination

For the shoulder affections, examination from the cervical and cervicodorsal spine to the tip of the finger is essential. If any pathology is detected in this range, that part should be examined thoroughly. The regional lymph nodes (the supraclavicular and axillary groups) should also be examined.

Local Examination

Prerequisites

(i) Patient must be examined standing on the floor or sitting on a stool, (ii) Neck to the tip of fingers must be exposed fully from all sides, (iii) Opposite shoulder must be examined for comparison, (iv) The limb should be kept freely hanging by the side of chest in anatomical position, i.e. elbow extended and forearm supinated as far as practicable.

Attitude

Attitude of the patient in relation to the shoulder is sometimes typical. The position of the neck, the shoulder point and the supported or unsupported upper limb should be noted. Many a times the attitude itself is diagnostic, e.g. patient with *fracture clavicle* inclines his neck to the affected side and supports the elbow in opposite hand keeping the arm by the side of the chest. Patient with *anterior dislocation of shoulder* loses the contour of shoulder, develops flattening of deltoid bulge, drooping of axillary fold and keeps the elbow away from the chest (Fig. 4.1). In luxatio erecta, the arm is kept widely abducted and sometimes internally rotated. In *Erb's palsy* the child keeps the arm abducted and internally rotated, elbow extended, forearm pronated, wrist partially flexed, thumb in palm and fingers semiflexed, i.e. position of the policeman receiving tip (Figs 16.2A and 16.2B, page 388).

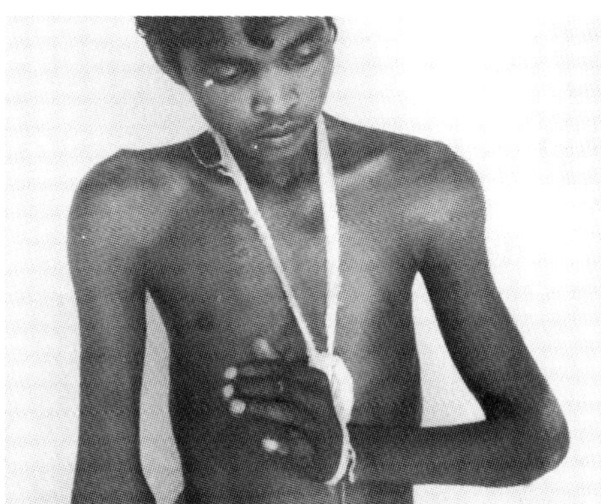

Fig. 4.1: The typical attitude of anterior dislocation of shoulder.

Contracture of the deltoid muscle may develop secondary to congenital fibrosis (Fig. 4.2A and B), intramuscular injection or trauma leading to fibrosis of the muscle. Abduction contracture of shoulder and winging of scapula due to the deltoid contracture should be differentiated from abduction contracture of shoulder due to other causes, e.g. brachial plexus palsy (it usually involves the infraspinatus and teres minor muscles and abnormal involuntary movement—dyskinesia—is a prominent feature); prescapular space occupying lesion, e.g. abscess, osteochondroma, etc. (Figs 4.2G and 4.2H).

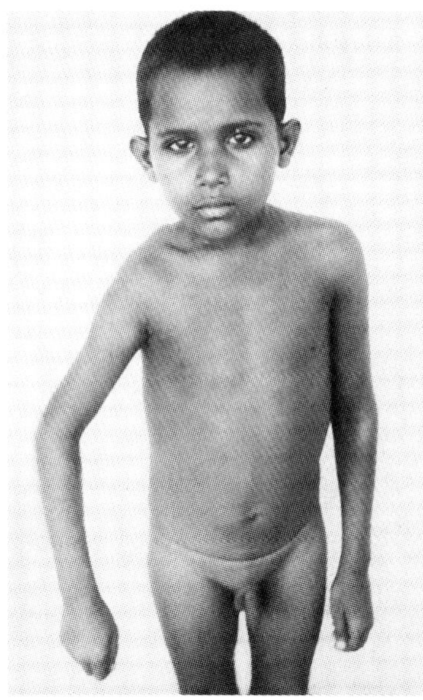

Fig. 4.2A: Fixed abduction deformity of shoulder due to congenital contracture of intermediate fibres of deltoid

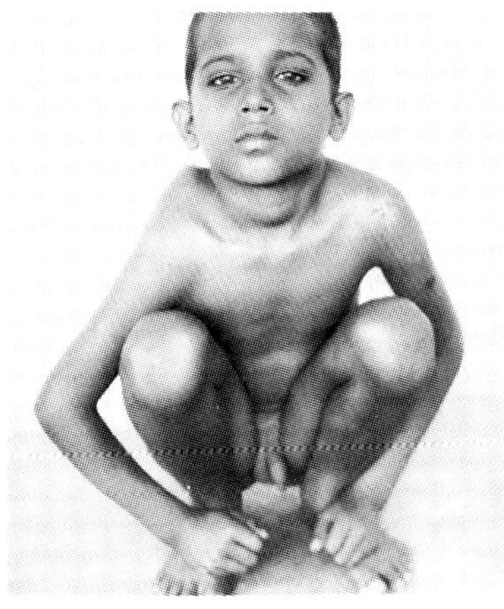

Fig. 4.2B: Same patient (Fig. 4.2A) in sitting posture. Note the projecting scapular acromion process on deltoid contracture side

In Klippel-Feil syndrome *(congenital webbed neck)*, hairline lies almost on shoulder level with or without high-placed scapula (Fig. 4.3C). In Sprengel's shoulder—*congenital elevation of scapula*, upper border of which may lie well above the shoulder (Figs 4.3A to C). In deltoid contracture, there is fixed abduction deformity at the shoulder (Figs 4.2A and 4.2B).

In gross congenital malformations, examination should be done on the lines pertinent to that particular case (Fig. 4.4).

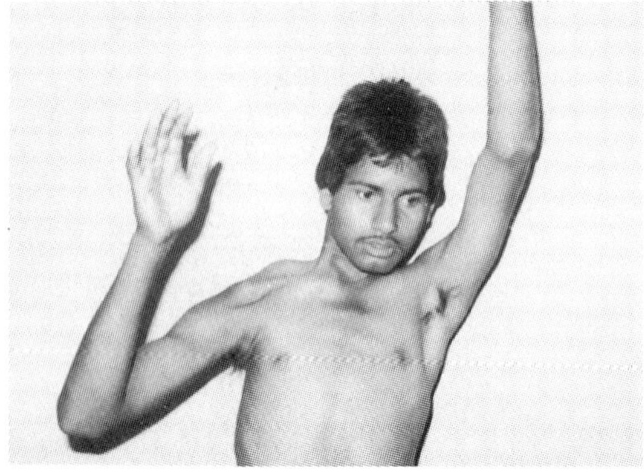

Fig. 4.2C: Fixed abduction deformity of right shoulder due to congenital dislocation of shoulder

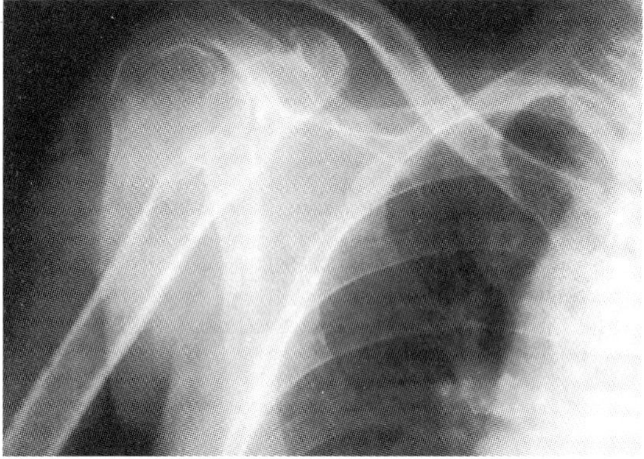

Fig. 4.2D: Fixed abduction deformity of shoulder due to neglected fracture subluxation/dislocation of shoulder

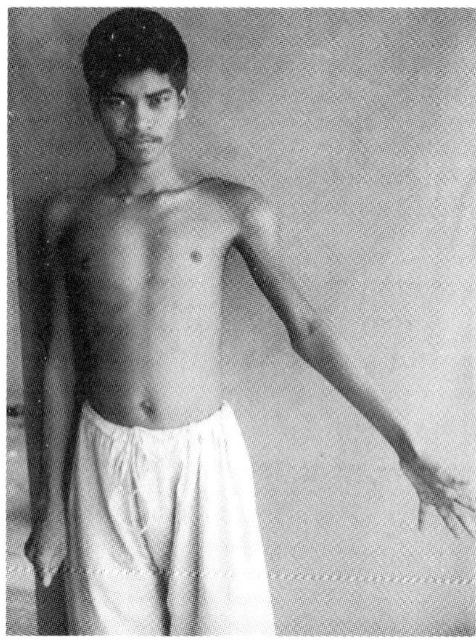

Fig. 4.2E: Fixed abduction deformity of shoulder due to haemangioma in deltoid muscle

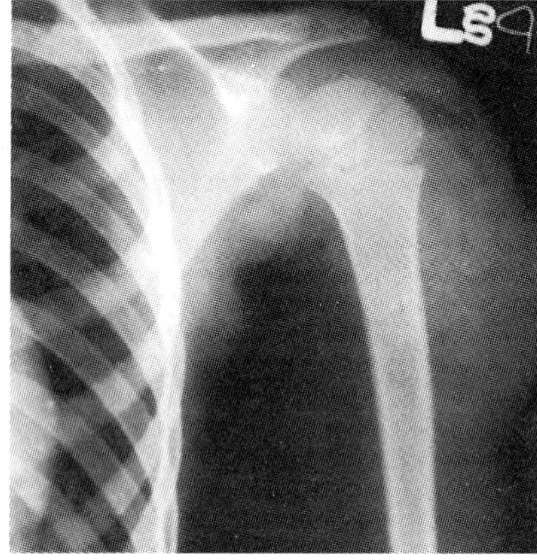

Fig. 4.2F: X-ray of same patient. Note the shadow of haemangiomatous mass in deltoid muscle

Inspection

Inspect from the front, side, back and the top simultaneously comparing with the opposite side. Note the condition of skin, its vascularity, presence of any swelling (Fig. 4.5), abnormal pulsation, wasting, fasciculation, etc.

From the front—Relation of the two clavicles from the sternoclavicular to acromioclavicular joints, anterior deltoid bulge, supraclavicular fossae, infraclavicular fossae, pectoral bulge, anterior axillary line and folds, contour of the shoulder and approximation of the elbow to the chest.

From the sides—The deltoid bulge and the side of the arm.

From the top—Acromioclavicular elevation and angle of acromion, the bulge of the shoulder.

From the back—Right from midspinal line, medial border of scapula and scapular prominence, scapular (supra- and infraspinatus)

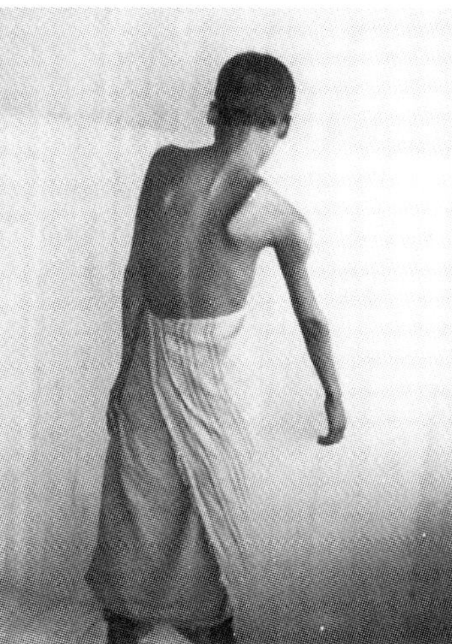

Fig. 4.2G: Fixed abduction deformity of shoulder due to 7 weeks old prescapular abscess which is also encroaching upon the posterolateral aspect of shoulder

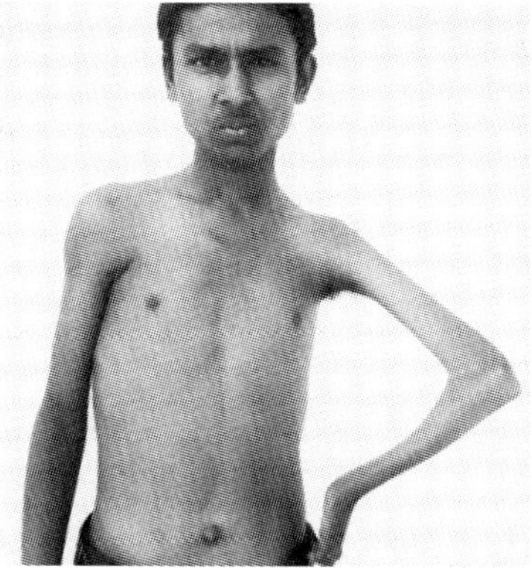

Fig. 4.2H: Fixed abduction deformity of shoulder due to axillary abscess

fossae, level of inferior angle of scapula, posterior deltoid bulge, posterior axillary line and folds. Any abnormality in comparison to the other side must be noted (Fig. 4.3).

Palpation

(a) Superficial—(As in the chapter on Introduction)

(b) Deep—Besides the common points as noted in the chapter on 'Introduction' locate and palpate the following, and note any abnormality. Palpate (i) clavicle from sternoclavicular to acromioclavicular joint, (ii) tip of the coracoid process, (iii) angle of acromion, (iv) the body and angles of scapula, (v) hollowness of the base of axilla, (vi) hollowness or fullness of infraclavicular fossae, (vii) palpate the supraclavicular region for pulsation or any other abnormality of the subclavian artery and upper medial aspect of the arm for the brachial artery, (viii) palpate the different groups of lymph glands in axillary and supraclavicular regions, (ix) in acute traumatic cases palpate for any dislocated articulating end or displaced bony fragment, and in late ones for any myositis or myositic mass.

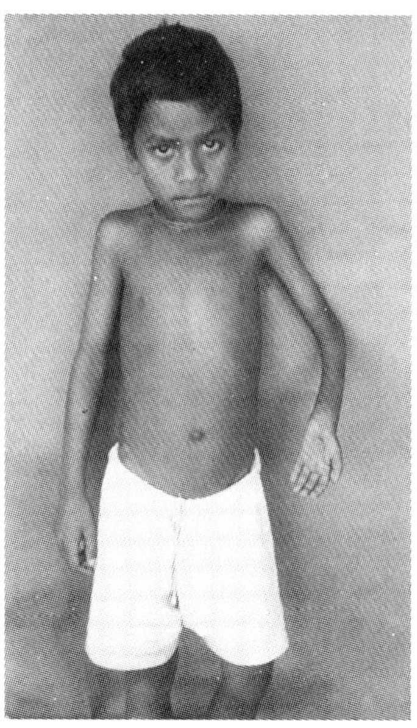

Fig. 4.2I: Fixed abduction contracture of shoulder due to neglected chronic septic arthritis of shoulder

Tenderness of the shoulder joint is mainly elicited at two regions; just lateral to the coracoid process anteriorly, and just below and behind the acromial angle posteriorly. In bicipital tendinitis, tenderness is along the biceps tendon on the anterosuperior slope of the shoulder bulge. Tenderness over the region of glenoid, head of humerus, tuberosities and upper humeral shaft should be noted separately.

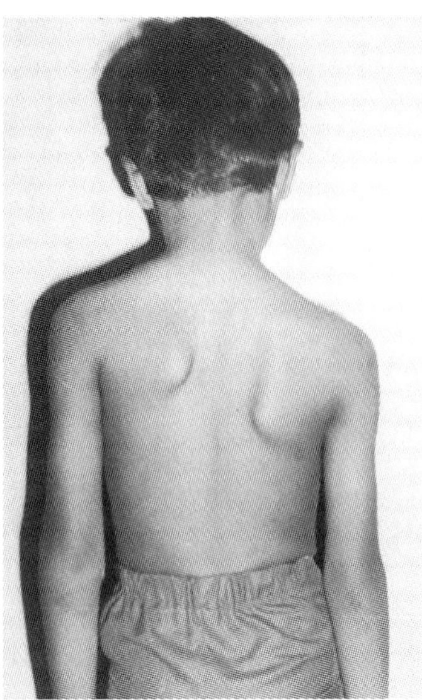

Fig. 4.3A: Sprengel's shoulder

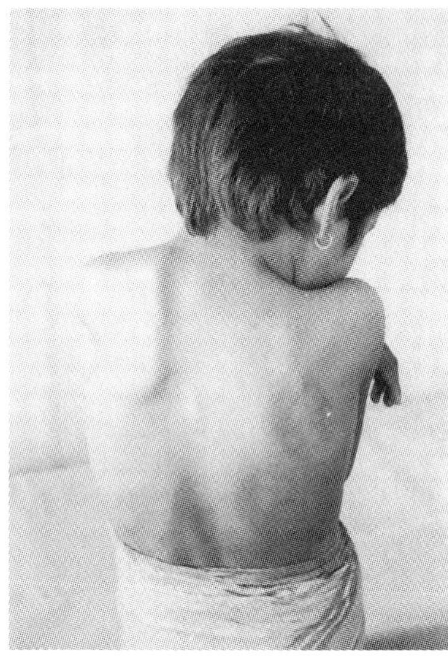

Fig. 4.3C: Sprengel's shoulder in embracing position

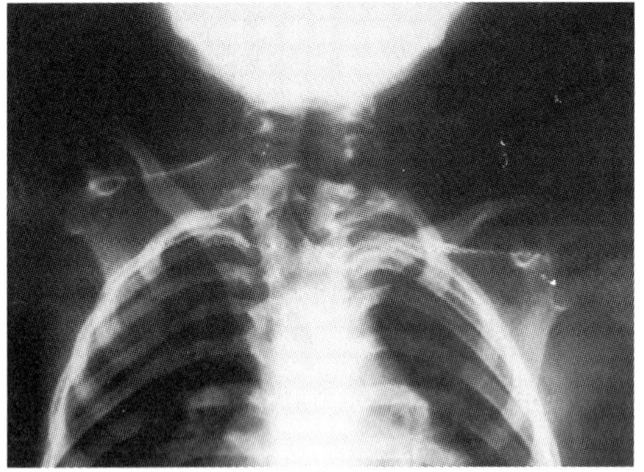

Fig. 4.3B: X-ray of the same patient (Fig. 4.3A)

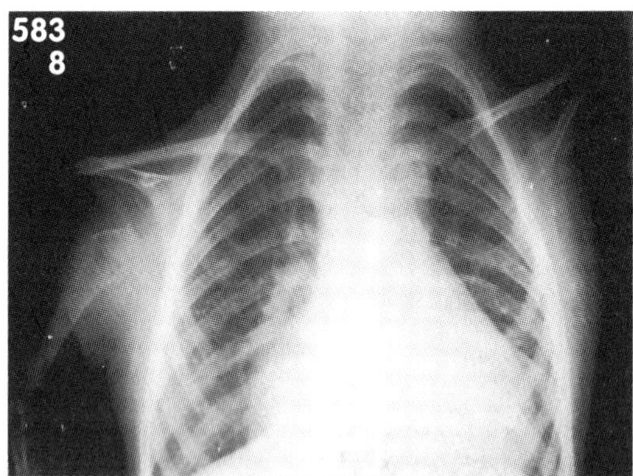

Fig. 4.4: Gross congenital malformations in the cervical regions and absence of both upper limbs

A cystic (the word cyst is derived from the Greek word meaning bladder) swelling around the shoulder should be confirmed by the usual methods of demonstration. Collection in the shoulder joint is usually localised anteriorly, posteriorly or inferomedially. However, when the collection increases, cross-fluctuation (anteroposteriorly) can be demonstrated. A cystic hygroma, having typical compressibility and very clear transillumination, may manifest anteriorly.

In doubtful cases of fasciculation, tapping over or squeezing the deltoid muscles can be useful in initiating the bout.

Since the muscular padding is very thick almost all around, on palpation one gets very little clue about the fracture ends unless they are quite obvious. One should not attempt to elicit crepitus and abnormal mobility. Most of the fractures around the shoulder are generally impacted and require hardly any interference. Overenthusiastic attempts at demonstrating

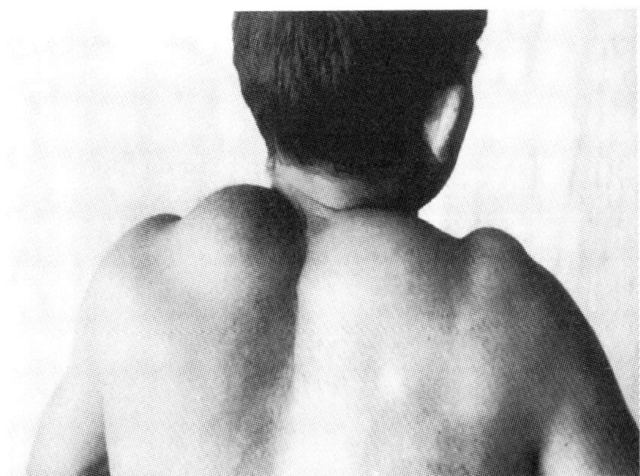

Fig. 4.5: Note the abnormal rounded swelling over the right shoulder and on both sides of root of the neck and also over the left shoulder top pseudolipoma due to repeated friction trauma in one who carries bamboo stick with hanging load on both sides.

crepitus and abnormal movements may disimpact the fractured ends.

If on inspection, the roundness of the shoulder is lost, search for abnormal position of the head of the humerus. In dislocations it usually lies in the infraclavicular fossa (anterior), and rarely just posteroinferior to the acromion or its spinous process (posterior) or the subglenoid region (inferior). In fresh cases of dislocations the finding of depressed contour should be enough to diagnose it. Any attempt to move the shoulder, to note the movement of the head under the palpating fingers, will initiate endless pain and spasm. In the paralytic shoulder, the deltoid mass thins out, the head of the humerus stands prominent much below the acromial process, thereby having a 'step' in between the acromion and the head of the humerus in which the finger can be well insinuated (Fig. 4.6). Atrophy of the deltoid, abnormal mobility of the shoulder (mainly passive) and the 'step sign' are diagnostic of paralytic subluxation or dislocation.

MOVEMENTS (Table 4.1)

Let the patient stand with his upper limbs hanging by the side of the chest in anatomical position, i.e. shoulder adducted, elbow extended and forearm supinated. Elicit the movements (active and passive) and note the results under the standard headings as given in the chapter on 'Introduction'. If the active movement is restricted, possible passive range of movement can be tested by holding the patient's hand by examiner's one hand, while his 90° flexed elbow is supported by the examiner's other hand.

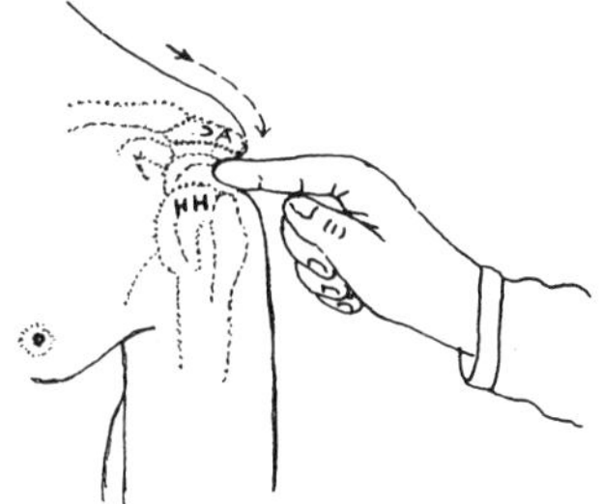

Fig. 4.6: Paralytic subluxation step sign

Measurements

a. Linear
b. Circumferential.

a. *Linear*
1. Apparent measurements
2. True measurements.

Segmental measurements should also be done.

1. *Apparent measurements:* Apparent measurement is not of so much value as in the lower limbs. However, it can give some idea.

Method: With the affected upper limb in a position as kept comfortably by the patient, the opposite upper limb is put parallel to it. Measure from the tip of the seventh cervical spine to the tip of the radial styloid on both sides while the trunk is aligned to the limbs.

2. *True measurements:* Prerequisites—Limbs must be kept in identical position at each joint, i.e. shoulder, elbow and wrist. Palpate and mark the angle of acromion (pass a finger laterally on the spine of scapula, at the extreme outer end posteriorly, an angle is formed known as

Table 4.1: Movements at shoulder

Movement	*Range*	*Prime movers*	*Assisted by*	*Root control*	*Limiting factors*	*Remarks*
1	2	3	4	5	6	7
Flexion Patient stands with arm hanging by the side, elbow extended and forearm supinated. Ask him to take hand towards the mid-line	0°-135°	Pectoralis major, pectoralis minor, anterior fibres of deltoid, coraco-brachialis	Biceps-brachii	C_5	Nothing specific except tension of posterior capsule	In extreme flexion internal rotation supervenes
Extension Diametrically opposite to that of flexion	0°-55°	Latissimus dorsi	Posterior fibres of deltoid, teres major.	$C_{5,6}$	Tension of shoulder flexor muscles. Contact of greater tuberosity of humerus with the acromion	
Abduction Extended elbow moving away from body. The glenohumeral and scapulothoracic components of abduction can be tested as follows. Stand behind the patient and hold the inferior angle of scapula firmly in between thumb and index finger of one hand. While doing abduction, so long as the movement is at glenohumeral joint, scapula will not resist. The moment scapulothoracic gliding starts, resistance is felt by the holding hand. Note the extent of each component (Normal: 90°+ 90°)	0°-almost 180°	While subscapularis steadies the humeral head in glenoid socket, initiation is by supraspinatus (15°-30°), by middle fibres of deltoid upto 90°, deltoid straps around the humeral head on the glenoid, making the gleno-humeral component into one unit. Beyond 90° the locked scapulo-humeral component glides over the chest wall till the extended elbow goes overhead. In this gliding mechanism, muscles involved are serratus anterior, trapezius, latissimus dorsi. The seat of this movement for all practical considerations; the initial 90° of abduction is at gleno-humeral joint, then gliding of locked scapulohumeral components over the posterolateral aspects of chest is supplemented by gliding movements of the clavicle at acromioclavicular and sternoclavicular joints. However, detailed work has shown that there may be involvement of the scapula or even the clavicle right from the beginning of abduction. (Turek, S.L. 1954)		C_5, Accessory nerve.	Upto 90°—none. Beyond 90°—at terminal stage by contact of the arm against the side of the head	(i) In extreme abduction, external rotation of the shoulder supervenes (ii) In terminal stage, some gliding movements occur at the sternoclavicular and acromioclavicular joints. (iii) Painful arc syndrome (pain in arc of 60°-120°) occurs in supraspinatus tendinitis, subacromial bursitis, partial supraspinatus tear, calcific deposits in subacromial bursa and rotator cuff, crack/fracture of greater tuberosity

Contd...

Table 4.1: Contd.

Movements	Range	Prime movers	Assisted by	Root control	Limiting factors	Remarks
1	2	3	4	5	6	7
Adduction Diametrically opposite to abduction	180°—0°	Pectoralis major, latissimus dorsi, teres major	Gravity	$C_{5,6}$	Contact of arm with chest wall	
External Rotation While arm is by the side of the chest, elbow flexed at 90° and forearm supinated, move the extended hand outwards	0°-70° to 90°	Teres minor, infraspinatus, posterior fibres of deltoid		C_5	1. Tension on internal rotators 2. Tension of upper portion of capsular ligament and coracohumeral ligament	Never try to demonstrate the rotational movement in extended position of elbow as rotational elements of forearm will be superadded
Internal Rotation While the position as above, move the extended hand towards the mid-body plane	0°-80° to 90°	Subscapularis, pectoralis major teres major, latissimus dorsi	Anterior fibres of deltoid	$C_{5, 6, 7, 8}$	1. Tension of external rotators 2. Tension of upper portion of capsular ligament	
Circumduction With the upper limb extended at the elbow and wrist, complete a circle starting from the adducted position of the arm	360°	Combination of all of the above		$C_{5, 6}$ Accessory nerve		If any of the above movements is affected, true circumduction will not be possible

the angle of acromion), lateral epicondyle of the humerus and tip of the styloid process of radius.

Total linear measurement of the upper limbs is done by measuring from the angle of acromion to the tip of radial styloid process. (Fig. 4.7).

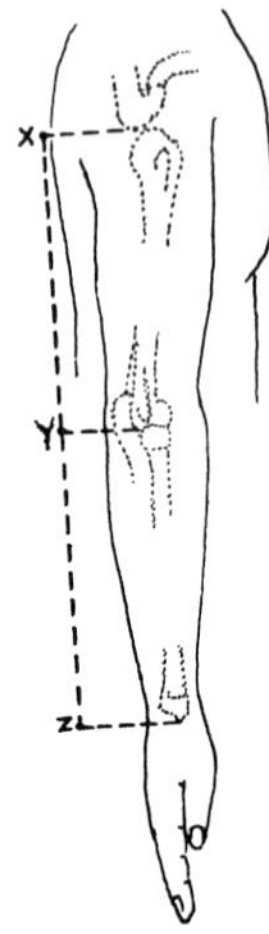

Fig. 4.7: True measurement of upper limb XY arm length; YZ Forearm length

Segmental measurements are for arm and forearm components. For the arm, measure from acromial angle to the tip of the lateral epicondyle and for the forearm, from the lateral epicondylar tip to the tip of the radial styloid process. If the lateral epicondylar tip is not discernible (e.g. in comminuted fractures, congenital absence, iatrogenic) identical fixed bony points can be taken for comparative measurement (e.g. medial epicondylar tips, radial head, olecranon tips).

b. *Circumferential Measurements*

Besides noting the wasting at the mid-arm level, or at equidistant from the acromial angles, circumferential measurements should also be done around the shoulder joint, i.e. across the base of axilla to the top of the shoulder. For all practical purposes, any increase in this measurement indicates an increase in the girth of the shoulder joint and *vice versa.*

The anterior and posterior axillary folds should be measured and compared with the other side (Fig. 4.8).

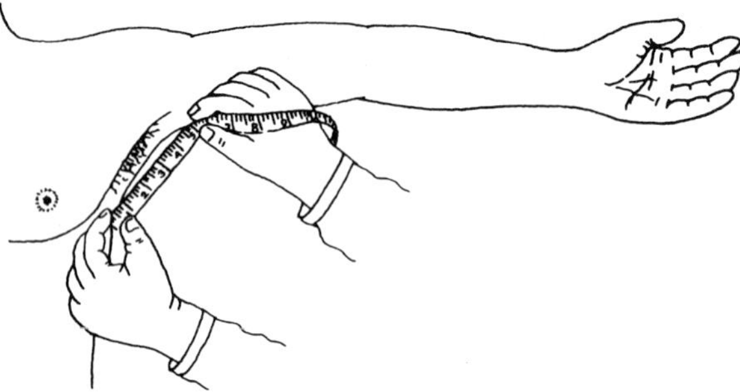

Fig. 4.8: Measurement of axillary folds

Method: Abduct the shoulder as far as practicable upto 90°. Keep the opposite shoulder in the same position. Axillary folds stand prominent. Measure from the junction of the axillary folds with the arm to their junction with the trunk (both anterior and posterior folds).

SPECIAL TESTS

1. *Hamilton Ruler Test* (Fig. 4.9)

In a normal shoulder, a straight ruler cannot touch the acromial process and lateral epicondyle of humerus at the same time (Fig. 4.9I) because of the prominence of the deltoid bulge, which is supported by the head of humerus. If the support is lost, the ruler can touch both the points (e.g. dislocation of the shoulder, congenital absence or iatrogenic excision of the head of humerus; complete paralytic atrophy of the deltoid, as in polio paralysis; dissolution of humeral head in septic arthritis) (Fig. 4.9II).

2. *Callaway s Test*

The girth from axillary base to shoulder top is symmetrical and same on both sides. If the head of humerus occupies an abnormal position, e.g. in dislocation, the girth increases on the affected side.

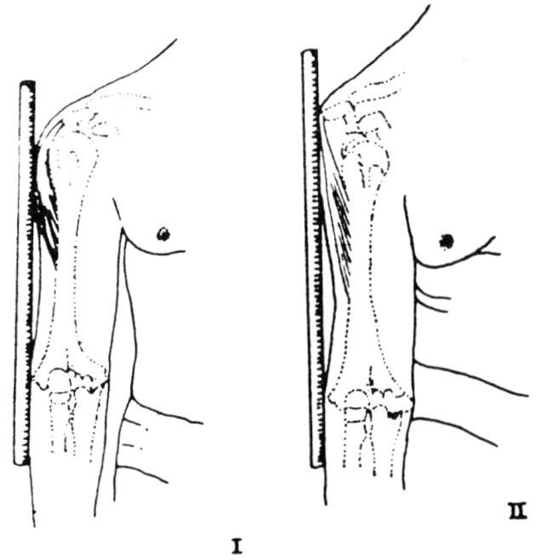

Fig. 4.9: Hamilton ruler test

(Fallacies—axillary abscess, huge lymphadenopathy, collection in the shoulder joint).

3. *Duga's Test* (Fig. 4.10)

Normally, after full flexion at the shoulder the elbow can be brought to near about the mid body plane and the hand to the opposite shoulder top. In dislocation of the shoulder joint, the full flexion of the shoulder cannot be achieved, the elbow therefore cannot be brought to the mid body plane and thus the hand cannot be taken to the opposite shoulder.

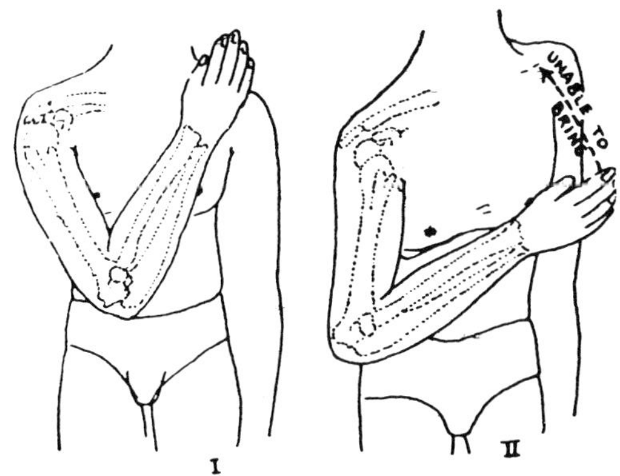

Fig. 4.10: Duga's test

4. *Bryant's Sign*

In anterior subcoracoid dislocation of the shoulder, the anterior axillary fold looks elongated and seems to be at a lower level.

5. *Test for Integrity of the Brachial Plexus*

Test for integrity of the brachial plexus is essential as it may be variably damaged in anterior dislocation of shoulder.

Erb's palsy (upper brachial palsy)—look for the typical attitude and test for the muscle supplied by $C_{5,6}$.

(See the chapter on Peripheral Nerve Injuries).

6. *Test for Integrity of the Axillary Nerve*

(See the chapter on Peripheral Nerve Injuries). It is manifested by loss of deltoid action, i.e. abduction of shoulder (though initiation is possible by the intact supraspinatus muscle) and sensory loss over the 'regimental badge' area at upper outer aspect of the arm.

7. *Radial Nerve*

Manifested by wrist drop (see Fig. 16.9A and B).

8. *Test for Thoracic Inlet Syndrome*

This syndrome comprises the pathologies in which there is compression of the subclavian artery and/or lower roots of the brachial plexus, e.g. scalenus anticus syndrome, costoclavicular syndrome, subclavian aneurysm, cervical ribs, Pancoast tumour, exuberant callus in fracture clavicle, etc. (See the chapter on Spine).

9. *Tests for Bicipital Tenosynovitis*

i. *Yergason's sign:* Patient flexes the elbow and then supinates the forearm against resistance. The resulting forceful contraction of biceps effects distal movement of the tendon and causes pain in the bicipital groove.
ii. The elbow is flexed 90° and examiner's three fingers are firmly placed along the anterosuperior slope of the deltoid bulge (line of bicipital groove); ask the patient to alternately rotate the shoulder externally and internally. Patient will complain of pain when the inflamed tenosynovitis will pass under the pressing fingers.

10. Test for Complete Rupture of Supraspinatus

It is difficult to categorically distinguish pure supraspinatus and other rotator cuff ruptures from any pathology of the subacromial region. However, in complete rupture, a gap may be felt beneath the acromion, which will be tender. Patient cannot initiate active abduction at the shoulder (glenohumeral joint), but once the arm is passively abducted to about 90°, he can sustain and further actively abduct the shoulder due to deltoid action.

Incomplete rupture of the supraspinatus and other rotator cuff muscles can be diagnosed by infiltrating local anaesthetic in the affected area, which abolishes the pain and spasm, allowing the patient to abduct the shoulder from the very beginning.

11. Test for Complete Tear of Rotator Cuff

Arm-drop-sign—Stabilising the scapula with one hand, the examiner passively abducts the patient's affected shoulder to 90° and asks him to sustain it. In case of complete tear, the patient cannot sustain the abducted arm and it drops by the side of the trunk.

12. Test for Detecting Subacromial Impingement of the Rotator Cuff

Painful arc syndrome (Fig. 4.26)—Patient is asked to abduct his/her internally rotated arm over his/her head. In case of impingement of rotator cuff in between the humeral head and the acromion, he/she starts getting pain at about 60° of abduction, which continues till about 120°, and then disappears.

13. Neer's Impingement Test

It is done to differentiate impingement syndrome (mainly subacromial pathology) from 'frozen shoulder' arthritis. Here the clinician prevents scapular rotation with one hand, while with the other hand he raises the affected arm in forced forward flexion and abduction, thus causing the greater tuberosity to impinge against the acromion. Pain is produced in all the above conditions. If the pain is primarily the result of impingement, it can be reduced or eliminated by injecting 10 ml of 1% lignocaine beneath the anterior acromion.

14. Apprehension (Sign) Test

It is performed to detect any instability of the shoulder (e.g. in recurrent subluxation/dislocation of shoulder). The suspected shoulder is gradually abducted and externally rotated pressing the shoulder along the long axis of the arm. In case of instability the patient becomes gradually apprehensive and tries to resist any further movement by his other hand and making the shoulder stiff.

INVESTIGATIONS REQUIRED FOR SHOULDER PATHOLOGY

Besides the routine X-ray, haematological investigations and urine analysis, some special investigations may also be required, according to indications.

i. X-ray

It is of great importance in any shoulder affection. It is always useful to take a comparative X-ray of the opposite shoulder. The shoulder girdle must be fully exposed along with a minimum of the upper one-third of the arm. In suspected referred pain around the shoulder, X-ray of cervical spine is necessary.

Anteroposterior X-ray—Patient lies supine with the arm adducted. The plate is kept behind the shoulder and beam is focussed from the front at the shoulder level. With any suspicion of subluxation/dislocation at the acromioclavicular joint, anteroposterior X-ray should be taken, while the patient stands, keeping his upper limbs hanging by the side of his chest, with some equal weight tied to his hands. Standing position X-ray should also be taken in case of paralysed shoulder.

Lateral axillary (transaxillary) view—The shoulder is abducted to about 90° and the plate is kept on the shoulder top. The X-ray is shot through the base of the axilla (Fig. 4.11).

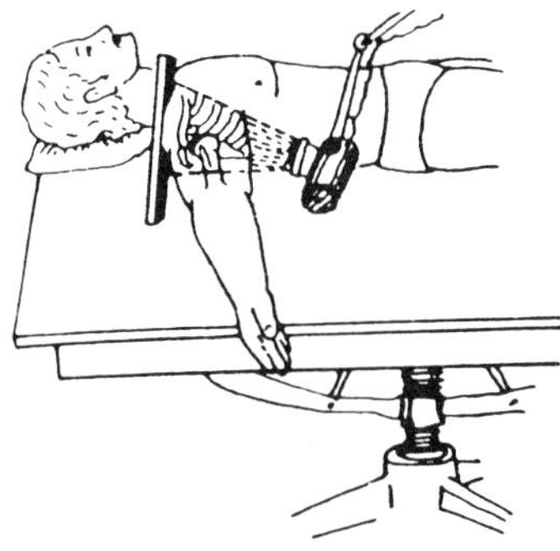

Fig. 4.11: Positioning for lateral axillary view

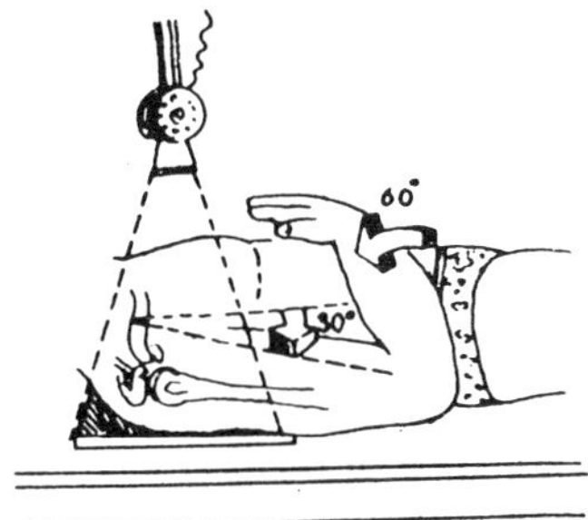

Fig. 4.12: Positioning for X-ray to demonstrate Hill-Sach's lesion

ii. *Special Anteroposterior Projection*

This special X-ray projection demonstrates the Hill-Sach's lesion in recurrent dislocation of the shoulder (Fig. 4.12).

While shoulder is abducted about 30° and internally rotated about 60°, the plate is placed behind the shoulder and the beam is shot from the front at the shoulder level. In certain recurrent anterior dislocations, a radiological step can be delineated on the posterosuperolateral aspect of the head of the humerus (Hill-Sach's lesion or Broca lesion) presumably due to repeated compression (impingement) over the postero-superior surface of head by impaction against the anterior margin of the glenoid, though it may also be congenital defect. A similar defect may be seen on the anteromedial sector of the head in recurrent posterior dislocation of the shoulder.

iii. *Aspiration of the Joint*

Whenever collection is suspected, aspiration should be done through anterior approach and the aspirate should be submitted to physical, biochemical, cytological, culture and chemo-sensitivity examinations.

iv. *Arthroscopy*

This investigation is being utilised to locate Bankart's lesion (the anterior margin of the glenoid cavity and capsule, with or without the glenoid labrum get torn off, presumably in the first traumatic dislocation, the non-healing of which has been blamed for recurrence), any foreign body, loose bodies, to study the condition of synovium and articular surfaces.

v. *Arthography*

Either utilising air or contrast dye, this investigation is useful for delineating the joint space, any filling defect, any leak of contrast medium into the surroundings (e.g. complete rupture of supraspinatus, Bankart's lesion).

vi. *Arthrotomy*

This step is seldom required for diagnostic purposes.

Key Diagnostic Points of Common Shoulder Affections (Table 4.2)

I. *Traumatic Conditions*

a. *Traumatic dislocation*
(Figs 4.13 to 4.17C) (Table 4.3)
- Young adult with comparatively good muscle built.
- History of comparatively severe injury.
- Loss of normal contour of the shoulder.
- Abnormal attitude of the upper limb, e.g. elbow held away from the side of the chest, loss of shoulder bulge.
- Globular bony swelling at abnormal sites around the shoulder joint, according to the type of dislocation.
- Axillary girth increases.
- Anterior axillary fold lowers down.

Table 4.2: Common affections of shoulder

Traumatic	*Paralytic*	*Non-traumatic*
Fracture surgical neck of humerus	Poliomyelitis	Periarthritis/frozen shoulder
Anterior dislocation of shoulder	Brachial plexus palsy	Subacromial bursitis/calcification
Avulsion fracture of greater tuberosity	Motor Neuron disease	Bicipital tendovaginitis
Fracture outer end of clavicle		Tuberculosis shoulder
Subluxation/dislocation of acromioclavicular joint		Septic arthritis
Fracture neck of scapula		

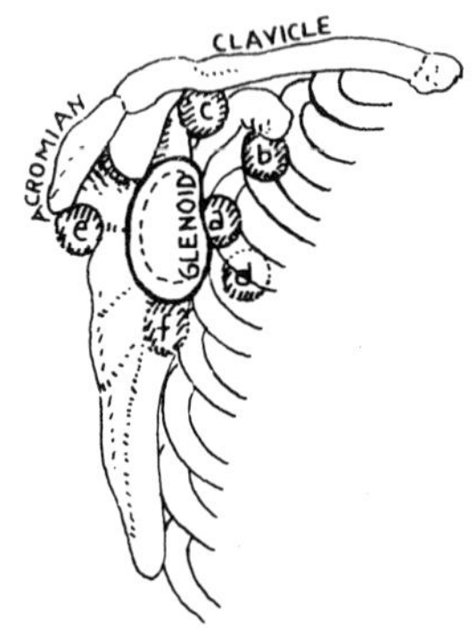

Fig. 4.13: Types of dislocation of shoulder. a = preglenoid, b = subcoracoid, c = subclavicular, d = intrathoracic, e = subspinous, f = infraglenoid (subluxatio erecta)

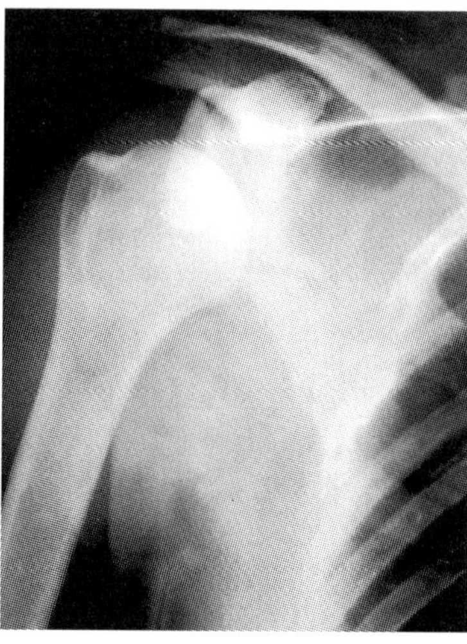

Fig. 4.14: Preglenoid dislocation of shoulder

— Ipsilateral hand cannot be brought to the contralateral shoulder.

— Look for possible neurovascular damage (axillary nerve, brachial plexus) (Fallacies—In (i) Fracture dislocation, (ii) Paralytic dislocation, where all above features may not be positive).

In dislocation of shoulder joint there is pseudolengthening (apparent lengthening) of the arm, and it appears as if the arm is originating at the lower level from the trunk when compared to other side.

b. *Recurrent Dislocation of Shoulder Joint*

— Recurrent anterior dislocation is more common while posterior is rare.

— Subjects are usually young adults with good musculature.

— History of recurrence even without significant trauma.

— No confirmatory clinical signs, however, subject may get apprehensive about dislocation with the limb put in a particular provocative position. While the shoulder is held in maximum external rotation and 90° or more abducted position and extension, the humeral head is pushed forward from behind. The patient becomes apprehensive and complains of pain in shoulder, and/or a sense of impending subluxation (*apprehension test*). By reducing or relocating the humeral head back into its normal position by manual pressure on the humeral head, the patient feels relieved of the apprehension symptoms (*relocation test*).

Table 4.3: Classification of shoulder dislocation

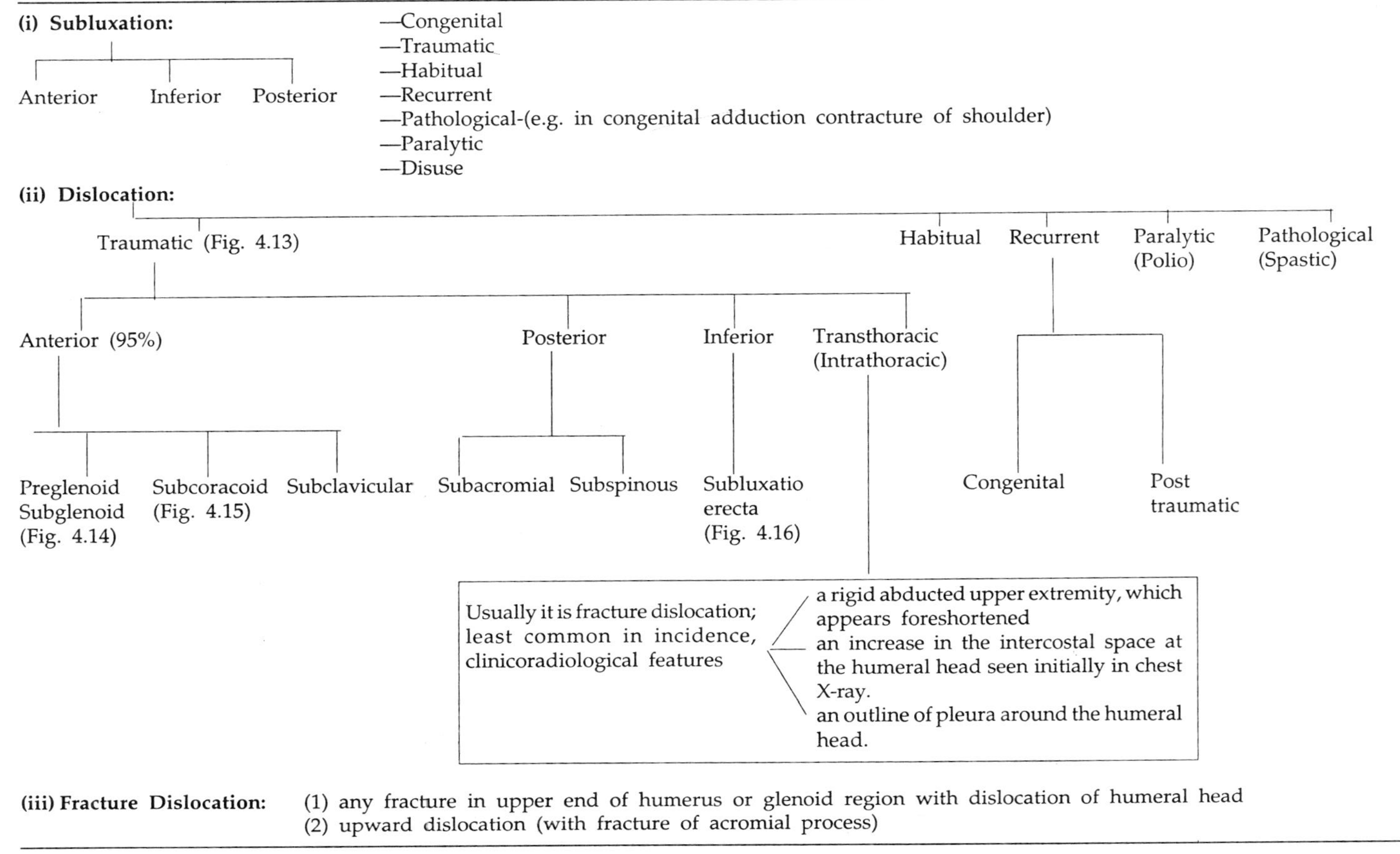

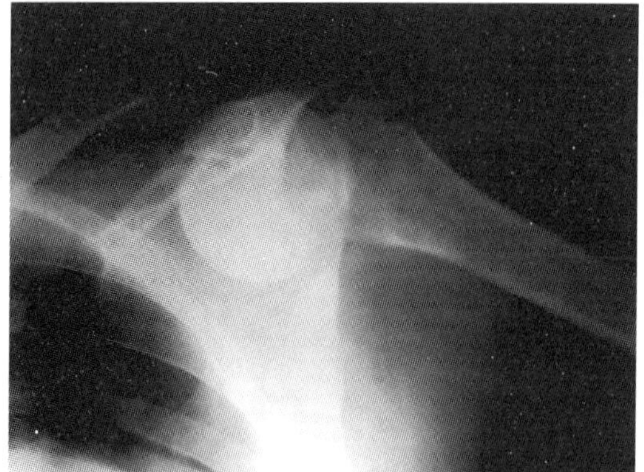

Fig. 4.15: Subcoracoid dislocation of shoulder

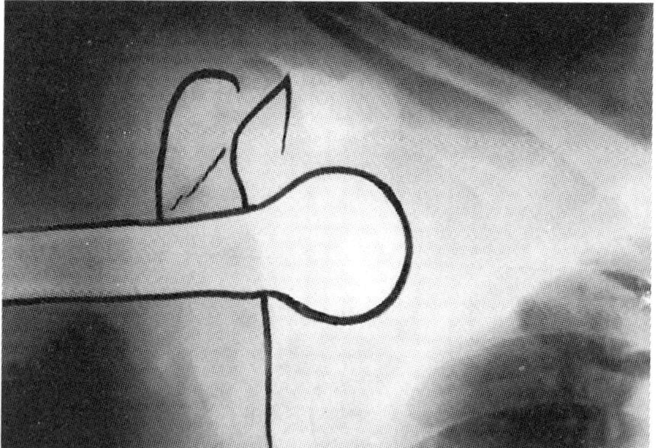

Fig. 4.16: Subluxatio erecta

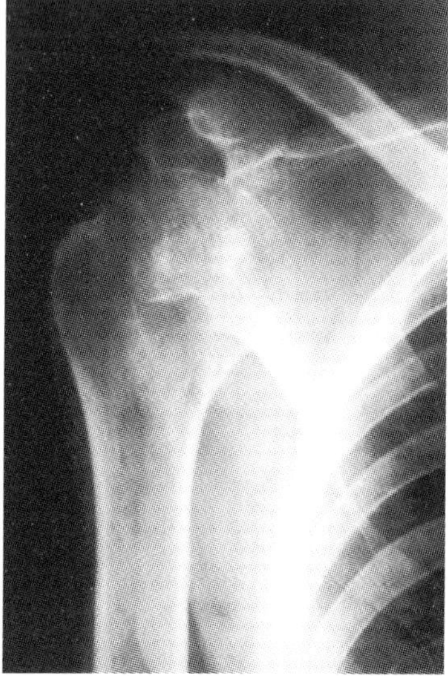

Fig. 4.17A: Posterior dislocation of shoulder

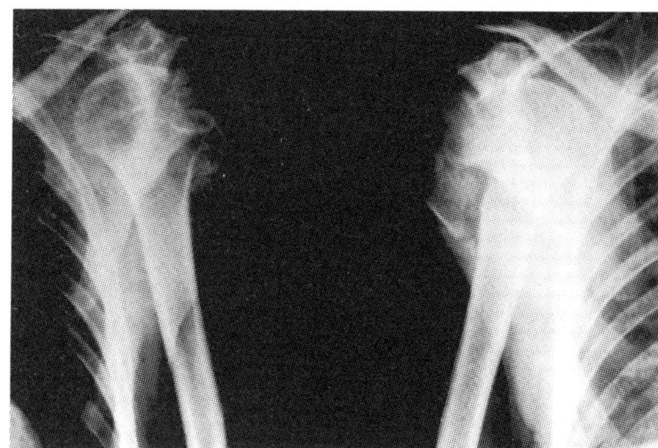

Fig. 4.17B: Fracture dislocation of shoulder bilateral

— A special X-ray may demonstrate Hill-Sach's lesion (anterior dislocation).
— Arthroscopy may demonstrate Bankart's lesion in anterior dislocation and reverse lesion in posterior recurrent dislocation.

c. *Fractures around the Shoulder: Most of the fractures can be accurately diagnosed only after taking the X-ray*

i. *The Most Common Fracture here is of the Surgical Neck of the Humerus* (Fig. 4.18).
— Elderly persons.
— History of fall on outstretched hand.
— Pain in shoulder region.
— In impacted fracture, fair/good range of passive shoulder movements.
— In unimpacted fractures, movements at the fracture site itself can be felt.
— Ecchymosis in arm.

ii. *Dislocation of Acromioclavicular Joint* (Fig. 4.23B)
— Usually due to fall on shoulder joint, resulting in either subluxation (coraco-clavicular ligament intact) or dislocation (coracoclavicular ligament torn).
— In subluxation—outer end of clavicle, which just projects under the skin, is tender, clavicle is stable.

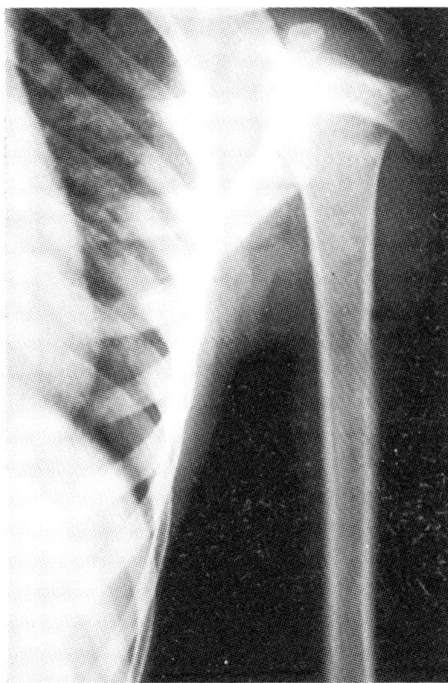

Fig. 4.17C: Upward subluxation (rather dislocation) of shoulder

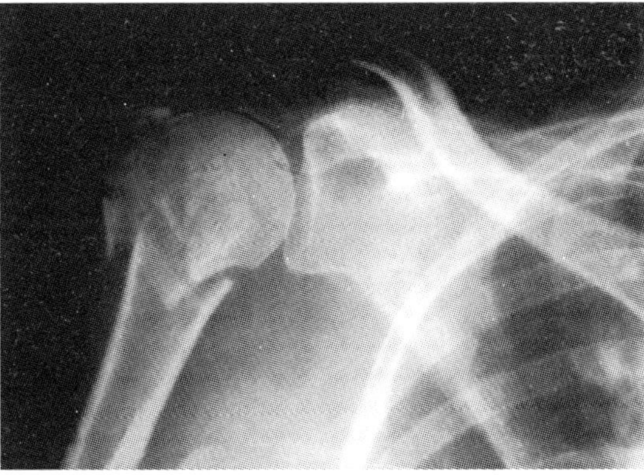

Fig. 4.18: Fracture of surgical neck of humerus

— In dislocation—outer end of the clavicle obviously ridden up, tender and the clavicle is unstable.
— X-ray is confirmatory.

iii. *Sternoclavicular dislocation* (Figs 4.19A to 4.20B)
— Comparatively uncommon injury produced due to fall on shoulder point or outstretched hand; or direct hit from the front.
— Sternal end of clavicle may subluxate/ dislocate forwards or backwards with upward shift.
— Local tender swelling at the joint.
— Rarely, clavicular end can be demonstrated to be mobile due to unstability (Figs 4.19A and B).
— X-ray is confirmatory.

iv. *Fracture clavicle* (Figs 4.21 to 4.23A)
— One of the commonest fractures in children and adults.
— Due to fall on outstretched hand and by direct hit.
— Typical attitude.
— Fracture of middle two-third common, may be of outer end (confused with acromioclavicular subluxation/dislocation (Figs 4.20A and 4.20B), may be of inner end (confused with sternoclavicular subluxation/dislocation).
— Common displacement of shaft fracture—medial fragment displaced and tilted upwards (due to pull of sternomastoid), and lateral displaced downwards by the weight of the arm.
— Locally fracture end felt as an irregularity, which is tender; in late cases as a bony swelling at the fracture site (exuberant callus).
— X-ray confirmatory.

II. *Nontraumatic Conditions*

a. *Pyogenic Arthritis* (Fig. 4.24)
— Acute onset with constitutional features.
— Inflammatory swelling all around.
— Pitting oedema.
— All movements restricted and severely painful.
— Lymph nodes enlarged.
— Polymorphonuclear leucocytosis
— Aspiration of pus.

b. *Tuberculous Arthritis* (Figs 4.25A and B)
— Chronic history (in adults usually confused with periarthritis shoulder). More or less constant pain, more on activities.
— Marked atrophy of muscles all around the shoulder.
— Marked tenderness all around joint line, even on the adjoining bone (in periarthritis/frozen shoulder adjoining bone not that tender; flexion, and adduction are

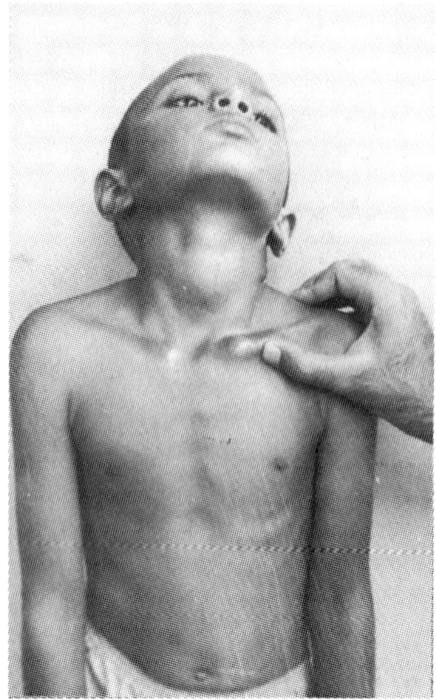

Fig. 4.19A: Sternal end of clavicle can be pushed up

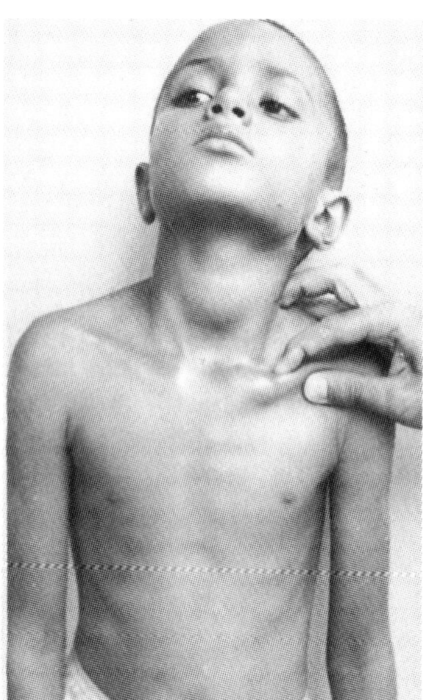

Fig. 4.19B: Sternal end of clavicle can be pushed down

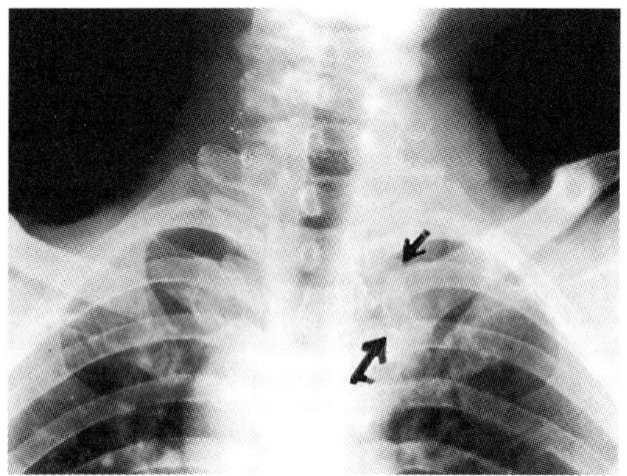

Fig. 4.20A: Subluxated sternoclavicular joint

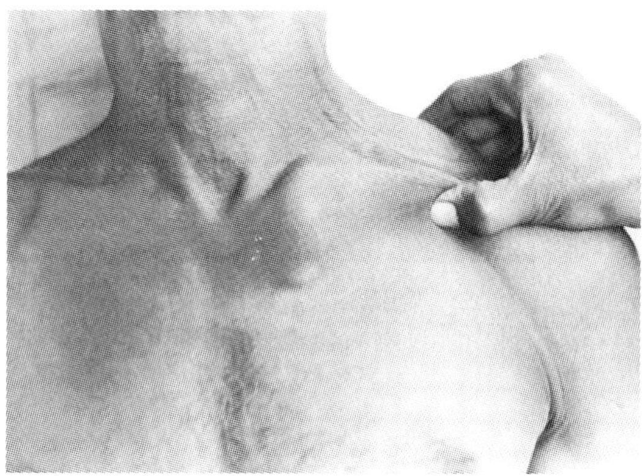

Fig. 4.20B: Dislocated sternal end of clavicle can be pushed up

free). Tenderness of the head can be easily elicited through the axilla.

— Movements painfully restricted in all directions (in periarthritis, flexion and adduction not limited).

— Cold abscess, usually not accompanied (shoulder tuberculosis is also known as caries sicca).

— Lymph glands may be enlarged.

— Radiologically: typical features of a tuberculous lesion. (joint space reduced; generalised rarefaction; irregular bony destruction; irregular bony collapse, etc.

c. *Periarthritis/Freezing Shoulder/Frozen Shoulder*

Periarthritis: It is the initial manifestation of an ongoing pathology which usually culminates in frozen shoulder. External rotation, terminal

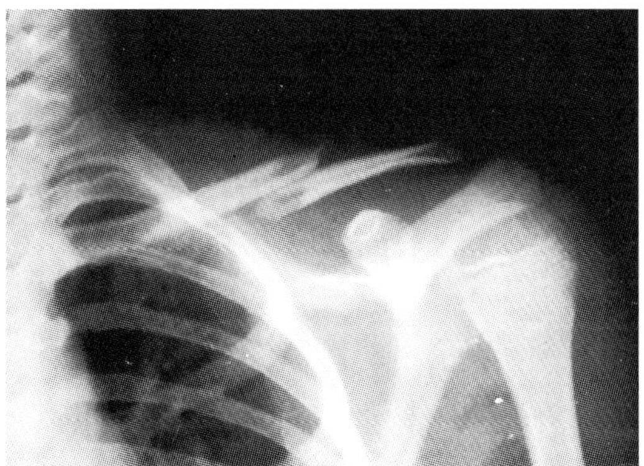

Fig. 4.21: Fracture clavicle with typical displacement

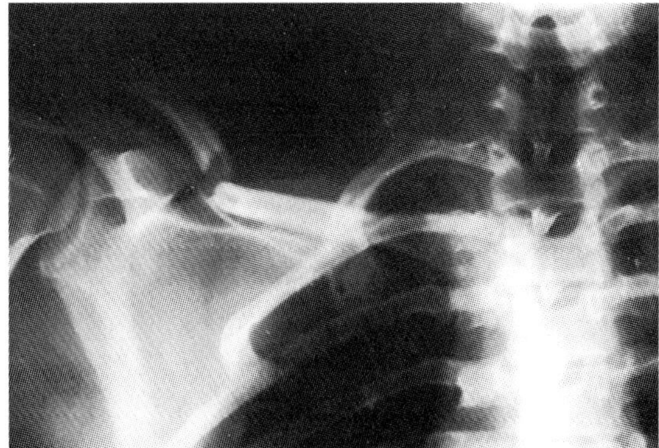

Fig. 4.22: Fracture clavicle with atypical displacement (medial fragment is displaced down)

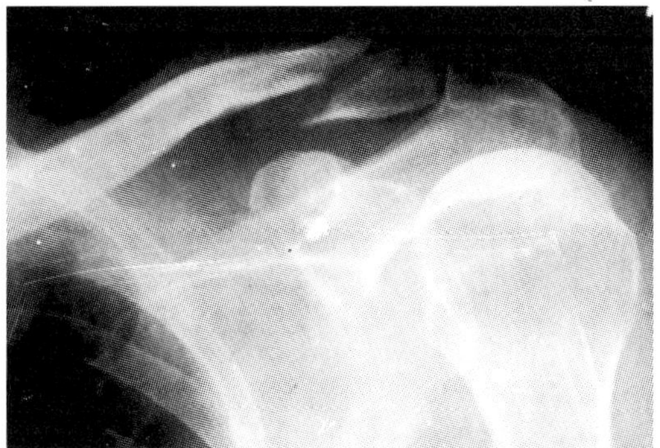

Fig. 4.23A: Fracture outer end of clavicle

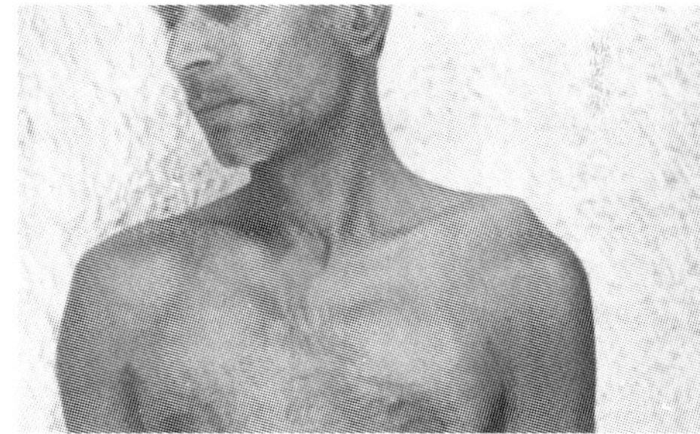

Fig. 4.23B: Acromioclavicular dislocation

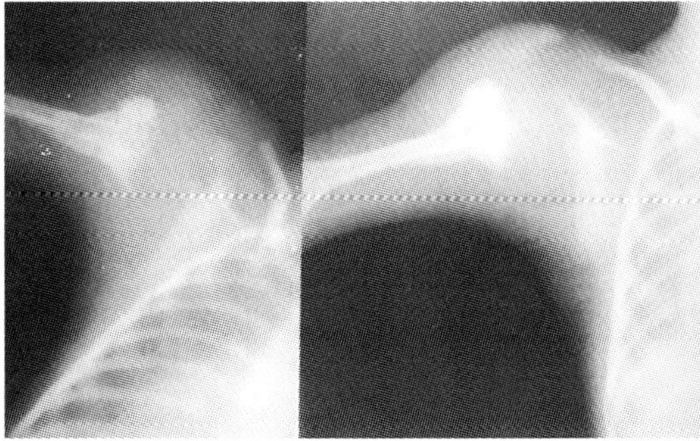

Fig. 4.24A: Primary septic arthritis of shoulder with osteomyelitis of upper part of humerus in an infant

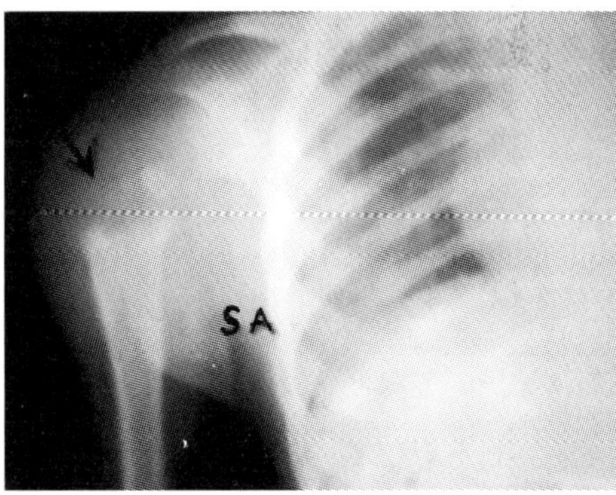

Fig. 4.24B: Septic arthritis of the shoulder and subacute osteomyelitis of upper region of humerus in an infant

internal rotation and terminal abduction painfully restricted.

Freezing shoulder: Painful restriction of rotational movements and abduction but shoulder can be abducted more than 90° (glenohumeral joint not completely frozen).

Frozen shoulder: Glenohumeral movements are frozen. Rotational and abduction movements

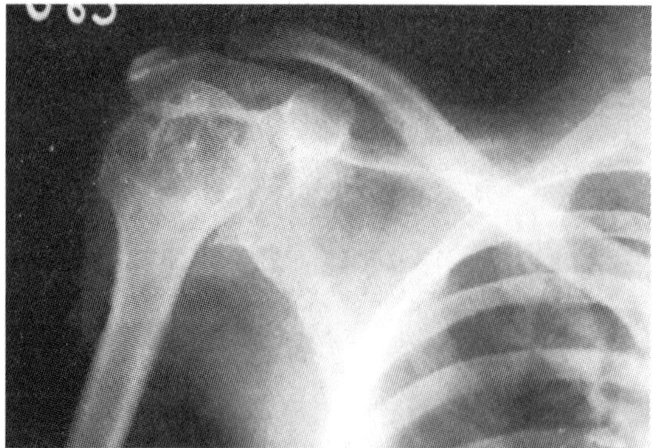

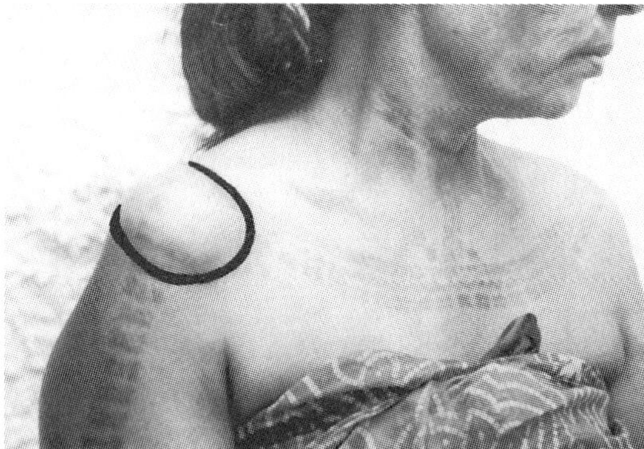

Figs 4.25A and B: Tuberculosis of shoulder with cold abscess

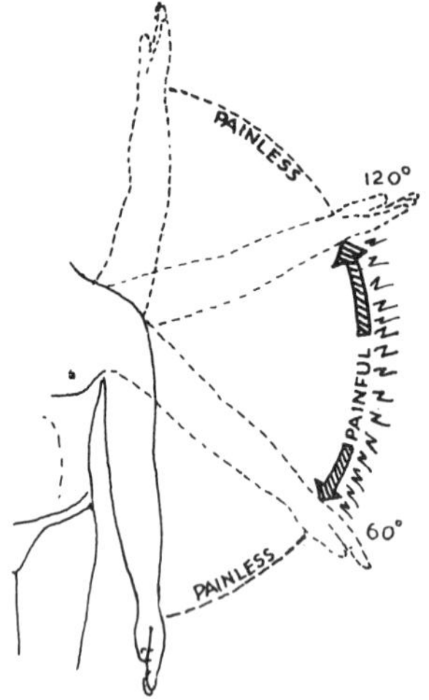

Fig. 4.26: Painful arc syndrome

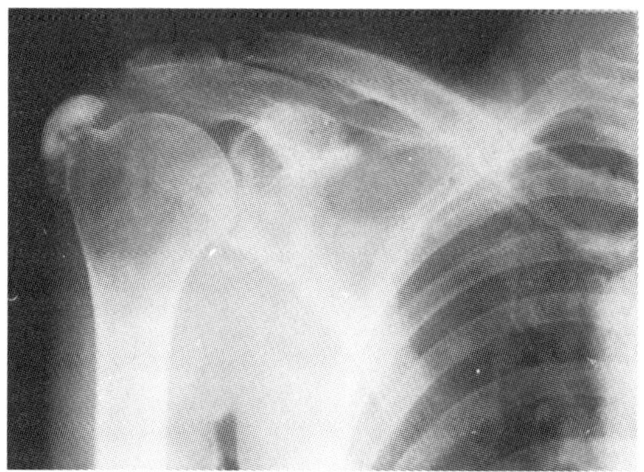

Fig. 4.27: Calcified subacromial bursa

are markedly painfully restricted. Less than 90° of abduction is possible by scapulothoracic gliding (glenohumeral joint completely frozen).

- —May be history of insignificant injury following which the symptoms develop.
- —Severe pain at rest (usually at night).
- —On right sided shoulder complaints, the right lower chest and upper abdominal pathologies must be excluded. On left sided shoulder complaints, cardiovascular system must be examined thoroughly.
- —Mild to moderate wasting of supraspinatus, infraspinatus and deltoid.

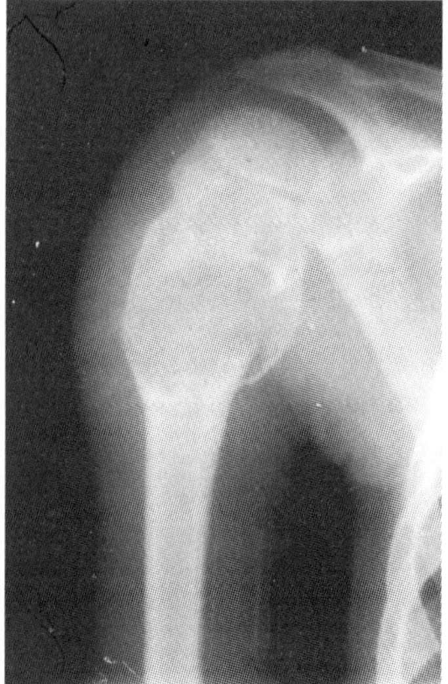

Fig. 4.28: Unicameral bone cyst

— Tenderness at anterior and/or posterior shoulder joint line.
— Gradual limitation of abduction and external rotation (when markedly advanced—frozen shoulder).
— Flexion and adduction are usually free, even in advanced cases.
— In late cases, rarefaction in surrounding bones, more of tuberosities.
— In elderly and even in adults, X-rays of shoulder must be taken to eliminate any hidden pathology (e.g. early giant cell tumour (GCT), secondary carcinoma, etc.).

(d) *Supraspinatus Tendinitis/Subacromial Bursitis*
— Typical history of pain at the shoulder in a certain arc of abduction movement (60°–120°) (Fig. 4.26).
— Tenderness below the subacromial area and over the greater tuberosity.
— X-ray may reveal abnormal subacromial calcification (Fig. 4.27).

(e) *Bicipital Tendinitis*
Patient complains of pain in anterolateral region of shoulder in abduction of shoulder and flexion at elbow simultaneously. Maximum tenderness on anterolateral slope of shoulder along the bicipital tendon. *Yergason's sign present.*

f. *Fibrous Dysplasia/Unicameral Bone Cyst* (Fig. 4.28)
— In young adolescent, more in males.
— Trivial injury producing pain in the upper arm or shoulder region.
— May be earlier history of pain off and on.
— X-ray reveals multicystic or monocystic expansion of the upper humeral end beneath the growth cartilage with or without pathological fracture.

BIBLIOGRAPHY

1. De Palma AF, Gallery C, Bennet C: Anatomy and degenerative lesions of the shoulder joint. *Ann Acad Orthop Surg Instr Course lecte* Ann Arbor: Edwards, **6**: 1949.
2. Simpson NS, Schwappach JR, Toby EB: Fracture-dislocation of the humerus with intrathoracic displacement of the humeral head. *J Bone Joint Surg* **80A**: 889-91, 1998.
3. Turek SL: The painful and stiff shoulder. *J Int Coll Surg* **22**: 695, 1954.

5

Elbow Joint

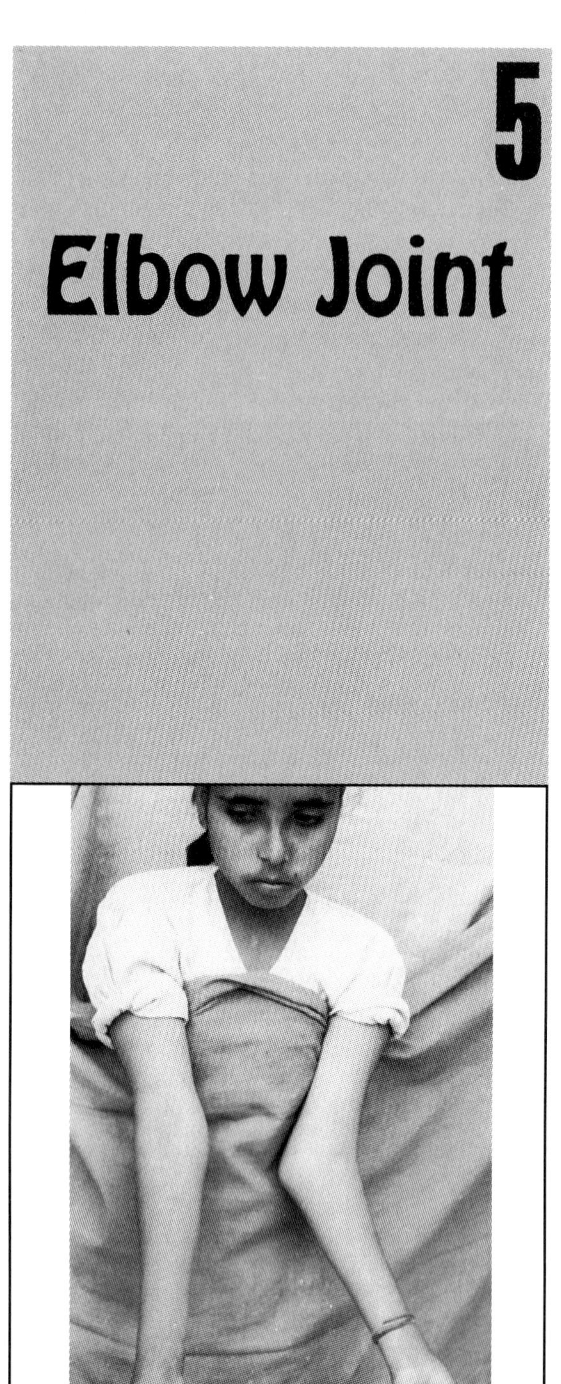

INTRODUCTION

The elbow joint (a hinge joint), is perhaps the main joint responsible for communicating the actions of the hand to the trunk. It is a compound joint having ulnohumeral and radiohumeral components. The upper radioulnar joint communicates with the elbow joint proper. The synovial reflections of these joints are also intercommunicating. The main articulation is in between the trochlear notch of the ulna and the trochlear region of the lower articular end of the humerus, the convex capitular portion of the humerus and the shallow concave top of the radial head, forming a passive articulation.

ANATOMICAL CONSIDERATIONS

1. The trochlear notch keeps its grip on the lower trochlear articular end almost throughout the full range of elbow movements. In the fully pronated position of the forearm, the trochlear notch assumes a wrenching grip over the trochlear portion of humerus and thus for all practical purposes the joint is locked. The main thrust is thereby directly transmitted in a straight line from the ulna to the lower end of the humerus.
2. The medial lip of the spool-shaped trochlea is more prominent and extends more distally (5 to 6 mm) than its lateral lip. This forms an oblique axis at the ulnohumeral joint, which results in the normal valgus angulation at the elbow—the carrying angle (10-15 degrees, more in females).
3. The lower articular end of humerus is placed about 40° tilted forwards in relation to the long axis of the humeral shaft.
4. The functional efficiency of elbow movements markedly improves in collaboration with the actions at the radioulnar joint.
5. Due to causes not well known, the elbow is very notorious for developing post-traumatic myositis ossificans (with or without massage).
6. In front of the elbow and a little above its level the brachial artery is very much

vulnerable, and can undergo spasmodic contraction following exogenic or endogenic stimuli. Therefore, Volkmann's ischaemic contracture is more likely to develop, following injuries in this region.

7. The three important peripheral nerves of the upper limb lie in close relation to the elbow joint. Of these, the ulnar nerve theoretically appears to be in a more vulnerable position, being placed in close association with the back of the medial epicondyle and then passing through a tight fibro-osseus tunnel. The median nerve, like the brachial artery, lies just in front and above the elbow level and is vulnerable in any injury, especially in supracondylar fracture. The radial nerve, lying closely related to the lateral supracondylar ridge, and the anterior capsule of the elbow is also likely to suffer in elbow injuries. In order of frequency, the median nerve (indicated mainly by pointing index and sensory loss in index finger), the radial nerve (indicated by wrist drop) and the ulnar nerve (clawing tendency and sensory deficit in the little finger and half of the ring finger) are affected in injuries around the elbow. The injuries—supracondylar fractures, Monteggia fracture dislocations, baby car fracture dislocations, elbow dislocations, fracture neck of radius, fracture medial epicondyle of humerus—are likely to affect the nerves, in that order.
8. The radial head, the lateral epicondyle and the tip of the olecranon forms a triangle over the posterolateral aspect of the joint. This space is occupied by the anconeus muscle overlying the joint capsule. With fluid collection in the joint, this 'anconeus triangle' bulges out.
9. The fascial compartments in front of the elbow are comparatively tight, therefore, any swelling in this region is likely to jeopardise the neurovascular bundles quite early.

OSSIFICATION AROUND THE ELBOW JOINT (Fig. 5.1)

METHODOLOGY

i. *History taking*: Besides detailed history taking as in general chapter, special attention must be paid to the following points: In cases of traumatic conditions—mode of injury; history of massage; number of attempts of manipulative reduction; history pertaining to impending features of Volkmann's ischaemia, *history for haemophilia:*
ii. *General and systemic examinations:* (As in the chapter on Introduction).
iii. *Regional examination:* As usual for the upper limbs (from the cervical spine to the fingertips).
iv. *Local examination*

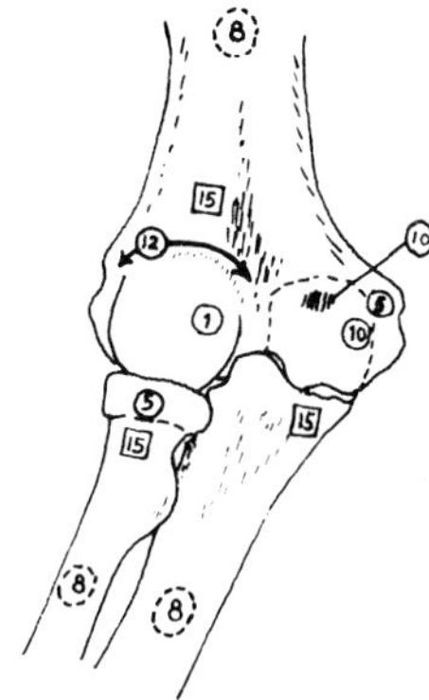

Fig. 5.1: Ossification around elbow: dotted circle denotes primary ossification centre in weeks (IUL), complete circle denotes secondary ossification centre in years, square denotes fusion of epiphysis in years

a. *Prerequisites*

1. Both the elbows must be examined in identical position.
2. The patient should either stand or sit on a stool.
3. The position of the shoulder, forearm and the hand of the normal side must be in identical position with that of affected one, preferably, with the arm lying by the side of the chest.

Attitude

Note the attitude of the elbow. The carrying angle of the elbow should be marked in supine and extended position of the forearm. The angle formed in between the extended long axis of the arm and the long axis of the forearm at the central point of the extended elbow axis is the carrying angle (Fig. 5.2—A position). It varies from 10-15° (more in females than in males). Exaggeration of this carrying angle is called cubitus valgus (Fig. 5.2—B position). Reduction, neutralisation or reversal of carrying angle is cubitus varus (Figs 5.2—C position and 5.3A and B). In most of the pathologies in and around the elbow, there is varying degrees of flexion deformity at the elbow. In an old, unreduced posterior dislocation of the elbow, the joint is flexed to about 45°, the triceps tendon stands prominent and the olecranon tip projects prominently.

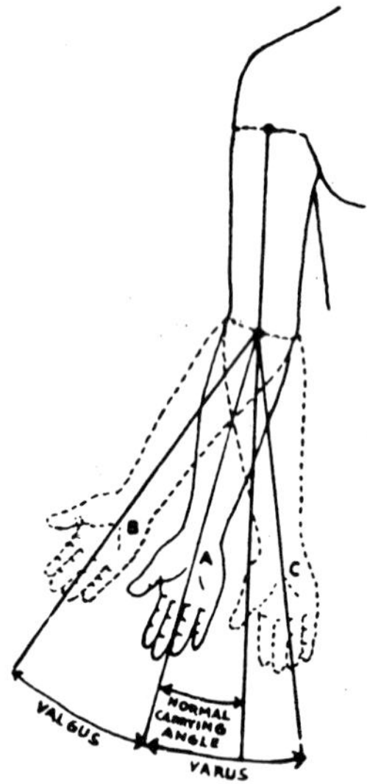

Fig. 5.2: (A) Normal carrying angle, (B) Cubitus valgus, (C) Cubitus varus

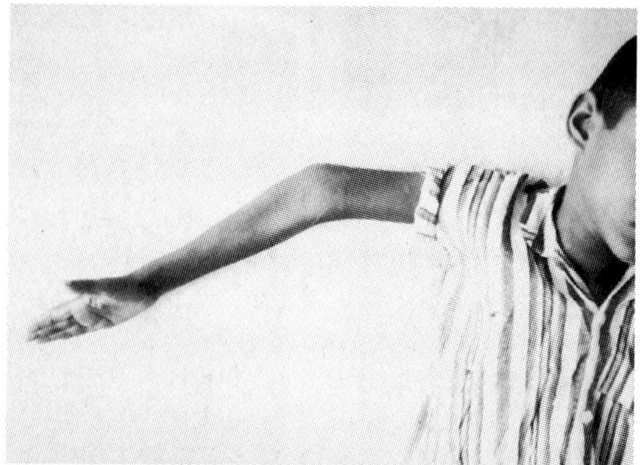

Fig. 5.3A: Photograph showing marked cubitus varus deformity following malunited supracondylar fracture. In prone position of forearm this deformity looks further exaggerated

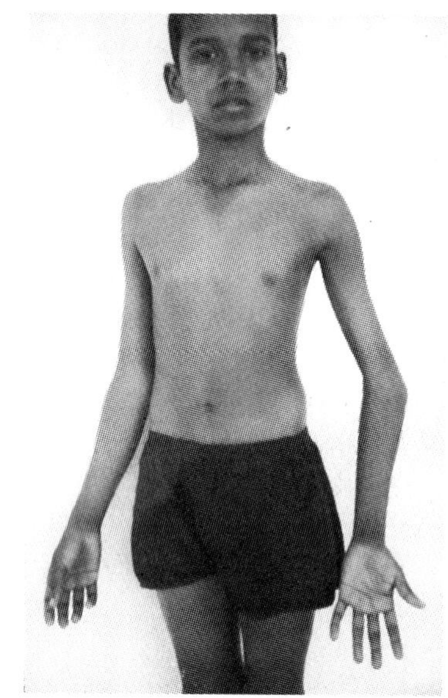

Fig. 5.3B: Cubitus varus deformity. Exact deformity should be assessed in supine position of forearm

Inspection

Assessment should be done in symmetrical position (in case of deformity the normal elbow should be kept in identical position to that of deformed one) from the back, the front and from the sides. Fixed bony and soft tissue points should be looked at.

From the front: Biceps bulge (Fig. 5.4), cubital fossa, upper forearm bulge, biceps tendon prominence, superficial veins, any fixed flexion deformity (Figs 5.5 A and B).

From the back: Triceps muscle bulge and tendon, olecranon process, callosity or any other swelling

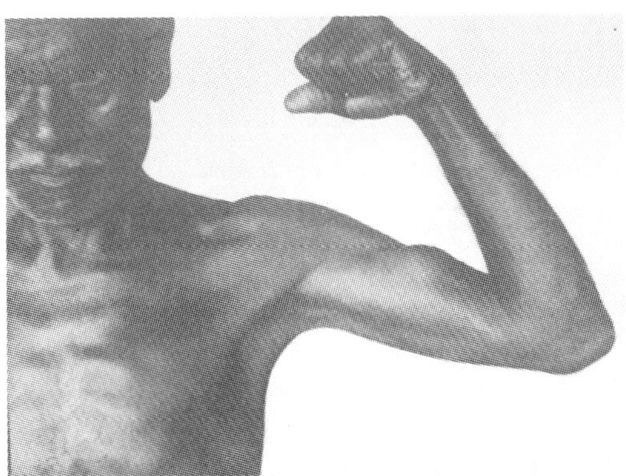

Fig. 5.4: Normal biceps bulge interrupted due to its tear; note that in performing active flexion of the elbow, the torn biceps mass stands markedly prominent

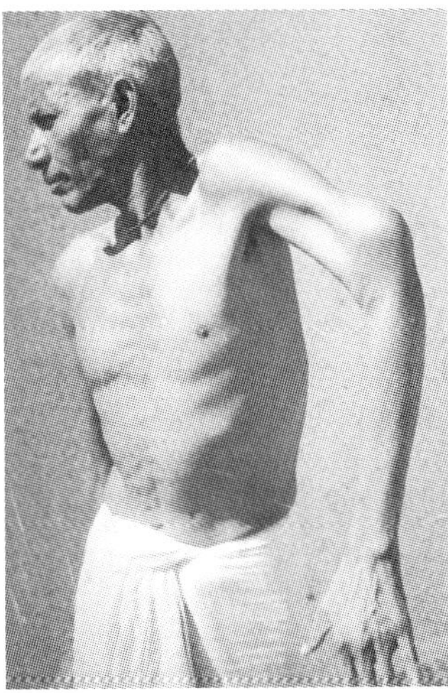

Fig. 5.5A: Photograph showing abnormal angulation above the elbow joint in attempt of flexing the elbow (double elbow) produced due to pseudarthrosis following fracture of lower humeral shaft

on the point of the elbow (e.g. in student's elbow), paraolecranon depression, anconeus triangle, upper end of the ulna, back of the medial and lateral epicondylar tips represented by depression on the surface.

From the side: From the outer side—the bulge of the brachioradialis and long extensors of the wrist, or any abnormality.

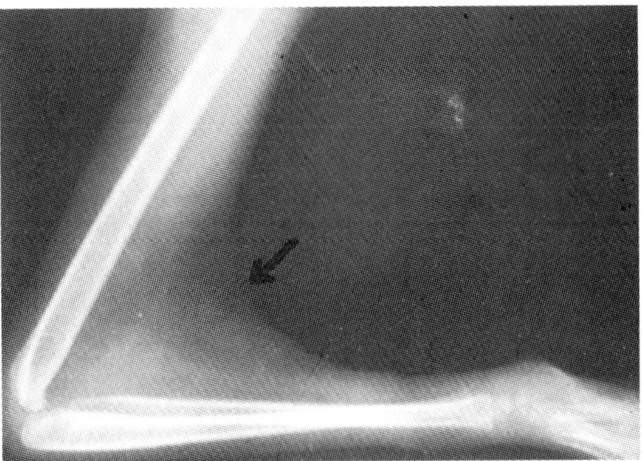

Fig. 5.5B: Congenital flexion contracture of elbow, leading to fixed flexion deformity

From the inner side: The medial epicondylar prominence, supracondylar depressions and the bulge of the common flexors.

Any abnormality, like swelling, sinuses, scars on any aspect should be noted clearly, as dealt with in the chapter of Introduction.

Palpation

Superficial palpation: Besides palpating as in the Introduction chapter, specially feel for any local rise of temperature and any superficial tenderness.

Deep palpation: Confirm the findings of inspection. Special points besides the general considerations are: The muscle around the elbow should be palpated for texture, bulk and pliability. In delayed traumatic cases, specially palpate for the presence of firm to hard bony plaques in the muscle mass (myositis ossificans). Feel the tips of the lateral and medial epicondyles, the supracondylar ridges, olecranon process, and head of the radius.

Palpation of Supracondylar Ridges

Method: Simultaneous bilateral palpation in symmetrical position of limbs is always helpful. Palpation will be convenient with the elbow semiflexed (about 45°) and the forearm supinated as far as possible (Fig. 5.6). The two epicondylar tips will stand out prominently. Hold the lower forearm in one hand, and use the thumb and middle fingers of the opposite hand to palpate the epicondylar tips. Proceed vertically upwards from the epicondyles along the shaft of humerus in the mid plane of the arm—the sharp bony supracondylar ridges are felt on the two sides (note any abnormality, like tenderness irregularity, and thickening, etc.)

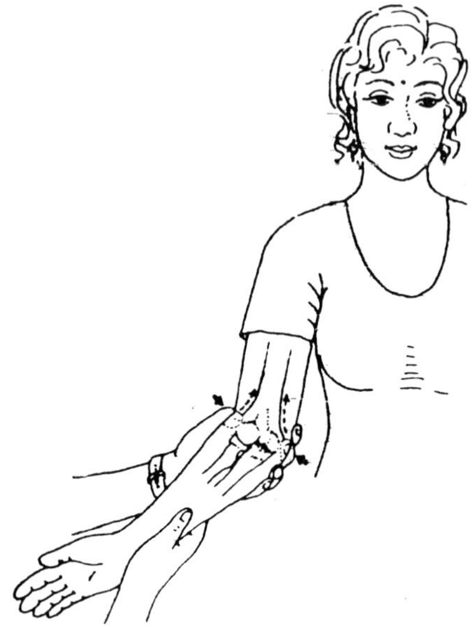

Fig. 5.6: Location of the epicondylar tips and palpating the supracondylar ridges

Three-Point Relationship

Confirm the normal relation of the epicondylar tips to the olecranon tip. Normally, in 90° flexed position of the elbow, they form more or less an isosceles triangle (Fig. 5.7), the interepicondylar line forms the base. If it is not possible to put the elbow in the desired position of palpation, palpation should be done in whatever position is possible. Comparison should be done with the elbow of the other side placed in similar postures, for assessing and comparing the correlation.

Fallacies in the three-point relationship: Fracture of the either epicondyle, fracture olecranon, excision arthroplasty of elbow.

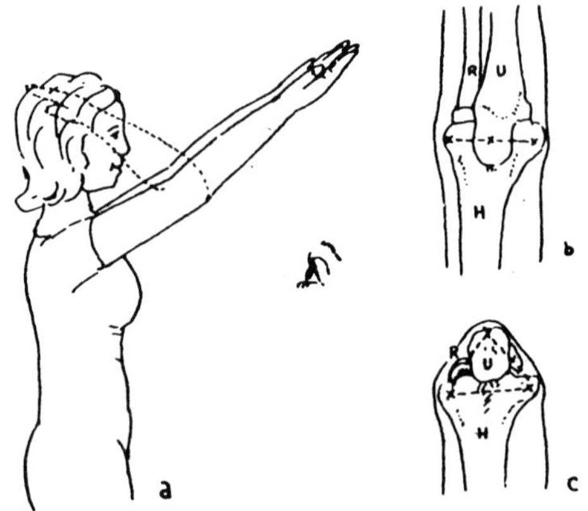

Fig. 5.7: (a) Position of the elbow in which the relation of the three bony points should be ascertained. (b) Relation of the three bony points in extension. (c) Relation of the three bony points in 90° flexion (H = humerus; U = ulna; R = radius)

Palpation of Epicondylar Region

Feel for bony tenderness—e.g. for lateral epicondylitis (tennis elbow) or medial epicondylitis (golfer's elbow or pitcher's elbow or Baseballer's elbow or javeline thrower's elbow, Little League elbow syndrome or manifestation of chronic tension stress injuries of elbow). Hold the distal forearm in one hand, with (your right hand holding the patient's right hand) the elbow of the patient in about 35° flexion. With the thumb and middle finger of your opposite hand, press the epicondylar areas. In lateral epicondylitis, there is maximum tenderness in the anteroinferior region of the lateral epicondyle. In medial epicondylitis, maximum tenderness is in the anteroinferior region of the medial epicondyle.

Both epicondyles lie in same line or slightly posterior to the supracondylar ridges. In case of internal rotation of the lower fragment in supracondylar fracture, the lateral epicondylar tip remains anteriorly in relation to the supracondylar ridge.

Palpate the *ulnar nerve* behind and above the medial epicondyle as far as possible and note its position, pliability, any thickening and/or beading, and tenderness.

Method: Support the lower forearm in the same position as above, using one hand. Gently roll the pulp of the middle finger of the other hand behind the medial epicondyle. The ulnar nerve can be felt like a slippery cord. Palpate the nerve as far above as possible, since in Hansen's neuritis its thickening is very marked in this region.

Palpation of Joint Line

The prominent brachialis and biceps muscle and their musculotendinous masses prevent the palpating fingers from reaching upto the joint line from the front. From the back, the olecranon process and the comparatively broad and tight tendon of the triceps do not allow the fingers to reach upto joint proper. However, on both sides of the main triceps tendon, the uppermost part of the olecranon notch of the humerus can be partially felt. On the outer side, the humero-radial joint line is felt as a transverse slit beneath the outer margin of the rounded capitulum.

Method: Bilateral palpation is always helpful. Flex the elbow at 35°– 45° for comparison. Hold the lower forearm in one hand (right hand holding patient's right elbow). The upper end of the patient's forearm is supported on the palm of the opposite hand, the thumb is placed on the outer side of the level of the elbow joint. The tip of the thumb can feel the rounded bulge of the outer margin of the capitulum. Keeping the thumb just below it, rotate the forearm. The head of the radius can be felt rotating. Just above the head of radius, a transverse slit can be felt (Fig. 5.8). For all practical purposes, this represents clinical palpation of the elbow joint. Since the elbow is a composite joint, tenderness in this region indicates tenderness in the elbow joint as well. However, when there is a synovial bulge (Fig. 5.9), the joint is grossly affected and it is difficult to palpate the joint line. Palpation along the interepicondylar line anteriorly will also demonstrate the elbow joint tenderness.

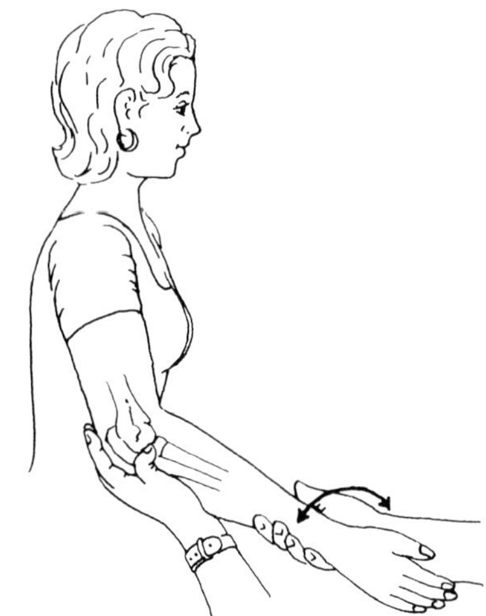

Fig. 5.8: Palpating the radiohumeral joint line and head of the radius

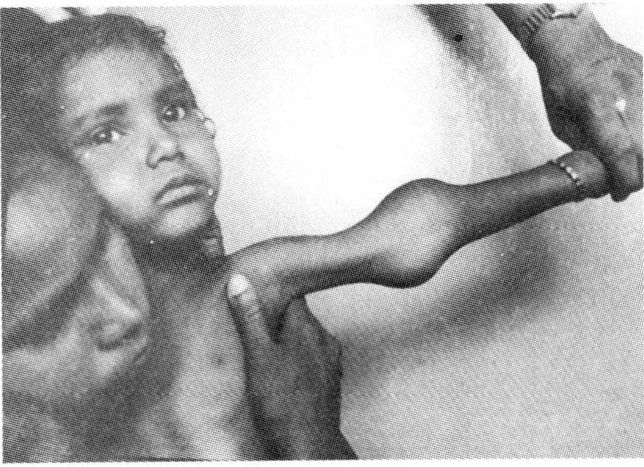

Fig. 5.9: Photograph of a patient of villonodular synovitis showing huge synovial swelling

Fluid in the Joint

Swelling of the elbow can be also due to any haemarthrosis or any pathological collection. On the whole it is difficult to clinically find out little or even moderate collections. However, fullness specially posterolaterally in the anconeus triangle, if it is not boggy in feel, is in all probability due to fluid in the joint. In such situations, the elbow is kept in semiflexed position, because then the joint capacity is maximum. Positive cross-fluctuation between the medial paraolecranon swelling and the posterolateral swelling indicates fluid in the joint. In huge collection, a tense bulge may be palpated in the cubital fossa.

A collection in the triceps bursa should be differentiated from any collection in the joint. In 45° flexed position of the elbow the bursal collection will stand as two identical sacculations on both sides of the triceps. Try to elicit cross-fluctuation, keeping both index fingers on both sides of the triceps. In triceps bursitis it is positive.

Palpate the supratrochlear lymph glands on the medial side of the elbow. Also palpate the axillary group of glands which drain this area.

MOVEMENTS (Table 5.1)

Movements should be tested at humeroulnar, humeroradial, and superior radioulnar joints. Besides assessing the flexion and extension movements occurring at the proper elbow joint (a hinge joint), movements occurring at the forearm joints should also be examined. These joints are true (synovial upper and lower radioulnar joints) and false (working through interosseous membrane) effecting rotational movements of the forearm.

Table 5.1: Movements of elbow and forearm

Movements	*Axis*	*Range of motion*	*Prime movers*	*Nerve supply*	*Assisted by*	*Limiting factors*
Flexion	At elbow joint—a line joining the two epicondylar tips	0° to 145°-160°	1. Biceps brachii 2. Brachialis	C-5, 6 (Musculo-cutaneous nerve)	Brachio-radialis	1. Contact of front of upper part of forearm with front of arm 2. Engagement of coronoid process of ulna into coronoid fossa of humerus
Extension (Reversal of flexion) Hyperextension	-do-	145°-160° to 0° 10°	Triceps	Radial (C-7, 8)	1. Anconeus 2. Gravity	1. Locking of olecranon process into olecranon fossa 2. Tension of anterior capsule of elbow (along with its reinforcement) 3. Tension of flexor group of muscles of the forearm
Supination	At radio-ulnar joints—a line passing through centre of head of radius to ulnar attachment of triangular disc	0° to 90°	1. Biceps brachii 2. Supinator	Musculo-cutaneus (C-5, 6) Radial (C-6).	Brachio-radialis	1. Tension of pronators 2. Tension of anterior radioulnar ligament and ulnar collateral ligament of the wrist 3. Tension of lowest fibres of interosseous membrane and the oblique cords.
Pronation	-do-	-do-	1. Pronator teres 2. Pronator quadratus	Median (C-8, T1)	Brachio-radialis	1. Tension on dorsal radiocarpal ligament. 2. Tension of dorsal radio-ulnar ligament. 3. Tension of ulnar collateral ligament. 4. Tension of lowest fibres of interosseous membrane

Elbow Proper

Movements occur from the zero position of full extension to terminal flexion (vide the Table 5.1 on movements).

Method of Assessing the Movements

Compare the movements on both sides. Though movements can be tested by making the patient sit or stand, it will be better to make her sit on a stool (Fig. 5.10). Let the patient lean over a table with arm fully supported over the table from shoulder to elbow (there should be no gap in between table surface and back of the arm). The forearm is kept in fully supinated position with wrist extended and fingers fully opened up. View from the side, ask the patient to touch the table from the back of the hand without lifting the shoulder at all. This will demonstrate extending back to zero extension position. From this position, ask the patient to approximate the front of upper forearm to the front of lower arm as far as possible, again without lifting the shoulder at all—this will be flexion.

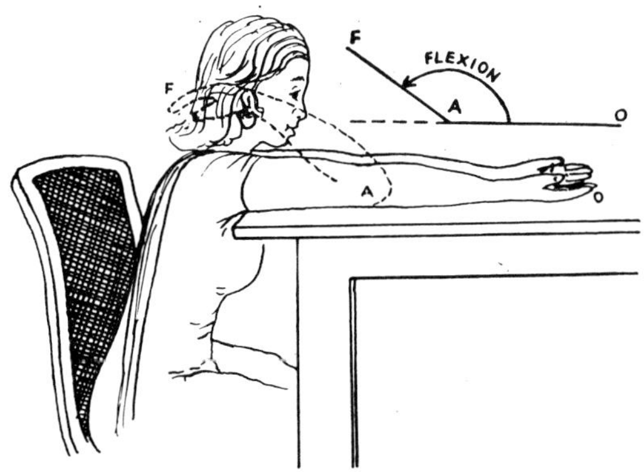

Fig. 5.10: Movements of elbow flexion and extension

Another method: If the patient cannot lean—let the patient stand or sit on a stool (Fig. 5.11) and view from side. Both arms are close to the sides of the chest with the elbow point being in vertical pendulum line to that of the shoulder. Ask the patient to keep the forearm in fully supinated position and extended at elbow as far as possible. In this position, hyperextension at the elbow can also be noted. Certain individuals have fairly varying extent of laxity. In them the elbow can be hyperextended upto 15°-20° (Figs 5.11-'H' position and 5.12A and B). From zero extension position he is asked to approximate the palm towards the shoulder—this will be flexion.

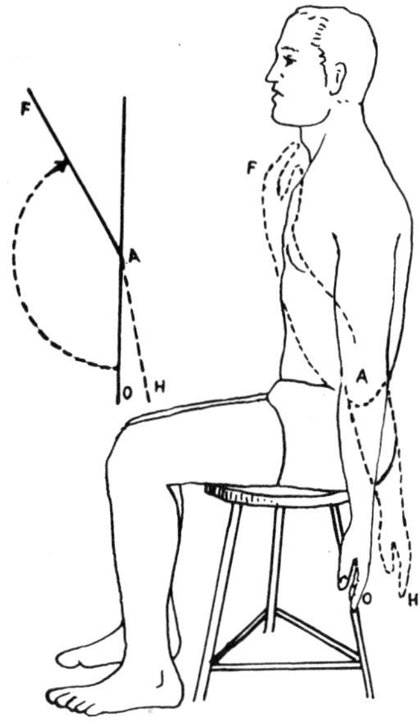

Fig. 5.11: With arms by the side (<OAF-flexion; <OAH hyper-extension) F = flexion, O = neutral position, H = hyperextension

Rotational Movements

Let the patient stand or sit on the stool with arm vertical and by the side of the chest. The elbow is flexed as far as possible upto 90° with wrist extended and fingers opened up. Ask the patient to rotate the palm towards the sky and towards the ground (Figs 5.13A to C). Movements should be measured from zero position of mid-prone either way.

Snapping elbow: Snapping elbow is mostly due to recurrent dislocation of ulnar nerve. However the medial head of triceps muscle or tendon also may dislocate over the medial epicondyle resulting in snapping while elbow is flexed from extended position or *vice-versa*. Dislocation of ulnar nerve and medial head of triceps tendon may co-exist producing the clinical

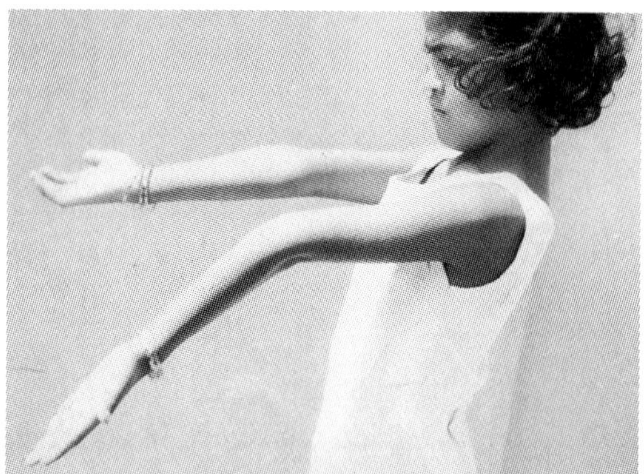

Fig. 5.12A: Photograph of a girl having abnormal hyperextension at elbow—cubitus recurvatum

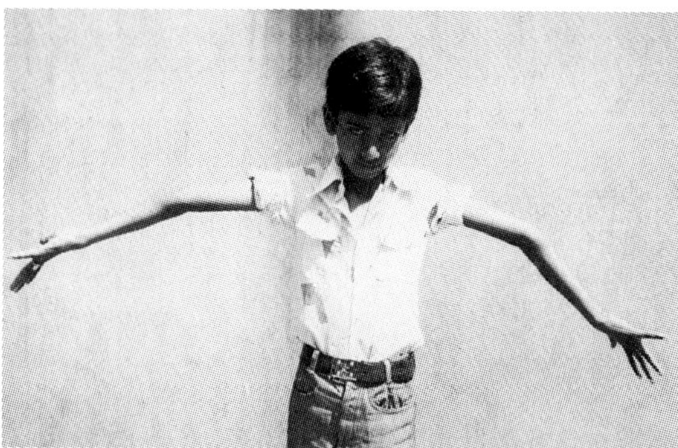

Fig. 5.12B: The boy is having hyperextension of both elbows

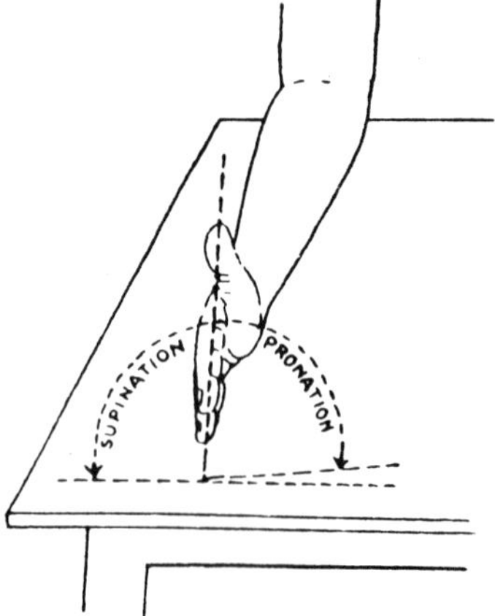

Fig. 5.13A: Rotational movements of the forearm (supination and pronation)

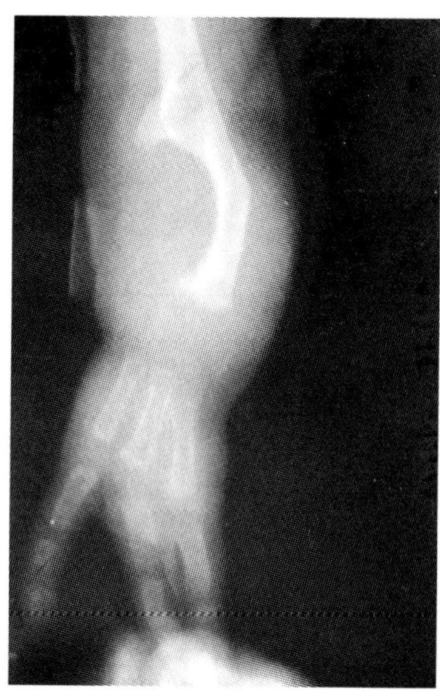

Fig. 5.13B: Congenital absense of elbow and ulna—no question of having any rotation in forearm or any movement in elbow region

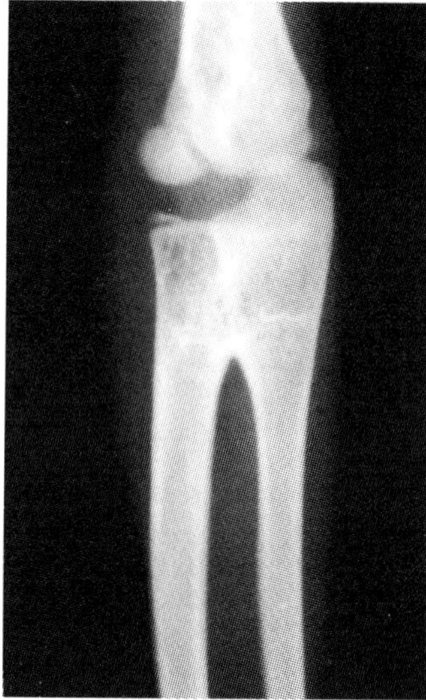

Fig. 5.13C: Congenital upper radioulnar synostosis—rotational movements not possible in such cases

finding of at least two snaps at the elbow. The condition may be asymptomatic or symptomatic (discomfort on the medial side of elbow with or without ulnar neuropathy—irritation or palsy). Snapping can be heard, seen, palpable, and reproducible.

The main cause of this condition is anatomical variations, e.g. shallow groove on medial epicondyle, hypermobility of ulnar nerve, abnormal configuration of the triceps (e.g. thickening of the fascial edge of medial head of triceps, accessory triceps tendon).

It should be differentiated from bicipital tendinitis, intra-articular abnormalities, medial epicondylitis, Little League elbow syndrome, recurrent dislocation of ulnar nerve itself. Non-symptomatic ones should be ignored, but symptomatic ones need operative management (exploration, dealing with the anatomical abnormality, anterior transposition of ulnar nerve).

As indicated in the Introduction chapter, note the following while assessing the movements: (1) Ankylosis (or congenital absence of joint or fusion of joint (Figs 5.13 B and C) or congenital flexion contracture of elbow joint (Fig. 5.5B) or post-burn (Fig. 5.14G) or post-infective ankylosis of joint, if any, (2) Fixation of zero position, (3) Lag of movement, (4) Fixity of movement, (5) Range of activity, (6) Range of possibility, (7) Limitation of terminal movement, (8) Pain during movement, (9) Achievement of critical arc (15° supination to 15° pronation), (10) Abnormal movements, (11) Achievement of ADL (Activities of daily living), (12) Abnormal sounds during movements, (13) Power of controlling groups of muscles.

MEASUREMENT

A. *Linear*

(i) As in shoulder joint, for arm and forearm, (ii) Locally, measure the distance between the lateral epicondyle to the olecranon tip, and medial epicondyle to the olecranon tip and compare with the corresponding measurements in the opposite elbow, kept in similar position. In posterolateral dislocation, the distance between the lateral epicondyle and the olecranon tip will be decreased. Similarly, in posteromedial dislocation, the distance between the medial epicondyle and olecranon tip will be decreased. In supracondylar fracture, these distances will be undisturbed. However, in comminuted supracondylar fracture, depending upon the displacement of the fragments, the measurements will be variable. One can have a rough estimation of displacements and rotation by these measurements, e.g. if the distance between the lateral epicondyle and olecranon tip is decreased it indicates external rotation of the outer fragments and vice-versa. Similar inferences can be had from the medial measurements too. These measurements will also be useful in assessing the displacement of epicondylar fractures, specially that of the medial. In lateral condylar fractures, in a few second and in all the third grades, it is difficult to palpate the epicondyle. In a medial epicondylar fracture beyond grade I, the distance between the medial epicondyle and the olecranon tip will be correspondingly decreased. Similarly, one can assess almost accurately the localisation and types of olecranon fractures. In fresh fractures of olecranon, one may feel the gap as an aid to diagnosis but in old fractures, the decreases in these aforesaid distances can be a guide to the displacements.

B. *Circumferential*

Measure the symmetrically aligned elbows (the normal limb aligned and put according to the diseased one) at the interepicondylar line and olecranon tip. For muscular girth, measure at points equidistant from the tip of olecranon, towards the arm and forearm.

Measurement of Cubitus Varus and Cubitus Valgus (Figs 5.2 to 5.3B)

Both upper limbs should be symmetrically extended at the elbow and supinated at the forearm as far as possible (affected elbow will be the guide). Join the mid point of the interepicondylar line to the mid point of the interstyloid line at the wrist. This will be the central axis of the forearm. Join the mid point of the interepicondylar line to the centre of a transverse line drawn outwards from the point, where the anterior fold of axilla meets the arm, to the upper outermost bulge of arm. This, for practical purposes is the central axis of the arm. Prolong this line downwards. The angle formed in between the long axis of the arm and the forearm is the "carrying angle" (normal 10 to 15°; more in females). If this angle is more on the affected side it denotes cubitus valgus deformity and the amount of increase in the carrying angle measures the extent of cubitus valgus. In cubitus varus, the forearm axis drifts towards, or even beyond the arm axis. Upto neutralisation of carrying angle, the normal carrying angle minus that on the affected side will be the measurement of cubitus varus. If the central axis of the forearm drifts further inwards, the cubitus varus will be measured as follows—carrying angle of the normal side + the angle subtended by the central axis of the arm with the medially drifted central axis of the forearm.

Cubitus varus deformity, the common complication of supracondylar fracture develops mainly due to uncorrected medial tilt and medial rotation of the distal fragment. The medial tilt can be confirmed as follows.

Ask the patient to bring both, about 90° flexed, elbows towards the mid-line. Note the position of the medial epicondylar tips. In case of medial tilt, it will be on a higher level.

Medial rotation of the lower fragment can be assessed as follows.

Both arms are kept close by the side of chest with elbows flexed at about 90°. Ask the patient to externally rotate both the upper limbs at shoulder. On the affected side, the external rotation will be limited more or less by the same degree as the medial rotation.

ASSESSMENT OF COMPLICATIONS DUE TO PATHOLOGY IN AND AROUND THE ELBOW

Besides any stiffness and deformity, look especially for any vascular (e.g. compartmental syndrome—VIC) or neurological complications (affections of peripheral nerves). If the patient can make a firm fist and open up the hand fully, all peripheral nerves are almost intact.

Test for Impending/Threatening Volkmann's Ischaemic Contracture

Following any injury in and around the elbow and the upper forearm, (e.g. war injuries, missile or high-velocity injuries, side sweep injury or bullet injury), any tight bandage/plaster in this area, after reducing any fracture or dislocation in this area, or after operating in this area—ALWAYS APPREHEND threatened vascular insufficiency (compartmental syndrome).

Increased tissue pressure is the key to compartmental syndrome. Once the pressure is raised, it can compromise the local circulation by decreased perfusion pressure, arteriolar closure, and reflex vasospasm.

LOOK FOR—(i) Pain—Disproportionate unrelenting pain is usually the earliest feature—believe your patient if he complains of pain (moderate to severe) especially in the forearm, (ii) Finger stretch test or passive muscle stretch test—passive stretching of the fingers aggravates the pain, which is progressive, it indicates that the muscle is ischaemic, (iii) Puffiness—swelling of the fingers, dorsum of the hand and palm, (iv) Pallor—earlier, there is cyanotic hue and then increasing pallor may develop, (v) Palpation of the muscular compartment elicits tender, which is one of the specific signs of compartmental syndrome, (vi) Pressing the nailbed—delayed capillary refilling, (vii) Pulse (radial) may be feeble, to absent, (viii) Paraesthesia—in the hand and fingers, (ix) Power—ask the patient to move the fingers. Earlier pain may have been the preventing factor in moving the fingers, but later actual neurogenic paresis supervenes, (x) Perception of temperature—ischaemic hand and fingers are comparatively colder.

Paralysis and pulselessness are the late findings. If the process has progressed to this point, the pathological changes are more likely to be irreversible (Figs 5.14A to F).

Warm and red skin overlying the affected compartment suggests cellulitis or thrombophlebitis.

Test for Lateral Epicondylitis

Lateral epicondylitis or tennis elbow is basically an overuse syndrome due to repetitive tension overloading of the wrist extensor origin at the

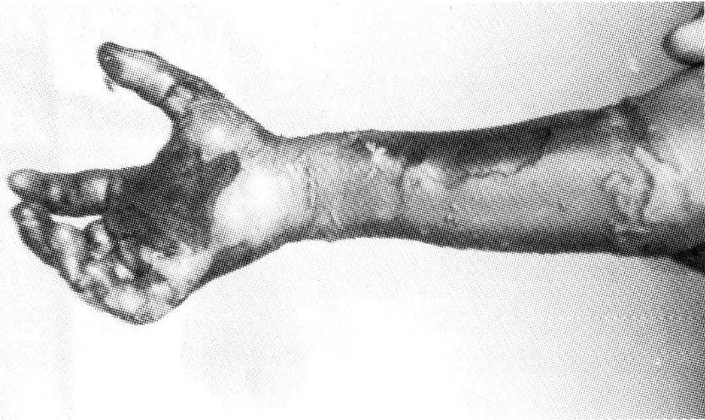

Fig. 5.14A: Volkmann's ischaemia

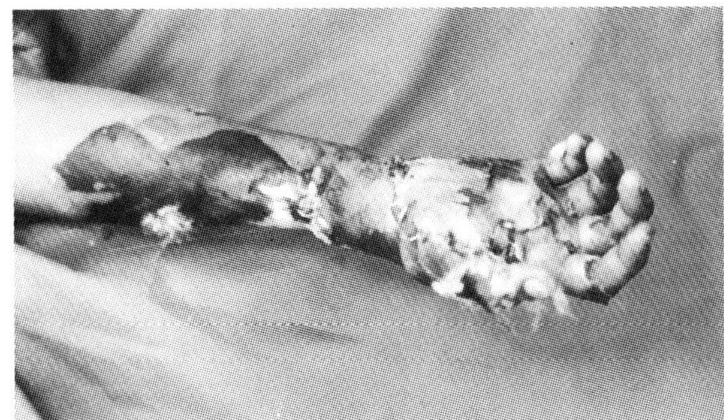

Fig. 5.14B: Volkmann's ischaemia

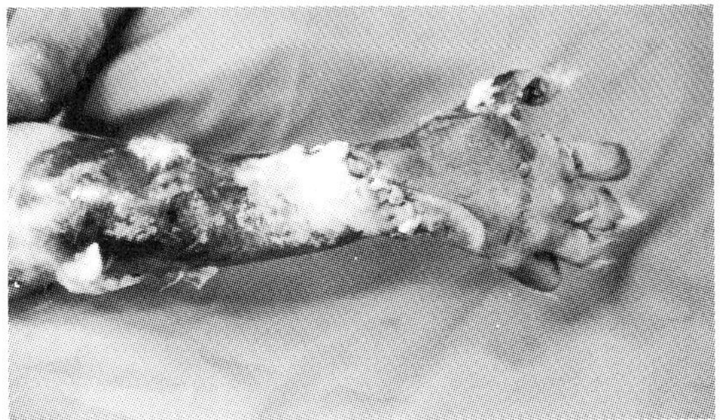

Fig. 5.14C: Volkmann's ischaemia

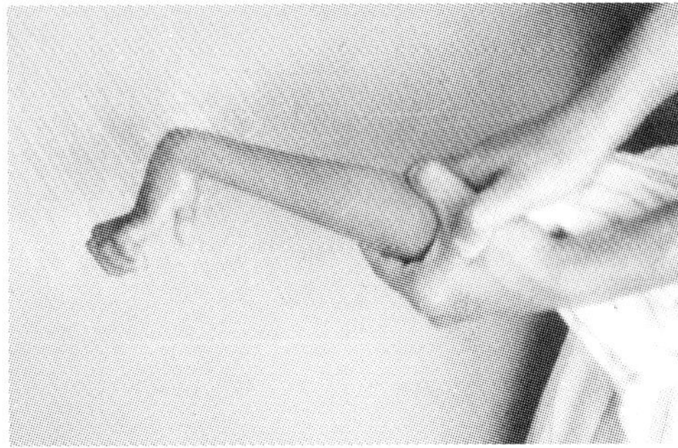

Fig. 5.14D: Severe Volkmann's ischaemic contracture

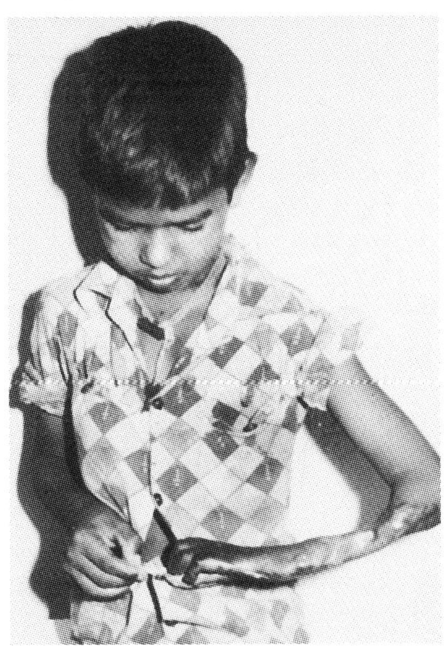

Fig. 5.14E: Very severe Volkmann's ischaemic contracture—After possible operative treatment the boy is trained to button his shirt.

N.B.: Note the swelling, blebs, necrosis and threatened gangrenous changes in forearm and hand following Volkmann's ischaemia in the Figs 5.14A to C

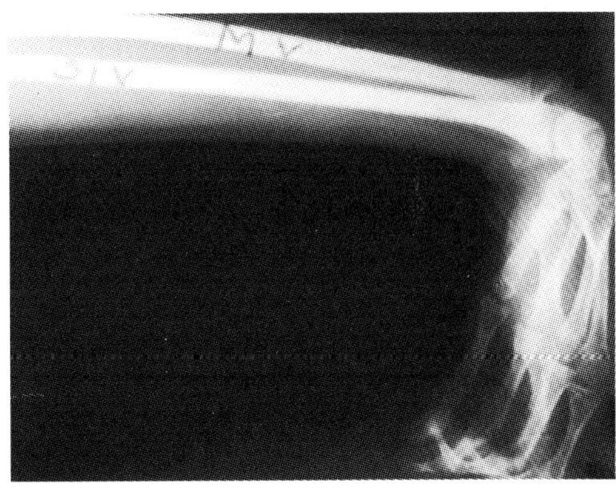

Fig. 5.14F: (Very severe) Volkmann's ischaemic contracture—the X-ray picture

lateral epicondyle. Resisted supination and pronation increase the stresses on the lateral epicondyle, which form the basis of the tests for lateral epicondylitis.

Traction or stress injuries or vascular causes induce osteochondritis of capitellum (Panner's

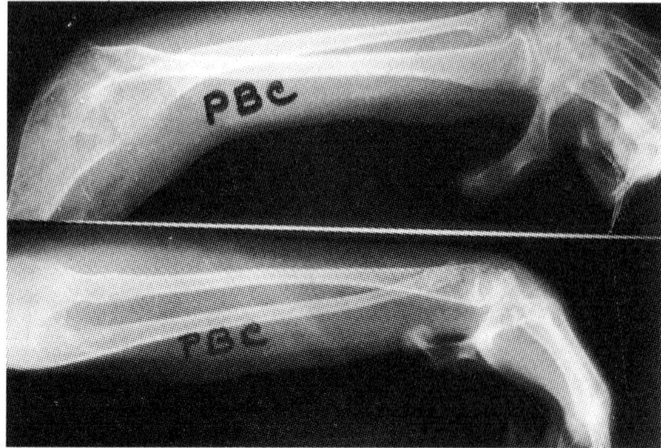

Fig. 5.14G: Post-burn contracture of wrist, thumb, fingers and forearm joints and ankylosed elbow

disease) which should be kept in mind while diagnosing the tennis elbow. Of course osteochondral fractures, ossification defects, avascular necrosis, accessory centre of ossification, and detachment of fragments have been suggested to be associated with osteochondritis dissecans.

1. *Wringing test:* Ask the patient to wring a towel—pain will be felt at the lateral epicondylar region (Fig. 5.15).
2. *Chair test:* Ask the patient to get up from a chair with both hands firmly gripping and pressing the arms of the chair. Pain is felt at the lateral epicondylar region, of the affected side.

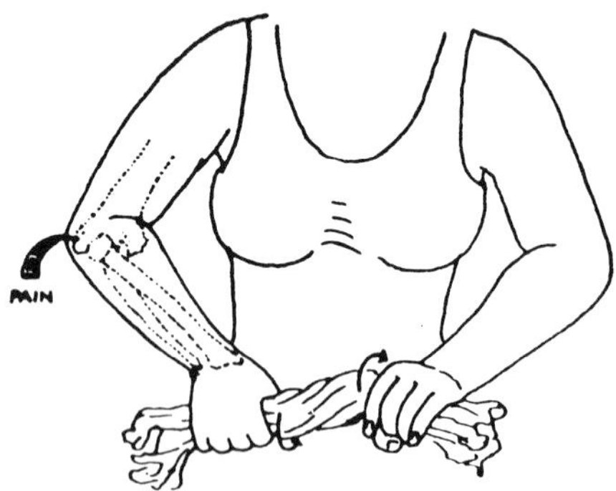

Fig. 5.15: Wringing test

3. *Jug test:* Ask the patient to lift a jug full of water, holding its mouth from above. Pointed pain will be felt at the lateral epicondylar region (Fig. 5.16).
4. *Cozen's test:* Ask the patient to make a firm fist. While the patient maintains this position, try to passively flex the wrist. Patient will feel pain at the lateral epicondylar region (Fig. 5.17).

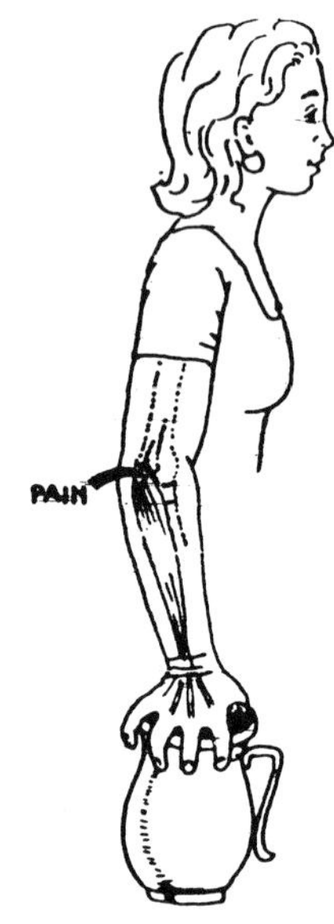

Fig. 5.16: Jug test

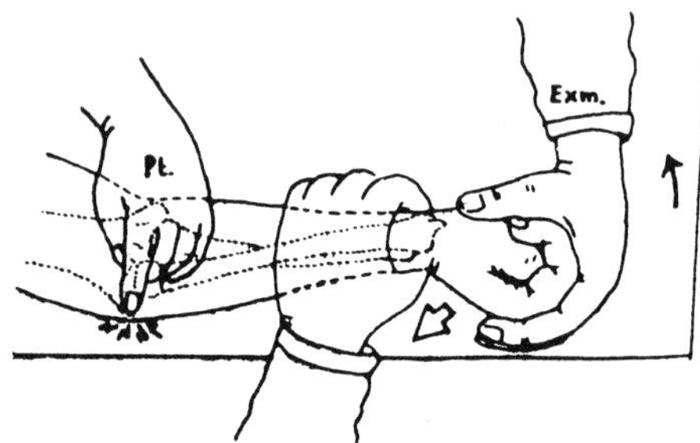

Fig. 5.17: Cozen's test

5. *Mill's manoeuvre:* While the patient keeps her elbow firmly straight and wrist flexed, pronation of the forearm initiates pain at the lateral epicondylar region (Fig. 5.18).
6. *Broom test:* Holding of broom firmly to sweep the floor initiates pains in the lateral epicondylar region. Ask the patient to hold

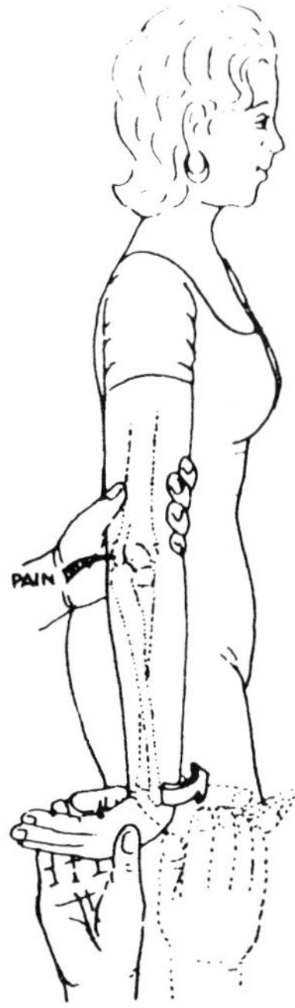

Fig. 5.18: Mill's manoeuvre

a broom firmly in her hand and attempt to sweep the floor, she will complain of pain in the lateral epicondylar region.

7. *Rolling-pin test:* Rolling the dough for preparing round bread, with firmly holding the rolling-pin (*belan*), initiates pain in the lateral epicondylar region and proximal portion of wrist extensors taking origin from lateral epicondyle.
8. *Stir-fry test:* While stir-frying in a pan, the patient feels pain in the lateral epicondylar region.

Test for Medial Epicondylitis (Fig. 5.19)

Medial epicondylitis or golfer's elbow is an overuse syndrome caused by repetitive tension overloading of the flexor-pronator muscle at or near its origin from the medial epicondyle. Resisted pronation and flexion of the wrist increase the stresses on medial epicondyle, which form the basis of the tests for medial epicondylitis.

With the elbow extended and the forearm supinated, ask the patient to make a fist and then flex the wrist against the examiner's resistance. The patient will complain of pain at the medial epicondylar region. Medial epicondylar pain is accentuated by a valgus stress to the elbow in extension.

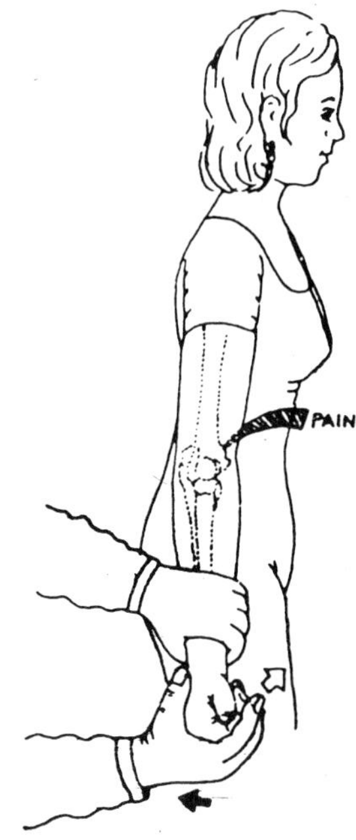

Fig. 5.19: Test for medial epicondylitis: White arrow showing active flexion at wrist by the patient and black arrow showing resistance offered by the examiner

Test for Cubital Tunnel Syndrome

Uninterrupted prolonged flexion attitude of elbow may lead to varied compression of ulnar nerve in the tight cubital tunnel (e.g. during sleeping), symptoms of which gradually improve after extending the elbow. Keeping the elbow acutely flexed for about five minutes precipitates the ulnar nerve compression symptoms, if the tunnel is tight (elbow flexion test).

INVESTIGATIONS REQUIRED FOR ELBOW PATHOLOGY

I. *General Investigations*

(As in the chapter on Introduction).

II. *Radiological Investigation*

If possible, comparative X-ray of both elbows helps in clearly delineating any pathological condition.

a. *Anteroposterior view:* Place the fully extended elbow along with the supinated forearm over the centre of the plate. The beam is to be focussed vertically, on the centre of the cubital fossa.
b. *Lateral view:* Plate is placed vertically on either medial or lateral side of fully extended elbow and fully supinated forearm. The beam is to be centred on epicondylar tip from either side on the plate. It is better to take a true lateral view of X-ray in maximum possible extension and flexion of the elbow in order to record the range of movement for future reference.

III. *Aspiration*

It is easy to aspirate the joint through the anconeus triangle.

Arthrography and arthroscopy: If carefully done, it can provide useful evidences.

Affections of Elbow

A. Congenital Conditions

- Agenesis
- Dysgenesis
- Congenital dislocation/subluxation of elbow (ulnohumeral, radiohumeral, radio-ulnar joints)
- Congenital single bone forearm
- Congenital contractured elbow
- Congenital radioulnar synostosis.

B. Inflammatory

i. *Infective*

1. *Acute*—Pyogenic (haematogeneous or after compound injury or iatrogenic)
2. *Subacute*
   - Gonococcal
   - Pyogenic
   - Variolar
   - Tuberculous
3. *Chronic*
   - Tuberculous
   - Pyogenic
   - Variolar
   - Syphilitic

ii. *Collagen-arthropathy*

- Rheumatoid arthritis
- Rheumatic arthritis
- Ankylosing spondylitis

iii. *Metobolic*

- Gouty arthritis.
- Chondrocalcinosis (calcium pyrophosphate arthropathy)

C. Traumatic

See Table 5.2.

Key Diagnostic Points for Common Elbow Pathologies

1. *Supracondylar Fracture* (Figs 5.20 and 5.21)
   - Commonest injury around the elbow in children (more in males, 5-8 years).
   - Mostly history of fall on outstretched pronated hand.
   - Tenderness around supracondylar region.
   - If there is no swelling, irregularity of supracondylar ridges can be felt (in acute and subacute cases, this irregularity is difficult to feel because of gross swelling and organising haematoma).
   - Passive movements at the elbow possible to a variable extent.
   - Active movements disturbed because of pain and mechanical reasons.
   - Arm is shortened (*not* the forearm) depending upon the amount of displacement and overriding. In late cases, cubitus varus deformity may develop if medial displacement, medial tilting and medial rotation have not been fully corrected.
   - Median, radial and ulnar nerves may be affected in that order.

Table 5.2: Corresponding injuries of elbow in children and adults

	Children	*Adults*
	1	*2*
1.	Pulled elbow	Strained or sprained elbow
2.	Supracondylar fracture (a) Posterior Posteromedial (Figs 5.20A and B) Posterolateral (b) Anterior Anterolateral Anteromedial. (Figs 5.20A and 5.21) (c) 'T' Fracture very rare (0.8%)	Comminuted supracondylar fracture (T and Y fracture)
3.	Fracture-separation of lower humeral epiphysis (a very rare injury)	X
4.	Dislocation— rare in children (a) Posterior (b) Anterior	Common in adults (a) Posterior, posterolateral and posteromedial. (b) Anterior (c) Lateral (d) Medial (e) Divergent (f) Isolated dislocation of radial head or olecranon
5.	Fracture dislocation	Fracture dislocation — Accompanying fracture may be as in baby car or sideswipe fracture dislocation. (i.e. fracture dislocation of the elbow with forward displacement of both forearm bones, fracture upper ulnar shaft, fracture olecranon, fracture lower humerus). Other accompanying fractures may be: — Radial head fracture — Capitulum fracture — Olecranon fracture — Coronoid fracture — Medial epicondyle avulsion fracture (adolescent) Supracondylar fracture — Posterior marginal fracture of condyles
6.	Fracture separation of upper radial epiphysis	— Fracture head/neck of radius.
7.	Fracture separation or avulsions of olecranon apophysis	— Fracture olecranon.
8.	Monteggia fracture dislocation	— Also in adults.
9.	Fracture lateral condyle (Figs 5.28A and B)	— Fracture capitellum.
10.	Avulsion fracture of the lateral epicondyle (very rare)	Hardly seen
11.	Avulsion fracture of the medial epicondyle.	Rare
12.	Floating elbow: Ipsilateral fracture of upper or middle third forearm, along with supracondylar fracture	Floating elbow, usually in RTA

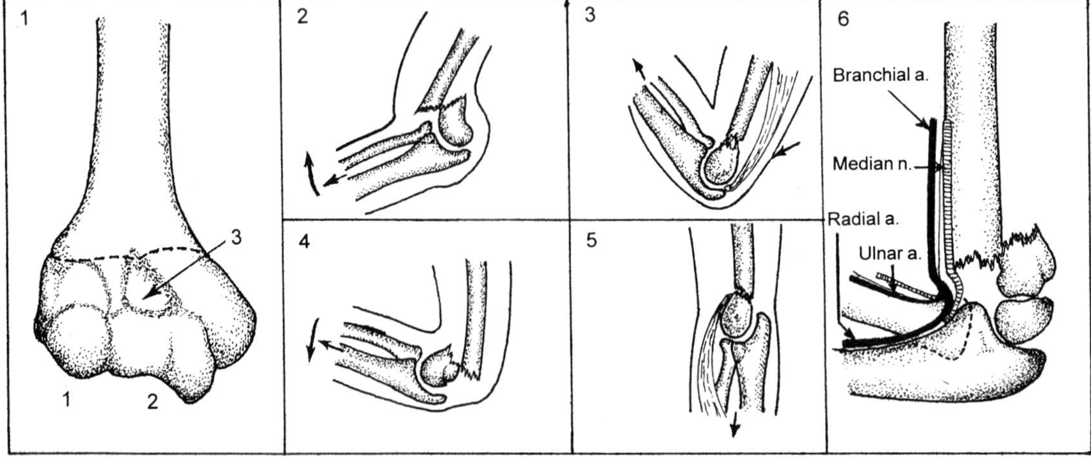

Fig. 5.20A: (1) Normal relation lower humeral end, (2+3) pre- and post-reduction of supracondylar fracture with posterior displacement, (4+5) same with anterior displacement, and (6) vulnerable neurovascular bundle

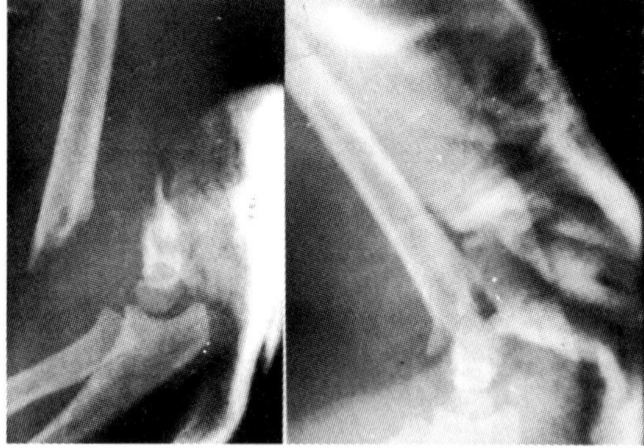

Fig. 5.20B: On the left supracondylar fracture with gross posteromedial displacement. On the right same after closed reduction

- Threatened or established Volkmann's ischaemic contracture must be looked for (Table 5.3)

— The relationship between the three bony points on the back of the elbow is *not* disturbed.

- Myositis ossificans is a common complication.

— In adults, supracondylar fractures are usually comminuted (communicating with the elbow joint 'T' or 'Y' fracture). Therefore, movements are grossly affected initially as well as later on.

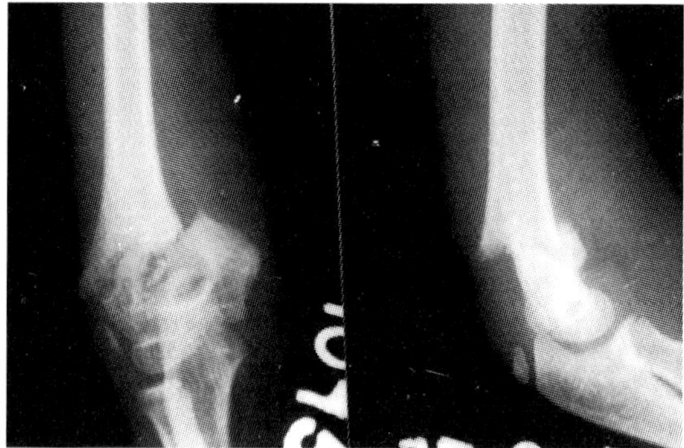

Fig. 5.21: Supracondylar fracture with anteromedial displacement

2. *Dislocation Elbow* (Fig. 5.22)

— Posterior dislocation is more common.

— Young adults are the usual victims.

— Olecranon stands out prominently on the back of the lower arm.

— The cubital fossa is occupied by a globular convex bony mass (the lower humeral articular part).

— Posterior dislocation of elbow constitutes 90 per cent of all elbow dislocations. Rarely lateral, medial, anterior, and divergent dislocations, as isolated dislocation of radial head or olecranon may occur anteriorly or posteriorly.

Table 5.3: Assessment of established Volkmann's ischaemic contracture

Clinical features	Mild	Moderate	Severe	Very severe
1	2	3	4	5
1. Deformity—				
(i) Tendency of clawing.	Negligible	Appreciable	Marked	Well marked
(ii) Flexion contracture of interphalangeal joint	+	++	+++	++++
M.P. joint	-	+	++	+++
wrist joint	-	-	+ to ++	+++
(iii) Correctability of deformities	With slight tendency of flexing the wrist —fully corrected	With full flexion of wrist —fully corrected	Even with full flexion of wrist —marked deformity	Wrist contracted in flexion —almost negligible effect on contracted deformities
(iv) Stretchability	Stretchable in all cases	Stretchable in majority of cases but prolonged endeavour required	Not stretchable	Not at all stretchable
2. Skin and subcutaneous tissue	Normal	Almost normal	Atrophic changes, may be patchy anaesthesia. Not freely pliable	Advanced atrophic changes, anaesthetic areas, adherent and parchment-like skin
3. Fingertip	Pulp normal	Stiffness of pulp	Stiff, tapering pulp	Atrophic, quite stiff pulp
4. Nailbed	Almost normal	Tapering atrophic tendency of nail	Dry look, tapering	Marked dry look, tapering, may be deformed
5. Palm	Normal	Almost normal, tendency of crowding	Crowded, atrophied thenar and hypothenar eminences	Contracted, atrophied, deep adherent creases
6. Wrist	Normal	Almost normal	Flexion contracture evident, subluxated carpals, extension not possible	Marked flexion contracture subluxated or even dislocated carpals—stiff wrist
7. Forearm	Normal	Wasted forearm specially on flexor aspect. Comparatively firm in feel in mid forearm area	Marked wasting of —forearm flexors+++ —extensors++ Firm feel of —flexor muscle+++	Negligible muscle mass in forearm (specially in lower 4/5th). Firm in feel

Contd.

Table 5.3: Contd.

Clinical features	*Mild*	*Moderate*	*Severe*	*Very severe*
1	*2*	*3*	*4*	*5*
			—extensors++ (muscles undergoing yellow degenerative and fibrotic contractures)	
8. Tendon	On hyperextension of wrist contracted long flexors become obvious —Otherwise normal	Long flexors remain contracted. Contraction gradually gets exaggerated as the wrist is extended. Extensors of wrist and fingers start losing power due to less use	Both groups suffer, flexors contracted but power not completely lost. In contracted position action can be demonstrated. Extensors suffer stretch weakness, may even appear to be markedly weak	Both groups markedly suffer; are contracted and powerless. Develops adhesions at places of ulcerations
9. Radial pulse	Normal	Nearly normal	Feeble	Very feeble/absent
10. Joint	Almost normal at all levels	Palmar capsule of inter-phalangeal joints and metacarpophalangeal joints contracted. Dorsal capsule has tendency of stretching	Palmar capsule of interphalangeal, metacarpophalangeal and wrist contracted. Dorsal capsule stretched. Mild tendency of sublu-xation at interphalangeal, metacarpophalangeal and wrist joints. Mild to moderate atrophy of synovial tissue	Palmar capsule contracted and adherent. Dorsal capsule stretched and atrophied. Marked subluxation at all levels Synovial tissue markedly atrophied

Contd.

Table 5.3: Contd.

Clinical features	Mild	Moderate	Severe	Very severe
1	2	3	4	5
11. Bones	Normal	Normal; in old cases terminal phalanges rarefied	Marked rarefaction especially near the joints. Thinning and tubular tendency of even the forearm bones	Marked rarefaction of bones of hand and forearm. Thinning of the forearm bones
12. Nerves- (either suffer from some vascular pathology as muscles do and/or also undergo pressure changes due to entrapment and consequent pressure within the fibrotic mass	All normal	All normal	May be features of affection of median nerve	All nerves may be affected
13. ADL— (Activities of daily living and functions)	Almost all functions possible	All ADL possible. Finer functions may be affected to variable extent	Very limited functions possible May carry on ADL anyhow	No function possible. Even ADL not possible
14. Gross management	—Reassurance —Supported guarded stretching —Dynamic splint	—Supported guarded gradual stretching —Dynamic splintage —Surgery for the residual deformities (soft tissue surgery—on muscles, tendons, capsule)	—Preoperative supported stretching Surgery, first on soft tissues (muscles, tendons, capsule); neurolysis: For the residual—on joints (carpectomy, arthrodesis, arthroplasty) and/or bones (shortening of forearm bones). —Dynamic splint if needed	—Preoperative stretching —Surgery on soft tissues (muscles, tendon, neurolysis, capsule), mostly on joints (carpectomy, arthrodesis) and or bones (shortening of forearm) —Dynamic splint

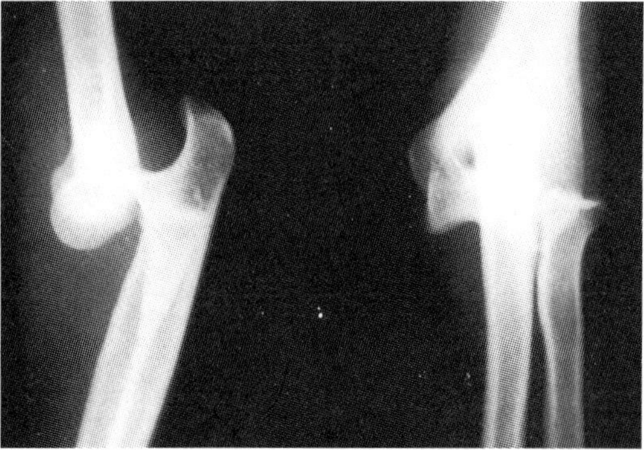

Fig. 5.22: Posterolateral dislocation of elbow joint

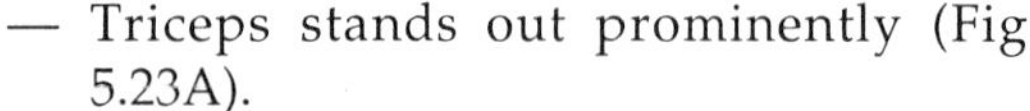

— Triceps stands out prominently (Fig 5.23A).
— Movements markedly restricted initially. Later on, variable range of movements may occur.
— Shortening of the forearm, (not of the arm.)
— Relationship of the three bony points *is* disturbed.

- Myositis ossificans is quite common complication.

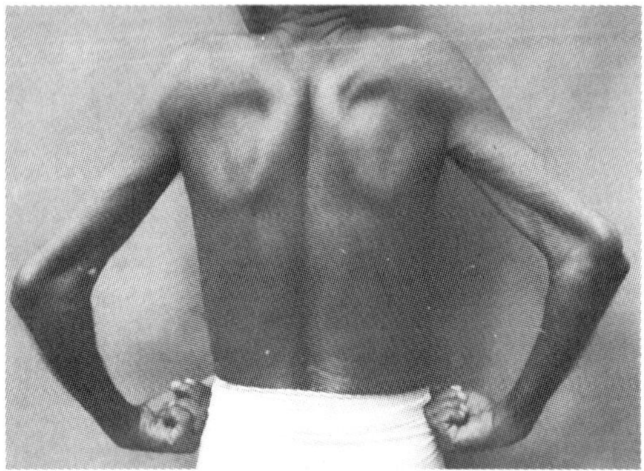

Fig. 5.23A: Photograph showing bilateral unreduced posterior dislocation of elbow—note the prominent triceps

In fracture dislocation of elbow (also called complex dislocation against simple dislocation, where there is no associated fracture) dislocation is associated with fracture (or fractures) of the articulating bone (s). When there is fracture of coronoid process, the threat of recurrent and chronic instability of elbow increases. Dislocation

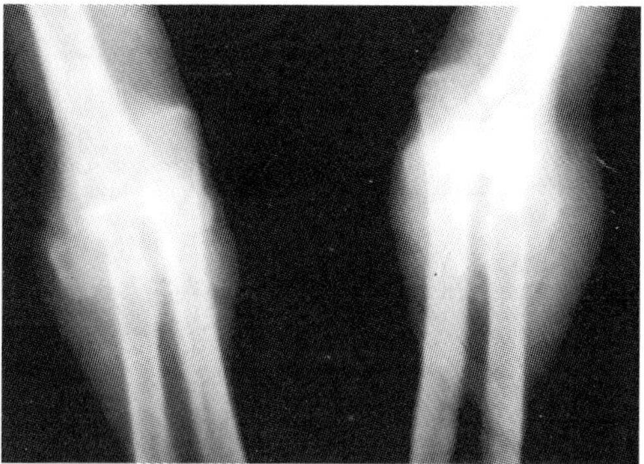

Fig. 5.23B: X-ray of the same patient (Fig. 5.23A)

of elbow associated with fracture of radial head, and coronoid process has been named as *"terrible triad of the elbow"* by Hotchkiss and is prone to acute redislocation and chronic instability.

3. *Myositis Ossificans* (Figs 5.24 and 5.25)

(Also refer to the chapter on 'Examination of Long Bones page no. 45).

— A common complication following injuries around the elbow.
— Usually there is a history of massage or repeated manipulations.
— In the early stage, the skin is warm all round the elbow, specially anteriorly.
— Firm to hard feel of the muscles in front of the elbow.
— Later on, reactive warmth may not be felt but hard bony plaques may be felt.
— Movements initially grossly restricted, (due to spasm and myositic activity) but gradually improves to variable extent.

4. *Medial Epicondylar Fracture* (Fig. 5.26)

Degrees of medial epicondylar fracture.

Degree I— Slight separation with minimal displacement.
Degree II— Avulsed fragment pulled down to joint level.
Degree III— Avulsed fragment entrapped in the elbow joint.
Degree IV— Avulsion of medial epicondyle with lateral dislocation of the elbow.

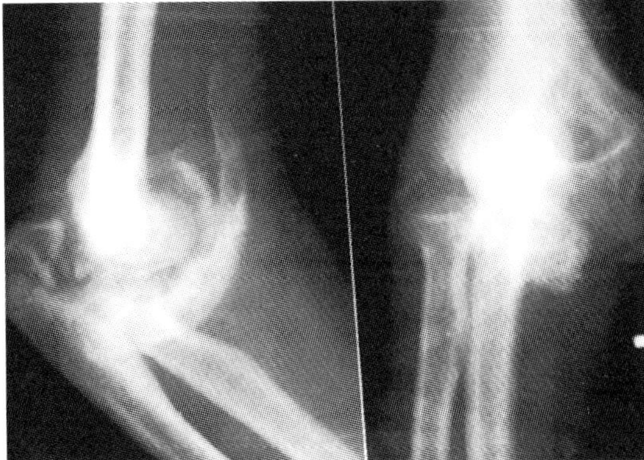

Fig. 5.24: Myositis in the cubital fossa in old dislocated elbow

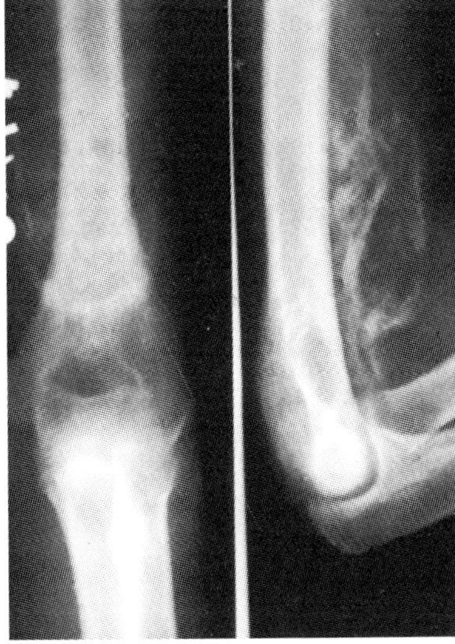

Fig. 5.25: Myositis in front of lower humerus in old injury of elbow

— Swelling, tenderness localised to medial epicondylar region of humerus.
— Extension movements mainly limited, and in grades III and IV both movements of the elbow may be grossly limited.
— In late cases, friction neuritis of the ulnar nerve may develop.

5. *Fracture of Head and Neck of Radius*

— Usually in adults.

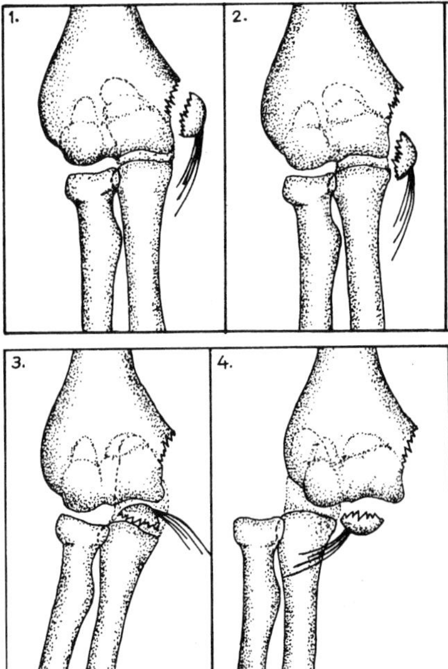

Fig. 5.26: Different degrees (types) of avulsion fracture of medial epicondyle

— History of fall on pronated outstretched hand.
— Rotational movements of forearm markedly restricted.
— Tenderness localised to just below the lateral epicondylar eminence.

6. *Monteggia Fracture Dislocation* (Fig 5.27)

GB Monteggia of Milan published about the combined injury of the fracture of proximal third of ulna with anterior dislocation of radial head in 1814. Much later J L Bado coined the term 'Monteggia lesion' to include the entire spectrum of such injuries in 1967.

In few cases there may be combined displacements (angulations) and dislocations (e.g. anterolateral)

— Comparatively more common in children (7-12 years) but can occur in adults also.
— History of direct blows over ulnar aspect of the forearm or fall on pronated hand.
— Rotational movements markedly restricted.

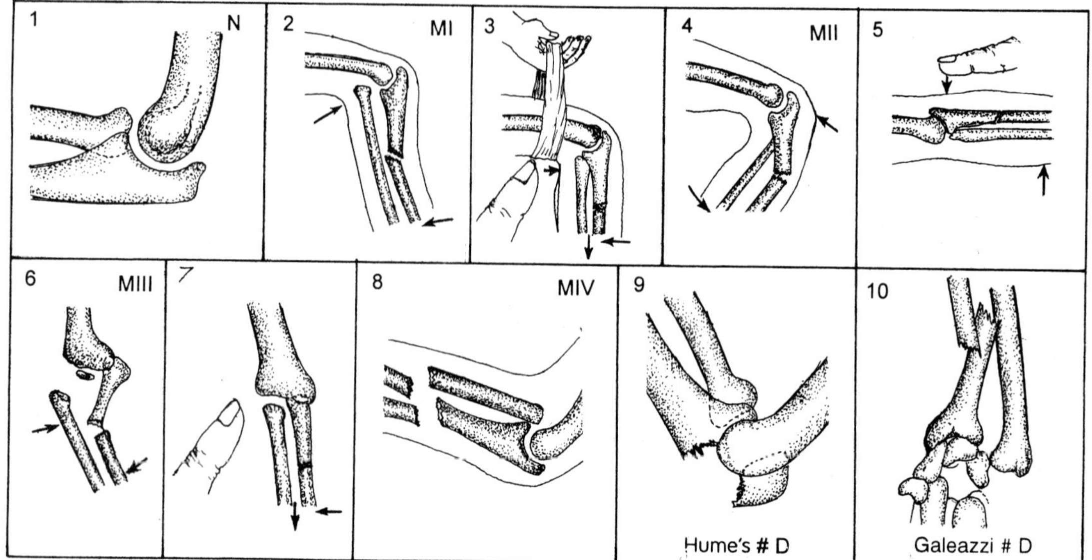

Fig. 5.27: Line sketch of 4 types of Monteggia fracture-dislocation with method of reduction

Classification of Monteggia lesions (Monteggia fracture dislocations) (after Bado, Hume's 1967)

Type I (Extension type) or Anterior type —60% of cases	Fracture in upper or middle third of ulna with anterior angulation	+ Anterior dislocation/subluxation or radial head
Type II (Flexion type) or Posterior type —15% of cases	Fracture in upper or middle third of ulna with posterior angulation	+ Posterior or posterolateral dislocation/subluxation of radial head + Often a fracture of the head of radius
Type III or (Lateral type) —20% of cases	Fracture in upper or middle third of ulna (usually just distal to coronoid process	+ Lateral or anterolateral dislocation/ subluxation of radial head
Type IV —5% of cases	Fracture in upper or middle third of ulna with anterior angulation	+ Anterior dislocation of radial head + fracture in upper third of radius

— While rotating the forearm, a rounded bony mass moving under the fingers is felt either anterior, posterior or lateral to the normal radial head position, depending upon the type of Monteggia fracture dislocation.

— Angulation, tenderness and swelling in the upper/middle third of the forearm depending upon the site of fracture.

7. *Fracture of the Lateral Condyle of Humerus* (Figs 5.28A to 5.30B)

Degrees of lateral condylar fracture:

Degrees

i. Lateral condyle displaced laterally but not rotated.
ii. Lateral condyle displaced laterally and downward (with or without some rotation).

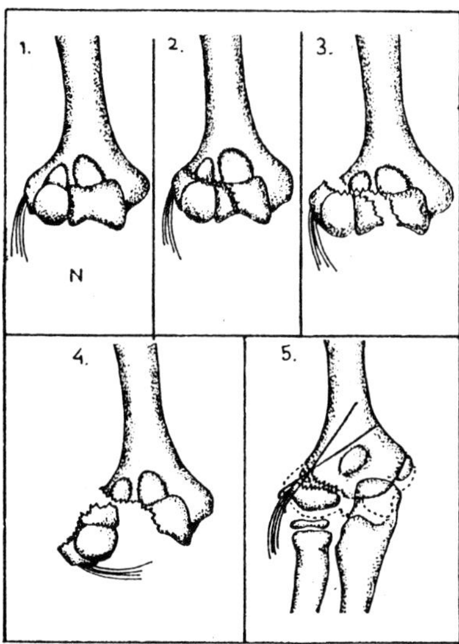

Fig. 5.28A: Line sketch of different types of fracture lateral condyle of humerus; 5-ORIF of No. 4

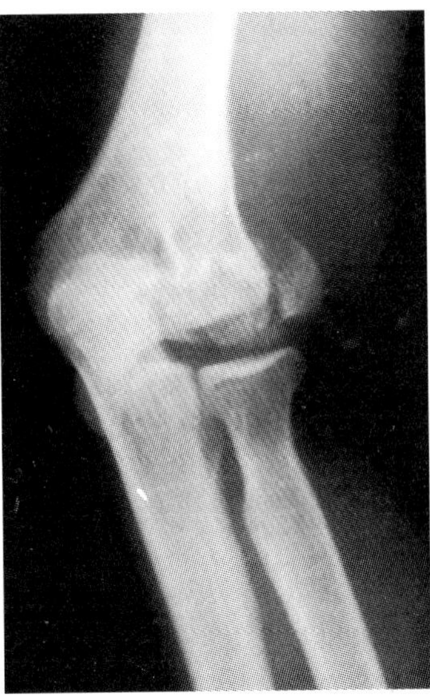

Fig. 5.28B: Fracture lateral condyle of humerus type II

iii. Lateral condyle displaced and rotated around the horizontal and vertical axis. May be associated with dislocation of the elbow.

— More common between 5-10 years of age.
— Tenderness and swelling localised to the lateral side of the lower humerus.
— In Grade III—a globular, bony chunk felt on the outer side of the elbow. In early cases, the outer rough surface can be felt, although later it gradually becomes smooth.
— If neglected, it mostly goes for delayed or non-union, which leads to gradually increasing cubitus valgus with or without tardy (tardy = tarde = slow) ulnar nerve palsy. Ulnar nerve gets gradually stretched and undergoes repeated friction with extension and flexion movements of elbow leading to slow friction neuritis palsy.
— Mobility of the fragment can be demonstrated by the following method:

Method: (Fig. 5.31) Hold the lower arm and elbow from the medial side in one hand while the

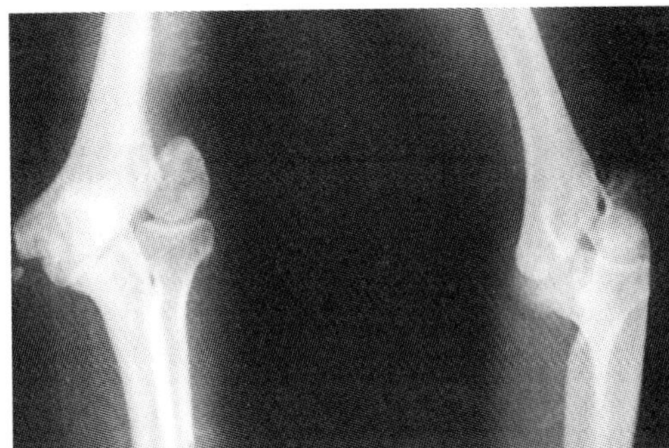

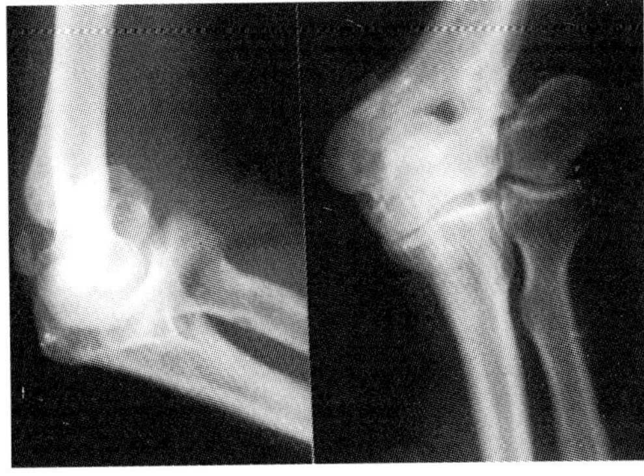

Figs 5.29A and B: Old ununited fracture of lateral condyle of humerus with marked cubitus valgus deformity

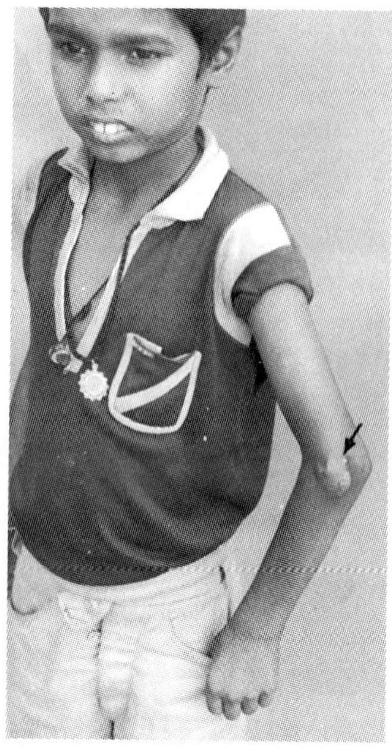

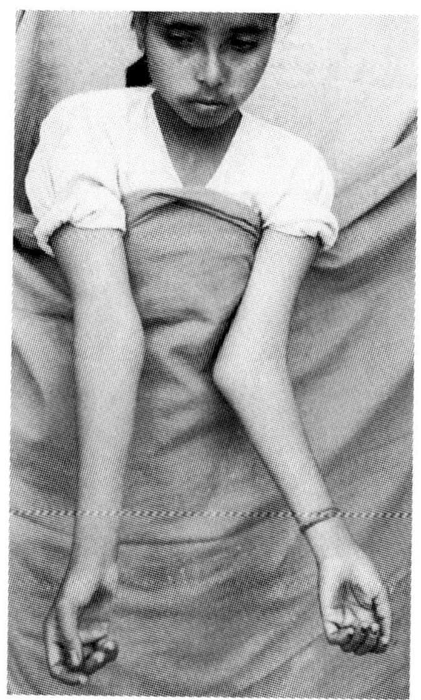

Figs 5.30A and B: (a) Photograph of a boy having displaced unreduced fracture of the lateral condyle. (b) Typical cubitus valgus deformity following ununited fracture of lateral condyle of humeurs

elbow is kept flexed at 45° or at maximum possible angle in a relatively stiff elbow. With thumb and index finger of the other hand, hold the distal, displaced bony mass. In ununited fractures, this mass can be slightly moved over the parent bone.

— Medial supracondylar ridge is normal but lateral disturbed.
— Movements at the elbow are fairly free, may be even complete in late cases.
— Rotational motions limited to a variable extent.
— In X-ray, this displaced mass appears quite small (in comparison to its clinically assessed size) because only the central ossified mass casts a shadow, the rest being cartilaginous.

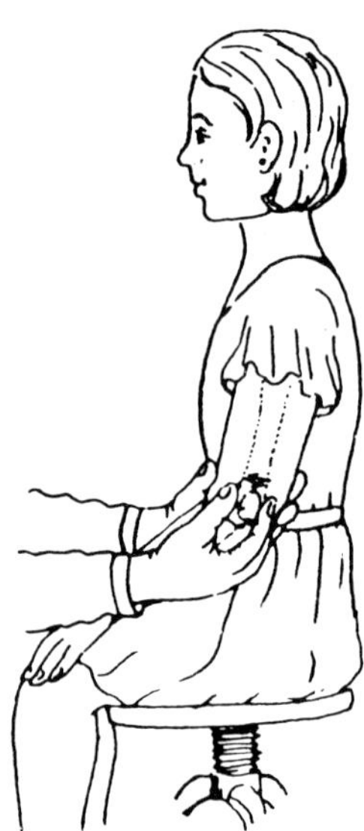

Fig. 5.31: Method of demonstrating mobility of the displaced fractured lateral condyle

8. *Fracture Olecranon* (Fig. 5.32)

— Common fracture in adults.
— Bruises may be seen on the back of the elbow.
— Irregular, tender surface of the olecranon, with or without a transverse gap. Since in most of the fractures, the olecranon process is avulsed—a transverse gap is felt at the upper end of the ulna. Patient has difficulty (even inability) in actively extending the elbow.
— In late cases, triceps get contracted.

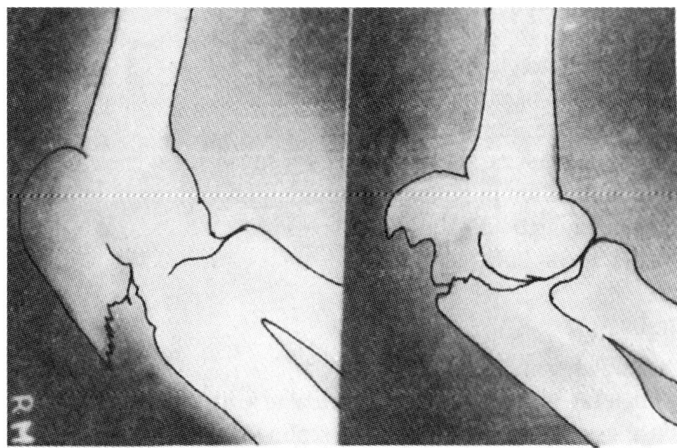

Fig. 5.32: Common varieties of fractures of olecranon (Left oblique fracture through base; Right transverse fracture)

Non-Traumatic

1. *Tennis Elbow*
   — Common amongst ladies between 25-40 years of age.
   — Complains of pain in wringing movements of the forearm or lifting an object by gripping it in between the thumb and fingers or while getting up from a chair with the hands firmly pressing over the arm of the chair.
   — Tenderness is more or less around the lateral epicondyle.
   — Confirm by tests: Cozen's tests, Mill's manoeuvre, Jug test, etc.

2. *Golfer s Elbow (Little League elbow syndrome/ chronic tension-stress injuries)*

- Common in young persons due to chronic tension stress injuries, e.g. baseball pitchers, javeline throwers, golfers, etc).
- Complains of pain in medial epicondylar region usually in valgus stress to the elbow in extension.
- Significant local tenderness and mild swelling over the medial epicondylar region.
- X-ray—Chronic stress leads to density of the bone in the distal humerus; the physeal line (if present) is irregular and widened; the skeletal age of elbow appears greater than the patient's chronological age.
- Clinical tests as given on page 93.

3. *Tuberculosis of Elbow* (Figs 5.33A and B)
   — Comparatively chronic history.
   — Slightly warm swelling around the elbow.
   — Typical tuberculous sinus.
   — Tenderness more at the joint line.
   — All movements are restricted.
   — Wasting of the muscles of the arm and forearm.
   — Flexion deformity to a varying extent.
   — May be fluctuant collection anywhere in relation to the elbow—usually anteriorly or a little below the elbow, even in the forearm, depending on the site of cold abscess.
   — Bony tenderness according to site of primary, focus i.e. usually the olecranon region, radial head, trochlear and capitular regions.
   — Regional lymph nodes enlarged with or without matting and tenderness.

4. *Rheumatoid Arthritis*

— Rheumatoid arthritis is a chronic progressive polyarthritis affecting about 0.75% of the population.
About 70% of these patients can develop erosions in the joint and disabilities.
Rheumatoid arthritis patients are on the average underweight.

— Chronic history, with remissions and exacerbations.

— Usually affects ladies in their 3rd and 4th decades.

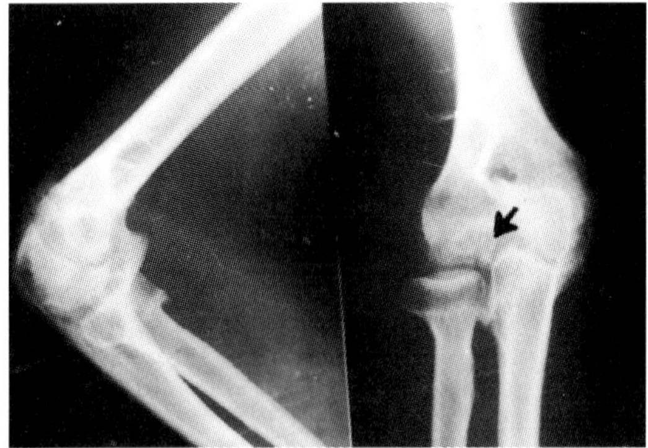

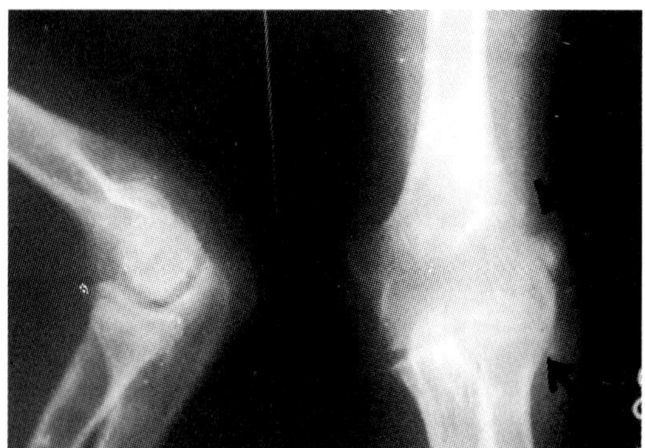

Figs 5.33A and B: Tuberculosis of elbow

— Other joints, specially smaller joints of hands, wrist and foot involvement (but very rarely the distal interphalangeal joints). Joints involvement is usually bilateral.
— Swelling/affection of three or more specified joints.
— Flexion deformity to varying extent.
— Decreased triceps skin fold thickness.
— Varying restriction of movements.
— Significant reduction in upper arm muscle circumference.
— Mild swelling all around the elbow.
— As the disease advances, ankylosis (usually fibrous—in late cases may be osseous).
— Associated with different typical rheumatoid deformities, especially in hand, wrist and foot.
— Subcutaneus rheumatic nodules over the olecranon.
— Repeated olecranon bursitis.
— Rheumatoid cachexia has been reported in patients with elevated serum levels of tumour necrosis factor-Q (TNF-Q)
— X-ray changes—periarticular osteopenia or erosion.

5. *Septic Arthritis of the Elbow*
— In young children.
— Usually with other septic foci in the body.
— Acute onset.
— Constitutional features present.
— Varying swelling depending upon collection in the joint.
— Acute inflammatory features in the elbow.
— Gross limitation of movements in all directions (due to pain).
— Aspiration of frank thick pus clinches the diagnosis.
— Regional lymph nodes enlarged, and tender.

6. *Post Viral Arthritis*
— Legacy following smallpox.
— Usually bilateral, more or less symmetrical affection of the elbow.
— Acute stage usually corresponds to the scaling stage of smallpox.
— In late stage—painless, ankylosed elbow or with gross limitation of functional movements, like old septic arthritis.

BIBLIOGRAPHY

1. Laurence, W: Supracondylar fractures of the humerus in children, a review of 100 cases. *Br J of Surg* **44**:143,1956.
2. Watson-Jones, R: Primary nerve lesions in injuries of the elbow and wrist. *J of Bone and Joint Surg* **12**:121,1930.
3. Bado, JL: The Monteggia lesion. *Clin Orthopaedics* **50**:71,1967.
4. Takahara M, Shundo M, Kondo M, *et al:* Early detection of osteochondritis dissecans of capitellum in young baseball players. *J Bone Joint Surg* **80A**: 892-97,1998.

6 Wrist Joint

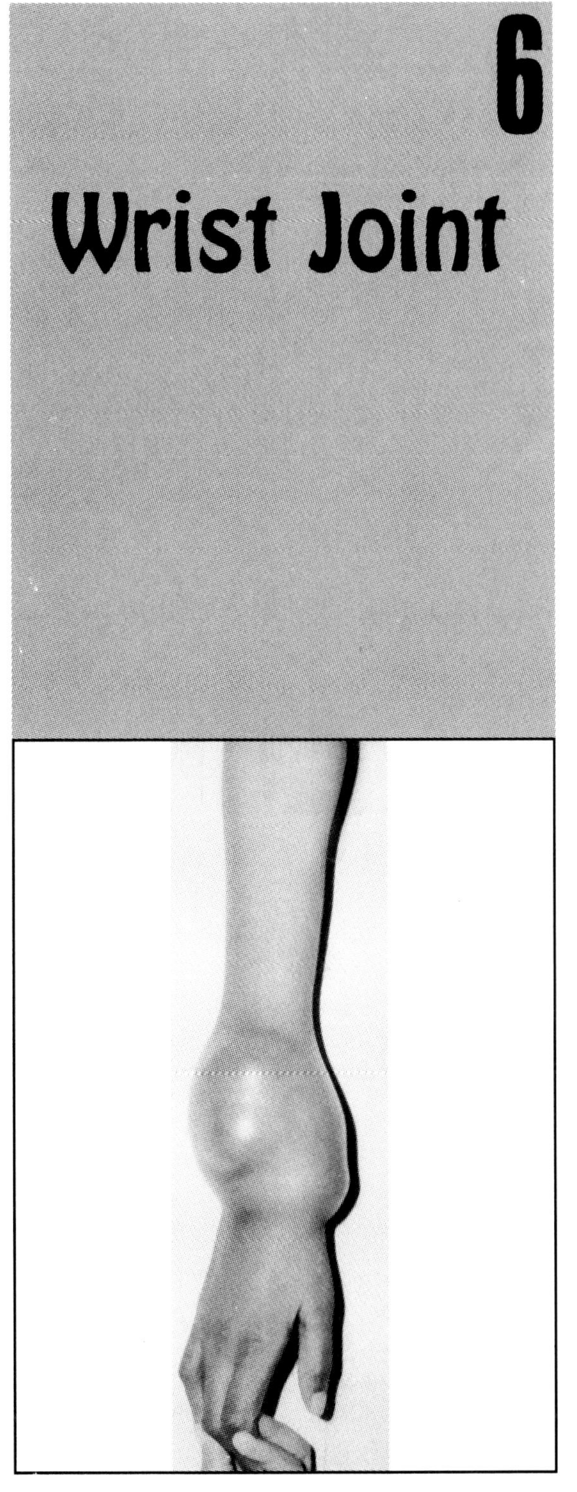

INTRODUCTION

The movements at the wrist are mainly oriented to facilitate the grip and finer movements of the hand.

For all practical purposes, in clinical assessment the local examination of the wrist includes the forearm and the hand.

ANATOMICAL CONSIDERATION

The wrist joint proper is the articulation of the lower articular end (concave in anteroposterior as well as lateral directions) of the radius and the inferior surface of the triangular fibrocartilage (extending from the medial margin of the lower end of the radius to a pit on the lateral surface of ulnar styloid process above its tip—i.e. from the rim of the sigmoid notch of radius to the ulnar styloid process) at the proximal end and the proximal articular surfaces of scaphoid, lunate and triquetral at the distal end. However, the intercarpal articulations (carpals arranged in two rows in first row scaphoid, lunate, triquetrum and pisiform and in second row trapezium, trapezoid, capitate, and hamate) participate in all movements of the wrist joint.

The synovial reflections of the wrist and the intercarpal joints are intercommunicating. As around the ankle, the wrist also has important hand-controlling tendons around it, but for a difference that on the palmar aspect, just above the wrist level, the stamp-like stout pronator quadratus muscle binds the lower ends of the radius and ulna.

The lower ends of the radius and ulna articulate as a pivot joint to form the inferior radioulnar joint. Here, the lower end of the radius along with the triangular fibrocartilage revolves around the head of ulna. This synovial joint has its continuity with the wrist joint, therefore, this joint is likely to be affected simultaneously in all affections of the wrist proper.

The articular surface of the distal aspect of radius tilts 21 degrees in the anteroposterior plane and 5 to 11 degrees in the lateral plane.

The scaphoid, trapezium, first metacarpal, and thumb phalanges function conjointly as an independent unit—like 'a jointed strut'. The joints of this strut are vulnerable to degenerative arthrosis.

The dorsal cortical surface of the radius thickens to form the Lister tubercle and osseous prominences which support the extensors of the wrist in the second dorsal compartment.

On the dorsal aspect of the wrist, just beneath the extensor retinaculum (more or less blended with the dorsal capsule of the wrist joint) the following tendons are arranged in a definite order. There are six fibro-osseous compartments lodging the following tendons (from dorsolateral to dorsomedial direction) (Fig. 6.1).

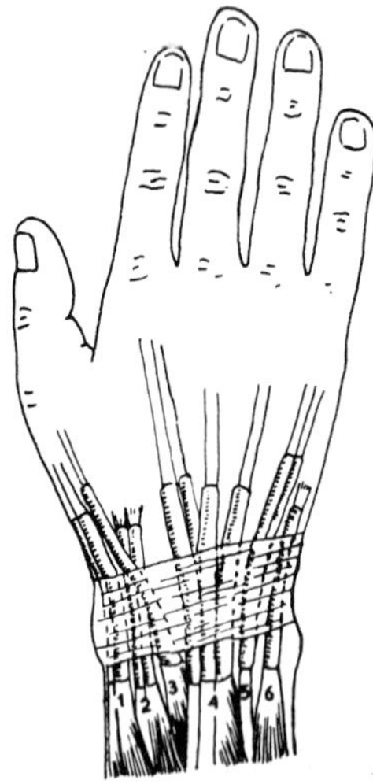

Fig. 6.1: Showing the fibro-osseous compartments on the dorsal aspect of the wrist with their contents

1. abductor pollicis longus and extensor pollicis brevis,
2. extensor carpi radialis longus and brevis,
3. extensor pollicis longus,
4. extensor indicis, extensor digitorum, anterior interosseous artery ending and posterior interosseous nerve ending in pseudoganglion,
5. extensor digiti minimi,
6. extensor carpi ulnaris

- First compartment—Abductor pollicis longus and extensor pollicis brevis;
- Second compartment—Extensor carpi radialis longus and extensor carpi radialis brevis;
- Third compartment—Extensor pollicis longus;
- Fourth compartment—Extensor indicis and extensor digitorum;
- Fifth compartment—Extensor digiti minimi;
- Sixth compartment—Extensor carpi ulnaris;

In the fourth compartment, deep to the tendons, the posterior interosseous nerve ends as a pseudoganglion and the anterior interosseous artery ends anastomosing with the fine local articular arteries. Each compartment has a double blind ending synovial sheath around the tendon. Proximally, the sheaths extend to a variable extent and distally they end beyond the retinacular extension.

On the palmar aspect, however, none of the tendons are directly bound to the wrist surface (as on the dorsal surface) because of: (i) intervention by pronator quadratus, (ii) concave surface of the lower end of radius, and (iii) lack of separate fibro-osseous compartments which would prevent the tendons from bowstringing during flexion.

Of the nerves, the median nerve is in closer relation to the wrist than the ulnar. The median nerve lies in between the tendons of the flexor carpi radialis and flexor digitorum sublimis and on the posterolateral aspect of the palmaris longus tendon. This nerve is likely to suffer with any encroachment of the space in between the flexor retinaculum and the wrist joint, i.e. the carpal tunnel. Normally *carpal tunnel contains the median nerve and nine flexor tendons*—the four sublimis, four profundus and the flexor pollicis longus tendons.

The ulnar nerve becomes superficial at the wrist level. At about 5 cm above the wrist joint proper, after sending a dorsal cutaneous twig, it passes in front of the flexor retinaculum on the lateral side of the pisiform bone and posterolateral to the musculotendinous mass of the flexor carpi ulnaris where it divides into a superficial and a deep branch. The deep branch continues under cover of the hook of the hamate into the palm (Guyon's canal). Guyon's canal is triangular and lies immediately ulnar to the carpal tunnel in the wrist region. Ulnar nerve and artery traverse the canal, which may be site of ulnar nerve entrapment.

The radial nerve more or less divides into 4 or 5 dorsal digital branches at about the wrist level. Clinically, it is not of much importance, as its cutaneous supply is ultimately limited to a stamp-shaped area on the back of the first web.

The creases around the wrist run almost circumferentially. The radial artery lies quite superficial on the anterolateral aspect of the lower forearm and wrist and it is not likely to be affected in common wrist affections, except for infiltrative neoplasms, glass pan cut and suicidal injuries.

The dorsal or Lister's turbercle lies on the dorsum of the lower end of the radius just lateral and proximal to the central point of the wrist. It provides a pulley-like surface on its medial aspect for the extensor pollicis longus tendon. This tendon, by passing a circuitous route around this tubercle becomes more effective in subserving its important function of extension of the thumb. On the other hand, this tendon, lying in such a close proximity to the bony tubercle, is likely to be affected in any roughness in this area (e.g. rupture of this tendon in Colles fracture).

Fracture separation of the lower radial epiphysis (cf. Colles fracture in adult) is a very common injury around the wrist in children. Due to seen or unseen damage of the growth plate, it may lead to various deformities in this region.

METHODOLOGY

History Taking

In case of trauma, ask about the mode of injury and the part of the limb which first bore the impact of violence. Usually, the wrist is involved in indirect injuries, seldom by direct violence.

General and Systemic Examinations

(See the chapter on 'Introduction')

Regional Examination

It includes overall assessment of the forelimb of the affected side with its connections to the central axis, both anatomically and neurologically. It is obligatory to examine the cervical spine, supraclavicular region, shoulder girdle, supracondylar region, elbow, forearm and upto the tip of the fingers while assessing the wrist joint.

Local Examination

Prerequisites: Both wrists must be fully exposed and examined simultaneously keeping them in identical position as far as possible, while the patient sits comfortably on a stool.

Attitude

Note any fixed attitude of the wrist and hand (Figs 6.2 and 6.5A and B). Certain typical attitudes are significant, e.g. dinner fork deformity of Colles fracture; congenital manus valgus of Madelung's deformity (forward and ulnar curving of lower end of radius due to growth disturbance at the ulnar-palmar aspect of distal radial physis)—(Otto Madelung, 1878—Figs 6.4A and B), arrow head deformity in diaphyseal aclasia (usually seen in X-ray (Fig. 6.3), flexion and ulnar/radial deviation of the wrist and ulnar deviation of the fingers in rheumatoid arthritis; hourglass swelling on the palmar aspect both above and below the flexor retinaculum in compound palmar ganglion (Figs 6.11A and B); wrist drop (radial nerve palsy. In established

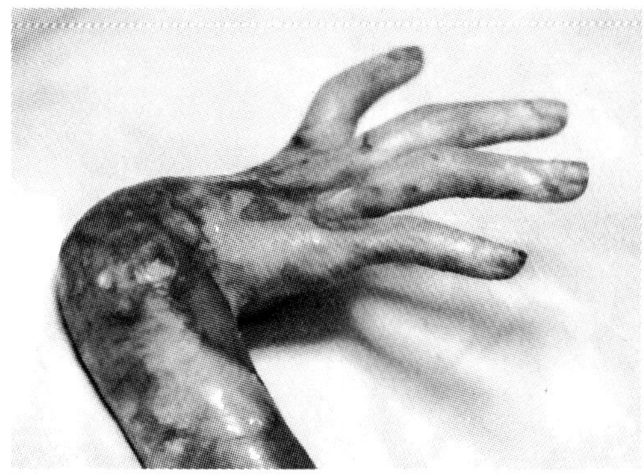

Fig. 6.2: Post-burn contracture of wrist

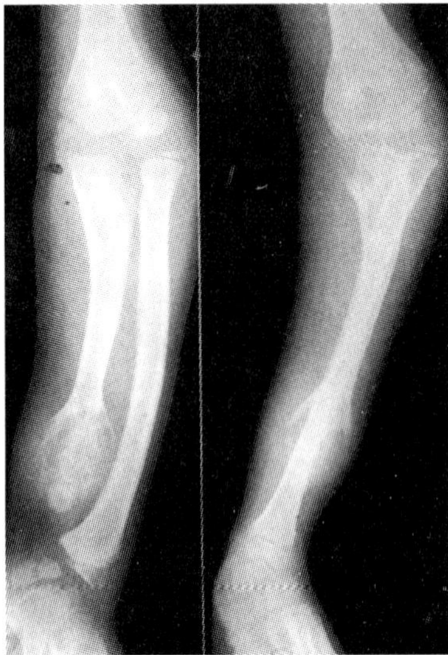

Fig. 6.3: Arrow head deformity of ulna in diaphyseal aclasia

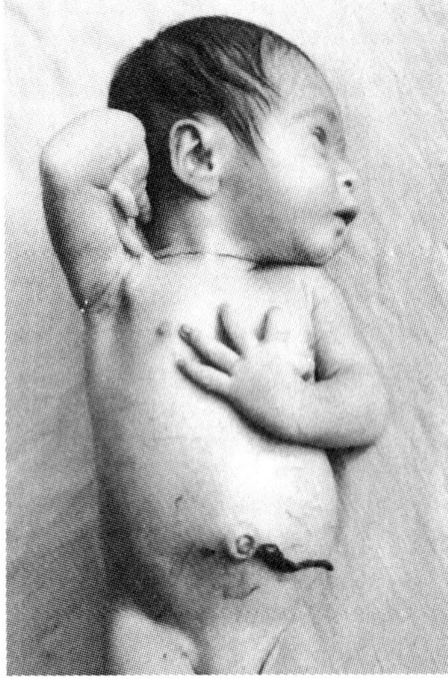

Fig. 6.4A: (Congenital) Madelung s deformity

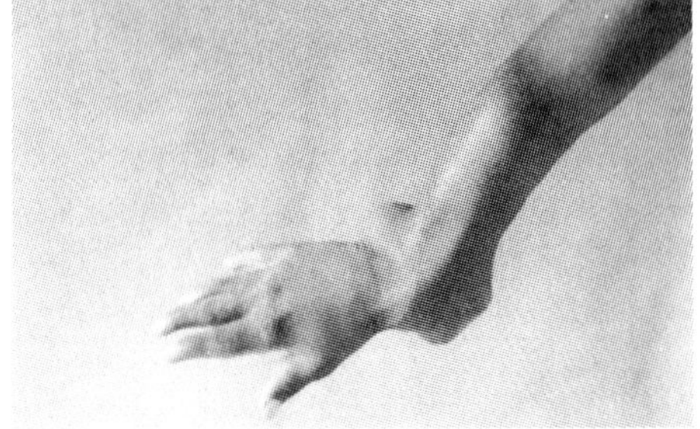

Fig. 6.4B: Photograph of Madelung s type deformity due to osteochondroma of lower end of radius and ulna

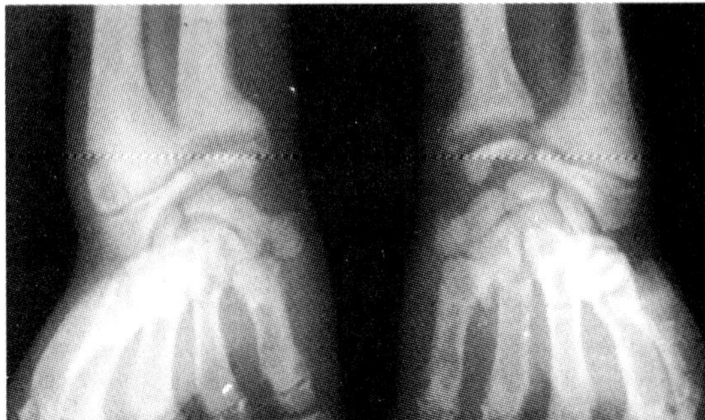

Fig. 6.4C: Madelung s type deformity

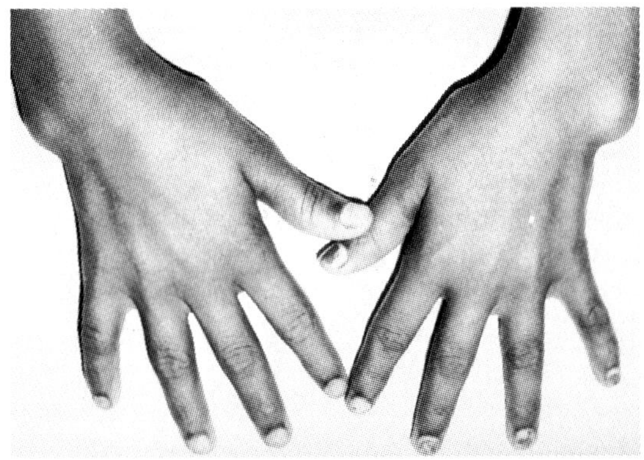

Fig. 6.4D: Madelung s type deformities

severe Volkmann's ischaemic contracture there is a striking flexion contracture of the wrist and fingers due to the shortening of the fibrotic forearm flexor muscles.

Inspection

Inspect from the sides, dorsal and palmar aspects.

On the dorsal aspect: Note the normal bony and soft tissue points in systematic order, while the fingers are opened up and the patient attempts to make a fist. Look at the contour of the region, any swelling, skin condition, venous prominence, ulnar styloid prominence, creases around the joint, any swelling in relation to any tendon or the wrist joint (e.g. ganglion) and

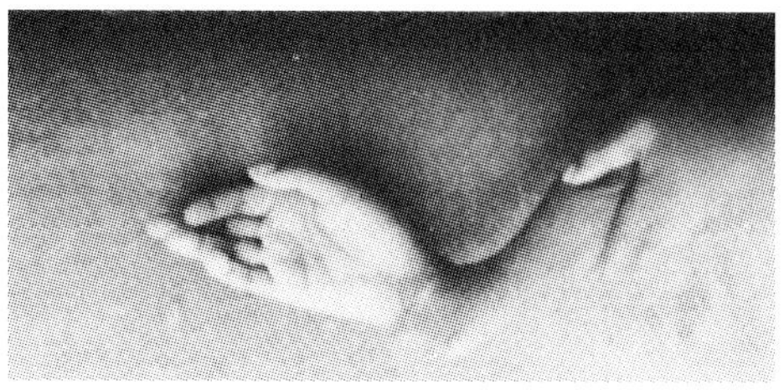

Fig. 6.5A: Old epiphyseal injury of lower end of radius leading to premature closure of growth epiphysis and overgrowth of ulna

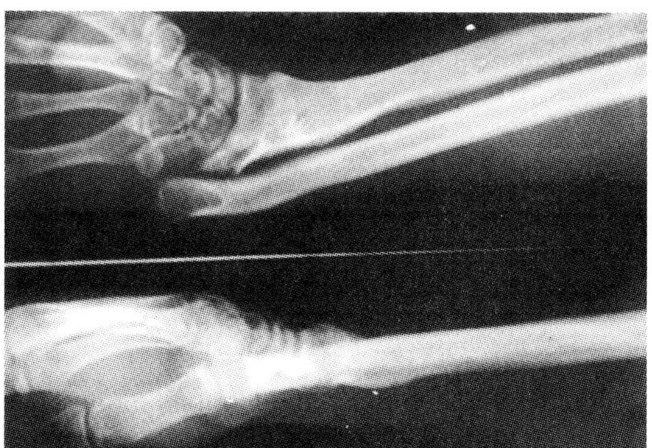

Fig. 6.5B: Old epiphyseal injury of lower end of radius premature closure of growth epiphysis and overgrowth of ulna

back of the forearm, any sinus, and skin contractures.

On the radial side: Ask the patient to extend the thumb and inspect the *snuffbox* (bounded by abductor pollicis longus and extensor pollicis brevis on the radial side, and extensor pollicis longus on the ulnar side) for any fullness. Note any abnormal prominence on this side of the lower radius (a typical site for de Quervain's disease and giant cell tumour).

On the palmar aspect: Look for the skin creases in relation to thenar and hypothenar eminences and at the wrist level, and note any abnormal finding—e.g. swelling, sinus, atrophy, hypertrophy, discolouration (in cervical rib syndrome), fullness in the lower forearm (compound palmar ganglion or Parona's space affections).

On the ulnar side: Look for the hypothenar eminence and muscular bulge of the lower forearm above the wrist. Most of the affections of the wrist, specially injuries, are associated with swelling of the hand components.

Palpation

Superficial palpation: Note the temperature, condition of the skin, any hyper or hypoanaesthesia, any bony projection, or any other abnormal feature. Note the radial pulse with any variation, if present.

Deep palpation: Certain normal relations must be confirmed before searching for any abnormal findings. Localise the tips of the ulnar and radial styloid processes. Note their levels and compare with the other side. Normally, the tip of radial styloid process lies about 1 cm distal to that of ulnar styloid process.

Method of palpating the styloid processes (Fig. 6.6) with the patient's forearm pronated and the wrist in as much neutral a position as possible, support the palm in one hand. Put the thumb and index fingertips of the opposite hand on the two sides of the wrist from the dorsal aspect. In case of the right hand of the patient your right index fingertip should be in the snuffbox and the thumb tip should be distal to the head of the ulna. Gently squeeze within and at the same time shift your fingertips proximally. The pointed bony projections will be felt (the tips of the radial and ulnar styloid processes). Reverse the position of your thumb and index finger for the patient's left hand.

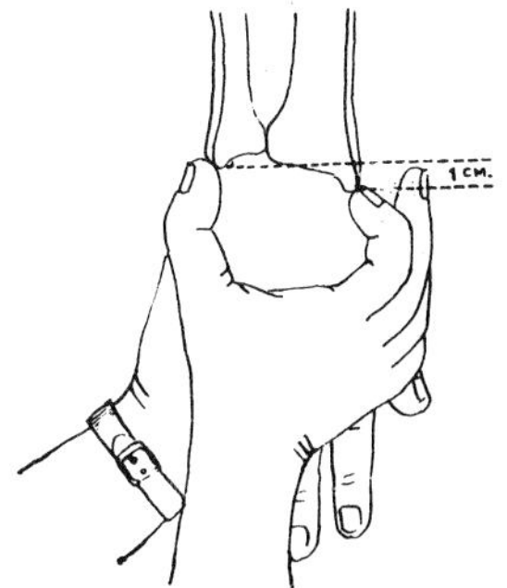

Fig. 6.6: Palpating the tips of radial and ulnar styloid processes

Method to localise the joint line on the dorsum of the wrist (Fig. 6.7) Support the patient's wrist on your one hand and put the tip of the index or middle finger of the opposite hand in about the centre of the interstyloid line. You will feel a gap. Confirm by gently dorsiflexing and palmar-flexing the wrist as far as practicable, the gap will slightly close and open up accordingly. Extend the fingertips along the interstyloid line while gently moving the wrist joint, and you will assess the wrist joint line. Now, palpate for the presence of any abnormal finding, especially those which you have seen on inspection.

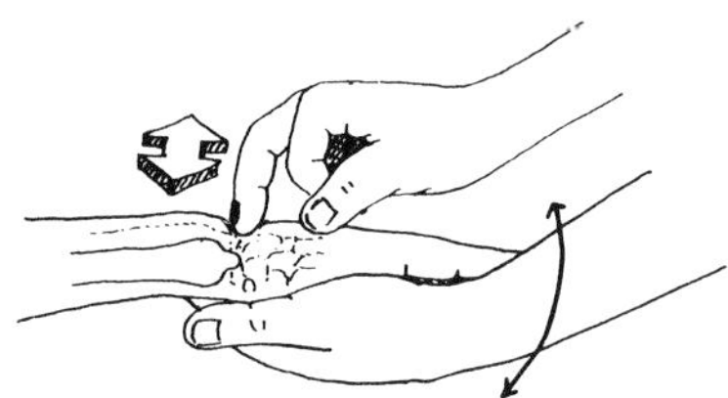

Fig. 6.7: Localisation of wrist joint line

Bony components: Note for any bony irregularities at the lower end and posterolateral surface of the radius and the lower end of the ulna. Any abnormal swelling or bony prominence in front of the wrist should be palpated for its temperature, tenderness, size, shape, texture, consistency, relation to deeper structures and mobility.

THE COMMONER SWELLINGS AROUND THE WRIST JOINT

A. Traumatic

Initially diffuse, soft to hard swelling, later localise as a bony swelling.

B. Non-traumatic

i. Diffuse swelling (soft to cystic):
   - — tuberculosis (Fig. 6.24)
   - — Rheumatoid arthritis (Fig. 7.10)
   - — Septic arthritis (Fig. 6.8)

ii. Localised swellings (either communicating with wrist joint or in relation to any tendon sheath).

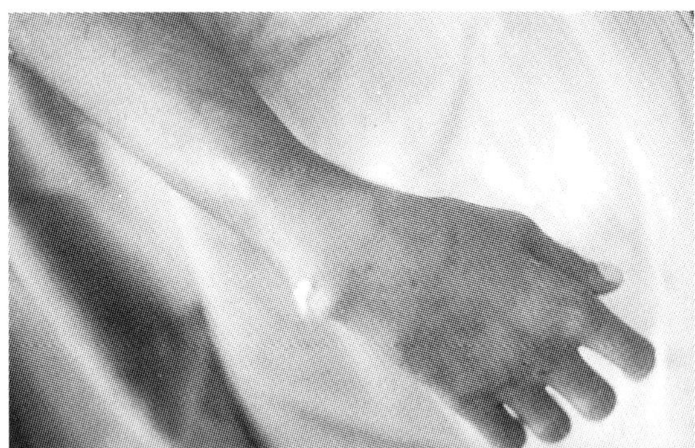

Fig. 6.8: Septic arthritis wrist with collection projecting below the ulnar stylodoid process

— Ganglion—round, tense, tender cystic swelling containing clear gelatinous. fluid usually on dorsal, radial-palmar and ulnar-palmar aspects of the wrist. (Figs 6.9A and B).

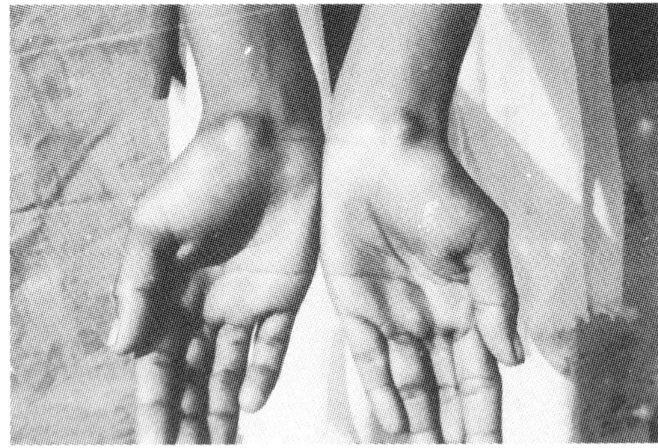

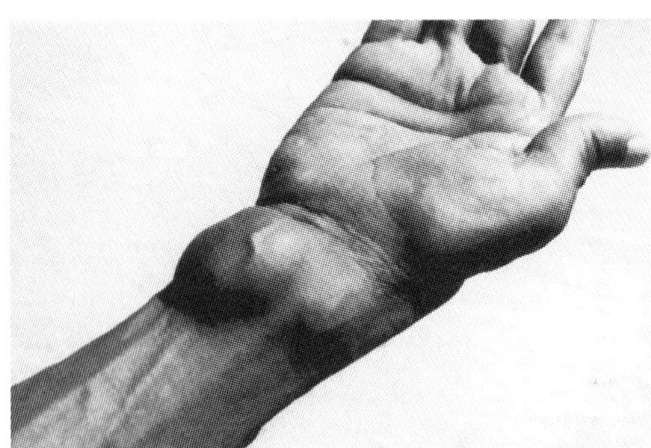

Figs 6.9A and B: Ganglion

— de Quervain's disease—a firm tender swelling about 1.5 cm proximal to the radial styloid process (Figs 6.25A and B).

— Giant cell tumour—expanded soft to bony hard swelling from lower outer aspect of the radius (Figs 6.10A and B).

— Compound palmar ganglion—diffuse bulge above and below the flexor retinaculum (Figs 6.11A and B).

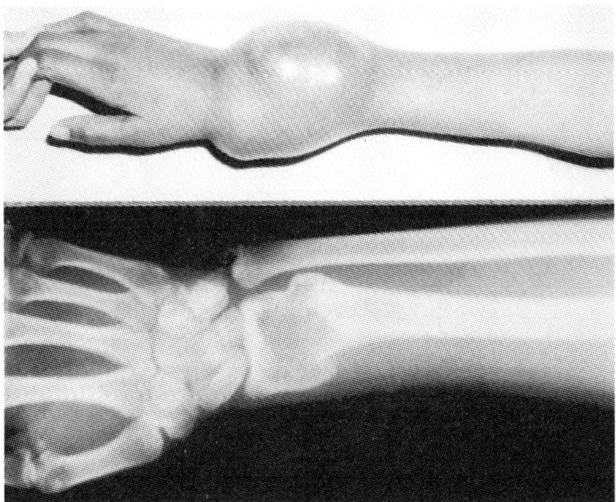

Figs 6.10A and B: Giant cell tumour from lower end of radius with pathological fracture

Egg Shell Crackling

The lower end of the radius is a common site for giant cell tumour. One of its cardinal clinical sign is egg shell crackling, which is tested by the method of palpation. Again this demonstration should not be done (reasons discussed in the chapter on Bone Tumours).

Step Sign

In case of injury, note for the step sign (Fig. 6.12). Pass down your index finger on the outer aspect of the forearm over the rounded radial shaft. In case of outer shift of the lower fractured fragment, your finger will suddenly step over the hard underlying structure. This 'stepping' can be felt in similar circumstances on the dorsal aspect too. This 'step sign' is of special importance in ascertaining the shift in *Colles* (posterior stepping up) and *Smith's* or *reverse Colles fracture* (posterior stepping down).

Palpation of the Snuffbox

Snuffbox lies just distal to the radial styloid process. Its radial border is formed by the abductor pollicis longus and extensor pollicis brevis tendons and ulnar border by the extensor pollicis longus tendon. The floor of snuffbox is the scaphoid bone.

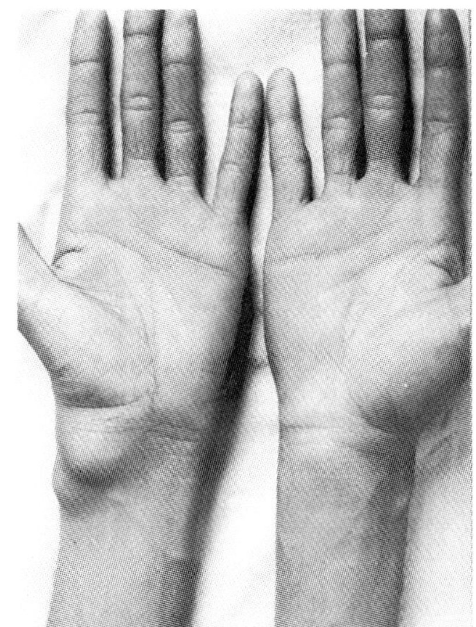

Fig. 6.11A: Compound palmar ganglion on the right side and (simple) ganglion on the left side

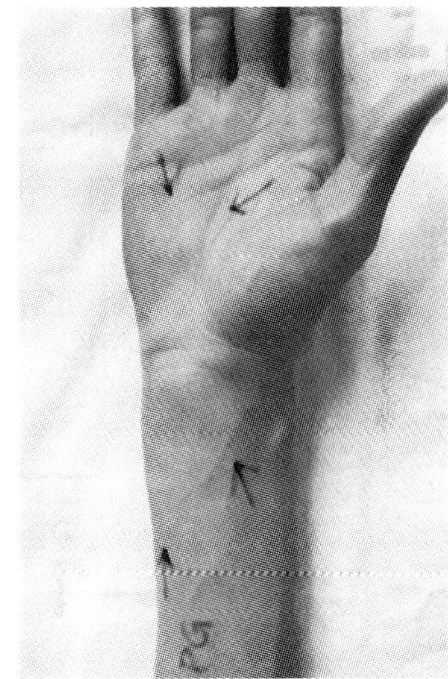

Fig. 6.11B: Compound palmar ganglion more marked in oblique position of the wrist

Palpate carefully the snuffbox, specially in case of fall on outstretched hand. Ask the patient to extend and abduct the thumb as far as possible (thumb up position). Supporting the wrist from the ulnar side in one hand, press deeply at the floor of the snuffbox, in between the prominent tendons, and note for tenderness which usually occurs in scaphoid fracture (in case of trauma) or osteoarthritis of the wrist or intercarpal joints.

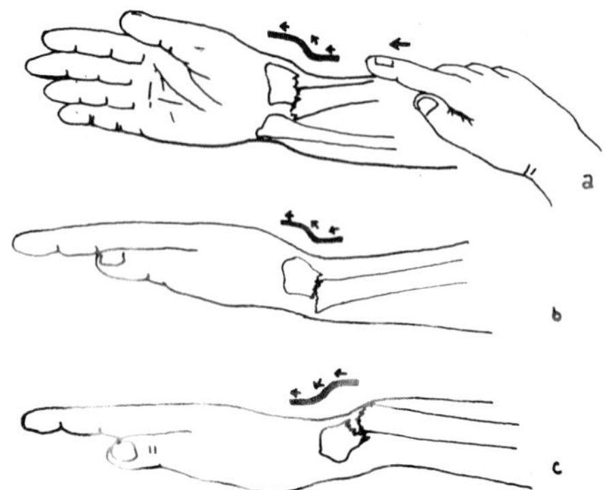

Fig. 6.12: (a) Lateral step up, (b) Posterior step up Colles fracture, (c) Posterior step down Smith s fracture

Crepitus

In a suspected case of fracture of the lower end of radius or ulna, note, if per chance crepitus is felt. Do not try to demonstrate it, even though it is diagnostic of fracture.

Test for de Quervain s Disease

Any suspicious swelling existing at the lower outer end of forearm, may be due to de Quervain's disease. Palpate for the local tenderness. Ascertain the relation of pain with strained movements of the thumb. Test as in Figure 6.13.

i. Ask the patient to make a firm fist, keeping the thumb in palm. The patient will complain of pain just above the radial styloid process (Fig. 6.13a).
ii. In demonstrating Finkelstein's test, the patient makes a fist keeping thumb in palm. Now the hand is pressed into ulnar deviation. There should be pain over the radial styloid process or even towards the thumb and/or elbow, if the test is positive. However, even without de Quervain's disease, variable pain can be felt in that region in this manoeuvre.

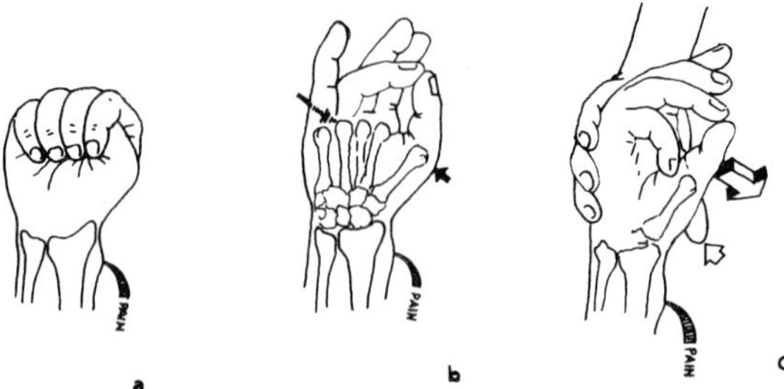

Fig. 6.13: Tests for de Quervain s disease. (a) Closing firm fist triggers pain, (b) Springing over 1st and 4th metacarpal head triggers pain, (c) Active abduction and extension of thumb against resistance triggers the pain

iii. While the patient keeps his thumb in opposed position towards the ring finger tip, press over the heads of 1st and 4th metacarpals with a springing action—the patient complains of pain on the outer surface of the radial styloid (Fig. 6.13b).
iv. In the same position, ask the patient to extend and abduct the thumb against resistance. The patient will feel pain at the same site (Fig. 6.13c).

MOVEMENTS (Table 6.1)

Movements of the Forearm

The movements of the forearm joints result in pronation and supination of the hand. In pronation, the radius, carrying the hand with it crosses obliquely the front of ulna, so that radial upper end remains lateral, and medial end goes medial to ulna. In supination, the movement is reversed so that radius lies lateral to and parallel with the ulna. These movements occur at the radio-ulnar joints: (1) proximal synovial uniaxial pivot radio-ulnar joint where the radial head rotates in fibro-osseous ring formed by radial notch of ulna and the annular ligament, (2) Middle radioulnar union, in which shafts of radius and ulna are connected by oblique cord and the interosseous membrane of the forearm, (3) Distal

Table 6.1: Movements at wrist

Movement	*Range of movement*	*Prime movers*	*Nerve supply*	*Assisted by*	*Limiting factors*
Palmar flexion	0° to 70°-90°	(i) Flexor carpi radialis (ii) Palmaris longus (iii) Flexor carpi ulnaris	Median nerve C_6 Ulnar nerve C_8, T_1	Flexor digitorum profundus, flexor digitorum superficialis	Tension of dorsal radiocarpal ligaments
Dorsiflexion	0° to 70°-90°	(i) Extensor carpi radialis longus (ii) Extensor carpi radialis brevis. (iii) Extensor carpi ulnaris	Radial nerve C_6, C_7.	Extensor digitorum, extensor indicis, extensor pollicis longus, extensor digiti minimi, extensor pollicis brevis	Tension of volar radiocarpal ligaments Contact of dorsal surface of distal row of carpals to the posteriorly projected lower end of radius
Ulnar deviation	0° to 25°-35°	(i) Flexor carpi ulnaris (ii) Extensor carpi ulnaris	Ulnar nerve C_8, T_1 Radial nerve C_6, C_7		Tension of lateral collateral ligament of wrist joint. Contact of ulnar styloid process to the hamate
Radial deviation	0° to 15°-25°	(i) Flexor carpi radialis (ii) Extensor carpi radialis longus (iii) Extensor carpi radialis brevis	Median nerve C_6 Radial nerve C_6, C_7	Abductor pollicis longus, extensor pollicis brevis	Tension of ulnar collateral ligament of wrist Contact of tip of radial styloid process to the scaphoid

synovial uniaxial pivot radioulnar joint where there is articulation between the convex ulnar head and the concave ulnar notch on the lower medial aspect of radius.

For pronation—pronator quadratus (supplied by anterior interosseous branch of median nerve, C8, TI) aided by pronator teres (supplied by median nerves, C6-7) is responsible for rapid movement and movements against resistance.

Supination—In extended elbow for slow and unresisted supination movement, supinator may be sufficient but in flexed elbow, fast movements and movement against resistance biceps brachi (supplied by musculocutaneous nerve, C5-C6) assists the supinator (supplied by posterior interosseous nerve, C5-C6).

Palmar-Flexion and Dorsiflexion (Fig. 6.14)

Method of Demonstration

The patient sits with both mid-pronated forearms supported on the table on their ulnar sides and kept parallel about 10-12" apart. The thumb and fingers are fully extended, while the forearms are firmly fixed on the table. The patient is then asked to bring his fully extended fingers towards each other in the mid line as far as practicable. The outer angle subtended between the axis of the forearm and that of the hand is the angle of maximum palmar flexion. Bringing back to the zero position, the patient is asked to move the hand with fully extended fingers away from each other as far as practicable. The inner angle between the axis of the forearm and that of the hand is the angle of maximum dorsiflexion.

A quick method of comparison of dorsiflexion and palmar-flexion is as follows:

Oppose the fully stretched up hands (finger to finger contact) and lift the elbows as far as possible. The angle sustained between the axis of the forearm and that of hand is the angle of maximum dorsiflexion. Next, the backs of the stretched hands are opposed while the elbows are depressed as far as possible, together. The angle subtended between the axis of the

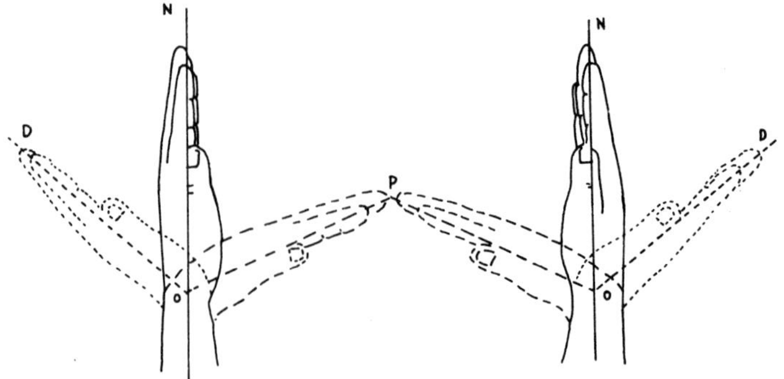

Fig. 6.14: Movements of wrist joint palmar-flexion (<NOP), dorsiflexion (<NOD)

forearm and that of the hand will be the angle of maximum palmar-flexion. However, in these manoeuvres, movement is not only at the radiocarpal joint but also includes the intercarpal and carpometacarpal joints.

Radial and Ulnar Deviation (Fig. 6.15)

The patient sits with both forearms and hands kept parallel and fully pronated about 12" apart on the table, the fingers and thumbs being kept fully extended. From this zero position, ask the patient to approximate the tips of extended middle fingers towards the midline as far as practicable. The outer angle between the axis of the forearm and that of the extended hand will be the angle of maximum radial deviation.

Ask the patient to move the extended fingers away from the midline as far as practicable. The inner angle between the axis of the forearm and that of the extended hand will be the angle of maximum ulnar deviation.

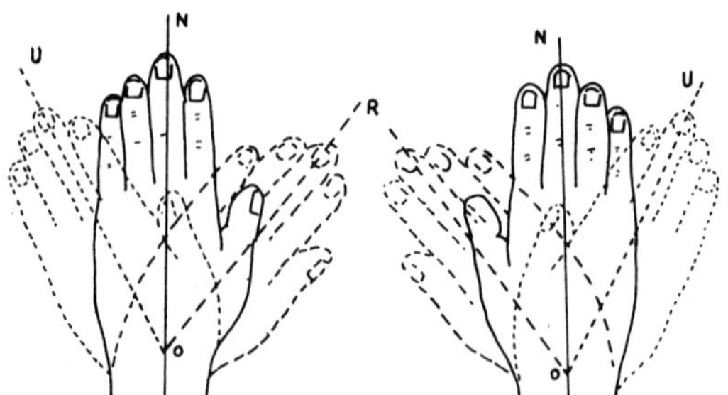

Fig. 6.15: Movements of wrist joint Radial deviation (<NOR), Ulnar deviation (<NOU)

Circumduction

Support the patient's pronated lower forearm from the flexor surface. Ask him to make a fist and circumduct (make a circle) in the air. This will be circumduction (Fig. 6:16).

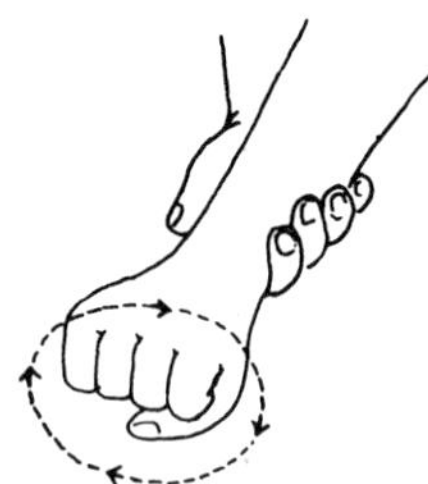

Fig. 6.16: Circumduction at the wrist joint

Test for Function of Important Tendons

You can perform group testing as well as individual testing.

On cursory examination, if the patient can make a firm fist and perform circumduction, probably all tendons and nerves associated with the wrist and hand are normal. However, individual testing of certain tendons is important.

The flexors, extensors, radial deviators and ulnar deviators will be tested in groups when testing for these movements at the wrist joints. Important tendons to be tested are:

i. *Extensor Pollicis Longus* (Fig. 6.17A)
While supporting from the flexor surface, the lower end of the forearm, wrist and proximal palm, kept in fully pronated position, ask the patient to extend the interphalangeal joint of thumb from fully flexed position as far as possible. This will be mainly by extensor pollicis longus tendon, which will stand out on the ulnar side of the snuffbox.

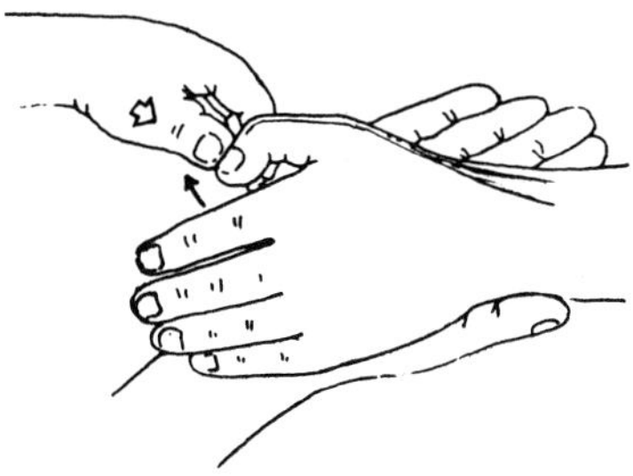

Fig. 6.17A: Extensor pollicis longus

Ask the patient to extend the thumb both backwards and outwards. This will be by extensor pollicis brevis, abductor pollicis longus and extensor pollicis longus as a conjoint effort.

ii. *Extensor Digitorum* (Fig. 6.17B)
Supporting the wrist and hand as above, the patient is asked to extend the fingers, especially the middle and ring fingers, from a flexed position at the metacarpophalangeal level. In this movement, the index and little fingers are also assisted by extensor indicis and extensor digiti minimi respectively.

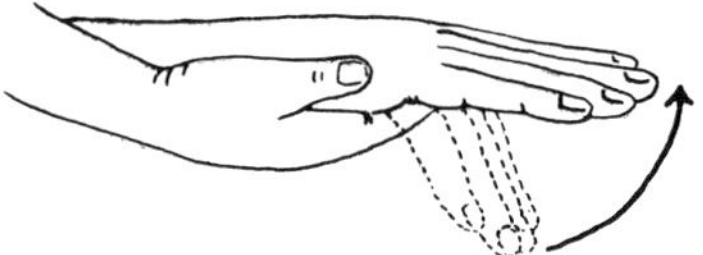

Fig. 6.17B: Extensor digitorum

iii. *Palmaris Longus* (Fig. 6.17C)
The fully supinated forearm and hand are placed firmly on the table. Put resistance by your hand over the palm and ask the patient to firmly flex at the wrist. Palmaris longus will become prominent near the midline of the lower forearm. About 1 to 1.5 cm radialwards, the tendon of flexor carpi radialis will also stand out. Keeping the wrist in zero position and interphalangeal joints of thumb and fingers fully extended with flexion at metacarpophalangeal joints, ask the patient to firmly flex the wrist against the self-imposed resistance—the three prominent flexors of the wrist will stand out, i.e. palmaris longus in the centre, flexor carpi radialis laterally and flexor carpi ulnaris medially (Fig. 6.17D).

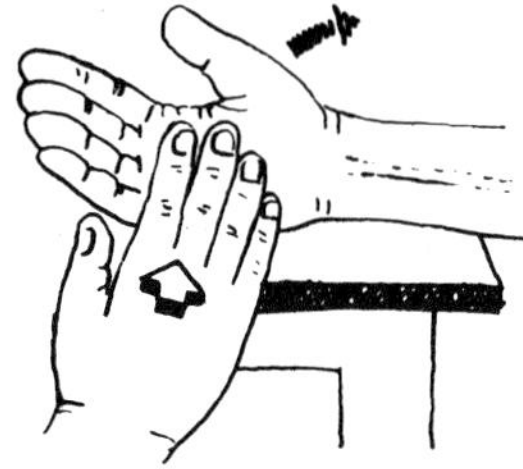

Fig. 6.17C: Palmaris longus

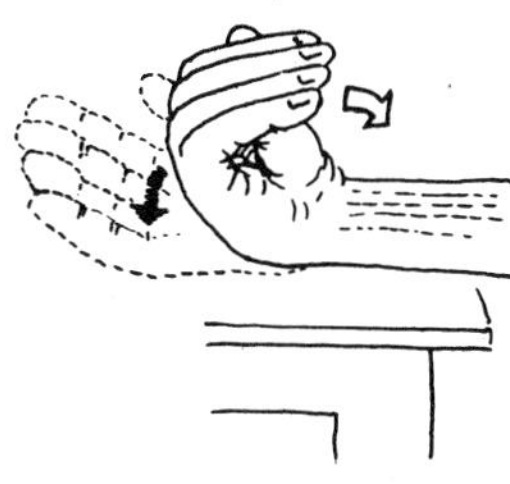

Fig. 6.17D: Three prominent flexors of the wrist palmaris longus, flexor carpi radialis and flexor carpi ulnaris

iv. *Flexor Carpi Ulnaris*
With the position of the forearm of the patient as described above and your hand giving resistance over the palm, ask the patient to flex with ulnar deviation tendency at the wrist level. Feel for a prominent longitudinal tight tendon—the tendon of the flexor carpi ulnaris.

MEASUREMENTS

Linear Measurement

The linear measurement of the wrist region is more or less the same as for that of the upper limb (both total and segmental measurements, i.e. for the arm and forearm). The measuring points are:

For total limb length—Acromion angle to tip of radial styloid process.

For the arm—From acromion angle to tip of lateral epicondyle of humerus.

For the forearm—From lateral epicondyle of the humerus to the tip of the radial styloid process.

The measurement must be comparative and both limbs must be in a symmetrically aligned position (guideline will be the affected limb).

Circumferential Measurement (Fig. 6.18)

It should be done at the joint level, i.e. the tape passing around both the styloid tips. The other circumferential measurement will be for increase/decrease of girth of muscle—to be measured at mid-forearm level.

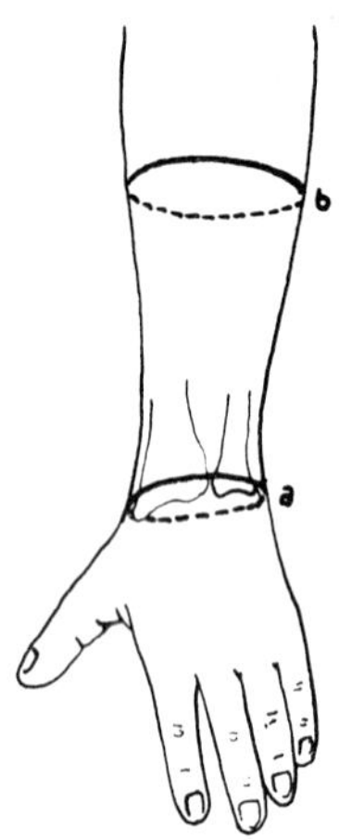

Fig. 6.18: Circumferential measurement, a = at wrist, b = at mid-forearm

Distally, the measurement of girth and size of palm will be considered in the examination of the hand.

Tests for integrity of peripheral nerves in relation to the wrist joint (median, ulnar, and radial nerves). (See chapter on Peripheral Nerves).

Look for the possible complications following trauma or disease in and around the wrist.

Investigations Required for Wrist Pathology

For lesions or injuries about the wrist, routine investigations more or less suffice. However, of the injuries about the wrist, a carpal fracture or dislocation or subluxation may sometimes be missed in routine posteroanterior and lateral radiograph. An oblique and 45° semipronated oblique views are essential for such lesions, specially for the scaphoid (the most common of the carpal bones to be involved in fractures). Hence, to diagnose even a hair line fracture of the scaphoid (which unless diagnosed and treated properly has a notorious reputation of going for non-union), it is mandatory to have 45° semipronated oblique views of the wrist region with contrast exposure and development.

The differently shaped carpal bones, arranged in rows create complex relationship with one another and with the distal forearm bones and metacarpals, which make their thorough evaluation difficult in only two views. Hence minimum views of exposure should include posteroanterior, lateral, posteroanterior in ulnar deviation and 45 degrees semipronated obliques.

Positioning of the Part for Oblique Projection (Fig. 6.19)

While the forearm and hand rest on its ulnar border on the X-ray plate, at an inclination of about 45 degrees (with palm looking down) the beam is centred to the ulnar styloid process OR from the lateral position, rotate the hand backwards by 45° and centre the beam to the ulnar styloid process.

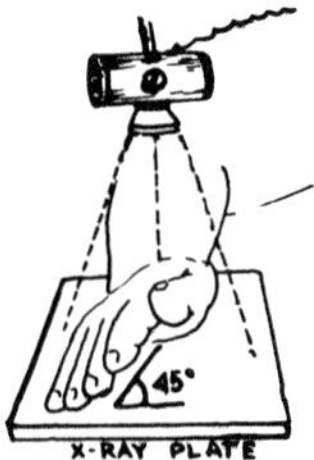

Fig. 6.19: Positioning the part for oblique view X-ray of the wrist joint

KEY DIAGNOSTIC POINTS OF COMMON WRIST PATHOLOGY

A. Traumatic

i. *Colles Fracture* (Abraham Colles, 1814)

— (In children before skeletal maturity, akin injury may produce 'fracture separation of lower radial epiphysis' with almost all clinical features of a Colles fracture).
— Commonest injury around the wrist.
— Usually elderly ladies with history of fall in courtyard or bathroom on an outstretched hand. The female:male ratio is 4:1.
— Immediate pain and swelling in the wrist region.
— In typical Colles fracture typical 'dinner fork' deformity develops (Fig. 6.20B).
— Radial styloid process recedes upwards, posteriorly and laterally.
— Step sign (step up) positive.
— Besides the radial fracture line, tenderness is also marked in the ulnar styloid region.
— In X-ray (Fig. 6.20A), three typical displacements (distal fragment displaced backward, upwards and outwards), and two typical tilts (distal fragment tilted backwards, outwards and impacted upwards into the proximal fragment). The lower fragment also supinates. The lower radial articular surface looks backwards and downwards [normally looks slightly forwards (7°) and downwards].
— If patient is taken into full confidence, variable wrist movements can be demonstrated.
— Shortening of forearm.
— Late cases may also be associated with Sudeck's osteodystrophic (Sudeck's atrophy, reflex sympathetic dystrophy, algodystrophy) changes in the hand and fingers. (probably due to sympathetic or parasympathetic disbalance or unknown aetiology—burning pain, hyperaesthesia of skin, heaviness, and puffiness in the hand; thin shiny skin, spindle-shaped tender swelling and stiffness of the fingers' joints with varying atrophic changes in fingertips and nails, excessive hair growth).
— In late neglected cases, shoulder and/or hand becomes stiff—shoulder hand syndrome.

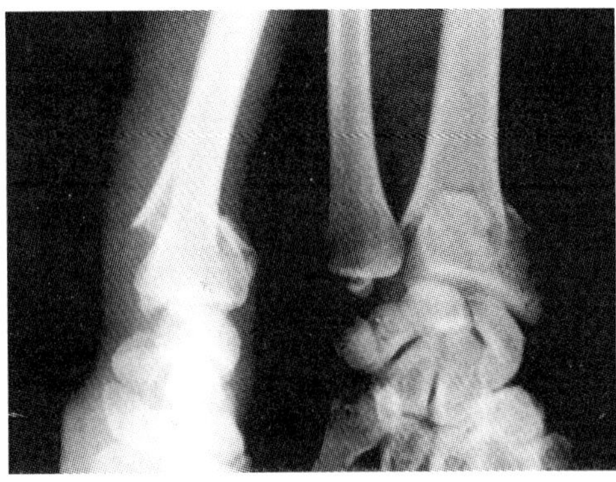

Fig. 6.20A: Colles fracture

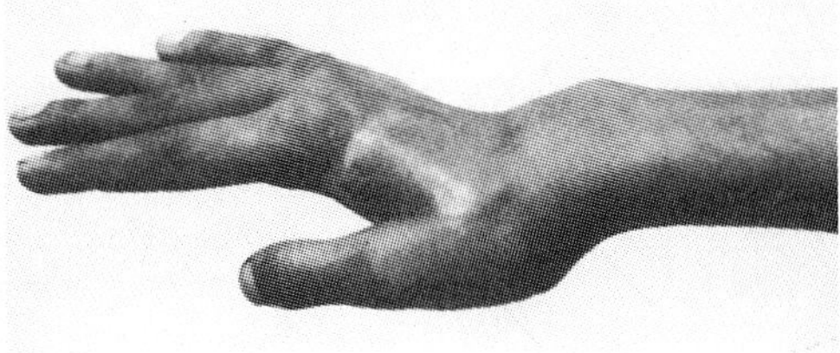

Fig. 6.20B: Typical dinner fork deformity of wrist and hand in Colles fracture

ii. *Smith s Fracture* (Robert William Smith, 1847, Figs 6.21A and B)

— Usually due to fall on the dorsum of a flexed wrist.
— Comparatively younger age group.
— The distal fragment displaces outwards, upwards and forwards.
— The distal fragment tilts outwards and forwards, therefore, lower radial articular surface looks more anteriorly and downwards than the normal one.
— Clinically, many a time it is difficult to distinguish it from Colles fracture, specially when gross swelling is present. However, in fresh cases, the look of the hand (absence of dinner-fork deformity), and presence of reverse posterior stepping, i.e. finger, passing from above downwards, steps down at fractured site (cf. steps up in Colles fracture) are suggestive.

—With patient taken in full confidence, wrist movements can be demonstrated to a variable extent.
—Shortening of forearm.
—Lateral view X-ray is confirmatory.

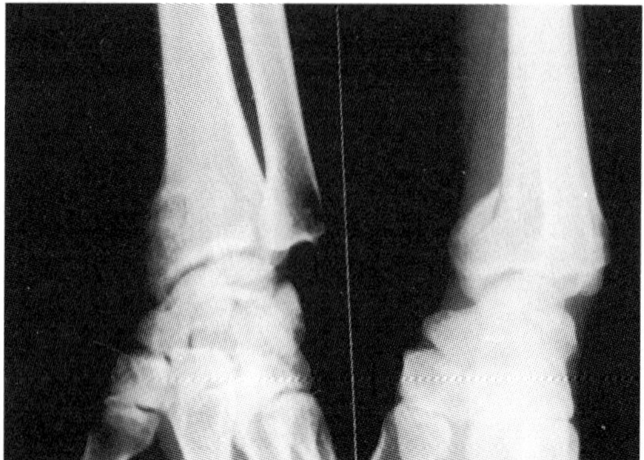

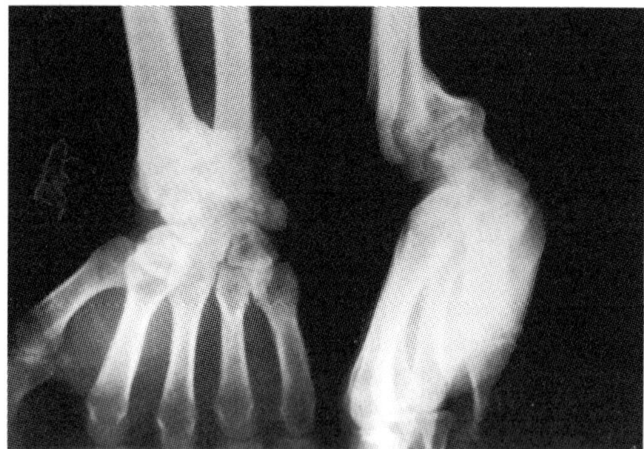

Figs 6.21Aand B: Smith s fracture (A) fresh fracture, (B) grossly displaced malunited fracture

iii. *Chauffeur s Fracture or Fracture Radial Styloid* (Fig. 6.22)

—History of injury—being backfire hit by recoiling car-handle directly over radial styloid process or fall on the ball of the thumb or similar injuries—commonly in young adults.
—Broadening of the lower end of the forearm at the radial styloid level.
—Feeling of irregularity or thickening at the junction of the radial styloid and lower radial shaft.
—Maximum tenderness in this region.
—Radial styloid process may recede up.
—X-ray is confirmatory—fracture line enters the wrist joint between the scaphoid and the lunate bones.

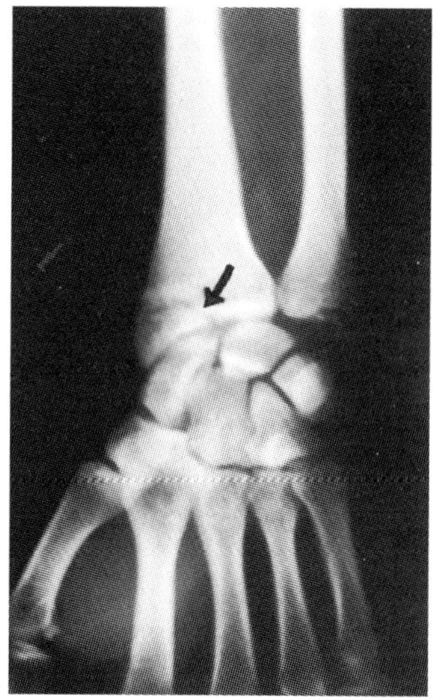

Fig. 6.22: Chauffeur s fracture (fracture radial styloid process)

iv. *Barton s Fracture* (J R Barton 1838) (Fig. 6.23)

—Clinicoradiologically, more or less exaggerated picture of either Colles or Smith's fracture—thus of two types: posterior and anterior (commoner).
—There is anterior marginal fracture of the radius.
—Subluxation, both of the wrist and inferior radioulnar joints.
—The fracture extends into the wrist joint and the carpus along with the hand displaces forwards with the anterior fragment.
—Wrist joint movements markedly painful, may be even difficult to initiate.
—X-ray is confirmatory.

v. *Fracture Scaphoid*

—May be missed initially unless and until carefully examined and X-rayed.
—History of injury, usually indirect (fall on outstretched hand or direct hit over the scaphoid region, specially when the hand is fisted).

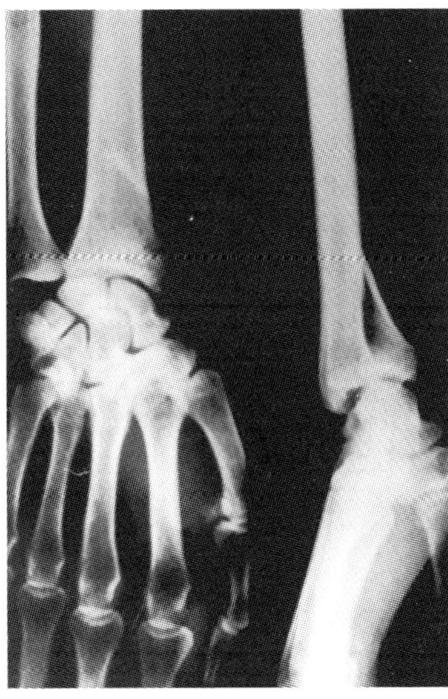

Fig. 6.23: Barton s fracture

— Maximum tenderness in the floor of the snuff-box, which may show comparative fullness. Snuffbox lies just distal to the radial styloid process. Its radial border is formed by the abductor pollicis longus and extensor pollicis brevis tendons and the ulnar border by extensor pollicis longus tendon.
— Patient (usually young males) feels pain in actively extending the thumb fully.
— Even with the slightest suspicion, oblique view X-ray of wrist region must be ordered for. In fact, in any injury of the wrist joint, it will always be rewarding to order for antero-posterior, lateral, and pronation and supination oblique views.
— Crack fracture is mostly missed in recent X-rays, hence these must be repeated after 3 weeks.

vi. *Lunate Dislocation*
(Most common among carpal dislocations)
— Indirect injury—the wrist assumes a variably dorsiflexed position.
— A bony mass is felt in front of the wrist.
— Median nerve may be involved.
— Lateral view X-ray confirmatory.
— Osteochondritis of lunate due to avascular necrosis (Keinbock's disease) is a prominent cause of pain in this region.

vii. *Post-traumatic Inferior Radioulnar Arthritis*
— It is a common accompaniment of late Colles fracture or other injuries around the wrist.
— Patient complains of pain in using the wrist as well as during rotatory movements of the forearm.
— Area of maximum tenderness lies just behind and below the ulnar styloid process.
— This tenderness further increases if attempt is made to displace the ulnar head forwards and backwards.

viii. *Post-traumatic Chronic Wrist Pain*
Two major causes are:

1. *Carpal instability*, which can be of two types—
   i. static instabilities can be identified on plain radiograph
   ii. dynamic instabilities need fluoroscopic examination for confirmation alongwith that of asymptomatic wrist for comparison.

Arthrography may be useful in demonstrating defects in the interosseous ligaments, joint capsule and triangular fibrocartilage.

Dissociated instabilities can be delineated by disruption of smooth carpal arcs.

2. *Osteonecrosis*: It affects the proximal scaphoid bone. Lunate is less commonly affected (Keinbock's disease) either due to trauma or abnormal repeated stresses.

Early osteonecrosis is negative on plain X-ray. It can be seen as a focal area of absent uptake on isotope bone scan. During healing it shows increased uptake.

Established osteonecrosis is seen on plain X-ray as increased bone density, flattening and fragmentation. MRI is very sensitive in demonstrating osteonecrosis which is seen as diffuse areas of decreased marrow signal intensity on both T_1 and T_2.

B. Non-Traumatic

i. *Tuberculosis of Wrist* (Fig. 6.24)

— More common in adults.
— Incidence not so uncommon.
— Slow onset.
— Pain in and around the wrist.
— Local temperature raised.
— Fullness around the wrist.
— Tenderness around the joint line.
— Gradual painful limitation of all wrist movements.

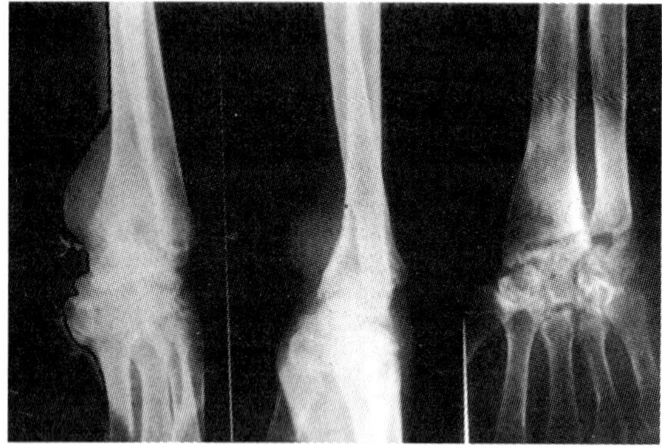

Fig. 6.24: Tuberculosis of the wrist joint with cold abscess

— Wasting of the forearm muscles, and to some extent, the hand muscles too.
— Supratrochlear and/or axillary glands may be enlarged and matted.
— In later stage, cold abscesses or sinuses may be present (Fig. 6.24).
— X-ray—as in typical tuberculous lesions.

ii. *Rheumatoid Arthritis* (see Fig. 7.10)

— Wrist is a common site, especially in ladies in their thirties.
— Wrist is swollen.
— Movements, specially extension, is painful. Gradually, flexion and ulnar/radial deviation deformities of the wrist develop.
— Smaller joints, i.e. metacarpophalangeal and proximal interphalangeal joints of thumb and fingers may be affected (not distal interphalangeal joints of fingers as in osteoarthrosis).
— May be typical deformity in thumb and fingers (e.g. swan-neck deformity, buttonhole or Boutonnièrs deformity).

iii. *de Quervain's Disease* (Figs 6.25A and B) described by de Quervain Fritz in 1895

— Basic pathology is idiopathic stenosing tenovaginitis, in which the sheath of a tendon thickens. Common sheath of the abductor pollicis longus and extensor pollicis brevis tendons, at the wrist, are most commonly affected.
— Usually observed in ladies in their thirties.
— Complains of painful swelling over the outer aspect of the lower end of forearm and with subjective weakness in thumb-pinch and grip.
— Pain more in squeezing type of movements by the thumb.
— Firm, tender swelling about 1.5 cm proximal to the radial styloid process.
— Stress tests for abductor pollicis longus and extensor pollicis brevis (as mentioned earlier) positive.

iv. *Giant Cell Tumour* (Figs 6.10A and B and see Figs 17.6 and 17.7)

— Commonest growth at lower end of radius.
— Gradual onset.
— Slowly expanding the lower radial end.
— Local temperature may be variably raised.
— Slight tenderness present.
— Yielding tendency of the expanded cortex.
— Movements of the wrist free till very late stage.
— Egg shell crackling—not to be demonstrated. However, in regular process of palpation, if one feels the crackling—it should be noted.

v. *Ganglion around the Wrist* (Figs 6.9A and B)

— Ganglions are common around the wrist, more in females between 20 and 40 years of age, and mostly appear insidiously.
— Patient presents with swelling and painful terminal movements of the wrist specially extension, however, the condition may be painless too.
— Local tense, tender swelling in the joint line, or along the tendon.

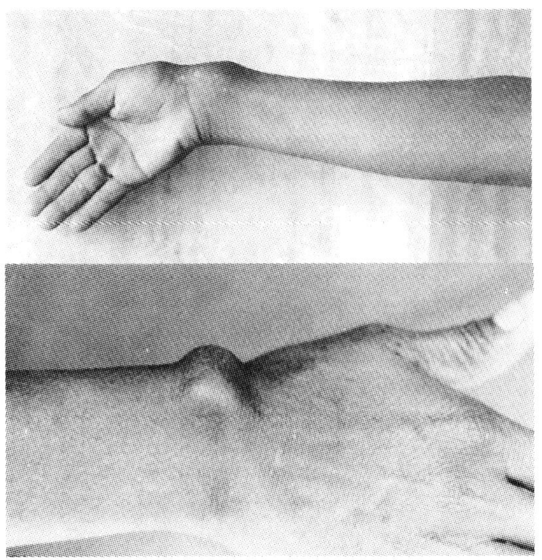

Figs 6.25A and B: Photograph of de Quervain s disease

- Though cystic, but very difficult to demonstrate fluctuation.
- Usually present on the dorsum of the wrist, disappears or reduces in size on extension of wrist and becomes more prominent on flexion of wrist.
- May also be related to the tendons of the wrist, more between the long extensor of thumb and extensor indicis—in that case they will not disappear on movement of the wrist, rather they may slightly move up and down with movements of the particular tendon.
- If the ganglion lies deeper to the tendon, its size reduces with contraction of the particular tendon, and *vice-versa.*
- When it lies superficial to the tendon, the position is reversed, i.e. becomes prominent with contraction of tendon and decreases in size with relaxation of the tendon.

vi. *Carpal Tunnel Syndrome (Tardy Median Nerve Palsy)*

- Most common compressive neuropathy of the upper extremity is the carpal tunnel syndrome in which the median nerve is compressed at the wrist in the carpal tunnel—a fibro-osseous canal rigidly bound by the carpal bones and roofed by the transverse carpal ligament. This tunnel contains the median nerve and nine flexor tendons of fingers and thumb.

  Causes of carpal tunnel syndrome:

  Non-specific tenosynovial proliferation, rheumatoid arthritis; degenerative arthritis; old trauma in that region; metabolic (hypothyroidism, gout, diabetes mellitus); alcoholism; acromegaly; pregnancy; tumours; connective tissue disorders (amyloidosis; haemochromatosis); idiopathic.
- Females in their fourty to fifties are the usual victims, complaining usually in the night or early morning of feeling of heaviness, vague pain, tingling, paraesthesia, numbness in first three digits and weakness in the hand in the distribution of median nerve, specially after doing fine work.
- Even without any history of earlier injury, patient complains of pain and/or tingling sensation or numbness in hand and fingers, specially in the index and middle ones.
- Clumsiness or lack of dexterity is a common complaint.
- Symptoms usually get relieved after rubbing the hand or hanging it over the side of the bed. However, if the hand remains in dependant position, there may be venous engorgement, which can exacerbate the symptoms.
- The symptoms get exaggerated when direct pressure is applied over the centre of the wrist from the front (this presses directly over the median nerve in that region), i.e. by compressing or percussing over the carpal ligament (Tinel sign).

Test for Carpal Tunnel Syndrome

Phalen's test: Patient is asked to keep both wrists in flexed position, keeping the forearm vertical. Usually, pain is felt on the affected side within a minute which dramatically disappears when the wrist is extended. However, this test is positive in 76% of cases only. There may be bulge of the flexor mass in the lower aspect of the wrist, which is characteristic of chronic tenosynovitis.

A *provocative test*, in which, the wrist flexion is combined with the median nerve compression appears to be clinically more useful. Here the elbow is extended, the forearm is supinated and wrist is flexed to 60°. The median nerve in the carpal tunnel is compressed evenly and constantly till numbness, pain or paraesthesia appears in the distribution of median nerve. If these symptoms occur within 30 seconds, the test is positive.

Tourniquet Test

When sphygmomanometer cuff is inflated above the systolic level, patient complains of pain and paraesthesia, more on the affected side usually within a minute (as against in 2-3 minutes in normal limb). If the pressure is continued further, the sensory loss appears in 5-8 minutes in the distribution of median nerve, as against 10 minutes in the normal limb.

Local anaesthetic infiltration about the median nerve, in the carpal tunnel, relieves the symptoms due to compression of the nerve here, but not if it is referred pain from anywhere else.

Demonstration of diminished median nerve conduction velocity across the wrist is almost diagnostic, of which the sensory nerve fibre conduction velocity (between finger to wrist) test is more sensitive than motor fibre conduction.

Local corticoid infiltration may provide variable relief.

Complete surgical decompression of the median nerve provides ultimate good results.

vii. *Madelung's Deformity* (Otto Madelung 1878—Figs 6.4A and B)

Congenital deformity manifesting during puberty, mostly bilateral and more in females, (at times a similar deformity develops following damage of inner third of lower radial growth plate due to trauma, infection or rickets). The components of this deformity are:

a. backward and outward bowing of lower part of radius,
b. backward subluxation of lower end of ulna,
c. shortening of radius,
d. forward and ulnar deviation of the hand,
e. limitation of dorsiflexion, abduction and supination with increased flexion of wrist,
f. dorsal bayonet-like deformity of radius.

In severe cases, pain, muscle cramps and weakness may be complained of.

viii. *Compound Palmar Ganglion* (Figs 6.11 A and B)

— In tuberculous diathesis or established pathology (?) or rheumatoid arthropathy.
— Painless mild swelling is main complaint, very rarely also manifests as carpal tunnel syndrome.
— There is chronic inflammatory collection in ulnar bursa, presenting as a dumb-bell appearance above and below the flexor retinaculum. There may be cross-fluctuation across the flexor retinaculum, and crepitus probably due to melon seed bodies present in the fluid. Swellings are usually not tender nor appreciably warm.

BIBLIOGRAPHY

1. Phalen GS: The carpal tunnel syndrome. *J Bone Joint Surg* **48A**: 211, 1966.
2. Tetro AM, Evanoff BA, Hollstien, Gelberman RH. A new provocative test for carpal tunnel syndrome. *J Bone Joint Surg* **80B**: 493-98, 1998.

7 Hand

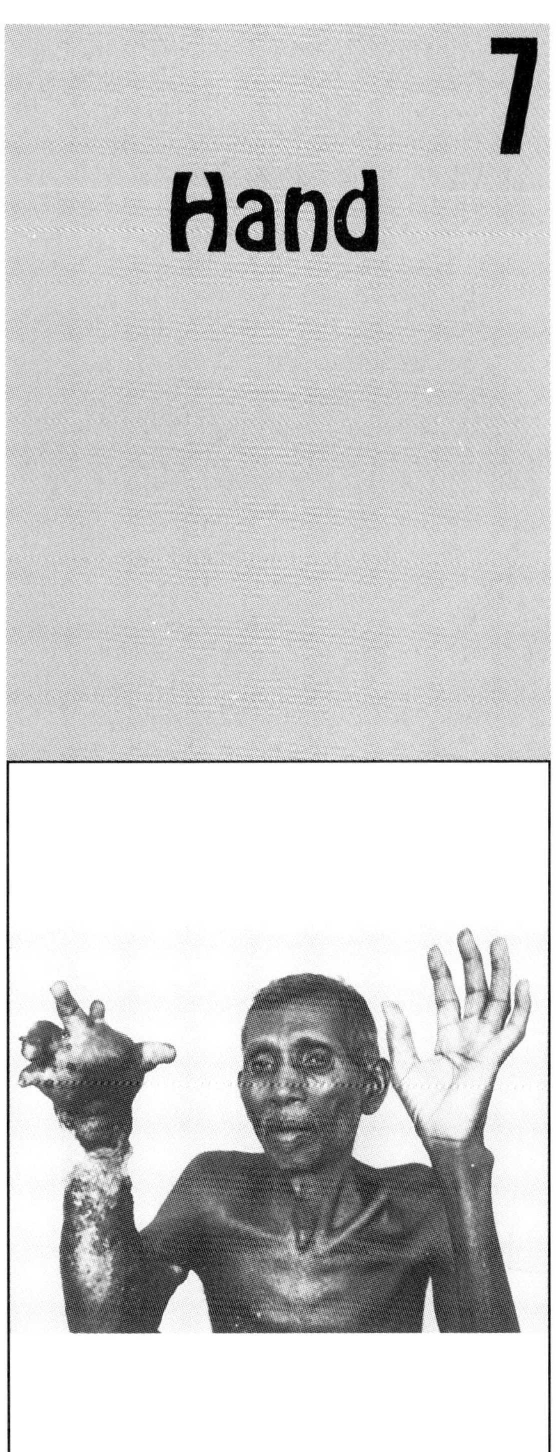

'The hand is an organ of grasp as well as an organ of sensation and expression'

—Sterling Bunnell

INTRODUCTION

The supremacy of mankind over the animal kingdom is decided not only by the use of the lower limbs, rather more by its superiority due to its psyche and hands.

The hand is the most developed part of the locomotor system in bipeds. It is not only meant for performing tough jobs, e.g. holding an object firmly, added to these are very fine and delicate manoeuvres, like painting, writing and fine adjustments. Along with these it also has an important role in sensory perception.

ANATOMICAL CONSIDERATIONS

In the process of morphological evolution, the main development in the hand has been the rotational adjustment of the thumb on the axis of the palm. This has helped in subserving the oppositional function with maximum accuracy. In human beings, the thumb does not lie in the same plane as that of the other fingers (cf, ape or chimpanzee), rather, it has rotated inwards, so that in the extended position it is placed at an angle of about 70°.

Crude movements of the hand are controlled by the long extrinsic tendons coming from the forearm. The basic controlling nerves for the crude functions are the radial nerve (posterior interosseous nerve), and the median nerve. The fine movements of the hand are basically controlled by the intrinsic muscles of the hand. The concerned nerve for this is primarily the ulnar nerve, in collaboration with the median nerve. The extrinsic long muscles, acting synergistically, extend at the metacarpophalangeal joints and flex at the interphalangeal joints. The attachment of the intrinsic muscles, specially the lumbricals and interossei, are such as to enable them to act in balanced antagonism to the main actions of the long tendons, i.e. flexing the metacarpophalangeal and extending the interphalangeal joints.

To subserve the important functions of the hand, like holding an object and/or doing fine work, the hand must be in a position of mechanical advantage. The moment the wrist is extended, grasp position of the hand starts appearing by automatic gradually increasing flexion from the little, to index finger. In this very position of the wrist, the thumb, along with the middle and index fingers, forms an important combination for fine/precision work and sensory perception. However, combined movements at the shoulder, elbow, and wrist are essential to place the hand in an optimal position for proper functioning.

In the hand almost no motion occurs at the third carpometacarpal joint. It forms the central stable post for the hand and its axis is used as a reference for adduction and abduction of the digits.

The fifth carpometacarpal joint (a saddle joint) is the most mobile of the all carpometacarpal joints.

Following any immobilisation, there is a chance of progressive fibrous contraction of the ligaments, leading to stiffness. Therefore, in immobilizing the hand, the position should be such as to keep the collateral ligaments of the metacarpophalangeal and interphalangeal joints taut. This is achieved by flexing the metacarpophalangeal joint to 90° while the inter-phalangeal joint is kept fully extended.

Palmar fascia and fibrous sheath: The deep fascia of the palm (palmar fascia) is divisible into three portions—the parts on both sides covering the thenar and hypothenar muscles, while the tough, triangular part covers the intermediate, central one. The central portion is attached proximally to the palmaris longus tendon, and transverse carpal ligament. At the level of the metacarpal heads it divides into four slips, one for each finger. The digital nerves, vessels and the lumbrical muscles pass distally in between these slips (lumbrical canal). Each slip divides into two processes, between which pass the flexor tendons. These processes diverge and proceed deeper and distally to be attached to:

i. The transverse ligament connecting the metacarpal heads.
ii. The tough fibrous flexor sheath extending from just proximal to the metacarpal heads to the distal interphalangeal joint. This sheath firmly encases the flexor tendons in the fibro-osseous tunnel in front of the phalanges. Any pathology in this tunnel affects the working of the tendon.
iii. The two borders of the proximal phalanx and the proximal half borders of the middle phalanx.

In Dupuytren's contracture, contraction of the palmar fascia produces acute flexion at the metacarpophalangeal and interphalangeal joints, but not at the distal interphalangeal joint (as this fascia does not extend upto it).

"NO MAN'S LAND" of the hand, first described by Bunnell, is the area where both the flexor tendons of the fingers pass through a tight fibrous tunnel. It extends between the distal palmar crease and the insertion of the flexor digitorum sublimis at the mid portion of the middle phalanx. Repair of the tendon injuries in this zone requires meticulous technique and care.

Spaces of the Hand

From the edges of the central portion of the palmar fascia, two septae dip down to the fascia over the interossei. Hence, three spaces are created:

i. Thenar space—encasing the thenar muscles.
ii. Hypothenar space—encasing the hypothenar muscles.
iii. Intermediate space (mid palmar space) containing the superficial palmar arch, long flexor tendons (sublimis and profundus), lumbrical muscles and the median nerve with its branches.

On the palmar aspect, the skin is tough, tight and inelastic but at the same time very sensitive, whereas that on the dorsum is delicate, loose and elastic, accommodating even the inflammatory exudates and collections due to palmar pathology (since the dorsal subcutaneous space receives most of the lymphatics from the palm).

Space of Parona

When the radial or ulnar bursa gets distended with pus, it bursts, and pus travels up the forearm between the flexors profundus anteriorly and the pronator quadratus and interosseous membrane posteriorly—the space of Parona. In this space a quantity of pus can remain collected with much swelling.

Ossification of Bones of the Hand (Fig. 7.1)

Carpal Bones

Each bone usually ossifies from one centre in order of appearance:

Capitate	—2nd month	Trapezium	—4-5 years
Hamate	—3rd month	Trapezoid	—4-5 years
Triquetral	—3rd year	Scaphoid	—4-5 years
Lunate	—4th year	Pisiform	—9-12 years

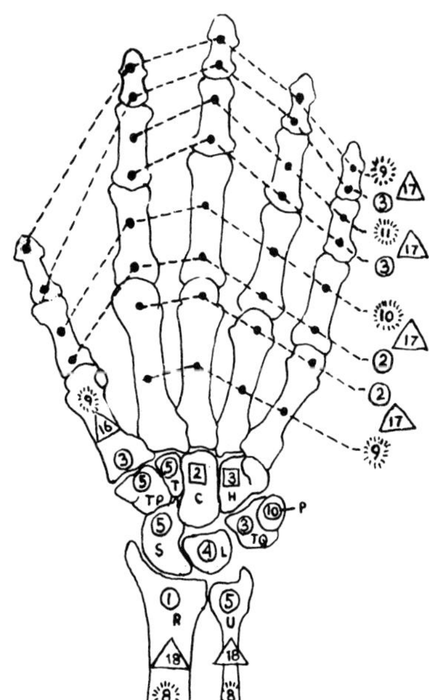

Fig. 7.1: Ossification of bones of wrist and hand, dotted circle denotes primary centre in week (IUL), complete circle denotes secondary centre in years

Metacarpal Bones

Each bone ossifies from 2 centres, one primary for the shaft, and other secondary centre for the base of the 1st and for the head of rest of the metacarpals (2nd to 5th).

Phalanges

Each ossifies from two centres, one primary for the shaft, one secondary for the proximal end.

Synovial Sheaths of Flexor Tendons (Fig. 7.2)

Synovial sheaths of the long tendons on the palmar aspect start 2.5 cm proximal to the flexor retinaculum. One, ensheathing the flexor digitorum sublimis and profundus, proceeds as common sheath upto half way along the metacarpal bones (ulnar bursa). Except for the little finger, in which it is continuous with digital synovial sheath, the rest of the sheaths end in blind diverticulae around the tendons of the ring, middle and index fingers at mid-palm level. Another sheath for the flexor pollicis longus continues along the thumb.

The hand is supplied by the radial and ulnar arteries, dominantly by the latter.

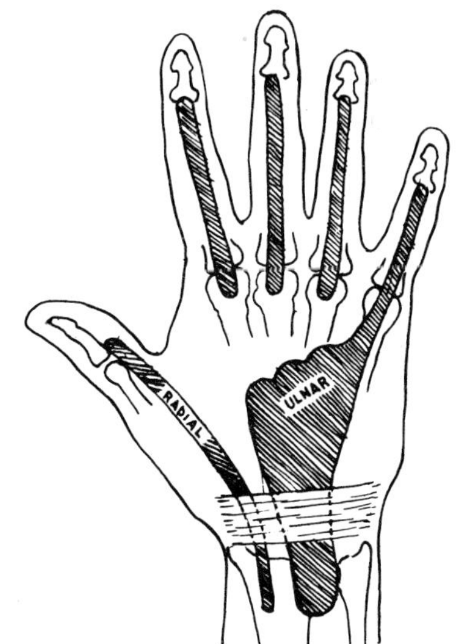

Fig. 7.2: The extent of the synovial sheaths of flexor tendons

METHODOLOGY

History Taking

(As in chapter on Introduction)

The common complaints concerning the hand are pain, stiffness, deformity, weakness, and abnormal sensation. The pain may be local or referred from anywhere from neck to the wrist.

Gross Assessment of Hand Functions (Figs 7.3A and B)

General and Systemic Examinations

General and systemic examinations—As described in the chapter on Introduction.

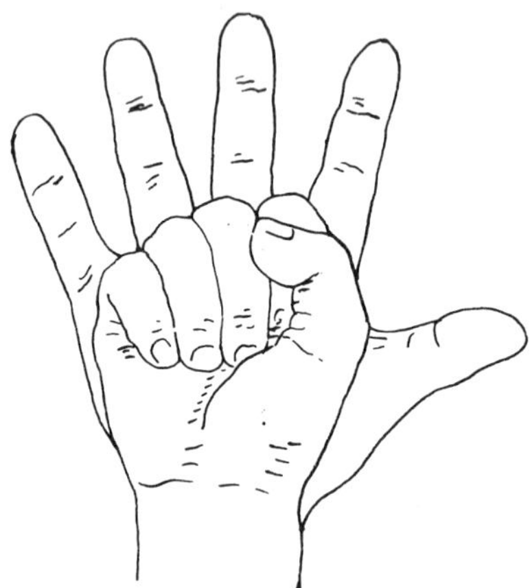

Fig. 7.3A: Making a firm fist and opening of the hand with thumb and fingers extended, indicates normal hand

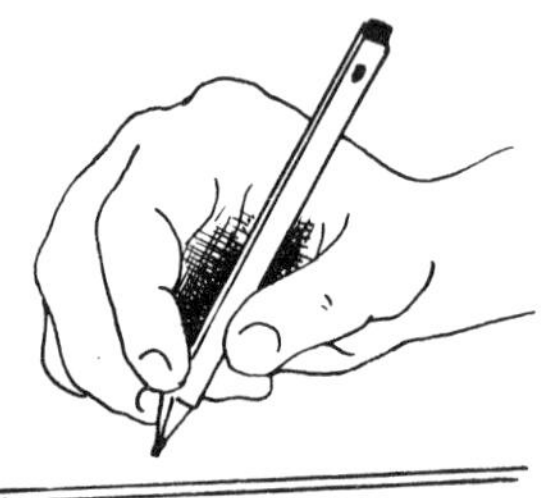

Fig. 7.3B: Normal holding a pen in writing position indicates normal intrinsics and good function of thumb and fingers

Regional Examination

The cervical region, supraclavicular region, shoulder girdle, arm, elbow, forearm and wrist must be examined in any examination of the hand.

Local Examination

At the outset, the integrity of the hand should be grossly tested for. If the patient is able to make a firm fist and open up the hand fully, and the fingers and thumb can be fully extended, it is probably a normal hand.

i. *Prerequisites*

Both the upper limbs must be comparatively assessed, in identical position, from the neck to the tips of the fingers.

ii *Attitude and Common Deformities*

1. Certain congenitally absent conditions (Fig. 7.4A) or deformities of hand and finger are quite obvious, like *polydactylism* (reduplication of fingers—preaxial (radial) polydactyly is commoner than the postaxial (which are 10 times more common in Negroes than Caucasians); *syndactylism* [(jointed fingers—it may be simple (fingers are joined by soft tissue only or complex (Fig. 7.4B) (when bone is involved as well)]; *arachnodactyly* (= 'in the form of spider'—the fingers and toes are very long and thin, e.g. in Marfan's syndrome) or dolichostenomelia; *brachydactylism* (shortened finger); *symphalangism* (fusion of interphalangeal joint); *congenital annular grooves;* cleft hand or *lobster-claw hand* (Figs 7.4C to E); *megalodactylism* (congenital hypertrophy) (Figs 7.23A and B), *macrodactylism* (enlarged digits); *camptodactylism* (fixed flexion deformity of the proximal interphalangeal joint, usually of little finger and mostly bilateral); *clinodactyly* [fixed contracture (usually of little finger) with angulation in radio-ulnar plane]; *Kirner's deformity* (there is radial and palmar curving of the distal phalanx).

Brachymetacarpia (congenital shortening of the metacarpal caused by premature closure of the epiphysis.

Cleft hand is usually bilateral, and is frequently associated with cleft foot, cleft lip, cleft palate and even non-cleft anomalies in cardiac and GIT systems.

Radial club hand (Preaxial radial hemimelia) (Fig. 7.4F) (absence of thumb, short index finger, entire hand deviating towards radial side, distal

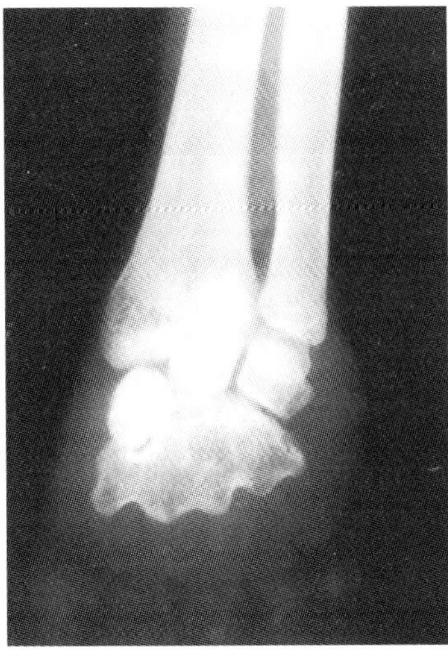

Fig. 7.4A: Congenital abscence of hand

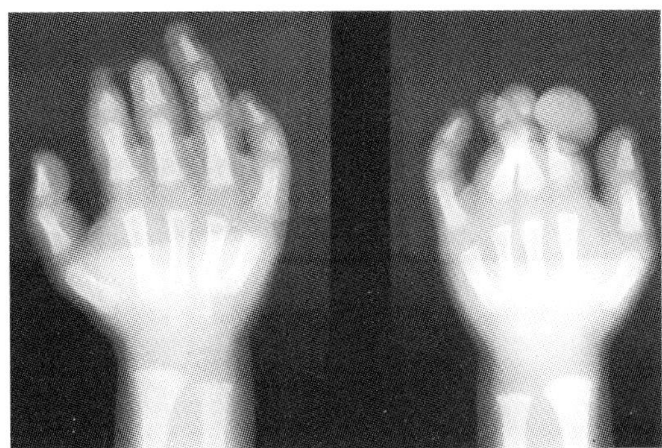

Fig. 7.4B: Congenital absence of terminal phalanges of index and middle fingers of left hand, and distorted fusion and malformations of the digits of right hand

end of ulna quite prominent, may be associated with defects in cardiovascular system, gastrointestinal tract, or genitourinary tract, aplastic anaemia and platelet defects (may be managed by centralisation of forearm and wrist and pollicisation); *ulnar club hand* (absence of small finger, ulnar deviation of the hand and wrist, short and ulnar-bowed forearm).

2. There may be spindle shaped swelling at the proximal inter-phalangeal joint (rheumatoid arthritis, rupture of collateral ligaments of the joint, gout).

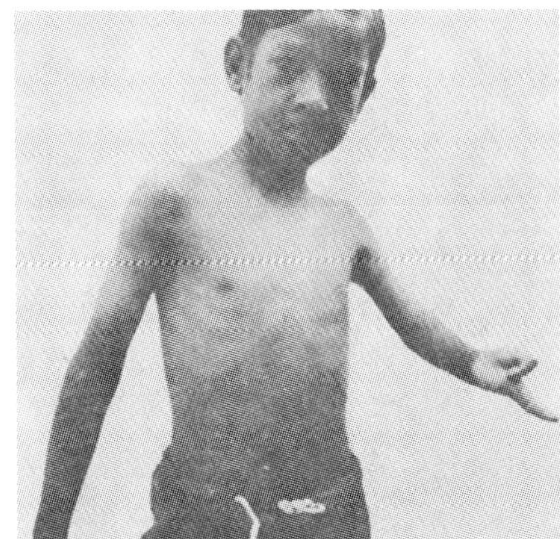

Fig. 7.4C: Typical cleft hand or lobster-claw hand

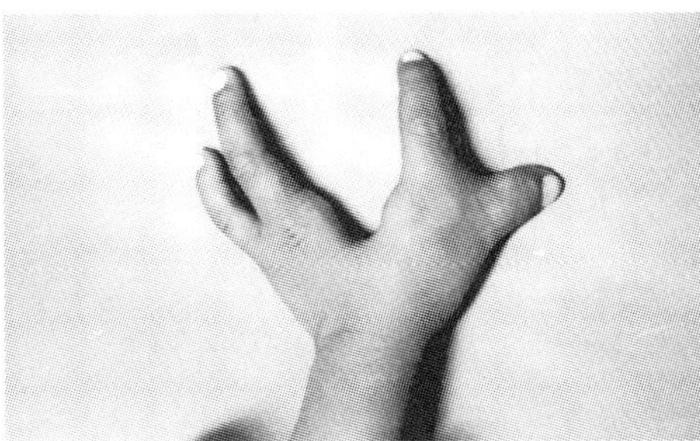

Fig. 7.4D: Same condition. Note the typical V shaped cleft and absence of 3rd ray

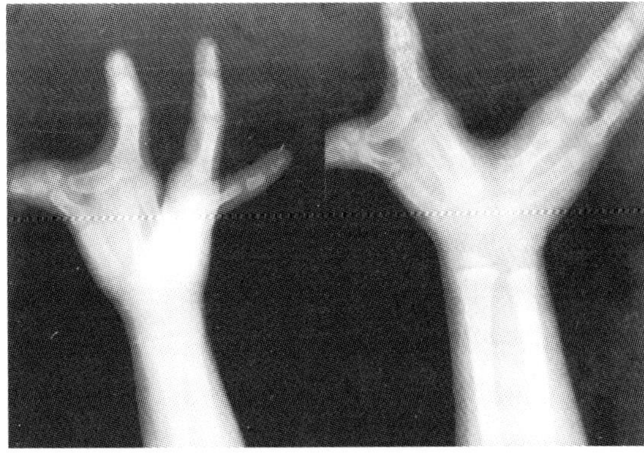

Fig. 7.4E: X-ray picture of cleft hand

3. Similar swelling may occur along the phalanx, which is called dactylitis e.g. tuberculosis (spina ventosa) (Figs 7.5A to E) pyogenic (Fig. 7.5F) enchondroma (Figs 7.5G and H), syphilis, Madura hand (Figs 7.6A and B).

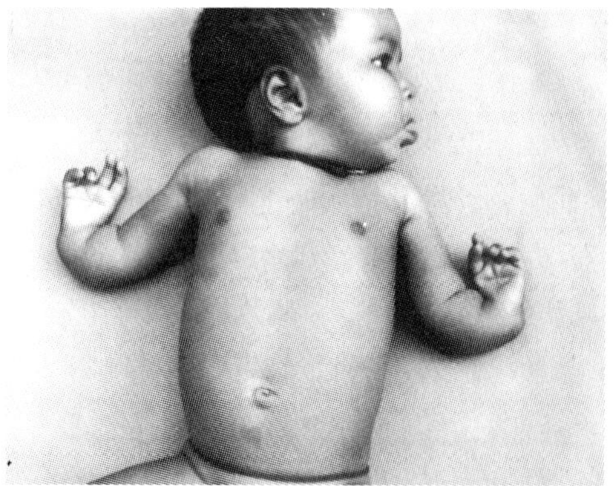

Fig. 7.4F: Bilateral radial club hand

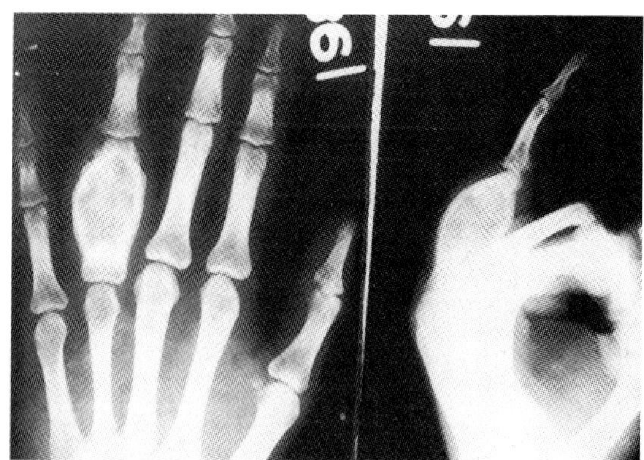

Fig. 7.5B: X-ray picture tuberculous dactylitis of ring finger (proximal phalanx)

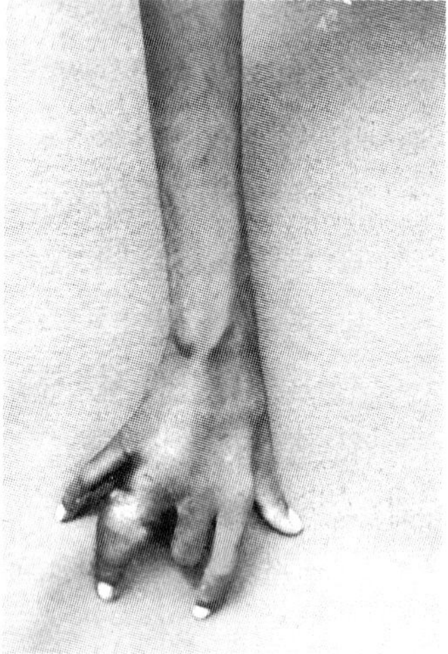

Fig. 7.5A: Tuberculous dactylitis of ring finger (spina ventosa)

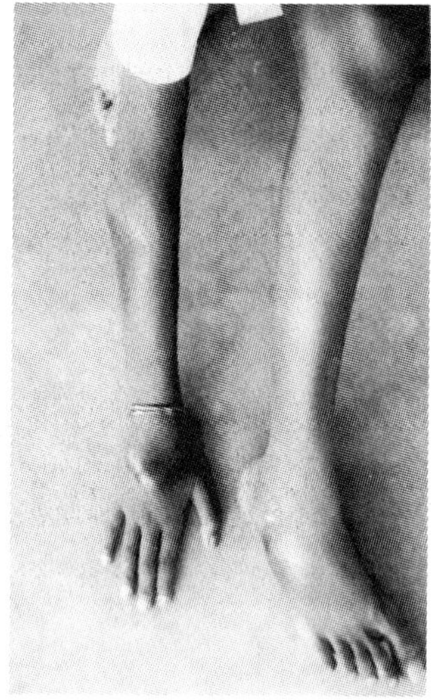

Fig. 7.5C: Tuberculosis of 2nd metacarpal, right elbow, right cuboid and right upper tibio fibular joint multifocal osteoarticular tuberculosis

4. The tips of the fingers may present a bulbous appearance (whitlow, osteomyelitis of the terminal phalanx, hyperparathyroidism). Sometimes nodular swellings are seen on the dorsum of distal interphalangeal joints (Heberden's node—Fig. 7.7) in osteoarthrosis [cf. psoriasis, xanthomatosis (Fig 7.8A and B), hypertrophic osteoarthropathy].

5. In tendon sheath infection, the finger assumes a semiflexed position and the patient will be hesitant to extend it due to pain.

6. Relation of the fingers with the thumb, and amongst themselves and the position of the metacarpophalangeal and interphalangeal joints must be noted clearly. To evaluate the rotational alignment of the fingers, ask the patient to flex the metacarpophalangeal and the proximal interphalangeal joints and look at the alignment of the fingers. Normally they should point towards the scaphoid bone. Subtle differences can be seen by looking at the semiflexed fingers'

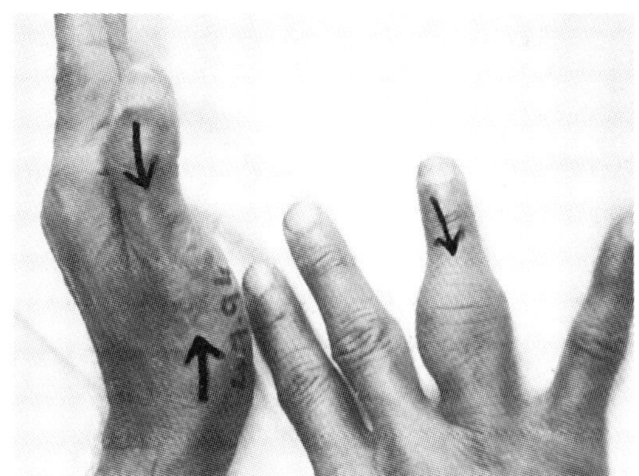

Fig. 7.5D: Tuberculous dactylitis of ring finger of right hand; 3 years back he was operated for tuberculosis of metacarpophalangeal joint of his left hand

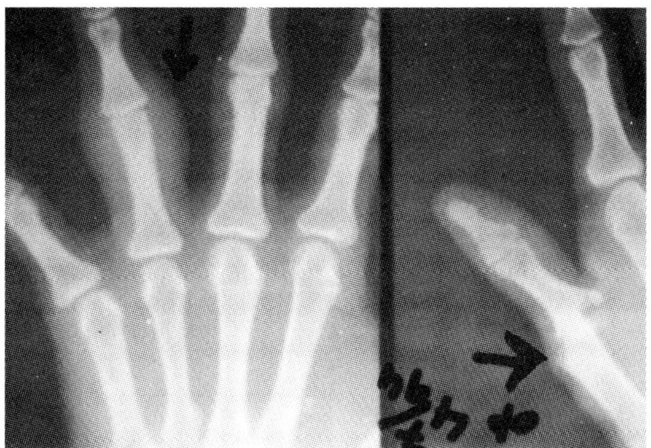

Fig. 7.5E: X-ray picture of the hands in Fig. 7.5D

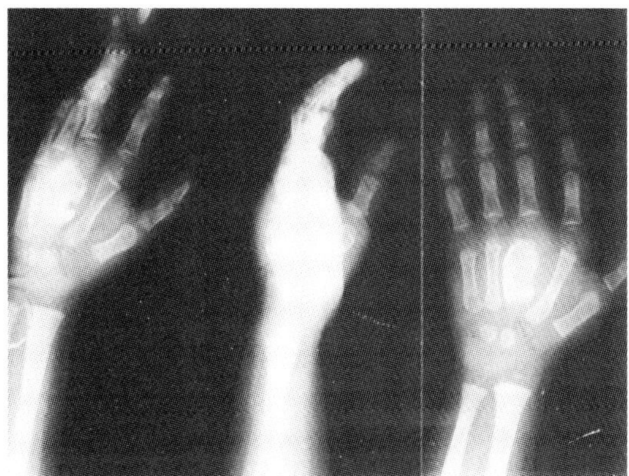

Fig. 7.5F: Pyogenic dactylytis (osteomyelitis) of 3rd metacarpal

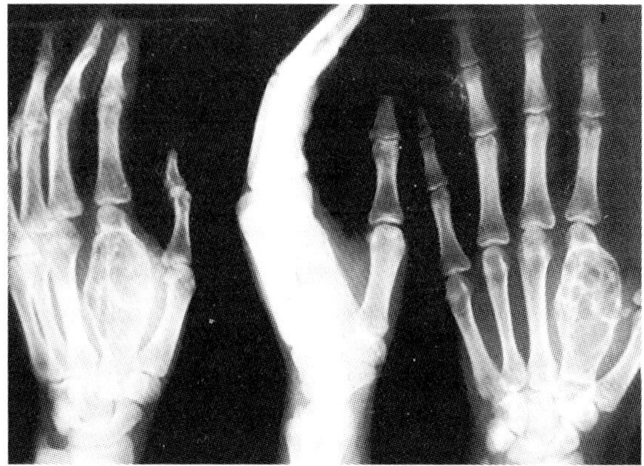

Fig. 7.5G: Enchondroma of second metacarpal

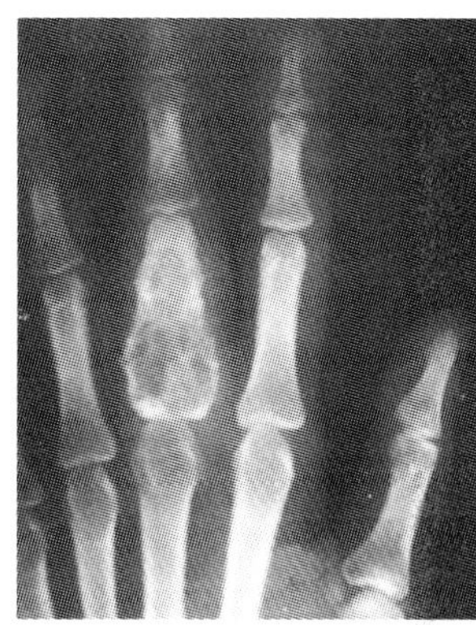

Fig. 7.5H: Enchondroma proximal phalanx of middle finger

ends and comparing the planes of the fingernails to those of the normal side. Even little rotational discrepancies at the base of the finger gets magnified at the finger tips leading to overlap or divergence of the digits with increasing flexion.

There are certain well described deformities of the fingers and thumb. Claw hand is the attitude of the hand in which the fingers become flexed at the interphalangeal joints and extended or hyperextended at metacarpophalangeal joints.

a. Typical claw hand develops due to paresis/paralysis of the intrinsics (ulnar (Fig. 7.9A) or ulnar-median paralysis (Fig. 7.9B). Here, overaction of the long

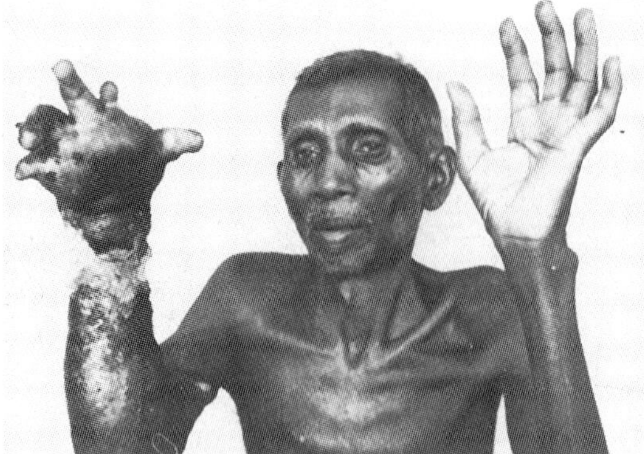

Fig. 7.6A: Mycetoma of right hand

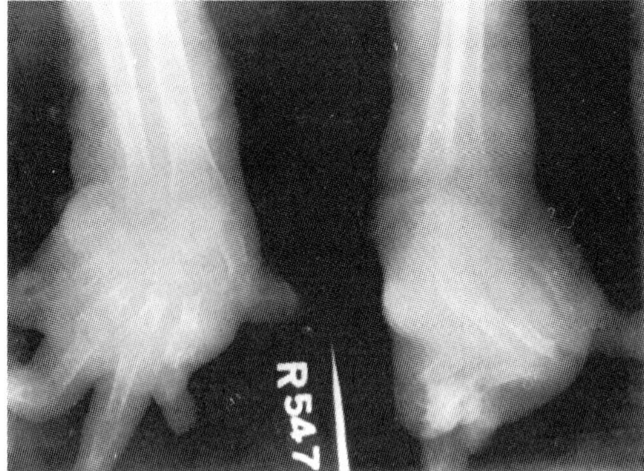

Fig. 7.6B: X-ray of the same hand (mycetoma)

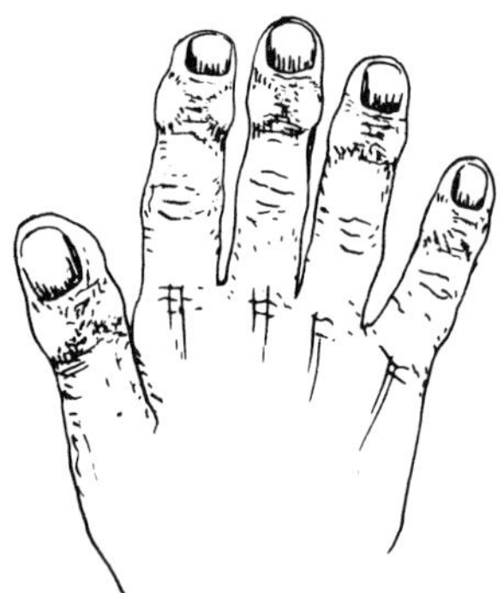

Fig. 7.7: The typical site and presentation of Heberden s node

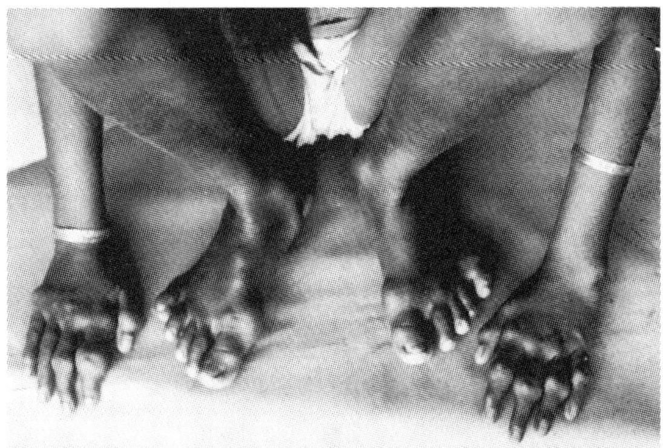

Fig. 7.8: Multiple xanthomatosis of both hands and feet

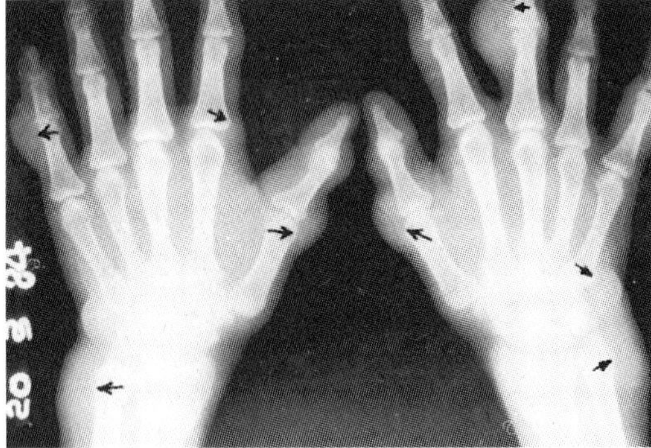

Fig. 7.8A: Radiograph showing synovial Xanthomas from various joints of hand and wrist

flexors and long extensors conjointly produce the claw hand which is of 'intrinsic minus' type (Figs 7.9B and C) e.g. in leprosy, Klumpke's paralysis, peripheral nerve injuries.

b. If the intrinsics are overactive, (in spasm or contracted), then the fingers present a picture which is due to overaction of the intrinsics (similar picture can be seen in less or loss of function of long tendons; skin or subcutaneous tissue contractures). The developing deformities produce an 'intrinsic plus' hand (Fig. 7.9D). Here, there will be flexion at the metacarpophalangeal joints, extension at the interphalangeal joints and adduction of the thumb with phalangeal extension e.g. in rheumatoid hand, Volkmann's ischaemic contracture, post burn contracture, cerebral palsy (due to spasticity), trauma, fibrotic contracture following infection, Dupuytren's contracture.

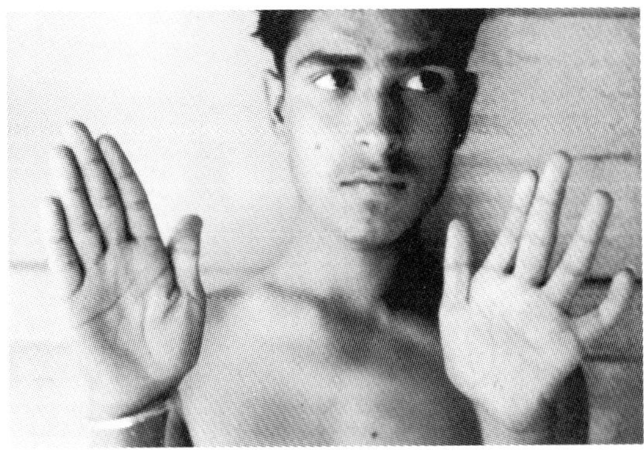

Fig. 7.9A: Clawing tendency of little and ring fingers (due to ulnar nerve paralysis) pateint is unable to adduct little and ring fingers

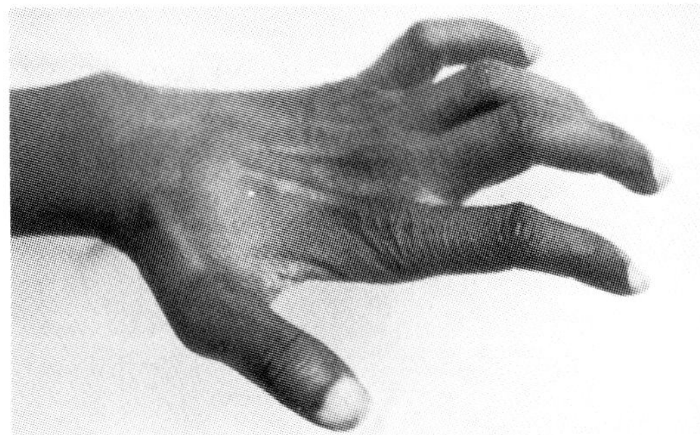

Fig. 7.9B: Intrinsic minus type of claw hand due to ulnar-median nerves paralysis

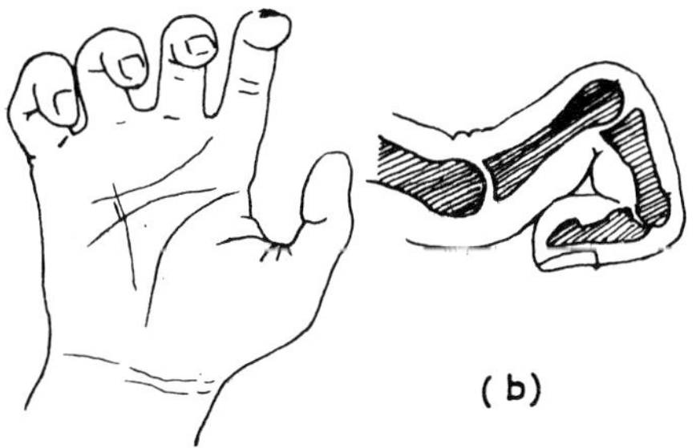

Fig. 7.9C: Intrinsic minus hand

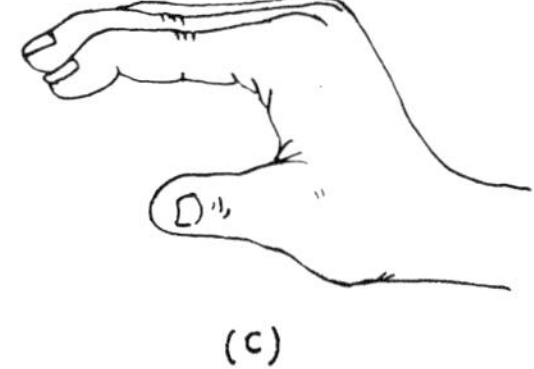

Fig. 7.9D: Intrinsic plus hand

c. A concept of 'intrinsic zero' has been developed (Srinivasan 1979), where both the lumbrical and interosseous muscles are paralysed. The extensor of the finger acts alone to produce both excessive extension of the metacarpophalangeal joint, and incomplete extension of the interphalangeal joint, thus resulting in a claw deformity.

Srinivasan (1979), has kept fingers, with paralysis of the interosseous muscle, but with functioning lumbrical, in the 'intrinsic minus' group.

Test for Intrinsic Plus Hand

The initial or mild 'intrinsic plus' hand, which may not be producing an obvious deformity can be tested by the following method.

Push the metacarpophalangeal joint into hyperextension to stretch the intrinsics. Now passively try to flex the distal interphalangeal joint. This will be very difficult, or even impossible.

Reverse Intrinsic Plus Test

In tightness of the extensor tendon or instability of the proximal interphalangeal joint, the central slip of the extensor attachment can be relaxed by hyperextending the metacarpophalangeal joint. This allows the lateral slips to descend, resulting in flexion of the proximal interphalangeal joint.

Typical, or similar to, claw hand deformity can occur in several conditions due to lesions in:

i. Cerebral cortex—cerebral palsy, tumours, hemiplegia.
ii. Spinal cord—poliomyelitis, syringomyelia, progressive muscular atrophy, motor neuron disease.
iii. Spinal roots (C_8 T_1) and brachial plexus—Klumpke's paralysis.
iv. Peripheral nerves—ulnar and median nerve paralysis.
v. Muscular affections—myopathy.
vi. Vascular affections—Volkmann's ischaemic contracture.

vii. Arteriosclerotic diseases—as in Raynaud's disease and in professionals using vibrating tools.
viii. Subcutaneous tissue and skin—congenital or burn contracture.
ix. Miscellaneous—disuse atrophy, rheumatoid arthritis, Sudeck's osteodystrophy, post-infective contractures, post-traumatic contractures.

7. Ulnar/radial deviation of the wrist and ulnar deviation of the fingers in rheumatoid arthritis (Figs 7.10A and B).

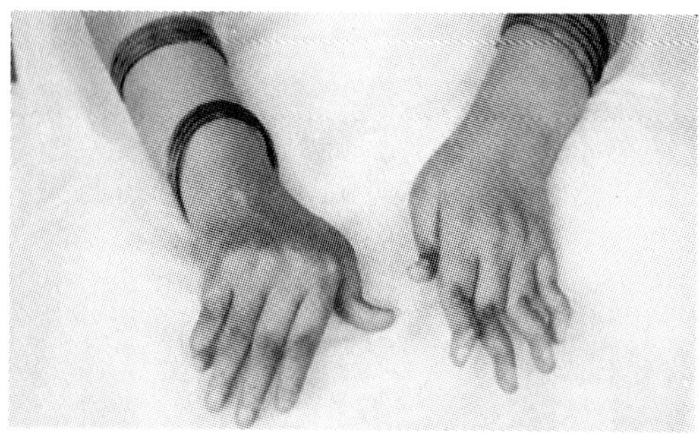

Fig. 7.10A: Typical rheumatoid hand. Note ulnar deviation at wrist, swan neck deformity of fingers, boutonniere deformity of right little finger, ulnar deviation of fingers

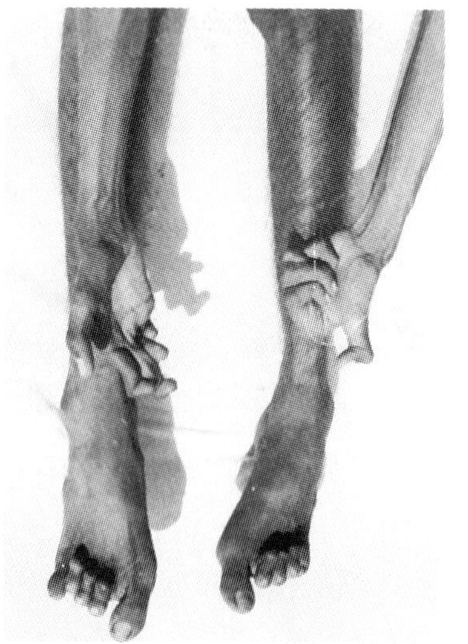

Fig. 7.10B: Sometimes bizarre deformities develop in hands and feet

8. Finger drop (Fig. 7.11) due to spontaneous rupture of the extensor tendon, usually at the wrist (e.g. rheumatoid arthritis).

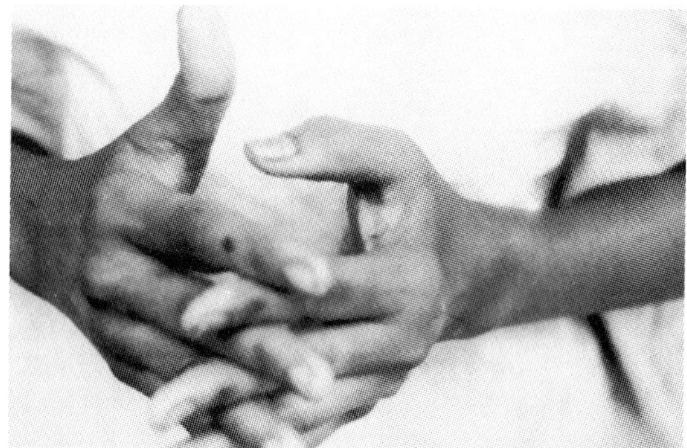

Fig. 7.11: Drop thumb deformity (left) due to rupture of extensor pollicis longus tendon in old rheumatoid arthritis. (also called *drummer's palsy* when it occurs in malunited Colles fracture due to friction attrition on the tendon)

9. Swan neck deformity: (Figs 7.10 and 7.12A) This deformity is common in rheumatoid arthritis in ladies. In this condition, there is flexion at the distal interphalangeal joint and hyperextension at the proximal interphalangeal joint.

10. Button hole or boutonniere deformity (Figs 7.10A and 7.12B): Due to rupture of the central slip, the lateral bands drop volar to the axis of the proximal interphalangeal joint. Then they become flexors of the proximal interphalangeal joint as the joint buttonholes through the rupture. Here there is flexion deformity at the proximal interphalangeal joint and hyperextension at the distal interphalangeal joint (e.g. rheumatoid arthritis).

11. Hooding deformity (in leprosy Fig. 7.12C): It consists of flexion at the proximal interphalangeal joint and either straight or hyperextended position of the distal interphalangeal joint.

Test for the presence of hooding deformity—Passively extend the fingers at the proximal interphalangeal joints and then attempt flexion of the distal interphalangeal joints. In the extended position, the distal joint presents marked resistance to flexion, whereas in flexed position of the proximal interphalangeal joint, it flexes easily.

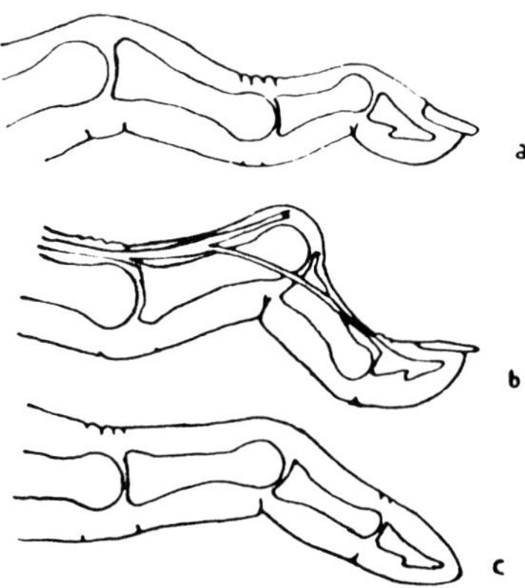

Figs 7.12A to C: Deformities of finger: (a) Swan neck deformity, (b) Boutonniere deformity, (c) Hooding deformity

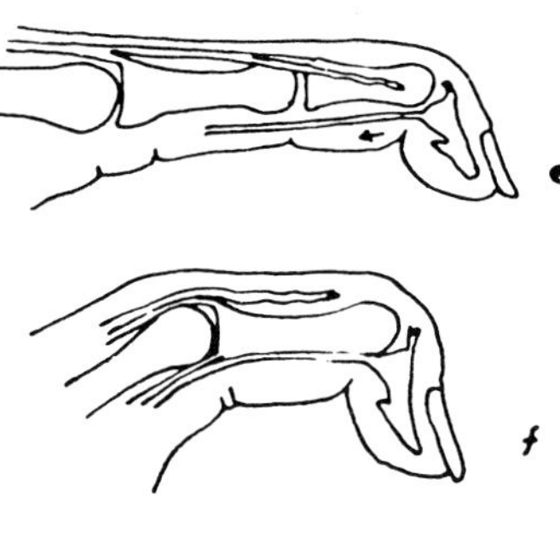

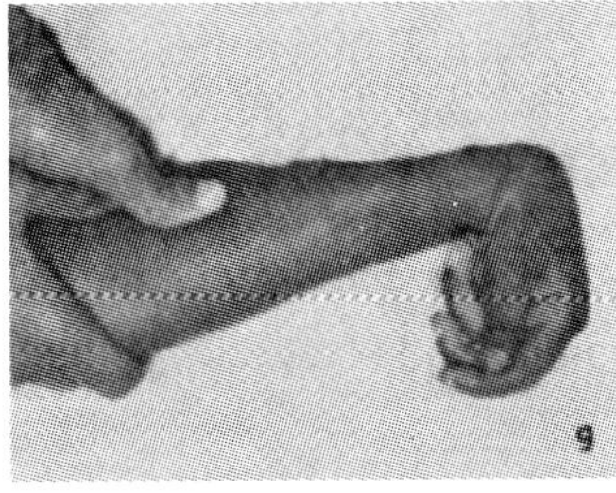

Figs 7.12E to G: (E) Mallet finger, (F) Mallet thumb, (G) Thumb in palm deformity due to cerebral palsy

12. Attitudes and deformities due to peripheral nerve paralysis:

a. *Wrist Drop*

In complete radial nerve paralysis, there is obvious wrist drop. Here the patient cannot dorsiflex the wrist; he cannot abduct the thumb, nor can he extend the thumb and the fingers

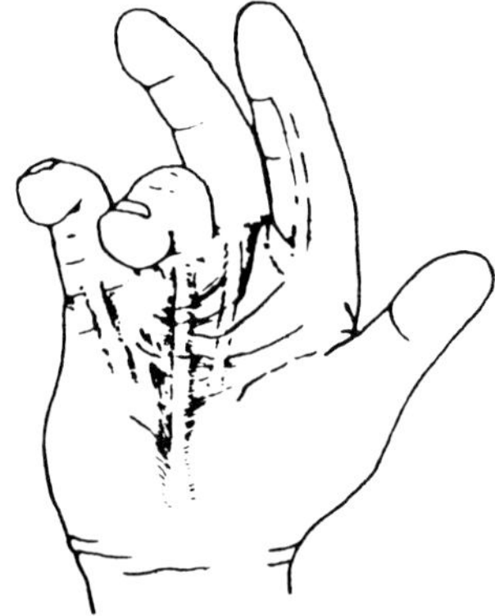

Fig. 7.12D1: Dupuytren's contracture

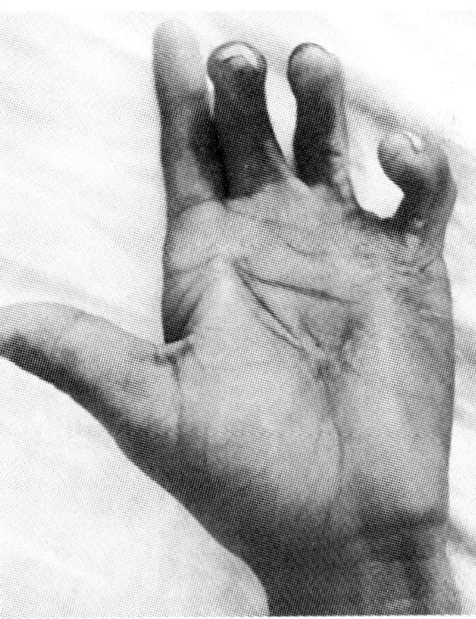

Fig. 7.12D2: Dupuytren's contracture of left hand with middle, index and little fingers markedly affected but affection of index finger is in early stage

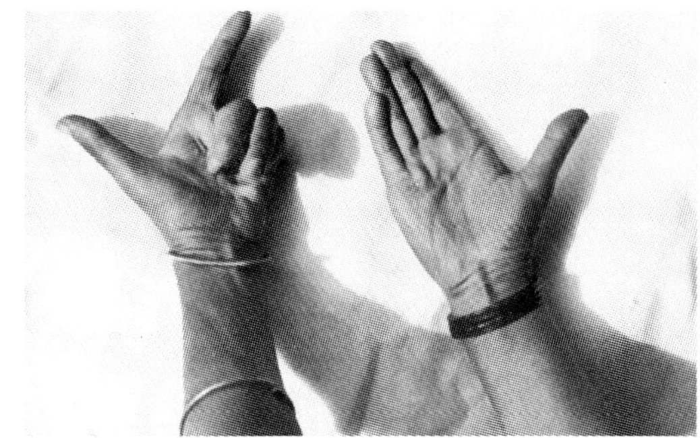

Fig. 7.12D3: Dupuytren's contracture in both hands—left is markedly affected with three fingers acutely flexed. On the right hand there is initial stage of affection of little, ring and middle finger

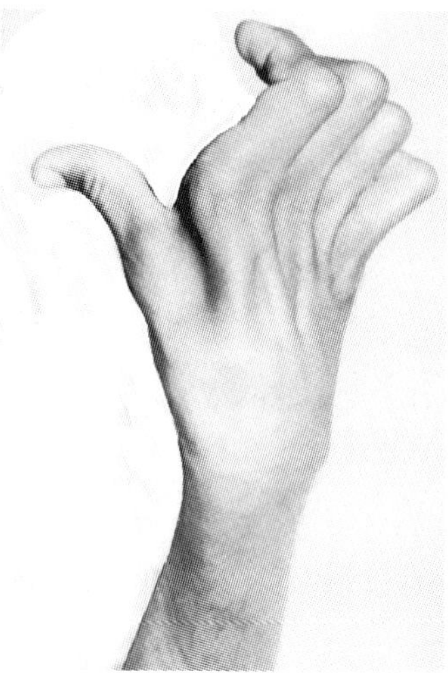

Fig. 7.13: Complete claw (combined ulnar and median nerve affections)

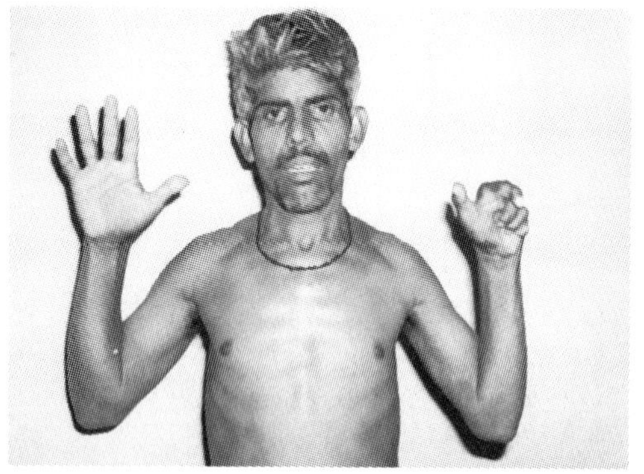

Fig. 7.14: Neglected spastic flexion deformities of fingers in residual hemiplegia

at the metacarpophalangeal joint. The attitude of the hand remains in palmar-flexion.

b. *Benediction Attitude*

In median nerve paralysis, the attitude of the hand may be typical. In long standing cases, there may be ape thumb besides wasting of the thenar eminence (Simian thumb). In this condition, the thumb lies in the same plane as that of the fingers and palm, like that of an ape. If the patient is asked to make a fist, the index finger remains prominently extended (Benediction attitude/pointing index).

c. *Claw Hand*

In ulnar nerve paralysis, besides wasting of hypothenar eminence, the webs, as well as the intermetacarpal spaces (which are prominent from the dorsal aspect of the hand) the typical attitude of 'claw hand' develops, affecting the little and ring fingers. When the affection of ulnar and median nerves are combined (e.g. in leprosy), clawing of all the four fingers develops (Fig. 7.13).

13. In *Dupuytren's contracture* (Figs 7.12D1 to D3): Dupuytren's contracture is the progressive contracture of the fingers due to contraction of the palmar fascia, Baron Dupuytren (1833) was the first to identify the cause and perform successful surgical release.

Dupuytren's contracture is more likely to occur in alcoholics and diabetics. It may be associated with *Peyrenei's disease* (fibrous contracture in plantar fascia leading to deformities—plantar fibromatosis), knuckle pads, *Ledderhose's disease* (fibrous contracture of penis, plastic induration of penis).

The initial stage can be apparent in *'table top sign'*—i.e. ask the patient to keep the palm flat on the table, the affected finger will not touch the table all through and stand's buckled back. There may be clawing tendency of the fingers but here the flexion element mainly prevails at the metacarpophalangeal joint and the proximal interphalangeal joint and rarely, the distal interphalangeal joint. This usually affects the ring finger but the little, middle, index or even thumb may also be affected in that order.

14. There is a typical attitude of the *hand in brachial palsy.* In the distal type (i.e. Klumpke's type (C_8, T_1) the hand is in intrinsic minus claw hand position. In the proximal type (i.e. Erb's palsy), the hand remains in policeman's tip position, i.e. shoulder adducted and internally rotated, elbow extended, forearm pronated, wrist partially flexed, thumb in palm and fingers semiflexed.

15. *Mallet finger* (Fig. 7.12E): It results from avulsion or rupture of the extensor digitorum

tendon at the base of the terminal phalanx. Due to unopposed action of the flexor digitorum profundus, the finger gets flexed at the distal interphalangeal joint.

16. *Mallet thumb* (Goose neck deformity) (Fig. 7.12F): Mallet thumb results from rupture of the extensor pollicis longus tendon (usually a late complication of Colles' fracture, rheumatoid arthritis).

17. *Trigger finger:* Due to fibrotic thickening and constriction of the fibrous flexor sheath of the long tendons, the patient (usually a female in her forties), complains of pain at the root of a finger (mostly ring and middle) or thumb with or without locking of the finger/or thumb in flexion. If hand is opened up from a clenched position, then the affected finger remains flexed. With more forceful effort or while passively opening by other hand, it may be extended with a jerky release and often with a palpable and/or audible click. A firm tender nodule is felt in front of the metacarpophalangeal joint. It may be bilateral. Trigger thumb has been seen to produce locked flexion effect in babies (misdiagnosed as dislocation).

18. *Jersey finger*: It results from avulsion of the flexor digitorum profundus (usually of ring finger, but any digit may be involved) from its insertion on the distal phalanx. It usually occurs in young males playing football and rugby. In an attempt of grasping the jersey of any opponent player, the distal interphalangeal joint is forcibly extended.

19. Thumb-in palm deformity (Fig 7.12G): It is usually seen in patients of cerebral palsy and stroke. The thumb is adducted and flexed into the palm, and this tendency is exaggerated by any activity.

Sakellarides and Mitall (1984) have classified this deformity into four types. Thus, it can be due to:

i. Weak or paralysed extensor pollicis longus.
ii. Spasticity or contracture of the adductor pollicis.
iii. Weakness or paralysis of the abductor pollicis longus.
iv. Spasticity or contracture of the flexor pollicis longus.

In neglected hemiplegia, there may be spastic flexion deformities of fingers (Fig. 7.14).

Inspection

The domain of the hand starts from the distal transverse crease in front of the wrist to the finger tips. Inspect both the hands in symmetrical position. Note the number (supernumerary fingers); relative length [(Marfan's syndrome—described by French paediatrician Marfan in 1896 who named it dolichostemelia (= long, thin limb)—and is characterized by long thin limbs, generalised joint laxity, dislocation of lenses, dissecting aortic aneurysm, prolapsed cardiac valves, increased prevalence of hernia,—spider fingers and toes—the fingers and toes are very long and thin—arachnodactyly (= in the form of a spider)]; achondroplasia—trident hand—fingers are short, stubby and equal in length); and size of the fingers (in gigantism, the hand and fingers are enlarged and elongated). Note the shape; size; normal anatomical bulges and creases, e.g hypothenar eminence, thenar eminence, hollow of the palm, creases across the palm (in Down's syndrome there is only one palmar crease), creases on the finger and finger pulps; the web condition (e.g. for syndactylism, club hand) and presence of any nodule. Skin should be inspected for its colour, texture and for presence of callosities. Inspect the tips of the fingers and thumb, regarding shape, presence of any deformity, atrophy, broadening, and also the nailbeds (shape, colour, brittleness, atrophy or degeneration of nails).

On the dorsum of the hand look for any swelling, condition of venous arches, knuckle (alignment and prominence when patient makes a fist), interosseous spaces and the webs.

The phalanges and joints of the fingers, and hand should be inspected from all aspects.

Inspect the hand with fully extended and fully flexed fingers. The fully flexed fingers normally point towards the scaphoid, and their nails lie in one plane. Note any abnormality.

Palpation

Superficial Palpation

Feel for the texture and, sensation of the skin (hypoaesthesia, hyperaesthesia, paraesthesia or anaesthesia).

Palpate the finger pulps for texture and/or tenderness and nailbeds for refilling of capillaries and for any tenderness.

Palpate the webs individually (specially the first web) and note its bulk, looseness and stretchability.

Deep Palpation

Feel for any abnormality, specially for thickening and deep tenderness in the palm, the webs, the metacarpals (from dorsal and palmar aspects), the metacarpophalangeal joints, the interphalangeal joints, the phalanges and the fingers and thumb tips. In *glomus tumour* there is excruciating pain if pointed pressure is applied on the overlying nail. Abnormal findings (like swellings, ulcers) must be examined thoroughly. Feel for presence of any nodule in the line of tendons, mainly at the base of the thumb and finger, specially ring and middle—trigger thumb or finger. To confirm regarding its fixity to the tendon, ask the patient to contract the concerned tendon and ascertain the fixity of the nodule to it. On deep pressure, the nodule is tender.

Infections of the hand may remain masked for varying periods. Since the fascial spaces are quite close and tight and the skin of the palm is quite thick and tough, pus usually takes a long time to come on the surface. The manifestations are usually:

i. Constitutional features.
ii. Swelling on the dorsum of hand.
iii. Throbbing pain in the hand.

Depending upon the place for pus collection, the site of maximum tenderness can be localised (Fig. 7.15) (in whitlow, Fig. 7.15a) pulp of the terminal phalanx; Felon (Fig. 7.15b) (an abscess of the finger tip pulp)—finger tip (Fig. 7.15a); in paronychia (infection of the eponychial fold)—on dorso-lateral aspects and proximal to the nail root; in infection of the flexor sheaths of the fingers—direct pressure on the centre of the finger from the palmar aspect; in web infection—about 1 cm proximal to the web margin on the palmar aspect; in ulnar bursa infection—near about the centre of the ulnar margin of the palm; in case of the radial bursa—at about the most prominent point of centre of thenar eminence).

Tenderness in the palm should be localised either by a match stick or by a blunt pencil point (Fig. 7.15).

It is not easy to demonstrate fluctuation in infections on the palmar aspect. However, in case of any suspicious swelling on the dorsum of the hand, fluctuation and induration must be demonstrated before labelling it as a pus collection. As such, any infection or trauma of the hand does manifest as swelling on dorsum of the hand. This is because the subcutaneous tissue on the dorsum is quite loose and the lymphatics of the palm drain into the dorsum.

MOVEMENTS (Tables 7.1 and 7.2)

For all practical purposes, movements of the hand mean movements of the thumb and fingers.

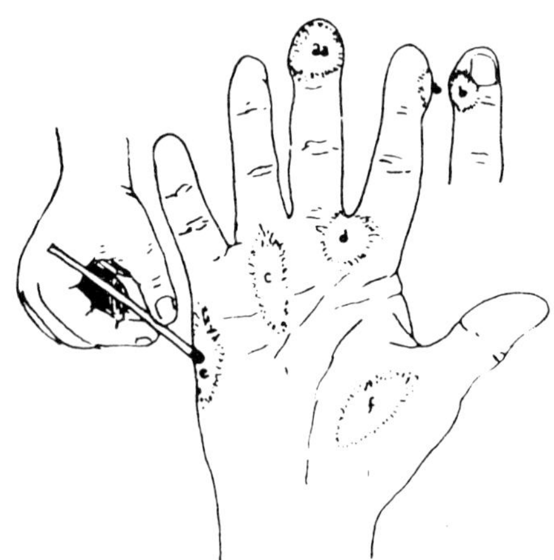

Fig. 7.15: Eliciting tenderness for infections of the hand. a = whitlow, b = paronychia, c = flexor sheath of finger, d = web infection, e = ulnar bursal infection, f = radial bursal infection

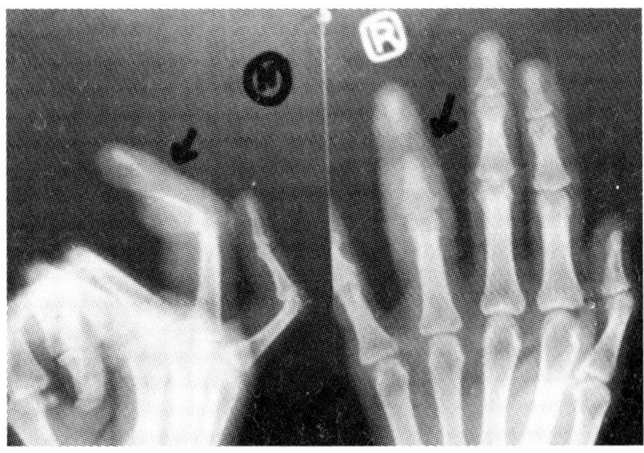

Fig. 7.15A: Pyogenic abscess of finger tip which led to pyogenic arthritis of DIP joint and osteomyelitis of middle and terminal phalanges

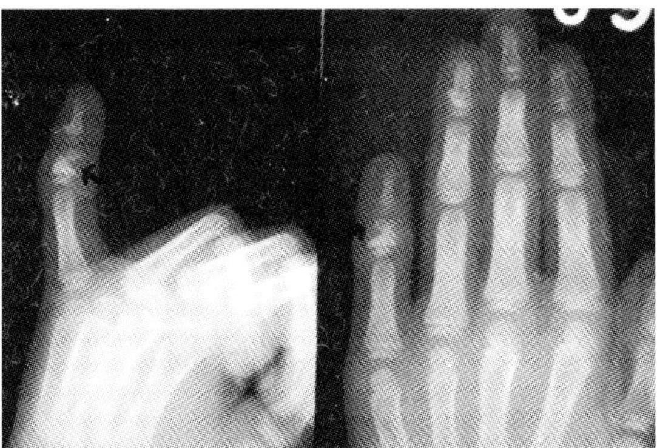

Fig. 7.15B: Destruction of middle phalanax of little finger due to pyogenic osteomyelitis in infant

The movements at the smaller intercarpal, carpometacarpal and inter-metacarpal joints are negligible from the clinical point of view.

GROSS ASSESSMENT OF MOVEMENTS OF THE HAND

Ask the patient to put both hands in the shape of a cup (cupping). They should be bilaterally symmetrical. Any lag in cupping may be due to:

(i) Wasting of the smaller muscles of the hand, especially at thenar and hypothenar regions.

(ii) Lack of movements at the intercarpal, carpometacarpal, intermetacarpal and metacarpophalangeal joints.

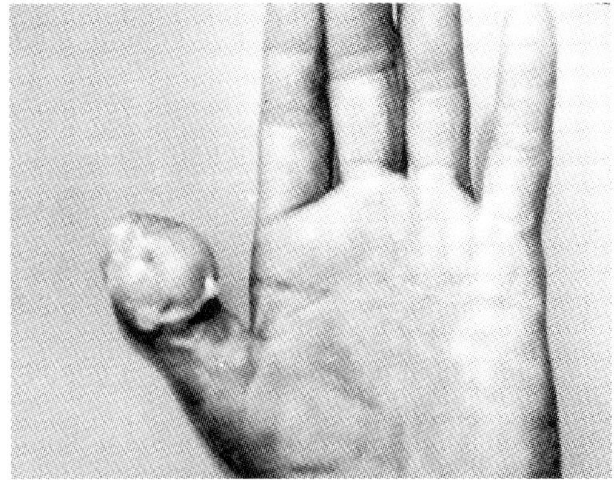

Fig. 7.15C1: Felon of thumb

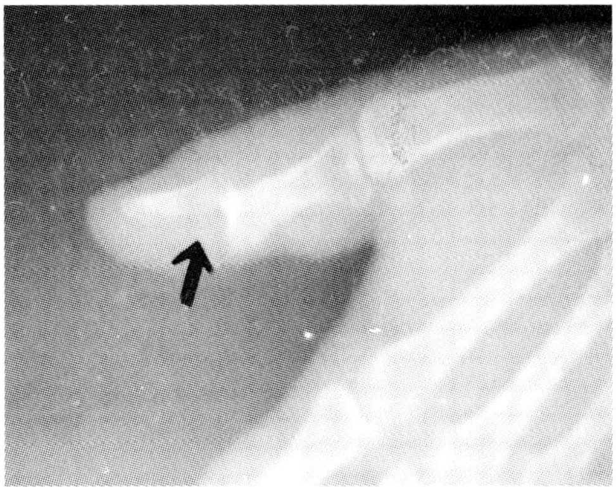

Fig. 7.15C2: Whitlow of thumb leading to pyogenic osteomyelitis of terminal phalanx and pyogenic arthritis of interphalangeal joint

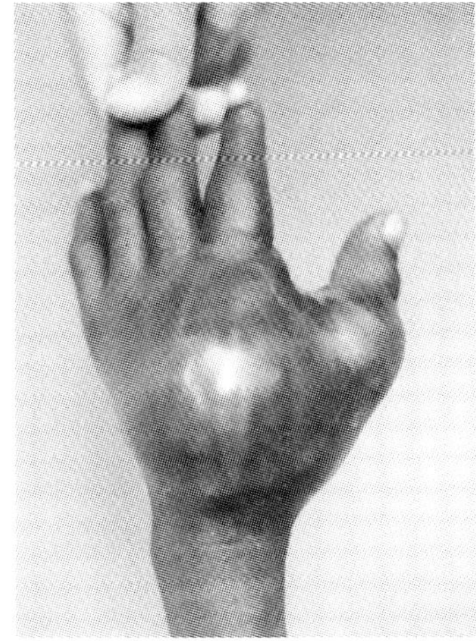

Fig. 7.15D: Pyogenic abscess along the extensor tendons of thumb and index finger

Table 7.1: Movements of the thumb

Movements	*Normal range*	*Muscle concerned*	*Root control*	*Factor limiting movement*	*Joint of action*	*How to test*
1	*2*	*3*	*4*	*5*	*6*	*7*
Abduction	0°-60°	Abductor pollicis longus, abductor pollicis brevis	$C_{6,7}$	Tension of skin between thumb and index finger and tension of first dorsal interosseous muscle	Primarily at carpometacarpal joint, also at metacarpophalangeal joint	From thumb lying close to radial border of palm, ask the patient to open the web without producing any stretch or squeeze of the palmar skin (Fig. 7.16A)
Adduction	60°-0°	Adductor pollicis (oblique and transverse heads)	$C_8.T_1$	The contact of ulnar border of thumb with radial border of palm	-do-	From fully abducted position, as in above, ask the patient to close the web without producing any tension or squeezing of the dorsal skin (Fig. 7.16A)
Flexion: Metacarpophalangeal joint	0°-60°	Flexor pollicis brevis	$C_{6,7,8}$	Tension of extensor tendons of thumb	Metacarpophalangeal joint	With patient's hand resting on a table gently press over the thenar eminence. Ask the patient to bring the first phalanx of thumb towards palm, from position of easy stretch. (Fig. 7.16B)
Flexion: Carpometacarpal joint Interphalangeal joint	0°-80°-90° 0°-15°	Flexor pollicis longus	C_8T_1	—	Interphalangeal joint	Hold the first phalanx from the sides. Ask the patient to bring pulp of thumb towards the palm (Fig. 7.16C)
Extension: Metacarpophalangeal joint	60°-0°	Extensor pollicis brevis	C_7	Tension of palmar and collateral ligaments of thumb	Metacarpophalangeal joint	From fully flexed position as in above, patient is asked to bring back the first phalanx towards stretched position (Fig. 7.16B)
Extension: Interphalangeal joint	90°-0°	Extensor pollicis longus	C_7	—	Interphalangeal joint	From fully flexed position, ask the patient to bring back the distal phalanx to extended position (Fig. 7.16C)
Opposition: Palmar aspect of pulp of thumb rests on palmar aspect of pulp of little finger		Opponens pollicis, Opponens digiti minimi	$C_{6,7,8}$	Tension of transverse metacarpal ligament, tension of extensor tendons of thumb and little finger	Metacarpophalangeal, Carpometacarpal and intercarpal joints.	The stretched thumb and little finger are brought across the palm to touch palmar aspects of terminal phalanx (Fig. 7.16D)
Circumduction: When all movements are free, then only possible						Ask the patient to rotate the thumb so as to make a circle in the air by its tip (Fig. 7.16E)

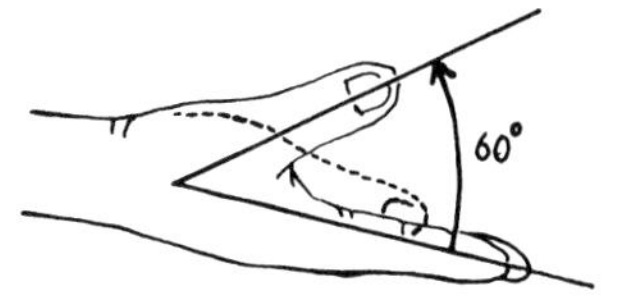

Fig. 7.16A: Abduction and adduction of thumb

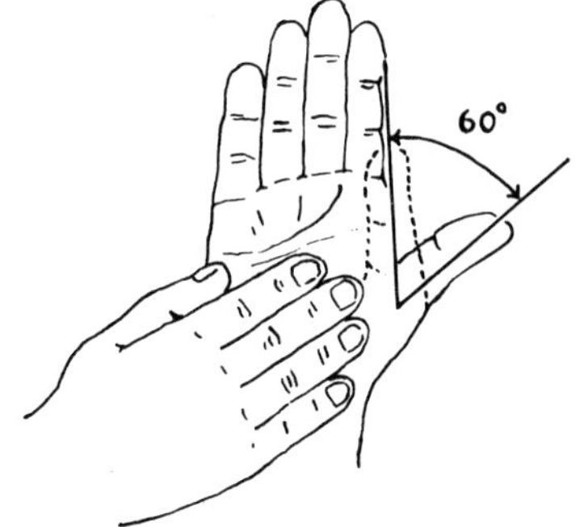

Fig. 7.16B: Flexion and extension at MP joint

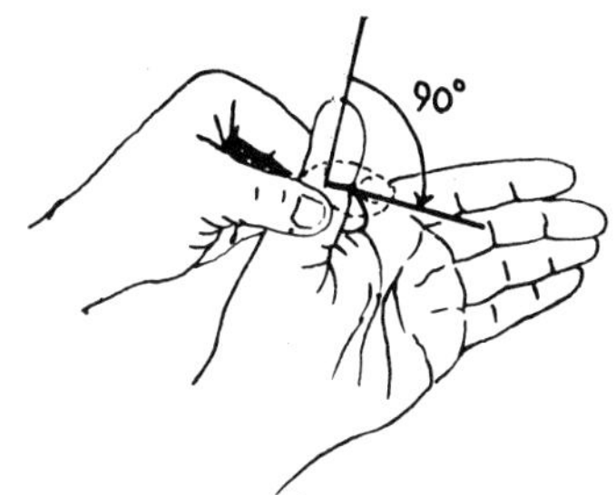

Fig. 7.16C: Flexion and extension at IP joint

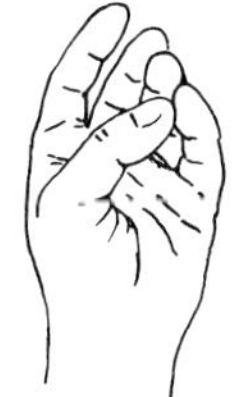

Fig. 7.16D: Opposition

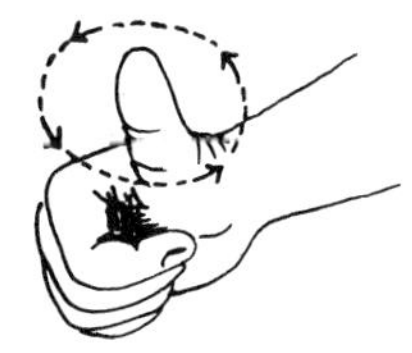

Fig. 7.16E: Circumduction

(iii) Mechanical obstruction due to lesions in the palm, either following trauma, infection or neoplasm.

Gross movements of the hand can be further tested by asking him to make a firm fist (Fig. 7.3A). A firm fist indicates almost normal movements of the hand.

Ask the patient to hold a pen (Fig. 7.3B) in writing position. A normal hold indicates normal functioning of the intrinsics as well as a fairly good range of motion of the thumb, index, middle, ring and little fingers in that order.

Movements of the Thumb (Table 7.1)

Clinicoanatomically, normal movements of the thumb may be grouped as:

i. Abduction
ii. Flexion
iii. Extension
iv. Adduction
v. Opposition
vi. Circumduction.

Some Important Points about Thumb

- In most of the movements of the hand, the thumb acts as an active partner (functionally thumb is 40% of the hand), while the other fingers along with the palm remain comparatively passive.
- Thumb has only one inter-phalangeal joint. Hence, most of its movements are subserved at its metacarpophalangeal and carpometacarpal joint. No wonder, these sites are predisposed to primary osteoarthritis.
- In an outstretched hand, the thumb is placed at about 80°-90° of abduction and some extension to initiate and facilitate grasp, catch, pinch and opposition movements.
- Zero position of the thumb will vary according to the axis of the movement concerned.
- The movements of the thumb and fingers should also be noted, as in the chapter of Introduction as far as practicable.

No examination of the hand is complete without repeated assessments for neurovascular integrity. Of course, sensibility to touch in the fingers is a most useful index of the adequacy of circulation.

Special Tests

1. Test for intrinsic plus hand—See page 133.
2. Test for hooding deformity—See page 134.

Table 7.2: Movements of fingers

Movements	*Normal range*	*Muscle concerned*	*Root control*	*Factors limiting movement*	*Joint of action*	*How to test*
1	*2*	*3*	*4*	*5*	*6*	*7*
Flexion: Metacarpophalangeal joint.	0°-90°	Lumbricals, dorsal and palmar interossei. Long flexor of fingers can also influence metacarpophalangeal joint to produce flexion.	$C_{6,7,8}$, T_1	Tension of extensor tendon expansion of the fingers	Metacarpophalangeal joint	Patient rests the dorsal aspect of the hand on table. Fix the metacarpals by your fingers at about proximal transverse palmar crease. Ask the patient to flex the extended finger to the maximum (Fig. 7.18)
Flexion: Proximal interphalangeal joint	0°-120°	Flexor digitorum sublimis and profundus	$C_{7,8}$, T_1	Tension of expansion of extensor digitorum tendons	Proximal interphalangeal joint	Fix the proximal phalanx between your thumb and index finger. Ask the patient to bend finger just beyond your thumb (Fig. 7.19)
Flexion: Distal interphalangeal joint	0°-80°	Flexor digitorum profundus	C_8, T_1	Dorsal ligaments of distal interphalangeal joint	Distal interphalangeal joint.	Hold the middle phalanx between thumb and finger. Ask the patient to bend the finger just beyond your thumb (Fig. 7.20)
Extension: Extension at metacarpophalangeal joint not possible beyond zero position. Hence range will be flexion to zero position. In certain individuals, probably, due to laxity of the ligaments, varying degree of hyperextension may be possible at MPJ and/or PPJ (Fig. 7.17)	0°-30° (hyperextension).	Extensor digitorum, extensor indicis for index finger and extensor digiti minimi for little finger.	C_7	Palmar and collateral ligaments Flexor muscles of fingers	Metacarpophalangeal joint.	Place the hand, resting on its ulnar border, on the table. Fingers being stretched more or less in the line of posterior surface of forearm. Fix the metacarpals (in between your thumb and fingers). Ask the patient to take extended finger (at interphalangeal joint) as far back as possible (Fig. 7.21)
Hyperextension—at distal interphalangeal joint.	0°-10°					

Contd.

Table 7.2: Contd.

Movements	Normal range	Muscle concerned	Root control	Factors limiting movement	Joint of action	How to test
1	2	3	4	5	6	7
Abduction	0°-25°	Dorsal interossei, abductor digiti minim: for little finger	C_8 T_1	Tension on skin and fascia in between the fingers	Metacarpo-phalangeal joint, carpo-metacarpal joint	Hold the tip of extended middle finger, with mild traction. Ask the patient to take finger (to be tested) away from middle finger in transverse direction (side ways), (Fig. 7.22). (Central axis of extended middle finger will be the zero position).
Adduction	25°-0°	Palmar interossei	C_8T_1	Contact of fingers	Metacarpo-phalangeal joint, car-pometacarpal joint.	After testing for abduction, ask the patient to approximate the fingers along the transverse axis (Fig. 7.22)

Testing for the flexor digitorum sublimis—Full flexion at the PIP, while other fingers are held in extension (which inactivates the flexor digitorum profundus) indicates intact flexor digitorum sublimis.

The flexon digitorum profundus muscles seperate for each finger more distally than the sublimis, whose individual finger bellies seperate higher. Hence profundus has mass action bellies.

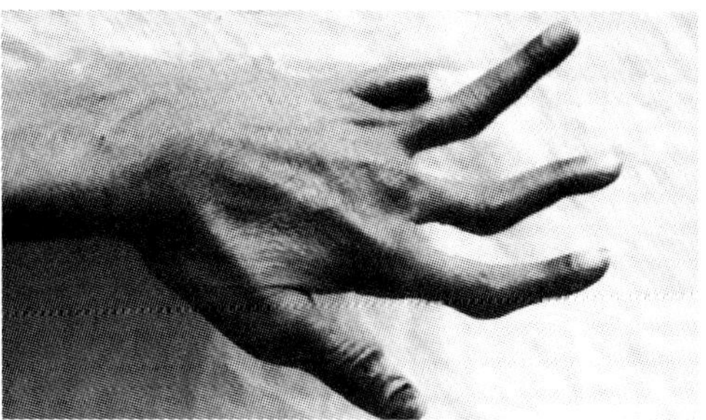

Fig. 7.17: Hyperextension at PIPJ

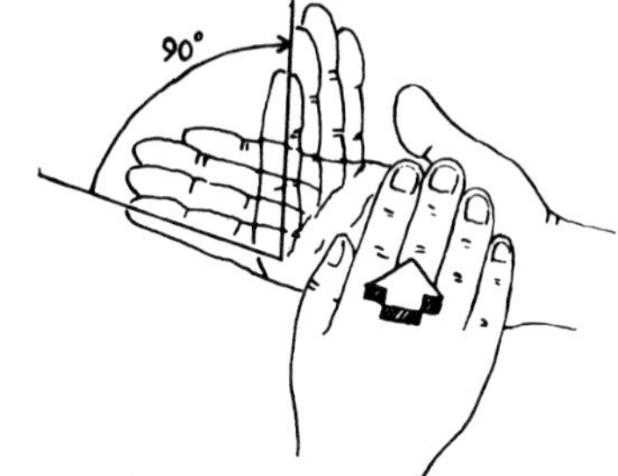

Fig. 7.18: Testing for flexion and extension at MP joint

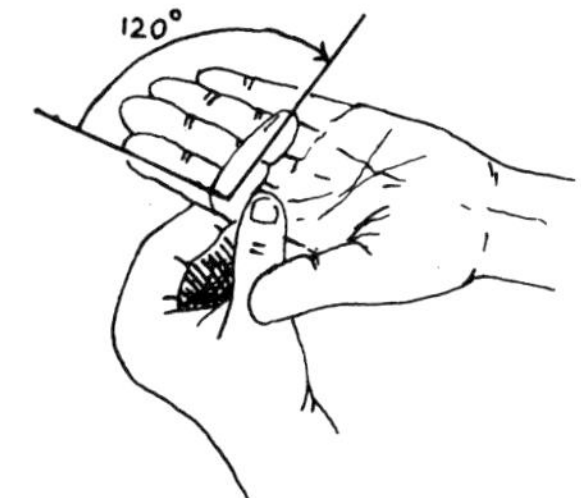

Fig. 7.19: Testing for flexion/extension at PIP joint

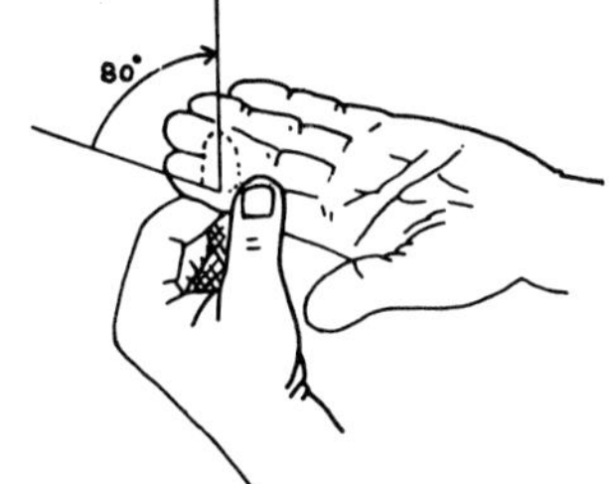

Fig. 7.20: Testing for flexion/extension at DIP joint

3. Test for intrinsic minus hand—as follows: Deficient intrinsic action is mainly due to weakness of the interossei.

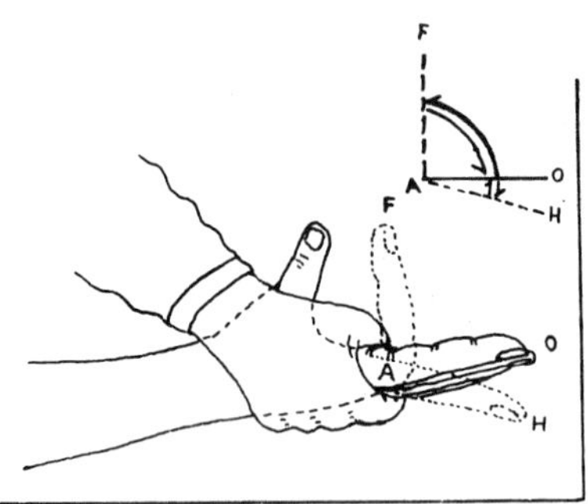

Fig. 7.21: Testing for hyperextension at MP joint

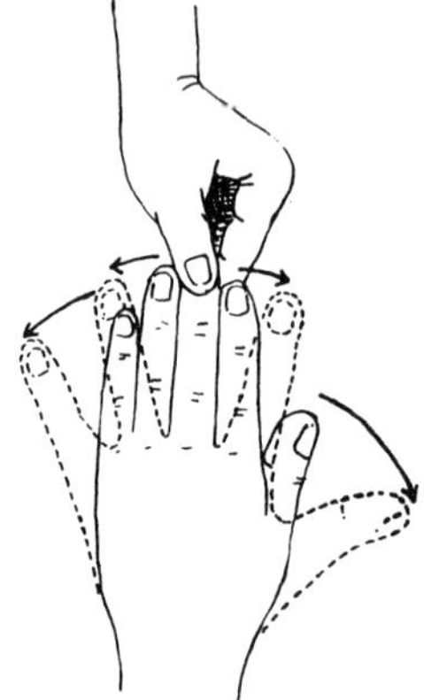

Fig. 7.22: Testing for abduction and adduction of fingers

Test: The patient will not be able to abduct or adduct the fingers (the middle finger being the axis).

Further, conjoint action of the lumbricals and interossei, i.e. flexion at metacarpophalangeal joint and extension at the interphalangeal joints will also be affected to a varying extent.

The patient is asked to stretch both his hands, keeping the fingers extended and closetted to each other, if possible (with deficiency of interossei there will be lag in adduction of the fingers). Further, he is asked to flex and extend the fingers at the metacarpophalangeal joints in quick succession. Any weakness of the intrinsics will manifest by lag in flexing the extended finger.

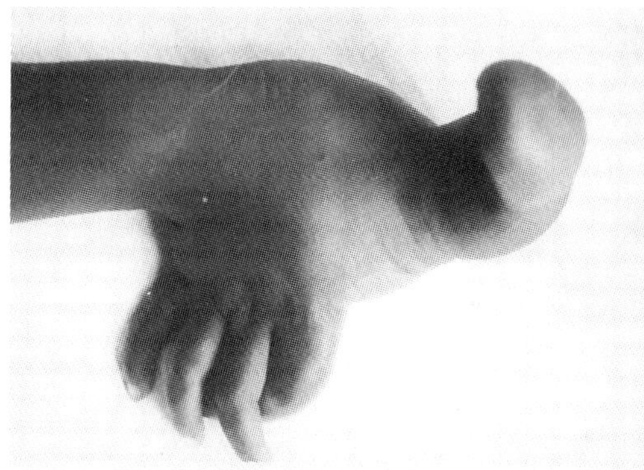

Fig. 7.23A: Hyperplasia of thumb

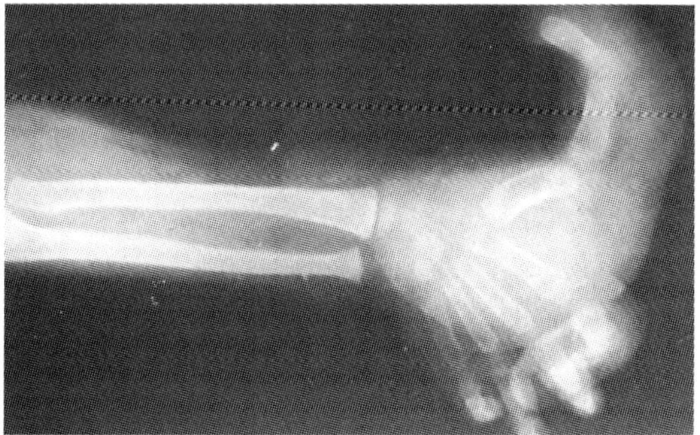

Fig. 7.23B: Radiograph of hyperplasia of thumb

4. Test for isolated division of flexor digitorum sublimis tendon:

Hold the adjacent fingers in full extension and ask the patient to flex the concerned proximal interphalangeal joint. This will not be possible, if the flexor digitorum sublimis is divided. The flexor dititorum profundus will not help in this action, since it gets anchored in extension with other fingers.

INVESTIGATION

1. General investigations.
2. Radiological investigations.

Antero-posterior and lateral views of hands and fingers, in maximum opened up position, are essential.

For taking a lateral view of the individual finger, the other fingers should be flexed into the palm as far as practicable, while the fingers

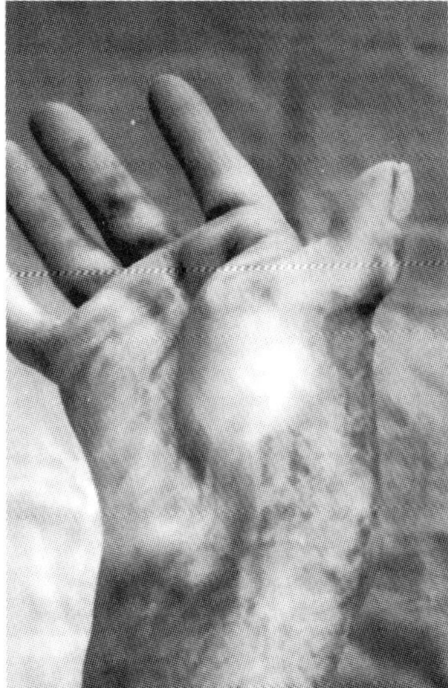

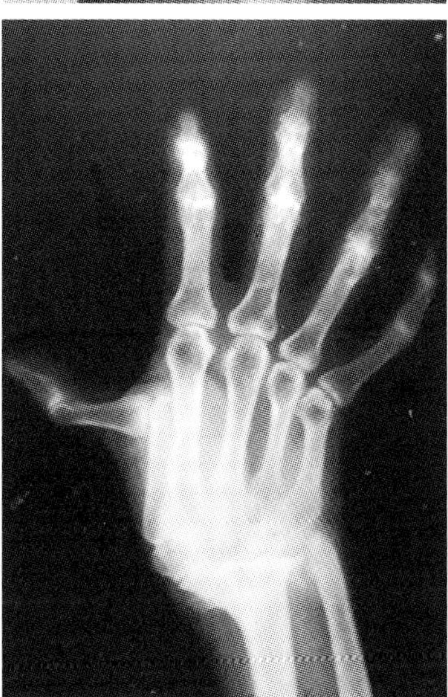

Figs 7.24A and B: Seven years old unreduced dislocation of thumb

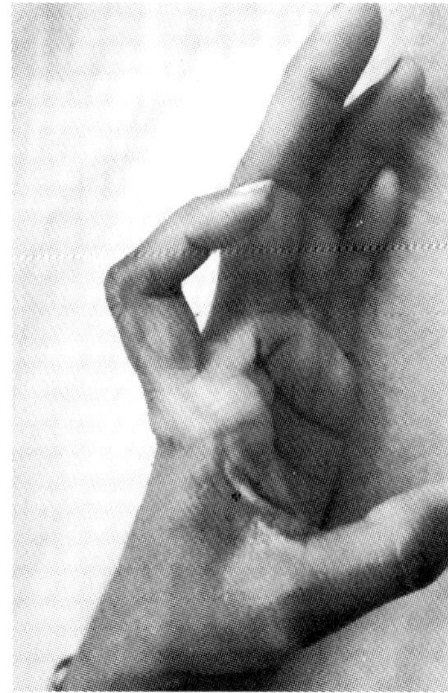

Fig. 7.24C: One year old unreduced dislocation of little finger

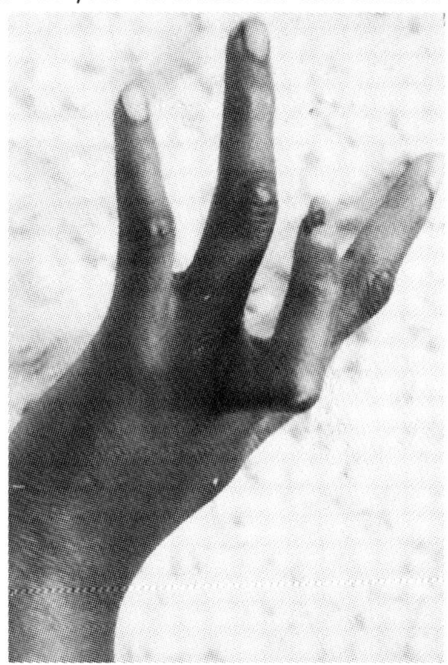

Fig. 7.24D: Three years old unreduced dislocation of middle finger

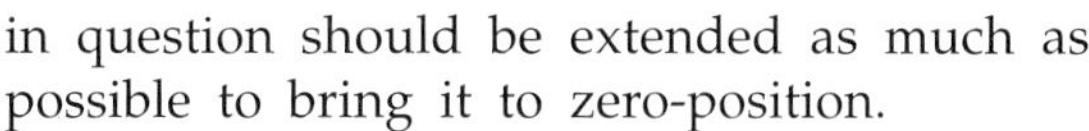

in question should be extended as much as possible to bring it to zero-position.

3. Hand print, as a whole and prints of the thumb and finger pulps:

These are not only important from genetic and medicolegal point of view, but also for medical records. They also demonstrate the shape and size of hand and fingers, along with any deformities.

Traumatic conditions of the hand need careful clinical evaluation and proper investigations (both for soft tissues and bony injuries). Several of them (e.g. dislocations of small joints, fractures of the phalanges, and metacarpals tender injuries etc) are likely to be missed initially due to post-traumatic gross swelling of the hand. If missed, they can produce various deformities which hamper the hand functions (Figs 7.24A to D).

BIBLIOGRAPHY

1. Bunnel S: *Surgery of the Hand* (5th ed) JB Lippincott: Philadelphia, 1970.
2. James, JIP: Assessment and management of the injured hands. *The Hand* **2**: 97, 1970.
3. Lampe EW: Surgical anatomy. Ciba Clinical Symposia **9(1)**: 3, 1957.

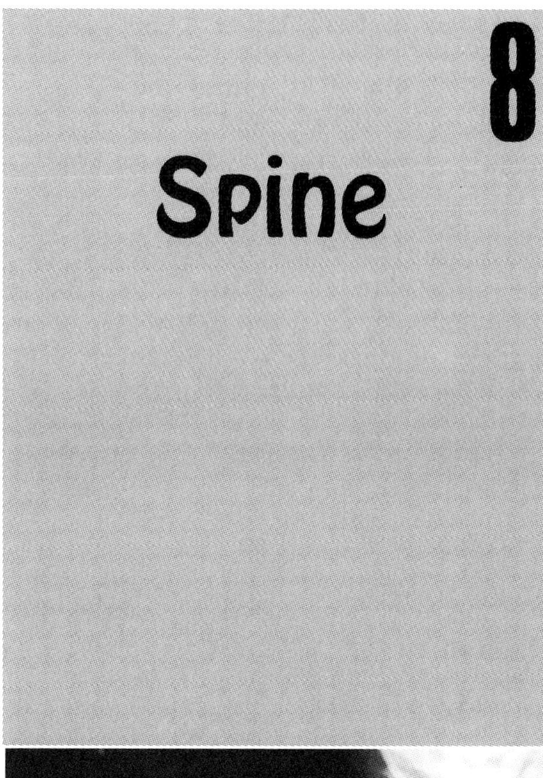

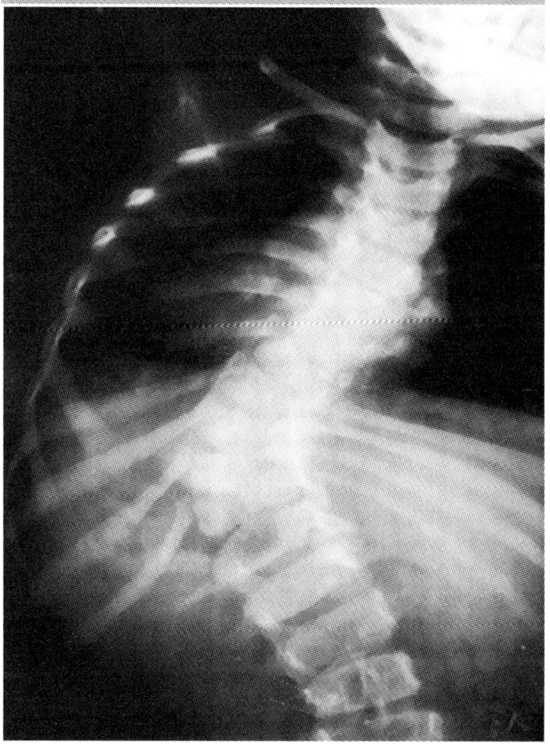

INTRODUCTION

Skeletal system basically comprises of:

A. Axial skeleton—consisting of axial structures, i.e. the cranium, vertebral column and allied bones (i.e. ribs and sternum).

B. Appendicular skeleton—consisting of bones of appendages in fins, limbs or wings.

The axial endoskeleton (earlier as notochord and then as vertebral column) is the basic distinguishing feature of the phylum chordata and its subphylum the vertebrata (e.g. mankind).

In bipeds, the spinal (vertebral) column assumes following important functions:

i. Encasement of the spinal cord.
ii. Transmission of the weight of head, neck and trunk to the lower limbs through the pelvis.
iii. Maintenance of posture.
iv. Forming a stout back support for the vital organs of the chest and abdomen.
v. Providing attachment to certain important groups of muscles responsible for the maintenance of posture.

According to the functional needs, the different parts of the spine have become modified in the process of evolution in bipeds, e.g. to effect the movements of the head, the cervical spine has the maximum mobility. On the other hand, at the caudal end, the coccyx represents more or less a vestigeal remnant.

Examination of the spinal column, automatically implies the examination of:

- The vertebrae
- The spinal cord, (with its meninges)
- The spinal roots.

ANATOMICAL CONSIDERATIONS

Development of the Spine

The spine develops in concurrently running stages which overlap each other.

First stage—Notochord—15 days of IUL (Intrauterine life).

Second stage—Membrane stage—21 days of IUL.

Third stage—Cartilage stage—5-6 weeks and continues throughout the foetal stage.

Fourth stage—Bony stage—2nd month of IUL.

The neural tube develops from the ectoderm in the second to third weeks of intrauterine life.

Notochord develops from endoderm. Around the notochord, which forms the primitive axial support, formation of thirty or more somites occur. The dorsomedial part of the somite forms the skeletal muscle and is known as myotomes. The ventrolateral portion forms the vertebral body and is known as sclerotome.

Congenital anomalies can occur in any stage but usually occur due to defects in the membrane stage, when mesenchyme first starts forming around the notochord.

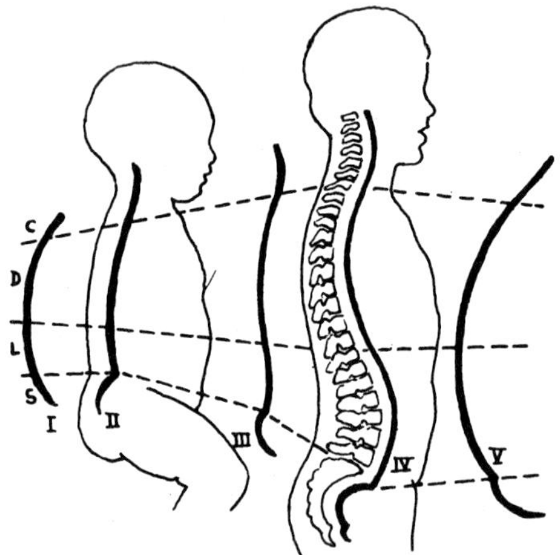

Fig. 8.1: Curvatures of spine at different ages; I-curvature in utero and early infancy; II curvature at early childhood; III curvature at late childhood; IV curvature at adulthood; V curvature of senile spine; C = cervical spine; D = dorsal spine; L = lumbar spine and S = sacral spine

CURVATURES OF THE SPINE (Fig. 8.1)

A graph for recording the curves of the spinal column should be plotted—RACHIGRAPH.

BLOOD VESSELS OF THE SPINAL CORD AND AROUND

Arteries of Spinal Cord

1. *Main arteries (branches of vertebral artery)*
   i. *Anterior spinal artery*: Runs in the anteromedial fissure (supplies anterior two-thirds of the spinal cord).
   ii. *Two posterior spinal arteries:* Run downwards on the dorsolateral surface, posterior to the spinal roots (supply the posterior parts of the posterior horn and column).

2. *Reinforcements:* Spinal branches of vertebral, inferior thyroid, intercostal, iliolumbar, sacral or radicular arteries (at different levels from above downwards), enter through the intervertebral foramina. Largest of the radicular arteries is the arteria radicularis magna or great spinal *artery of Adamkiewcz,* which originates from the left intercostal or lumbar artery between the 4th thoracic and 4th lumbar vertebrae, with special predilection for T_9 to T_{11}. These together contribute to the formation of anastomosing channels along the cord.

Arterial Supply of Vertebrae

The vertebral bodies receive the arterial supply in corresponding embryological pattern. The branches emerge from ascending cervical, intercostal and lumbar segmental arteries. Consequently on each side upper half of vertebrae below and lower half of vertebrae above (with its intervening intervertebral disc) receive arterial supply from the same segmental supply.

Veins

Veins are principally organised in the external and internal venous plexuses (Batson's plexus-1940).

External Vertebral Venous Plexus (Most Marked in the Cervical Region) consists of

i. The anterior plexus lies anterior to vertebral body and communicates with the basi vertebral and internal vertebral venous plexus.
ii. Posterior plexus lies around the posterior surface of the laminae, spinous and transverse processes, anastomosing freely with each other and with vertebral, posterior intercostal and lumbar veins.

Internal vertebral venous plexus This lies between the duramater and vertebrae, receiving tributaries from bone and cord and running in a vertical direction forming two anterior and two posterior veins.

The anterior internal venous plexus lies behind the posterior surface of the vertebral bodies and discs, on each side of the posterior longitudinal ligament, and are connected by transverse branches into which the basi vertebral veins open. The posterior internal venous plexus lies on each side of the median plane, in front of the ligamentum flava, and anastomoses with the posterior external plexus.

Veins of the Spinal Cord

These are situated in the piamater and form a plexus consisting of:

i. Two medial longitudinal veins.
ii. Two anterolateral longitudinal veins.
iii. Two posterolateral longitudinal veins.

These communicate with the internal vertebral venous plexus and intervertebral vein.

The Spinal Column

The spinal column is composed of vertebral segments (7 cervical, 12 dorsal, 5 lumbar, 5 fused sacral and 3-4 fused/unfused coccygeal). Each vertebral segment consists of an anterior solid vertebral body which has the responsibility of carrying the body load. The posterior appendages form a ring with the body of the vertebrae for encasing the spinal cord. The pedicles lie at the junction of the anterior and posterior segments. *Pars interarticularis* is the developmental region of fusion of the pedicles from front, the superior articular facets from above, laminae from behind, inferior articular facets from below and transverse processes from the sides.

In the spinal column, each vertebra has a pair of synovial joints on either side, i.e. the arthrodial joints formed by the superior articular facet of the vertebra below and the inferior articular facet of the vertebra above. These bilateral joints actually form the fulcrum of movements in between two vertebrae. However, a little movement does occur, also in between two adjacent vertebrae at the intervertebral disc level. Posteriorly, the corresponding processes of adjacent vertebrae are held together by stout ligaments.

Important Ligaments of the Vertebral Column

1. Anterior to the bodies—The anterior longitudinal ligament extending from basi-occiput to sacrum.
2. Posterior to the bodies—The posterior longitudinal ligament extends from basi occiput to sacrum, upper end is known as tectorial membrane (extending from axis to occiput).
3. In between adjacent laminae—The ligamentum flava.
4. In between adjacent spinous processes—The inter-spinous ligament.
5. Bridging the tips of the spinous processes—The supra-spinous ligament (from vertebra prominens to occiput, is known as ligamentum nuchae).
6. The spinal cord is more or less suspended in the vertebral canal by the denticulate ligaments of both sides.

The vertebral column is controlled by a complex group of muscles, which extend from the pelvis to the skull—the sacrospinalis—supplied by the dorsal rami of the segmental spinal nerves.

The articular facets and spinal appendages (transverse processes and spinous processes) of different regions may have different shape, size and directions according to their functions and required mobility (right from the atlanto-occipital zone to the lumbosacral zone).

The stability of spine depends upon three-column support (Denis 1983):

Anterior column consists of anterior longitudinal ligament, anterior portion of annulus, and anterior half of the vertebral body.

Middle column consists of posterior longitudinal ligament, posterior portion of annulus and posterior half of vertebral body.

Posterior column consists of posterior bony arch (comprising of the pedicles, facets and laminae) and the posterior ligamentous complex consisting of supraspinatus ligament, interspinus ligament, ligamentum flava, and facet joint capsules.

Spinal Cord

The spinal cord, starting as a direct continuation of the medulla oblongata at the lower border of the foramen magnum continues as far as the lower border of L_1 vertebra (in children upto L_3), where it forms the conus medullaris. Beyond this, the bunches of the emerging roots form the cauda equina (like the hairs arranged in a horse's tail). From the tip of the conus medullaris, a delicate band continues in the centre of the cauda equina to end at S_2 vertebra forming the filum terminale interna. The meninges of the cord (dura and arachnoid) blend around the filum terminale-interna at the S_2 level forming the filum terminale externa which runs upto the coccyx (Fig. 8.2). The spinal cord has two enlargements to accommodate the roots supplying the limb (cervicodorsal—C_3 to T_2, and lumbar—T_9-T_{12}).

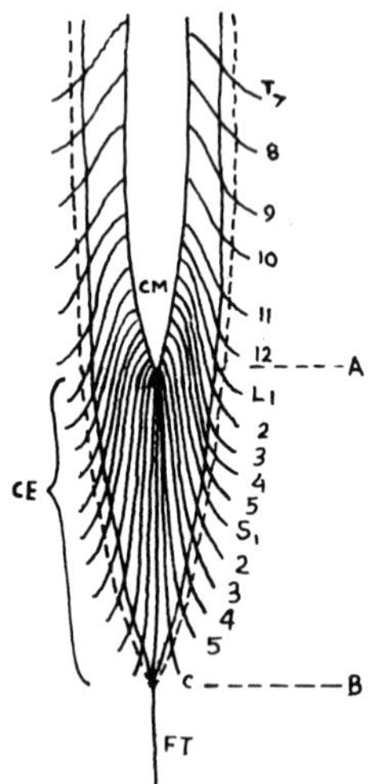

Fig. 8.2: Lower end of the spinal cord and cauda equina. CM = conus medullaris; CE = cauda equina; FT = filum terminale; A = lower border of L1 vertebra and B = lower border of S_2 vertebra

The Intervertebral Disc

Normally, 23 discs exist starting from 2/3 cervical intervertebral space to lumbosacral intervertebral space. The disc is thinner in the thoracic region and thicker in the lumbar region.

Functionally, this may be taken as a shock absorber in between two adjacent vertebral bodies. It develops from mesoderm (annulus fibrosis and cartilaginous plate) and endoderm, i.e. notochord (nucleus pulposus) and is adherent to the hyaline cartilage layer covering the adjacent surfaces of the vertebral bodies. Taken together, the discs occupy 1/5th of the total length of the spinal column with diurnal variation in thickness of 1 cm (in women) to 1.5 cm (in men). The discs are practically avascular by the age of about eighteen years and derive their nutrition by diffusion from adjacent cancellous bones.

The structure of the intervertebral disc—Each disc consists of an outer laminated part called the annulus fibrosus and an inner part called the nucleus pulposus. The narrower outer zone of the annulus consists of collagenous fibres and the wider inner zone of the nucleus pulposus is fibrocartilaginous. The nucleus pulposus is well developed in the cervical and lumbar regions. At birth, it is soft, gelatinous and comparatively large, containing about 88% water, mucoid material and a few multinucleated notochordal cells. By the first decade, the notochordal cells disappear and the mucoid material is gradually replaced by a fibrocartilaginous structure. With these changes, the nucleus pulposus becomes amorphous, its water binding capacity diminished to 70% and its elasticity reduces, due to the alteration in its mucopolysaccharide and protein components. Nerve bundles have been demonstrated ouside the anterior and posterior longitudinal ligaments, but not in the disc. After the second decade, degenerative changes are likely to occur, in the disc. Gradually the water content of the nucleus pulposus decreases, converting it into a granular and friable mass. Similarly, there is a softening and weakening of the annulus fibrosus. Following degeneration, even with minor strain, either the nucleus pulposus may be displaced eccentrically within the disc itself or it may bulge or burst through the annulus fibrosus, usually in a posterolateral direction. The former is responsible for unequal tension in the disc, leading to lumbago (severe acute pain and spasm) and the latter may lead to pressure upon the spinal roots.

WEIGHT TRANSMISSION ALONG THE VERTEBRAL COLUMN

Weight transmission along the vertebral column changes according to the posture or type/phase of mobility. In a normal stance phase, the weight is transmitted mainly along the anterior half of the spinal segments. The posterior half plays more or less a passive role and transmits very little weight (except C_1 and C_2). Anteriorly too, the main weight is transferred along the body surfaces. Partial weight transmission is along the diarthrodial joints. Very little weight transmission occurs along the posterior elements and processes.

APPLIED ANATOMY OF MOTOR AND SENSORY SYSTEMS

Motor System (Fig. 8.3) (Table 8.1)

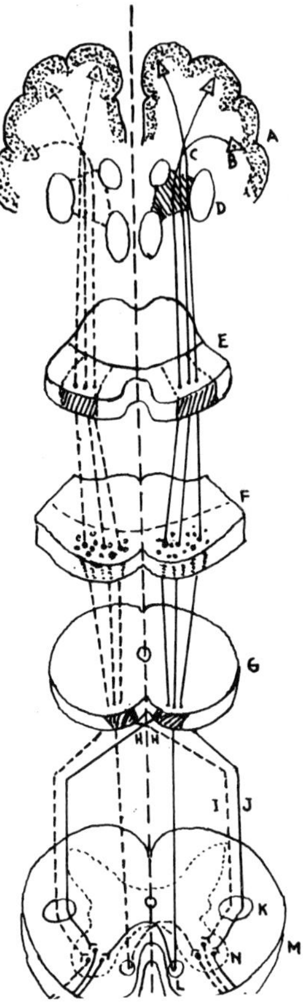

Fig. 8.3: Course of pyramidal fibres. A = motor cortex; B = pyramidal cells; C = corona radiata; D = internal capsule; E = mid brain; F = pons; G = medulla; H = medullary decussation; I = crossed fibres; J = uncrossed fibres; K = lateral white column; L = anterior white commissure; M = spinal cord; N = anterior horn cells; O = spinal nerves containing mostly crossed fibres

Sensory System (Fig. 8.4)

The first order sensory fibres for the appreciation of pain, touch and temperature terminate at the tip of the grey matter of the posterior horn. From there, second order neurons start. These fibres cross immediately, or a little above, to the opposite side in front and benind the central canal as the lateral spinothalamic tract to carry mainly pain and temperature extremes and the anterior spinothalamic tract for carrying crude touch. Both these groups of fibres terminate in the thalamus, from where the third order neurons carry impulses to the post-central gyrus.

The first order sensory fibres for the appreciation of sense of position, sense of movement, moderate temperature variation, vibration, size, shape, two point discrimination and light discriminative touch ascend directly in the posterior column and end in the nuclei gracilis and cuneatus situated in the medulla oblongata. From there, second order neurons start and terminate in the thalamus of the opposite side. The fasciculus gracilis carries fibres from the

Table 8.1: Applied anatomy of motor system

Motor System

Execution of movements of the limbs depends upon:

Cortico-spinal system	*Extrapyramidal system*	*Cerebellum*
(A) Intact higher centres (*upper motor neuron*)—for initiation of the impulses for voluntary movements, for maintenance of the posture		
Responsible for initiaing voluntary and skilled motor activities. The following sequence illustrates this pathway. Pyramidal cells of fifth layer of motor cortex, corticospinal tract, anterior 2/3rd of posterior limb of internal capsule, middle 3/5th of the peduncles of mid brain, pons, medulla (lower part). Majority of fibres decussate with those of opposite side in the lateral column of the spinal cord as crossed corticospinal tract, few fibres which do not decussate descend downward in the anterior column as the direct corticospinal tracts and they decussate at segmental levels. A few uncrossed fibres continue as uncrossed, corticospinal tract of same side and end in the anterior horn cells of same side. The corticospinal fibres terminate at different levels in the grey matter of brain stem and the anterior horn cells of the spinal cord. *Affection of the corticospinal system-is an upper motor neuron lesion* (signs—weakness, spasticity, increased tendon reflexes, extensor plantar response—except in the stage of neuronal shock; superficial reflexes are absent).	Responsible for control of posture and initiation of movements. Specially responsible for postural mechanisms e.g. turning to the sides, sitting, standing, walking, running, etc. *It consists of*—basal ganglia, subthalamic nuclei, substantia nigra, red nuclei and other structures in the brain stem. These centres are connected to the lower motor neurons in spinal cord by indirect tracts—dentorubro spinal, reticulo-spinal, vestibulospinal, and olivospinal. Affections of this system lead to: —Difficulty in initiation of voluntary movements, impairment of orientation and balancing reflexes —Alterations in muscle tone —Appearance of involuntary movements —Muscle weakness (rarely)	Receives afferents from the spinal cord, vestibular system, basal ganglia and cerebral cortex. It controls the lower motor neuron through its connections via thalamus with the basal ganglia and cerebral cortex. Lesions—cause muscular hypotonia, incoordination (ataxia).
(B) *Lower motor neuron:* Lower motor neuron consists of anterior horn cells, homologous cells in brain stem and their efferent nerve fibres, which pass through anterior spinal nerve roots and peripheral nerves upto the muscles.		

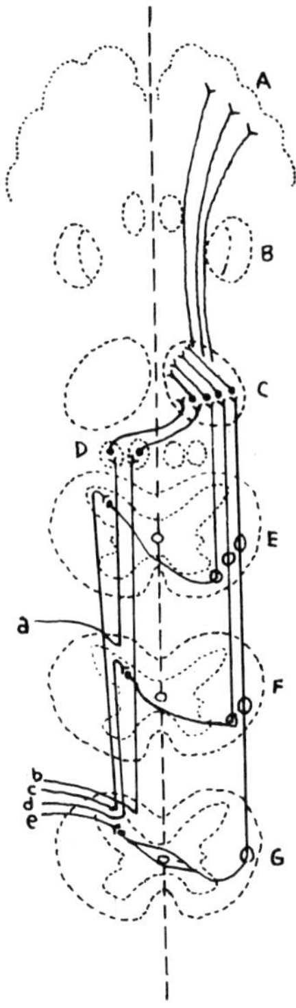

Fig. 8.4: Sensory pathways; A = posterior central gyrus; B = internal capsule; C = thalamus; D = nuclei gracilis and cuneatus; E, F and G = section of spinal cord at different levels; a = tract of Burdach; b = tract of Gall; c = touch fibres; d = thermal fibres; e = pain fibres

lower half of the body, whereas the fasciculus cuneatus (laterally situated) carries fibres from the upper half of the body. The third order neurons carry impulses to post-central gyrus through the internal capsule. Therefore, at any spinal cord level two major groups of sensory fibres exist.

i. Those carrying pain, temperature and crude touch sensations from the opposite side of the body,
ii. Those carrying appreciation of posture, weight, size, shape, vibration, moderate temperature variation and fine touch from the same side of the body.

Hemisection of the spinal cord results in loss of pain, thermal sensation and crude touch below the level of the lesion on the opposite side, while on the ipsilateral side there is loss of sense of position, vibration, recognition of weight, size, shape, and fine touch, besides spastic paralysis. This is called Brown-Séquard syndrome.

Bundle Arrangements and Tracts of the Spinal Cord (Fig. 8.5)

Innervation of the Urinary Bladder and its Clinical Importance (Fig. 8.6)

Nerve supply of bladder consists of three main groups:

Nerve fibre groups	*Root value*	*Action*
Parasym - pathetic	S_{2-4}	• Contracts detrusor muscle • Relaxes internal sphincter • Action on genitalia •penile erection • engorgement of clitoris
Sympathetic	L_1-L_2	• Relaxes detrusor • Contracts internal sphincter • Action on genitalia • ejaculation • orgasm
Somatic	Pudendal nerve	Relaxes the external sphincter

Sympathetics relax the detrusor and contract the internal sphincter. Urine collecting in bladder stretches the detrusor muscle. The sensation of filling passes through the sympathetic via the posterior column in the spinal cord—to higher centre. According to space and surrounding, there is either inhibition through sympathetic action, or release through parasympathetic action. When micturition is desired, parasympathetic contracts detrusor and relaxes the internal sphincter. Urine reaches the external sphincter, thereafter pudendal nerve relaxes the external sphincter.

Section of the cord above S_2 leads to "**cord bladder**" or "**automatic bladder**" or "**upper motor neuron type bladder**", that is, bladder emptying is controlled by spinal centres through a spinal reflex arc. In such bladder there is frequency and incontinence. The bladder is small

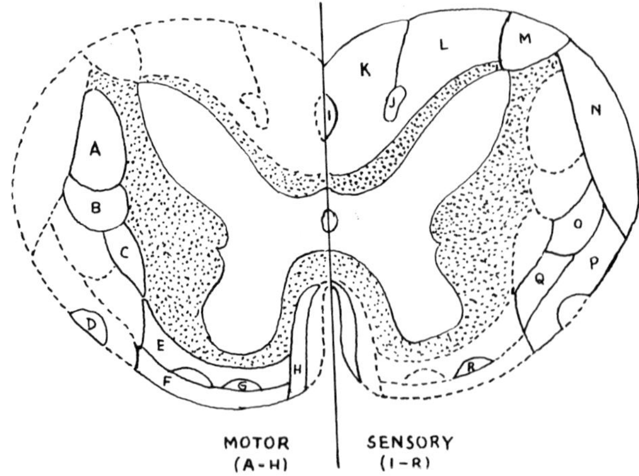

Fig. 8.5: Transverse section of spinal cord showing the motor (A to H) and sensory tracts (I to R) A = crossed pyramidal tract; B = rubro spinal tract; C = lateral vestibulospinal tract; D = oligospinal tract; E = reticulospinal tract; F = vestibulospinal tract; G = tectospinal tract; H = direct pyramidal tract; I = oval bundle; J = comma tract; K = tract of Gall; L = tract of Burdach; M = Lissauer s tract; N = dorsal spinocerebral tract; O = lateral spinothalamic tract; P = ventral spinocerebellar tract; Q = spinotectal tract; R = ventral spinothalamic tract

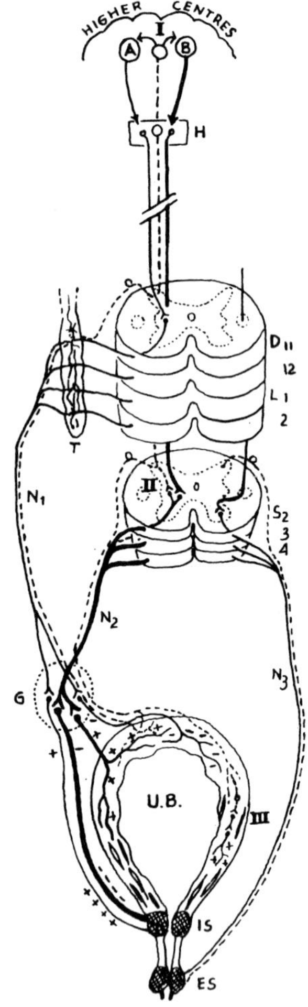

Fig. 8.6: Innervation of urinary bladder; A and B = higher centers; H = hypothalamus; T = Sympathetic trunk; G = hypogastric ganglion; N_1 = presacral nerve (sympathetic); N_2 = nervi ergentis (parasympathetic); N_3 = pudendal nerve (somatic); UB = urinary bladder; IS = internal sphincter; ES = external sphincter; + = shows the contraction; - = shows relaxation; sensory pathways have been shown by interrupted line

and usually sensitive to small changes in intravesical pressure-volume changes.

Section at and below S_2 leads to an **autonomous or lower motor neuron type or isolated or atonic bladder** controlled by local myoneural reflexes in the bladder wall.

In such bladder the urinary symptoms are produced usually by bilateral lesions. The bladder is flaccid, atonic and overflows without warning.

Failure of erection of penis (or engorgement of clitoris) and ejaculation (or orgasm) is caused by bilateral upper or lower motor neuron lesion, besides due to mental depression which may be commonly present in such a situation.

METHODOLOGY

History Taking

Besides the general mode of history taking in detail, certain important points should be given special consideration with special reference to specific pathology, e.g. (i) The patient may not have any symptoms in the spine, though the actual disease may be in it, (ii) When pain is complained of, with possible origin somewhere in the spinal column, the possibilities and course of root reference should be taken into consideration.

Patient may complain with a suggestion that he is suffering from 'sciatica' (pain along the course of sciatic nerve and its branches). Even the transfemoral amputated patient can complain pain in the sciatic distribution—phantom sciatica (Brown *et al* 1997).

General and Systemic Examination As Usual

Gait—If the patient can walk, the gait should be properly assessed (see page 177 to 180).

Regional Examination

This includes the whole spine and limbs.

Local Examination

Prerequisites: Ideally, the whole of the neck, back, chest and abdomen must be exposed. The patient should be examined in standing position, sitting on a stool and lying on a flat bed. Most of the examination is from the back. However, most of paraplegics and quadriplegics should be examined in supine and guarded rolling lateral position in traction (except in late cases) to avoid any further damage.

Examination of the spine includes examination from the atlanto-occipital region to the coccyx. However, for all practical purposes the sacroiliac joints examination must be taken as a part of the spinal examination.

Attitude: While standing, note the attitude of the patient. The posture of the patient while walking or standing can provide an important clue for reaching a diagnosis. A fixed statue-like, stooping posture is characteristic of ankylosing spondylitis; standing with the legs crossed and a tendency of equinus position may be seen in cerebral diplegia; and swaying of the body, especially while standing with feet close together is typical of cerebellar lesions.

Inspection

Ask the patient to stand as erect as possible. Note the position of head, the hairline, length of neck and the levels of shoulders, scapulae, and iliac crests.

Inspecting from the side and behind—note the spinal curvatures. In the midline of the back there is a longitudinal depression—the central furrow, which contains the tips of the spinous processes presenting as knob like projections. At the root of the neck, the seventh spinous process stands out quite prominently—the vertebra prominence. On both sides of the central furrow are the paraspinal bulges which are produced by the paraspinalis muscles. These muscles stand prominent when in *spasm* (Fig. 8.7), (nature's attempt to prevent movements which produce pain). If they look very prominent, increasing the median furrow at about the level of the 10th thoracic vertebra, it probably indicates early caries spine in that area (Jardine). On the outer side of sacrospinalis, the posterior surface of the chest wall and loin region continues. Note the levels of the medial and inferior scapular angles and the normal depression at the junction of the lower border of the 12th rib and the sacrospinalis muscle—the *renal angle*. The posterosuperior curvatures of the iliac crests stand prominent on both sides. The iliac crest ends posteriorly as the postero-superior iliac spine, represented on the surface by the *dimple of Venus*, whence a vague linear depression

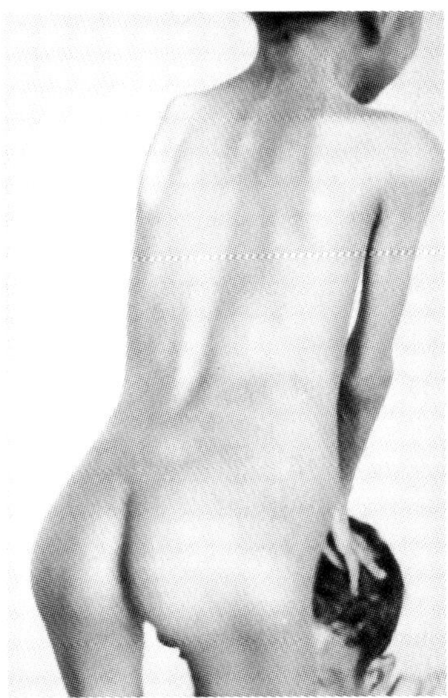

Fig. 8.7: Paraspinalis muscles go in spasm when the patient tries to flex the spine (A case of dorsolumbar caries spine)

runs downward with little outer inclination, which lies over the sacroiliac joint.

Note any deviation in the normal spinal curvature, the central furrow, the paraspinal bulge, slopes on the back of the chest, any bulge in the loin region, fullness over or below the iliac crest and any fullness or abnormality of the dimple of Venus.

Abnormalities in the Curvature of the Spine

The curvatures of spine should be recorded in a graph (*rachigraph*).

Torticollis (wry neck) (Fig. 8.8)

In this condition, there is side-ways bending of the neck with some rotational element resulting in head tilted to same side and chin to the opposite. It may be due to—a sternomastoid tumour (a congenital—firm mass in the sternomastoid); fibromyositis, spasm and contracture of one sternomastoid; trauma; bony anomalies (e.g. unilateral defect in the vertebral body); Klippel-Feil syndrome; squint; or an overlying soft tissue contracture (e.g. following burn).

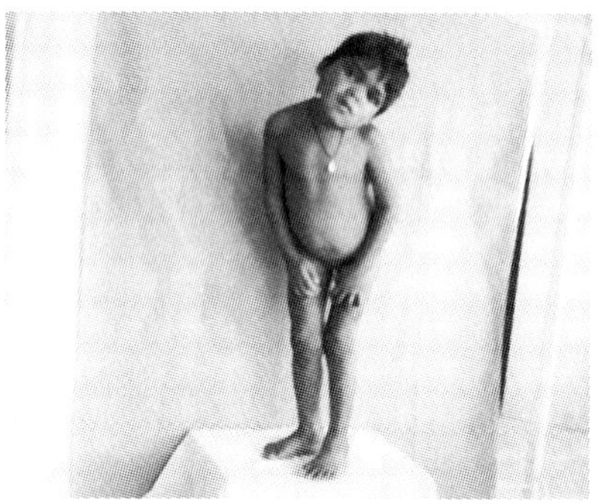

Fig. 8.8: Congenital torticollis on the left side

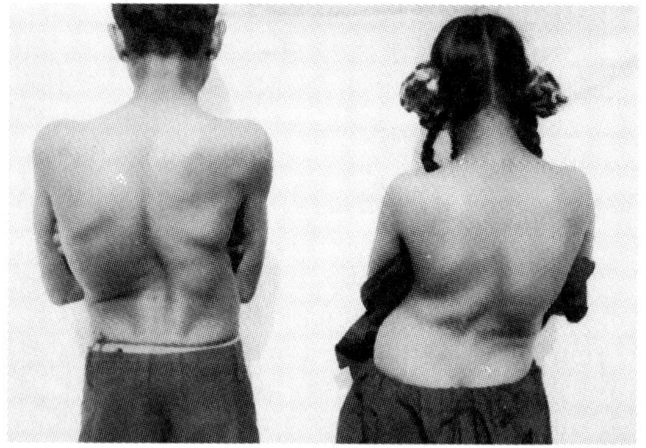

Fig. 8.9A: Structural dorsolumbar scoliosis in brother and sister

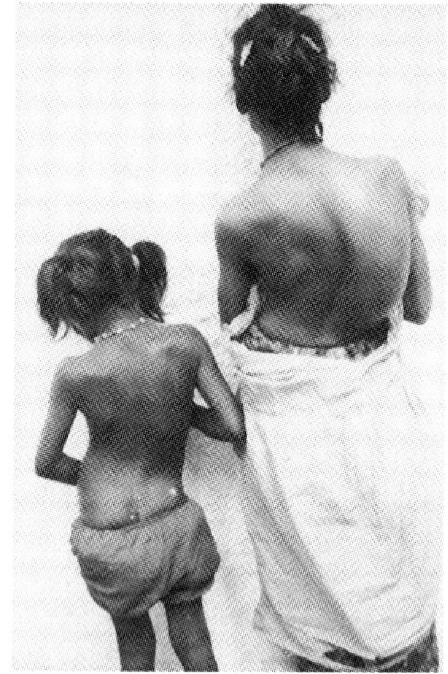

Fig. 8.9B: Structural dorsolumbar scoliosis in mother and daughter

Scoliosis (Figs 8.9A and B)

In scoliosis the spine bends sideways producing a lateral curvature but is usually accompanied by a rotational deformity as spinal column starts to buckle as it collapses (which is called scoliosis). If there is any scoliosis, note the following points: (i) the site, (ii) the persistence or disappearance of scoliosis in forward bending [functional scoliosis (sciatic, compensatory in leg length inequality, postural) disappears on forward bending and reappears when the patient becomes erect], (iii) the number of curvatures. Curves are primary (major) or secondary (compensatory) to the primary curve in an attempt to maintain spinal balance, (iv) approximate upper and lower limits of the curvatures and the most prominent level of the convexity, (v) the side of the convexity, (vi) association with other deformities like kyphosis

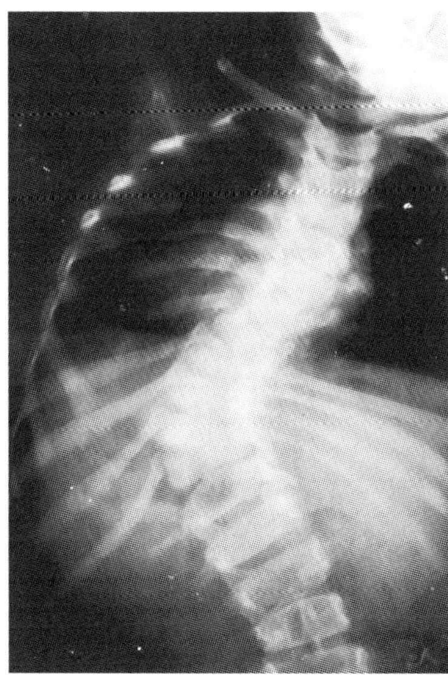

Fig. 8.10: Kyphoscoliosis following caries spine

(e.g. kypho-scoliosis, Fig. 8.10), (vii) the effect on the chest. The chest bulges out posterolaterally on the convex side of the scoliosis, since in the thoracic region the rotation of spinal column throws the ribs into prominence producing ***rib hump (razor back)***, which can be better assessed in forward bending position of the patient. On the concave side of the scoliosis, there is crowding of the ribs with the appearance of a transverse furrow in the flanks. Note the level of both iliac crests and the approximation of the last rib to the iliac crest, (viii) any change in the height of the patient due to abnormalities in the spinal curvatures, this can be assessed by the trunk/limb ratio, (ix) any facial asymmetry, deviation and prominence of the chin, squint, or difference in the level of the hair line, asymmetry in shoulder level as they may occur in certain cases of congenital or paralytic scoliosis.

The scoliosis is termed 'mobile', when normal spinal flexibility is preserved, and 'structural or fixed', when there is loss of normal mobility in the segment involved due to change in the shape of the vertebrae and adaptive changes in the allied soft tissue.

Aetiologically scoliosis may be: (1) Idiopathic (cause not known), (2) Congenital (due to congenital abnormalities in the vertebral e.g. hemivertebra) (3) Neuromuscular, e.g. in polioparalysis, cerebral palsy, spina bifida, muscular dystrophy (4) Neoplastic, e.g. in osteoid osteoma.

Idiopathic scoliosis is the commonest type and according to the age of onset it may be (i) infantile (0 to 3 years), (ii) juvenile (3 to prepuberty), and (iii) adolescent idiopathic scoliosis.

Kyphosis

There can be an abnormality in the anteroposterior curvature of the spine. Some amount of kyphosis is normally present in the thoracic region. If it becomes abnormally prominent (more than 45°) posteriorly, it is excessive kyphosis. These can be of two types:

A. Labile kyphosis—e.g. postural; due to muscle weakness (early stage of polio and myopathy), compensatory (in CDH).
B. Fixed kyphosis—they are of two types.
   i. angular kyphosis (knuckle or gibbus) (Figs 8.11A and B). This is due to collapse of one or two vertebrae, e.g. in tuberculosis, spinal fractures, congenital collapse, etc. Knuckle is sometimes referred as the prominence of a single spinus process indicating collapse of a single vertebra, e.g. in spinal injury, tuberculosis.
   ii. Gradual kyphosis (round kyphosis): This is due to partial or complete collapse of more than two vertebrae, e.g. in senile kyphosis, osteomalacia, adolescent kyphosis (Scheuermann's disease) and ankylosing spondylitis (Figs 8.13A to C). Sometimes tuberculosis of spine also produces acutely rounded kyphosis (Figs 8.12A and B).

Congenital kyphosis is a serious condition in which progressive deformity may result in paraplegia. Congenital kyphosis can be of three types: Type I (due to failure of formation

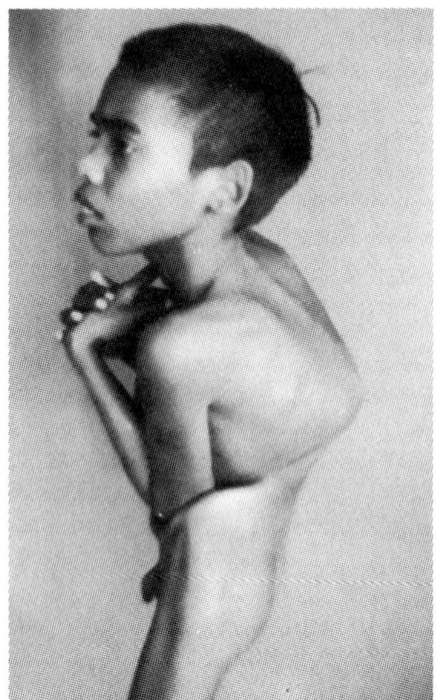

Fig. 8.11A: Angular kyphosis

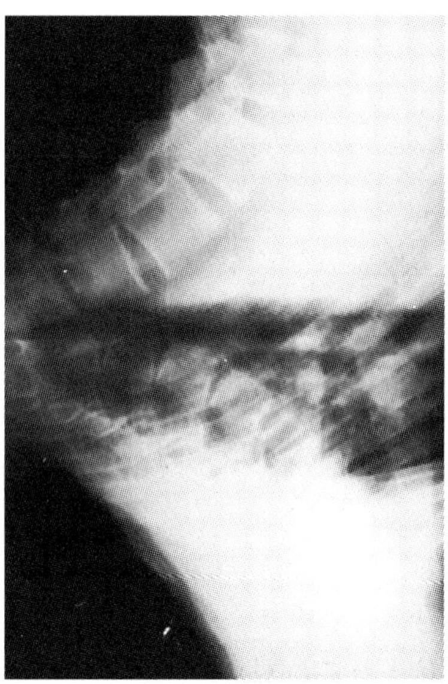

Fig. 8.11B: Acute gibbus of dorsolumbar region following old caries

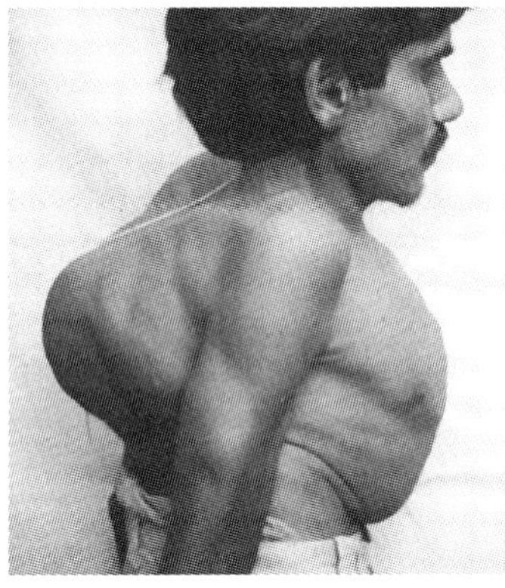

Fig. 8.12A: Acutely rounded kyphosis

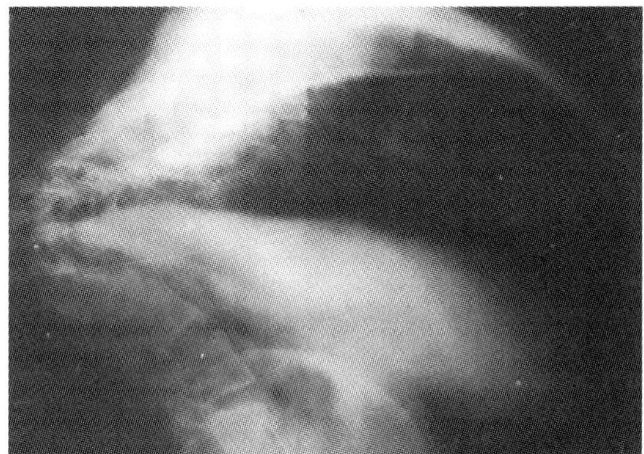

Fig. 8.12B: Acutely rounded kyphosis

of vertebral body) has the worst prognosis with greatest risk of neurological involvement; Type II (due to failure of segmentation of vertebral body); Type III (due to failure of formation and failure of segmentation of vertebral body).

Early detection and fusion of spine are the main management for avoiding the complications. Posterior fusion is adequate for children less than 5 years with a kyphosis less than 50°, otherwise combined anterior and posterior fusion is recommended.

In children, kyphosis is mainly due to tuberculosis and is rarely congenital. In adolescence, adolescent kyphosis [(Scheuermann's disease — kyphosis is associated with radiological changes) (irregular vertebral end plates, apparently diminished disc space, and wedging of one or more vertebrae by more than 5 degrees)] is the most common cause, followed by tuberculosis. In

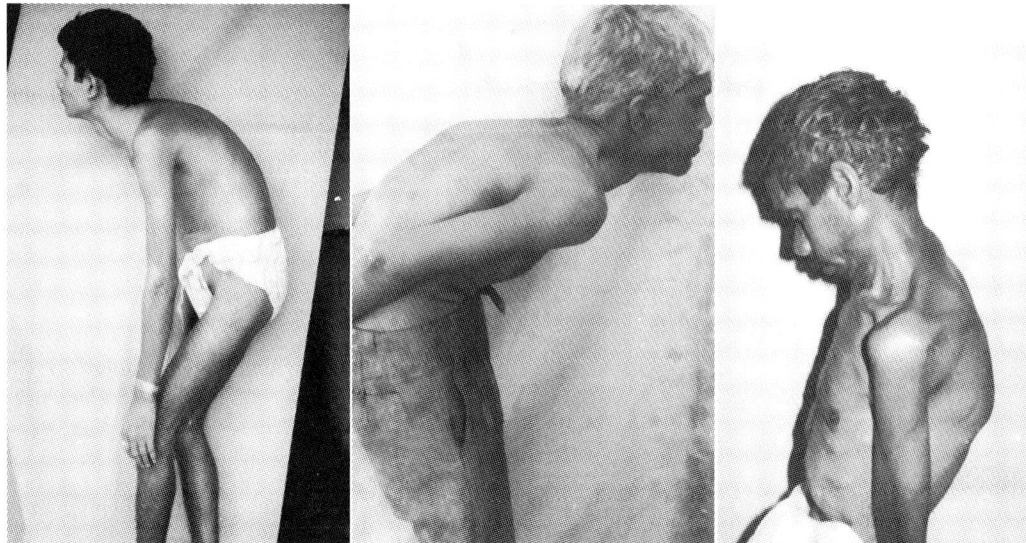

Figs 8.13A to C: Rounded kyphosis following ankylosing spondylitis. Note also the fixed flexed neck

adults, trauma, osteomalacia, caries spine and 'Kummell's disease account for most cases of kyphosis. In the elderly, senile kyphosis, senile osteoporosis, neoplastic collapse and Paget's disease are mainly responsible for kyphosis.

Lordosis

Kyrtorrhachic [Gr. kyrtos = curved + rhachis = spine) means spinal curvature with concavity backwards.

When the spinal convexity becomes abnormally prominent anteriorly, this is known as lordosis. (Fig. 8.14A). A slight amount of lordosis is normally present in the lumbar and cervical regions (In tetanus, the whole back curves posteriorly—opisthotonus). Rarely congenital cervical lordosis may be much marked (Fig. 8.14B).

In pathological lumbar lordosis, the abdomen becomes correspondingly prominent. The extent of lordosis can be assessed by visualising the central furrow. If it is deeper than normal—the lordosis is exaggerated. If it is about normal, the curvature is normal, if it is comparatively shallow—the lordosis is obliterating. If there is no central furrow, this is complete obliteration of the lordosis and flattening of the back; if the curvature reverses with the convexity backwards, this is kyphosis of the lumbar spine.

Any abnormal findings such as a swelling, sinus, depression, scar, naevus, tuft of hair, etc. should be noted.

In the lumbosacral region, or adjoining one or two spaces above, note for any sudden depression in the central furrow where it tends to end. This will give an impression of a "step". This step is due to forward slipping of one vertebra with the whole column above over the vertebra below—i.e. spondylolisthesis (Figs 8.15A to C and 8.16A). Spondylolisthesis also occurs in cervical region (Fig. 8.16B).

In certain conditions, there is a flattened appearance of the back especially the lower region. Ask the patient to bend forwards. The lower half of the back, or even the upper portion, may appear uniformly flat—board like. This is described as "boarding" and is produced by spasm of the sacrospinalis muscle (e.g. in intervertebral disc prolapse, early ankylosing spondylitis, acute back strain).

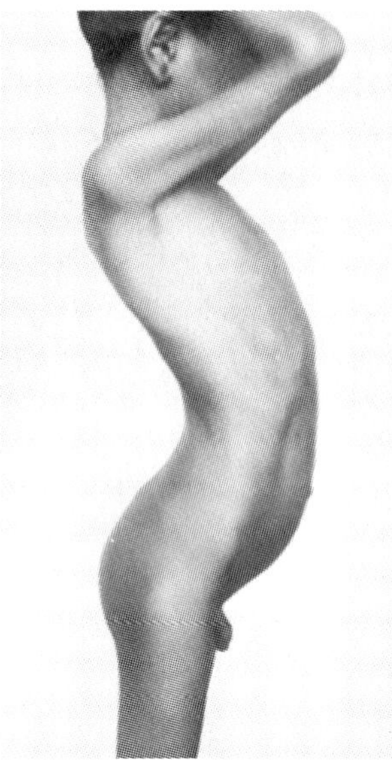

Fig. 8.14A: Marked lumbar lordosis

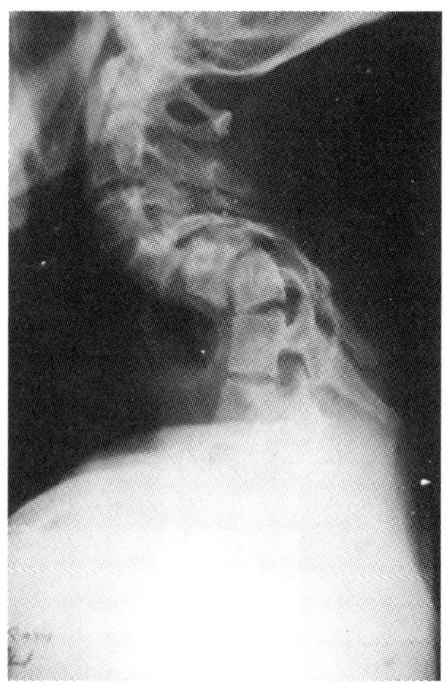

Fig. 8.14B: Congenital lordosis of cervical spine

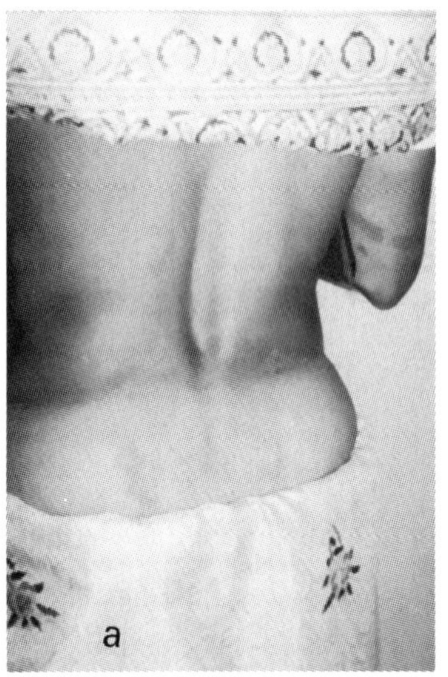

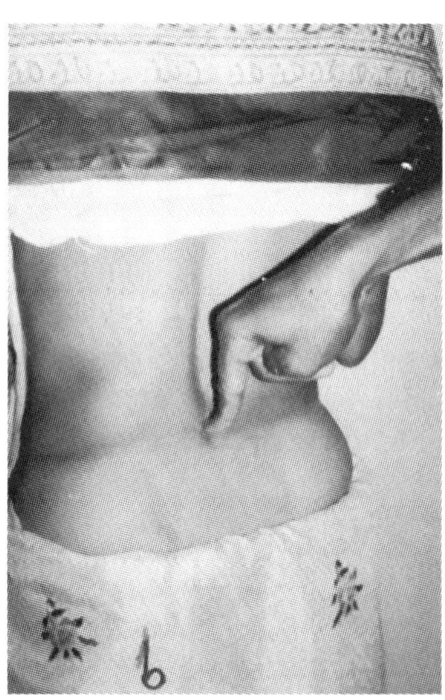

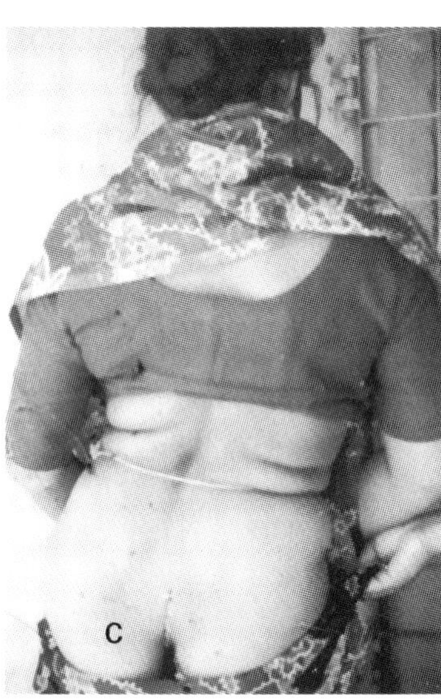

Figs 8.15a to c: Spondylolisthesis—note the marked deepened median furrow ending on a step. On the both flanks deep furrow are obvious

The spinal muscles may undergo segmental spasm as a protective mechanism to avoid pain. In cases of acute trauma, the posteriorly protruded vertebral column may give a kyphotic appearance, but the spasm of sacrospinalis will be much more apparent. Above and below this particular site, sacro-spinalis is mechanically stretched due to the posterior protrusion of the underlying bony projection. Hence there can not be local boarding.

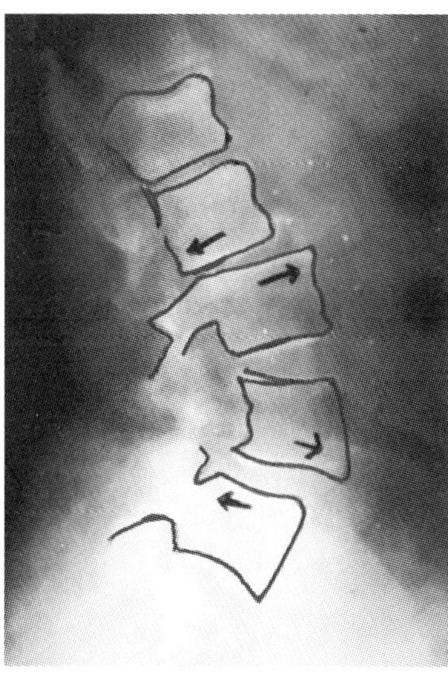

Fig. 8.16A: Spondylolisthesis at two levels: between L2 over L3 and L4 over L5

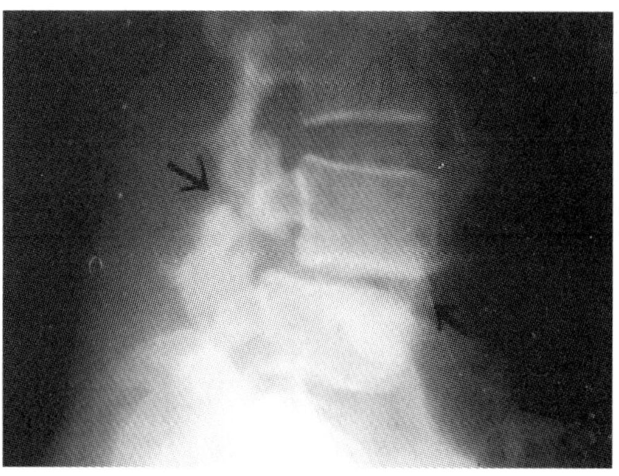

Fig. 8.16B: Spondylolisthesis (Gr II) of L4-L5 region. Note the complete dissolution of posterior spinal (skeletal) column

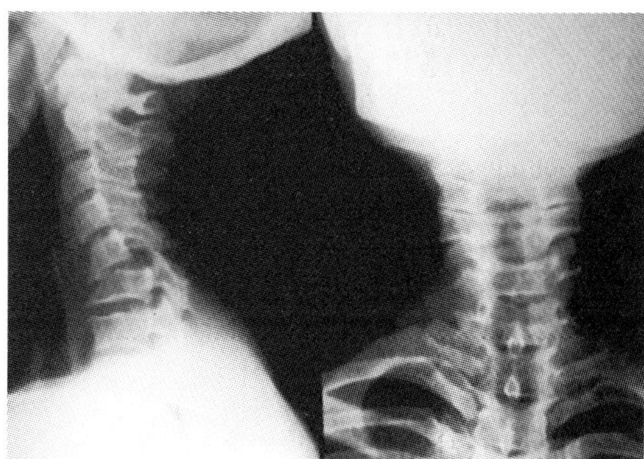

Fig. 8.16C: Spondylolisthesis of curvical 5 or 6th vertebra

Note any globular swelling, with or without a skin cover, especially in the lower lumbar region (*spina bifida manifesta*). Search the lumbosacral region for any bulge usually fibro-fatty mass, tuft of hair, hyperpigmentation of skin, depression or other signs of *spina bifida occulta*.

After inspecting the back, an examination must be done from the sides and front of the trunk. The shape of the chest, any abnormality of the abdomen and any bulge or swelling should be clearly noted along with its characteristics. In case of any apparent pathology, assess the possible level by inspection.

Palpation

Superficial palpation: Examine for hyperaesthesia, any abnormal prominence or depression, any pulsation, or any increase in temperature.

General palpation of the whole of the back should be done by passing the palm from above downwards, right from the external occipital protuberance to the tip of the coccyx. Then start palpating the central furrow, paraspinal bulge, sides of the cervical spines, sides of the chest, the loins, iliac crests, sacroiliac region and buttocks while the patient has his arms across his chest keeping the back in as neutral a position as possible. This makes the mid-spinal line, right from the nuchal furrow to the internatal cleft, comparatively prominent. Even a minor prominence of the spinous processes can be easily palpated if the hand is passed cautiously.

Central furrow—Here palpation is mainly for the spinous processes and interspinous gaps. In a patient having wasting of the paraspinal muscles, these processes stand more prominent. On the other hand, in presence of spasm of the muscles, these processes are less prominent. Any abnormality in the pattern of spinous processes (in terms of their feel, alignment and spacing) should be noted. To avoid missing even mild sideway deviation of spinous processes, it is better to mark each spinous process with a skin pencil. If any spinous process appears to be prominent, confirm its level, shape, size and tenderness. Tenderness of spine can be elicited by three methods (Fig. 8.17).

i. Direct pressure tenderness
ii. Twist tenderness
iii. Deep thrust tenderness.

i. *Direct pressure tenderness* (Fig. 8.17A): This is positive in any pathology in the spinous process or marked advanced pathology of the vertebral body. To elicit this tenderness, apply direct firm pressure with the thumb over the spinous processes, one by one, from cervical region to sacral region.

ii. *Twist tenderness* (Fig. 8.17B): This is positive even in early pathology of the vertebral body, besides affections of the posterior vertebral elements. To elicit this tenderness apply twisting pressure by the thumb of the hand on the side of the spinous process (as if trying to rotate the vertebrae) and proceed from above downwards.

iii. *Deep thrust tenderness* (Fig. 8.17C): This should be elicited only when the above methods have not indicated any tenderness and therefore the disease may be of chronic and/or less aggresive nature. It is done by applying a guarded thrust with the proximal part of the ulnar side of the fist over the spinous processes.

In younger children it is very difficult to elicit tenderness because of their general response of weeping to any stimuli. In such circumstances demonstration of indirect tenderness has been advocated in the form of the *'anvil test'*. This is not advisable as it may produce collapse of a pathologically osteoporosed vertebral body, e.g. in caries spine. In children, elicit tenderness as far as practicable after gaining their confidence.

In cases of spina-bifida manifesta, note the site, size, shape, content, and any impulse on coughing and perform the transillumination test.

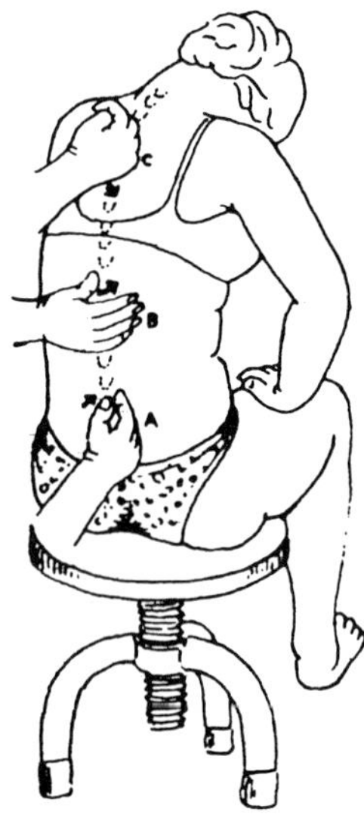

Fig. 8.17: Method of eliciting spinal tenderness. A = direct pressure tenderness (thumb directly over spinous process); B = twist tenderness (thumb twisting the spinous process from the side)(Fig. 7.15B) ; C = deep thrust tenderness

Palpate on both sides of central furrow to note the tone of paraspinal muscles. If they are tight, it means they are in spasm. On deep pressure the spasmodic muscle may even be tender. If the muscles are wasted, the bulge will be flattened and the feel will be soft. In marked wasting, it may be difficult to palpate the muscles as they are largely thinned out and the posterior portion of the ribs may be felt. In the cervical region, the sides of the neck should also be palpated. In the lumbar region the renal angle should also be felt. Pass your hands on both sides of chest and the abdomen to locate any abnormal swellings like cold abscesses. For *possible sites of cold abscesses.* See Table 8.2.

Palpate the posterior slopes of the iliac crests on both sides. It will end in the dimples of Venus. Pass the fingers more or less vertically down for about five centimeters. The edges of the sacro-iliac joints can be felt posteriorly. Note for any tenderness in this zone. Fibro-fatty nodules are usually felt in this region. Pressure over these nodules may elicit pain in distribution of sciatic nerve. This is called *pseudosciatica*. Deeper pres-

Table 8.2: Possible sites of cold abscesses in caries spine

Region	*Pathology*	*Site*	*Remarks*
1. Cervical	(i) Bursting through anterior cortex of bone as prevertebral abscess, beneath the prevertebral fascia	Retropharyngeal (central in position) may bulge in oropharynx	c.f. Acute retropharyngeal abscess which lies on one side and in front of prevertebral fascia—may burst in mouth
	(ii) Abscess tracking laterally behind the prevertebral fascia	In mediastinum.	—May mimic thyroid nodule —May produce mediastinal syndrome
	(iii) Along the posterior division of spinal nerves	At back of neck on one side of the midline.	
	(iv) From behind the prevertebral fascia	In posterior triangle of neck; in axilla; or even down to lower part of arm along the axillary/brachial artery; (Fig.8.20D) posterior mediastinum	—May produce mediastinal syndrome
2. Thorax	(i) Remains as prevertebral abscess.		
	(ii) May percolate on both sides of vertebral body in paravertebral gutters.	—Radiologically—paravertebral abscess (Figs 8.18A to C)	
	(iii) May perforate through parietal pleura.	—Pyothorax	
	(iv) From lower end of mediastinum, abscess may track:		
	(a) Behind the lateral lumbocostal arch in between anterior layer of lumbodorsal fascia and quadratus lumborum.	—Post-renal abscess	
	From here it may follow either of the three nerves lying behind the kidney i.e. 12th thoracic or ilioinguinal or iliohypogastric.	—Lower anterior abdominal parietal abscess or as rectus sheath abscess	
	Along the course of any thoracic nerve upto anterior end of intercostal space (Figs 8.19A and B and 8.20A to C).		
	(b) Through upper opening of psoas sheath, i.e. medial lumbocostal arch passing along the psoas muscle in the psoas sheath	In pelvis—as psoas or ilio psoas abscess or even around lesser trochanter	
	(c) Passing behind the median arcuate ligament along the aorta or any of its branches—branches of external iliac or branches of internal iliac	(i) Intraabdominal—in course of aorta (ii) Intrapelvic—may remain localised or present in gluteal region or in ischiorectal fossa	
	Along the course of one of the thoracic nerves (intercostal nerve).	— In thorax upto anterior end of intercostal space (Fig. 8.20C) — In abdomen—as rectus sheath abscess — Mid axillary line	
	Along posterior division of a thoracic nerve and its branches: medial branch—2.5 cm and lateral branch—7.5 cm from spinous process		

Contd.

Table 8.2: Contd.

Region	*Pathology*	*Site*	*Remarks*
3. Lumbar	Along aorta or its branches	—As in thoracic region i.e. iv (a) and iv (c).	
	Into the psoas sheath		
	Into quadratus lumborum sheath.		
	Following the course of a lumbar nerve:		
	—along femoral nerve	Infront of grion or thigh (anywhere	
	—along obturator nerve	along the course) (Fig.8.20F)	
	—along sciatic nerve	Back of the thigh (anywhere along the course)	
	Extending between the posterior part of abdominal wall muscle	Petit's triangle (Fig.8.20E)	—Abscess from thoracic disease cannot come in the Petit's triangle

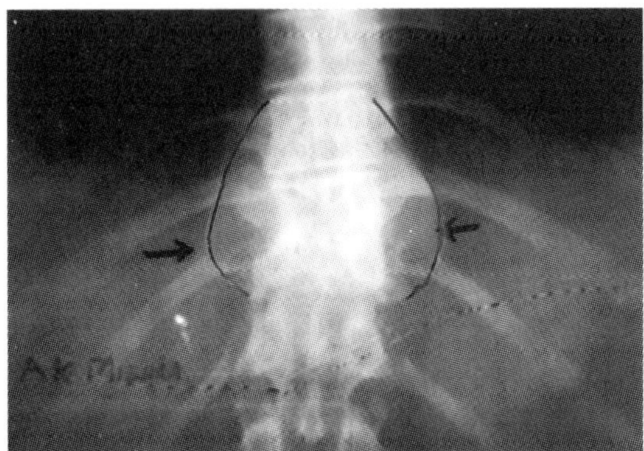

Fig. 8.18A: Caries spine of dorsal tenth vertebra, with bilateral paravertebral abscess

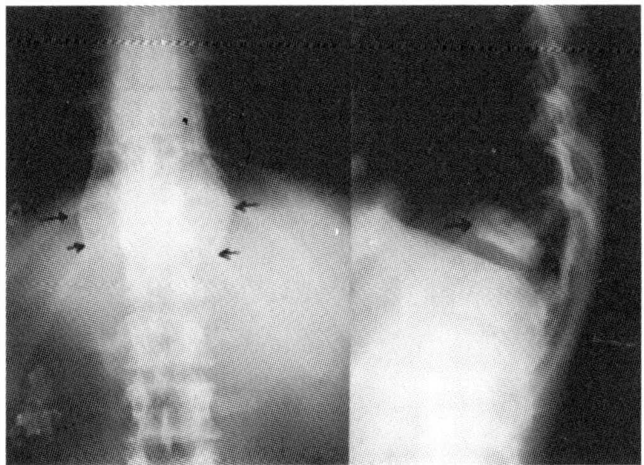

Fig. 8.18B: Caries spine dorsal 11-12 vertebrae with bilateral paravertebral abscess

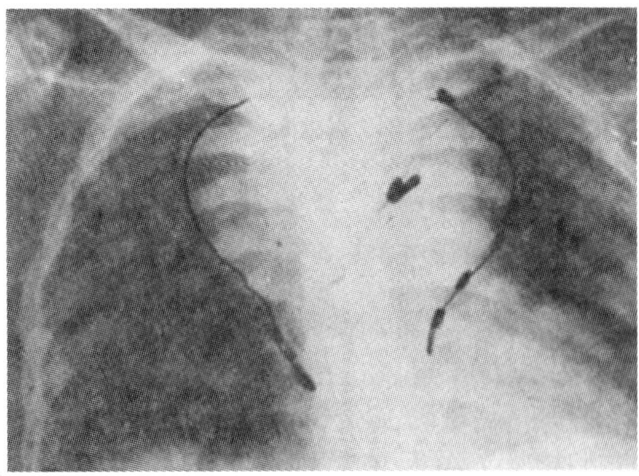

Fig. 8.18C: Caries spine of dorsal 5 with bilateral bird s nest abscess

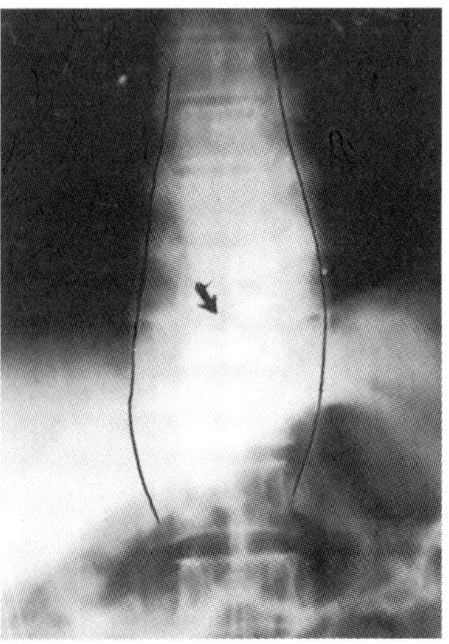

Fig. 8.18D: Caries spine of dorsal 9-10 region with spindle shaped cold abscess

sure is required to elicit the tenderness of sacro-iliac joints.

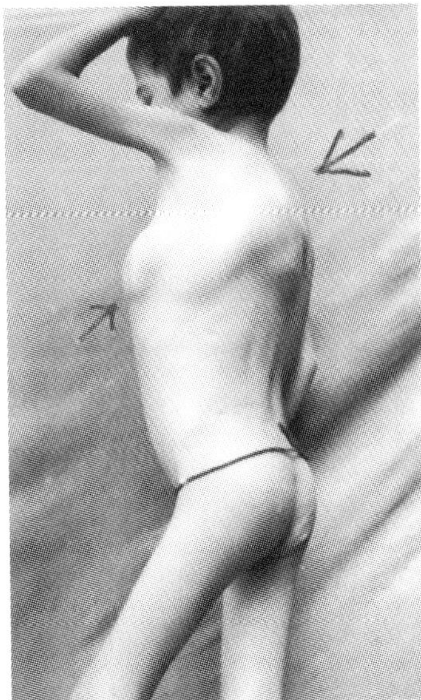

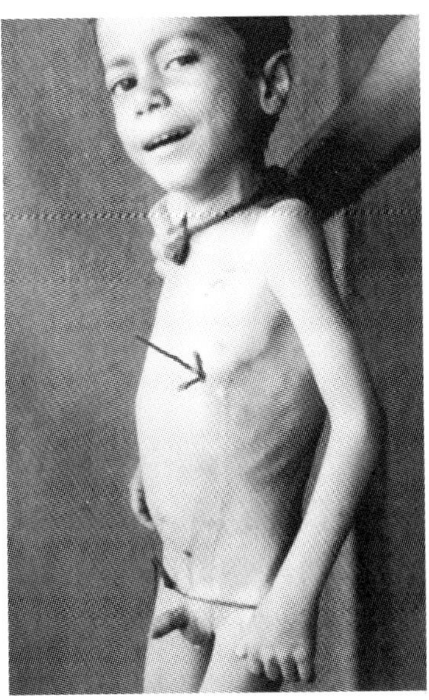

Figs 8.19A and B: Patient of caries spine with cold abscess, cold abscess tracking from dorsal 6 vertebra along the rib to front of the chest (a); same cold abscess bursted out spontaneously (b)

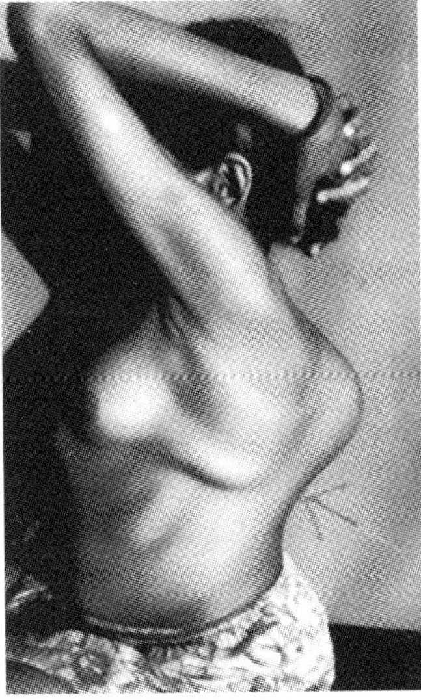

Fig. 8.20A: Tracking of cold abscess along the rib

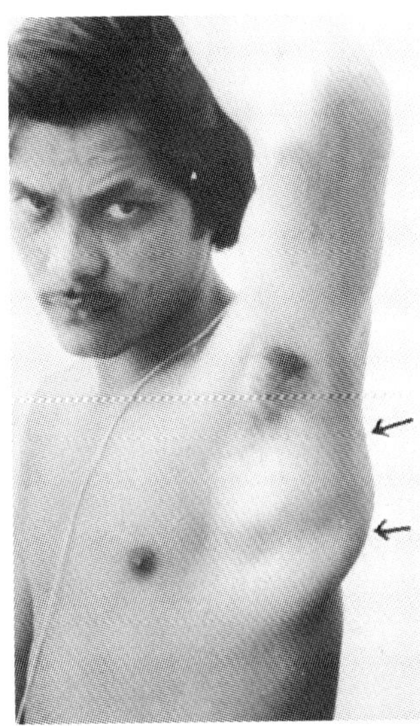

Fig. 8.20B: Patient presented with the tracking of cold abscess along the rib without any complain regarding spinal problem

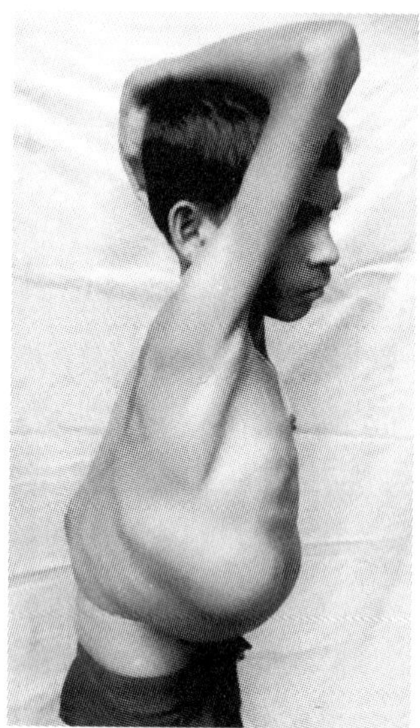

Fig. 8.20C: Tracking of cold abscess from caries spine (at two levels D5-6 and D11-12)

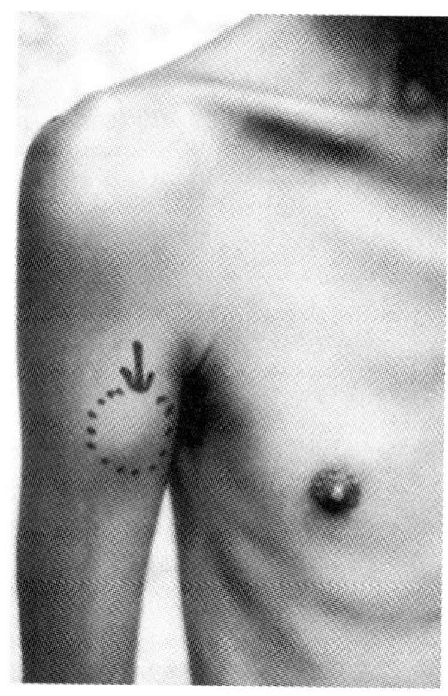

Fig. 8.20D: Tracking of cold abscess along the brachial sheath from cervical caries (C4-5)

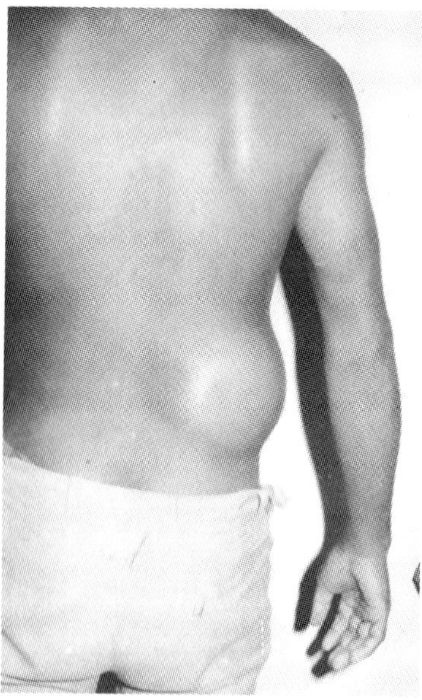

Fig. 8.20E: Tracking of cold abscess in the Petit triangle

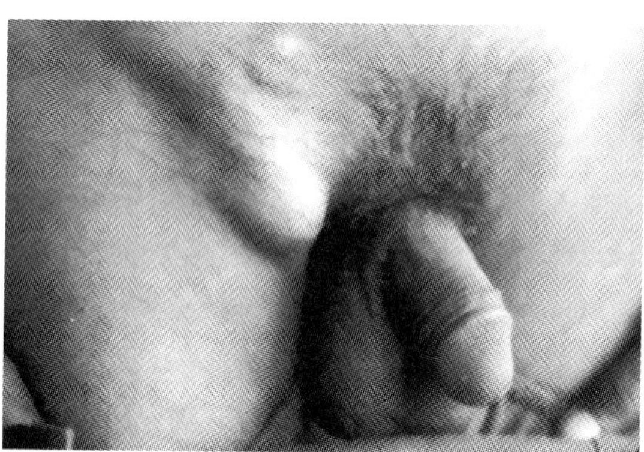

Fig. 8.20F: Tracking of cold abscess in the femoral triangle along inguinal sheath

Table 8.3: Movements at spine

Movements	Range of movement	Prime mover	Nerve supply	Assisted by	Limiting factors
At Cervical Spine:					
1. Flexion	With mouth closed, chin just touching manubrium sterni	Sterno-cleido-mastoid muscles	Spinal accessory C 2-3	1. Scalenus anterior 2. Sclaenus medius 3. Scalenus posterior 4. Longus capitis 5. Longus colli	1. Tension of posterior longitudinal ligament 2. Tension of supraspinous and interspinous ligaments 3. Tension of posterior cervical muscles
2. Extension	Till head comes in contact with posterior part of upper trunk	1. Trapezius 2. Semispinalis capitis 3. Splenius capitis 4. Splenius cervicis	Spinal accessory and C 3-4 Posterior rami of spinal nerve		
3. Side bending	0° to 45° on each side	Sterno-mastoid muscle	Spinal accessory C 2,3	1. Trapezius 2. Rhomboidus major 3. Rectus capitis lateralis	
At trunk					
1. Flexion	0° to 90°	Rectus abdominis	Lower intercostal nerve.	1. Internal oblique 2. External oblique	
2. Extension	0° to 30°	1. Sacro spinalis 2. Quadratus lumborum	Adjacent spinal nerve D 12, L1, 2	1. Semispinalis 2. Multifidus 3. Rotators of spine	
3. Trunk rotators	0° to 30°	1. External oblique 2. Internal oblique	Lower intercostal nerve 1. Lower intercostal 2. Ilio hypogastric 3. Ilio-inguinal		
4. Side bending	0° to 30°	Quadratus lumborum	T 12, L 1,2		

If there is any sinus, its edges, tract and deeper fixations should be palpated.

Percussion

Percussion Tenderness

With rubber hammer, apply brisk tap over the spinous processes and note the points of tenderness, if any. This should be done when the above methods have not elicited tenderness. Any tenderness denotes comparatively less acute pathology.

MOVEMENTS (Table 8.3)

The Movements Vary in Each Spinal Region

a. At the atlanto-occipital joint, normal movement is nodding. Movements occur at the condyloid joint formed by the condylar processes on the both sides on the base of skull articulating with the concave articular facets on the upper surface of atlas.
b. At the atlanto-axial joint side to side rotational movements occur at the pivot joint comprising of the odontoid process of the axis and fibro-osseous articular ring behind the anterior arch of the atlas.

However, initiating these movements at aforesaid joints, in extremes of these motions, all cervical joints do take part. The stress effects of rotational movements are more or less at the cervicodorsal region, it being the junction of comparatively mobile and fixed parts of spine.

Test for Active Movement at Cervical Spine

Method (Fig. 8.21): Cervical movements should be tested, while the patient sits erect on a stool. From behind, fix both shoulders in a horizontal plane. Then ask the patient to touch the front of chest with the chin while the mouth remains closed and to take back the extended head as far as practicable (Fig. 8.21); to touch ear on the shoulder top on each side (side bending Fig. 8.22); to look towards the right shoulder and then towards the left shoulder (rotations) (Fig. 8.23).

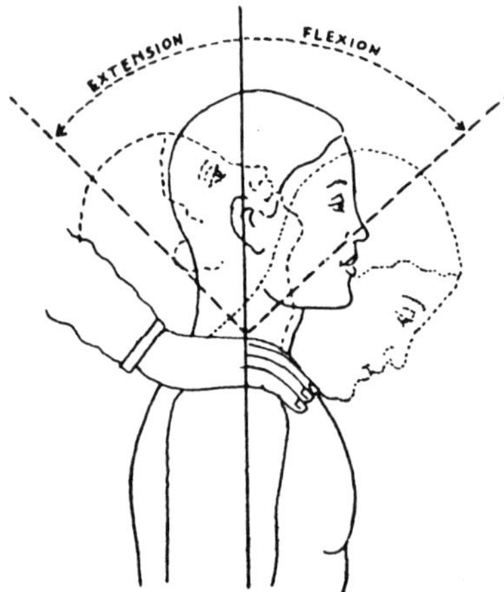

Fig. 8.21: Showing active flexion and extension at cervical spine

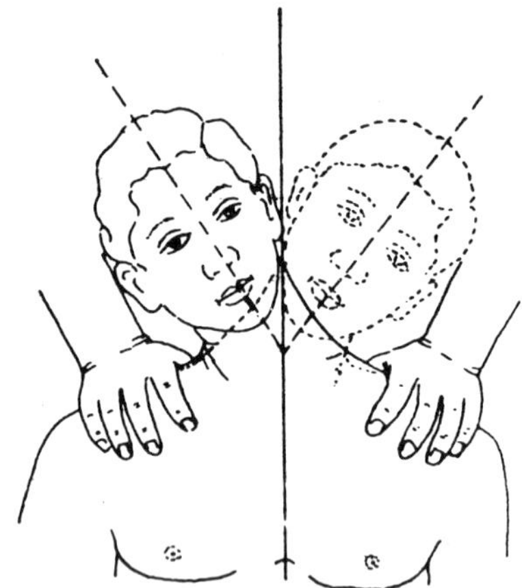

Fig. 8.22: Showing active side bending at cervical spine

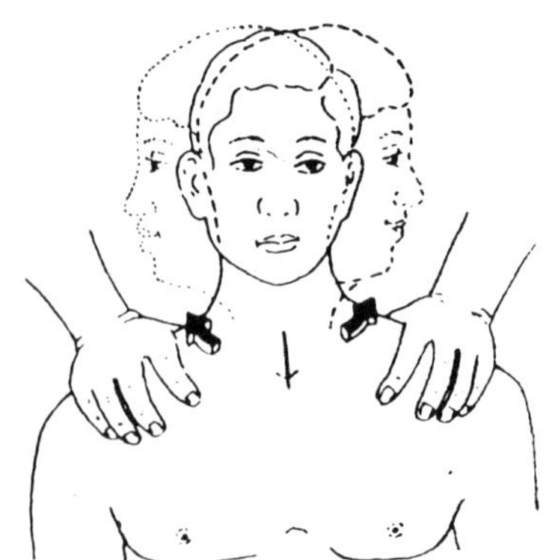

Fig. 8.23: Showing active rotations at the cervical spine

Generally speaking real movements of the spine are flexion and extension occurring at the facet joints. Other movements, like side bending are in the true sense—stretching of the opposite ligaments.

Perhaps, it is practically impossible to elicit movements of spine at single level. Whatever we see and assess is the sum total of smaller movements at each joint level. Therefore, it is worthwhile considering the movements zone-wise.

Even in zone-wise assessment of the movements, true assessment can only be done when other more mobile segments of spine are passively fixed (rather, it is difficult to actively fix the other part).

Passive testing of cervical movements (Figs 8.24 and 8.25): The patient should sit in maximum possible erect position on the stool. Stand behind the patient. The shoulder blades are stabilised in a horizontal plane by the left hand. Hold the chin in a neutral position, then test for backward bending and rotational movements. Now, support the chest from the front with one hand and press with the opposite hand over the occipital region to bend the cervical spine forward.

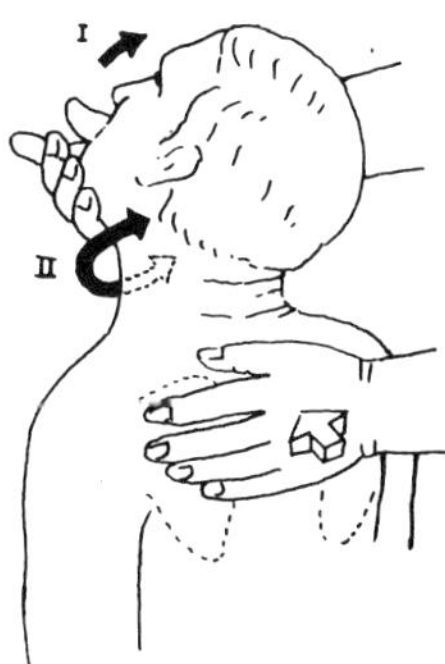

Fig. 8.24: Method of passive testing of backward bending and rotations; I = arrow showing backward bending; II = arrow showing rotations

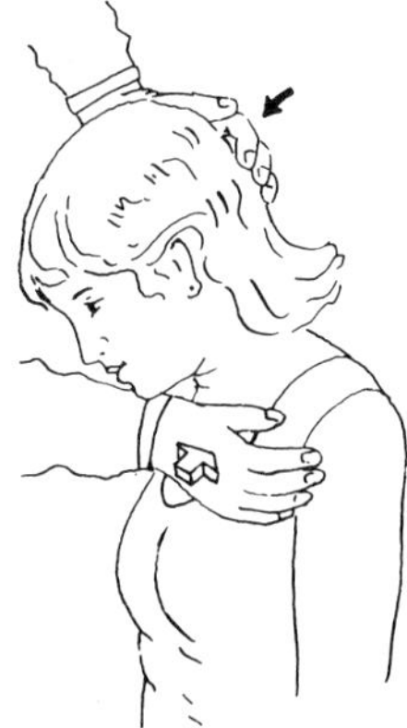

Fig. 8.25: Method of passive testing of forward bending of cervical spine

Movements of the Trunk

Dorsal spine: This portion of the spine is comparatively rigid, specially from cervicodorsal junction to D9. As such, all movements like flexion, extension, side bending, and rotational are possible but are much less as compared to other mobile portions of the spinal column. However, the augmented effect at each level along with the movements at the dorsolumbar spine provide an effective flexion and extension of dorsal and lumbar spines.

The dorsolumbar area (anatomically D 12-L1 but clinically for all practical purposes may be taken D 10-L2) is the transitional zone from a comparatively fixed to a mobile part of the spine. Hence, this area is subjected to more stress and strain by spinal movements. Effect of spinal movements at lumbar vertebrae get augmented at this level.

Lumbar Spine

Next to cervical, the lumbar region is the site where spinal movements are maximum possible. At the lowest part of the lumbar spine, i.e. lumbosacral region, again there is a transitional zone between the comparatively mobile lumbar vertebrae and the fixed sacrum. The movements in the lumbar region may not be to that extent as to which they appear. The comparatively fixed dorsal spines act like a lever-arm which gives an exaggerated effect to forward bending or backward bending. Skeletally, non-supported space below the lower costal margin provides an exaggerated effect of side bending. Here also,

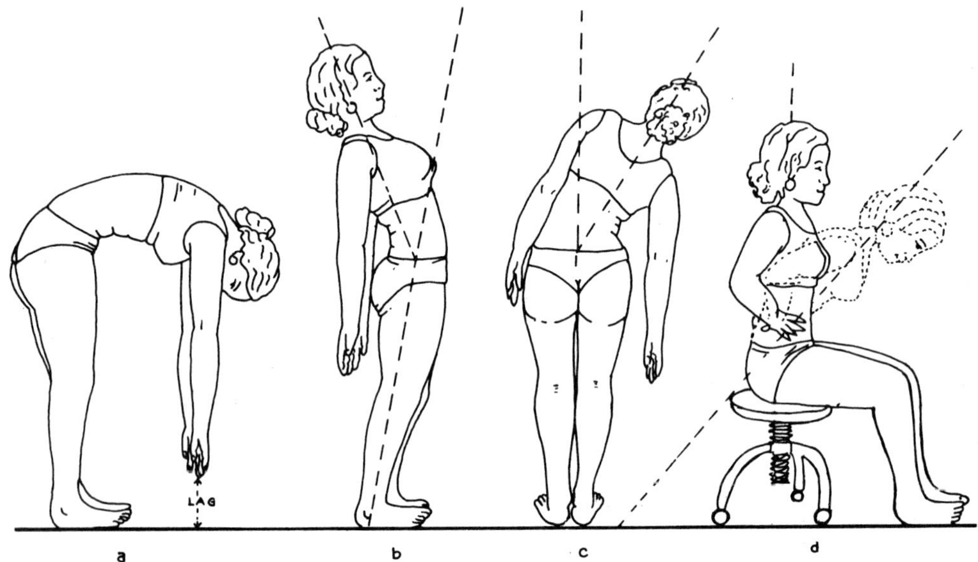

Fig. 8.26: Active movements of the trunk. a = Forward bending; b = backward bending; c = side bending; d = forward bending in sitting position

the dorsal spinal segment along with the chest cage provides a good leverage effect. Besides the above factors, one has to take consideration of movements at the hip in assessing movements of spines, specially lumbosacral and lumbars. Keeping the hip totally static, (e.g. bony ankylosed hips of ankylosing spondylitis) the effective forward, backward or side bending of the lower spinal column will be markedly limited. Very little gliding movements of sacro-iliac joints also play a small role in augmenting the spinal movements. Therefore, while assessing purely the movements of spine, one must obliterate the movements at hips and sacroiliacs.

Method (Fig. 8.26): For assessing the movements of spine in general—(these movements are the movements of utility in practical life) the patient is asked to stand erect with feet approximated together. He then has to bend forward, keeping the knees straight and touch the ground with the tips of both middle fingers. This will be full forward bending. Any limitation in this movement should be noted as distance lag from the ground to the tip of the longest finger (Fig. 8.26a).

For testing backward bending, standing in erect posture with feet approximated, the patient has to bend backwards and go as far as practicable towards heel. Normally, the fingers go up to about popliteal fossa level (Fig. 8.26b).

Side bending: The patient first stands in the same posture, i.e. erect with feet approximated and knee straight, he is then asked to bend towards lateral malleolus, while the other arm is diagonally opposite. Normally, the extended middle finger can reach up to about knee level. Change the arm for opposite side bending test (Fig. 8.26c).

Fallacies

Spinal movements vary to a great extent, depending upon the obesity, the elasticity of body and gymnastic activities.

How to test for pure movements at the lumbar, lumbosacral spine (Fig. 8.26d):

The patient will sit on the stool, keeping his both thighs approximated and fully opened first web of hand adapted on both iliac crests. The patient should then be asked to bend forwards with a tendency of taking his nose in between his two thighs without bending at hip. The movement occurs at the lumbar and lumbosacral region. From the erect sitting posture, he is then asked to bend backwards and sidewards alternately to assess these movements. While in this posture itself, the rotational movements of the spine can be tested very well. In the erect sitting posture on stool, ask him to look to his extreme right and that will be right rotation. Ask him to look extreme left which will be left rotation.

SACROILIAC JOINT

To complete the examination of spine, the sacroiliac joints must be examined. As such the movements of sacroiliac joints may be taken as invisible ones. In this joint, the bondage is mainly by tough interosseous ligaments. These ligaments are very short and allow very little of rotational movement in between the sides of the sacrum and the ear shaped articular facets of the iliac plates. In the physiomechanics of sacroiliacs, these motions are more or less involuntary (e.g. in defecation, raising the intra-abdominal pressure, during pregnancy and in locomotion).

Testing for these movements is done by indirect methods. The normal movements can not be seen and evaluated. But if any pathology exists in this joint, especially of inflammatory nature, pain in the joint is complained of on stress tests. They are of four types:

1. Straight leg raising test
2. Compression stress
3. Distraction stress
4. Axial rotational stress

} See the chapter on Pelvis

Measurements

Measurements of spine are not of that significance as they are for the limbs. However, in spinal deformities, specially kyphosis and scoliosis, special measurements are done to assess the degree of spinal curvatures.

Linear Measurement (Fig. 8.27A)

Distance from external occipital protuberance to the tip of coccyx will be the total length of spinal column. This should be measured if possible, in erect posture of the patient. This is of value for recording in the case sheet rather than comparing. The segmental measurement of the cervical and lumbar spines are sometimes of more value. In the cervical spine—in disease like Klippel-Feil-Syndrome, the distance between external occipital protuberance to vertebra prominence is markedly reduced (the lower hair line lies almost on cervicodorsal junction). In the lumbar region, the distance from dorso-lumbar spine to first sacral spine is reduced in spondylolisesis. Another linear measurement of significance is from tip of the last rib to the highest point of iliac crest (*ilio-costal distance*). In scoliosis or even in kyphosis these distances are accordingly reduced, while in lordosis these measurements are comparatively increased. These should be measured separately as record for the spinal deformities, localised in the upper region of lumbar spine.

The distance between external occipital protuberance to the highest point of iliac crests should be measured (*ileo-occipital distance*). They are equal on both sides. Any disparity will indicate the side bending of spine. In mild scoliotic tendency, these measurements may be of value.

Method: Ask the patient to stand or sit erect or lie prone in as much neutral a position as possible. Feel the external occipital protuberance at the highest point of central furrow. Pass your hands forwards over iliac crests from the dimple of venus. Stop at a point where the slope takes a downwards turn. Measure the distances between these points and compare with other side (Fig. 8.27A).

To assess the anatomical integrity in neutral position of cervical spine, oblique measurements are helpful, measured from the external occipital protuberance to acromian angle (Fig. 8.27A).

Linear measurements from vertebra prominence to S_1 point in full backward bending to full forward bending indicates the range of the spinal movements in anteroposterior directions (Fig. 8.27B). The measurement between these

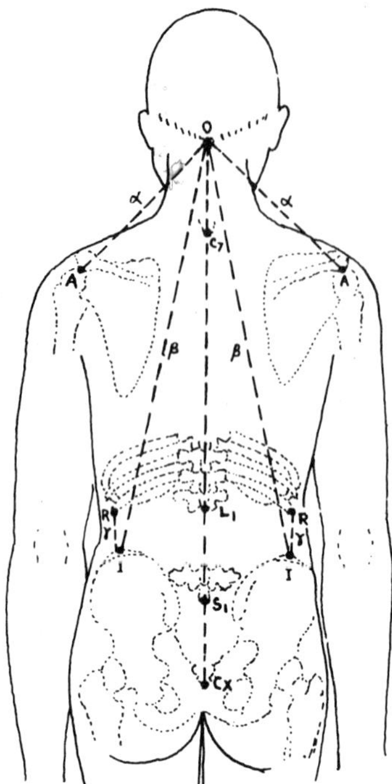

Fig. 8.27A: Linear measurement of spine. O = occipital protuberance; A = acromian angle; I = iliac crest; R = tip of the last rib

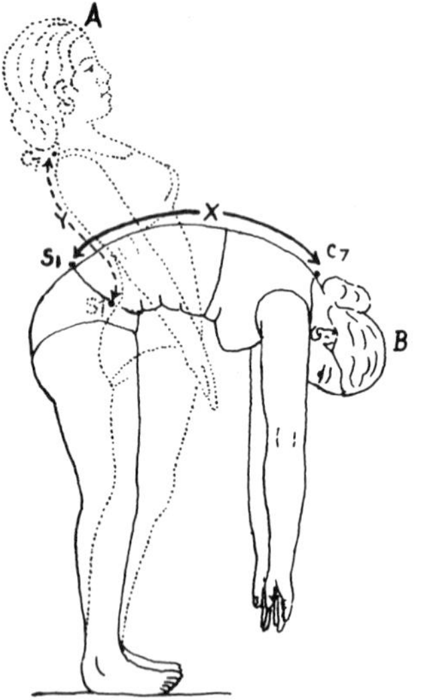

Fig. 8.27B: Method of measuring the anteroposterior spinal excursion (Ex). A = full extension; B = full flexion; X = distance between C_7 to S_1 spinous process; Y = distance between C_7 and S_1 spinous process in full extension, hence anteroposterior excursion, i.e. EX = (X-Y)

two points from the position of neutral erect posture to full forward bending allow an excursion of about 10 cm.

Measurement of Chest Expansion

In ankylosing spondylitis, this measurement is of paramount importance. In a normal individual, the expansion at the level of just below the nipple is allowed by about 5 to 8 cm. Limitation of this expansion to 2.5 cm in 4th intercostal space is highly suggestive of ankylosing spondylitis.

Auscultation

Auscultation in the spinal examination may appear to be of academic importance but at times, it is of immense value. There is no harm in putting the stetho bell on both sides of spinous processes as routine examination. In conditions like aortic aneurysm or highly vascular neoplasm, patient may complain of pain in the back as presenting symptom. In such conditions, clinically palpating and/or auscultatory bruit localised in that region of spinal column may be of immense value for further probe.

SPECIAL TESTS

1. Stress Test of Spine

In case of backache, especially in youngmen, this test is of significance in diagnosing ankylosing spondylitis. Ask the patient to fully bend the spine forwards, sideways and backwards, in sequence, for fifteen to twenty times. Then ask him to move about. He will feel relief in case of ankylosing spondylitis. However, in pathologies like, caries spine, disc prolapse, osteomyelitis and other infections of spine and spinal tumours, the patient feels his symptoms variably aggravated after the test.

2. Cervical Roots Stretch Test

Before performing these tests, one should rule out any instability in cervical region.

i. *Lateral Stretch Test*

In cervical spondylosis or cervical disc prolapse, lateral stretching of the cervical spine in opposite

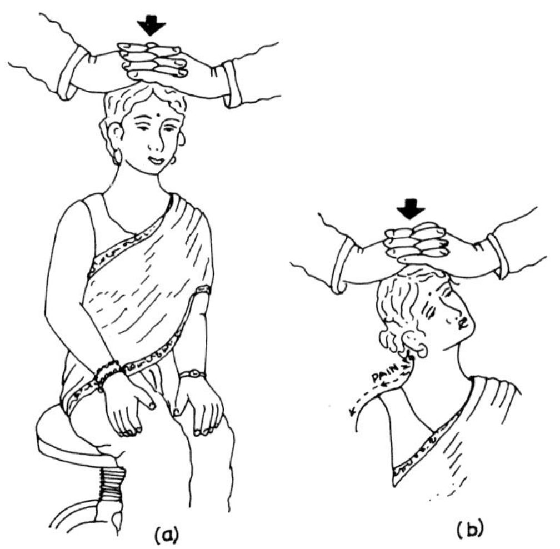

Fig. 8.28: Method of eliciting cervical compression test. a = in erect position; b = tilted and rotated position

direction may lead to pain along the affected nerve root.

ii. *Cervical Compression Test*

Even the initial stage of irritation of the roots can be tested by cervical compression test.

Method: Ask the patient to sit erect on the stool, keeping the head in as much neutral position as possible. Stand behind the patient with both hands placed over the vault of head, give a sudden brisk jerk in the line of spinal column (Fig. 8.28a). Note the reaction of the patient specially regarding pain in cervical region and referred area. Rotate the cervical spine to about 45° to each side and ask him to look to the ceiling. In each rotational position, repeat the brisk compression manoeuvre and note the patient's reaction (Fig. 8.28b). In positive cases, the patient will complain of augmentation of his typical symptoms in the area of root distribution which used to be felt off and on.

iii. *Distraction Test*

Passively distracting (stretch-elevating) the head in neutral position, by holding it at occiput and chin, relieves the symptoms of root irritation.

3. Test for Thoracic Inlet Syndromes

The vice like compression of the neurovascular bundle has bizarre manifestations like feeling of heat, burning sensation, tingling, numbness, heaviness, congestion, bluish discolouration and even weakness in affected-one, especially in the thumb and tips of the fingers. The vice compression can be clinically augmented by narrowing the angulation between the scaleni and first rib.

Method: Ask the patient to sit on the stool; stand on the side and behind the patient on which side the test has to be performed. Hold the wrist and palpate the radial pulse. Ask the patient to flex the neck on the affected side, while he elevates the chin and takes deep inspiration-OR-With palm of the opposite hand, press on the lateral side of neck towards the opposite shoulder as much as possible. At the same time, palpate the radial pulse of the extended limb. The latter is pulled downwards as far as possible (Fig. 8.29) while patient takes deep inspiration.

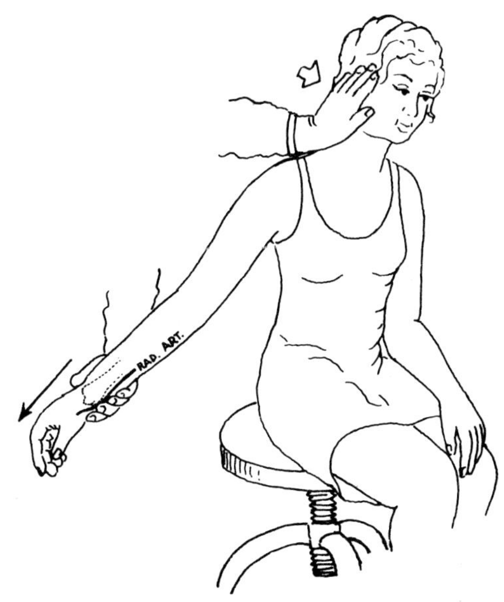

Fig. 8.29: Method of testing for thoracic inlet syndrome

There can be three manifestations:

i. No change in pulse and no complaint, except some feeling of stretch over root of neck—this is normal.
ii. Radial pulse may be weaker or even may get obliterated: This indicates that the subclavian artery is getting stretched and compressed.
iii. The patient may complain of re-appearance or augmentation of tingling and/or numbness in the affected area—this indicates that the brachial roots are stretched or compressed.

Second and third inferences should be taken as significant and corroborated with other clinical findings and investigation.

Tension Tests in Lumbar Disc Prolapse

Tension tests are based upon the manoeuvres which tighten the sciatic nerve and thus compress the inflammed nerve root against a herniated disc. The tests are:

1. Straight leg raising (SLR)
2. Well leg raising test (crossed leg raising)
3. Lasegue's (sign) test
4. Fajersztajn test
5. Lateral flexion test of spine
6. Sciatic stretch test } —including sudden
7. Figure of '4' test } sciatic stretch test
8. Bowstring test
9. Sitting root test
10. Femoral nerve stretch test is the tension test of the femoral nerve, mainly the L_4 root

1. *Straight Leg Raising Test*

The active straight leg raising in supine posture with extended knee, is normally possible approaching upto 90° (except in women, of Indian subcontinent, who remain very conscious in raising beyond 60° due to their clothing problems, as most of them do not use panty) without any pain. If patient can not lie supine (as in poker back, severe kyphosis), this test should be done in lateral position alternatively. In case of sciatic radiculitis, this manoeuvre elongates the course of the sciatic nerve, putting stretch on the sciatic root. Therefore, the patient complains of pain along the course of the sciatic nerve and its branches, if there is impingement on its root, (e.g. in intervertebral disc prolapse). By and large it has been seen that if the patient experiences pain in the course of the sciatic nerve by raising the leg upto 30°, it is diagnostic of intervertebral disc prolapse; if the pain is produced between 30°-70°, it is suggestive of disc prolapse and pain beyond 70° is equivocal.

This test is also of significance in assessing the stability of the hip joint, pathology of sacroiliac joint, integrity of hip flexors and quadriceps mechanism of the knee. However, acute/active pathology of lower lumbars and/or ipsilateral pelvis can also affect the straight leg raising.

2. *Well Leg Raising Test*

If raising of the unaffected extended leg produces pain along the sciatic distribution on the affected side, it is highly suggestive of disc prolapse, pressing on the root mostly from the medial side (well leg raising test).

3. *Lasegue's Test*

A similar test is done by elevating the straight leg by the examiner (Lasegue's test). If it is negative, one should be sceptical in diagnosing disc prolapse.

Method: While the patient is lying supine, the affected straight leg is elevated holding it with one hand above the ankle and pressing it by the other hand on the front of the thigh (Fig. 8.30). Normal leg can be elevated upto 90° without any pain. In case of sciatic root irritation, the patient will feel pain along the course of the sciatic nerve and the lower back much earlier. Measure the angle (between back of the thigh and the bed), at which pain just starts appearing.

4. This can be further confirmed by passively dorsiflexing the foot while the straight leg is kept at the same angle where pain has first appeared. This manoeuvre will accentuate the pain (Fajersztajn test) (Fig. 8.30).

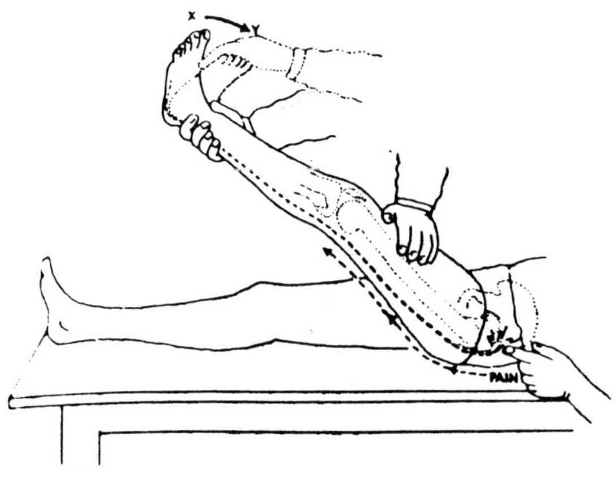

Fig. 8.30: Method of demonstration of Lasegue's test and Fajersztajn test

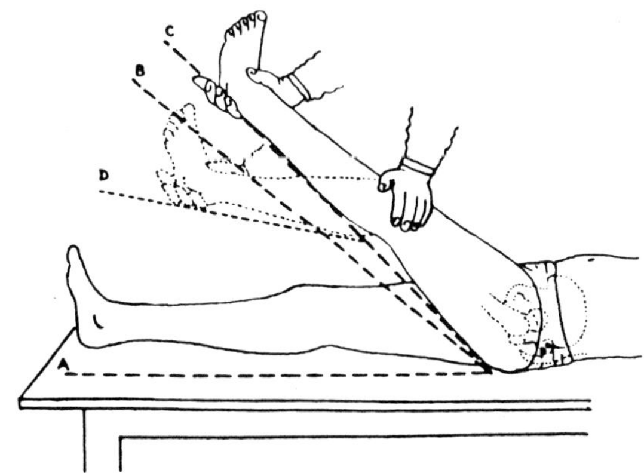

Fig. 8.31: Method of demonstration of sciatic stretch test. When limb was in position of 'A' there was no pain; in position of 'B' pain started appearing; in position of 'C' marked pain; in position of 'D' pain instantaneously disappears. 'P' indicates the site of pain at greater sciatic notch

5. *Lateral Flexion Test of Spine*

Ask the patient (standing or lying supine) with suspected disc prolapse to acutely flex the spine laterally on the affected side. Due to approximation of root to the protruded disc (from lateral side), the patient will feel a catching pain. If the symptoms are aggravated by flexing the spine on the opposite side, it indicates pressure over the root from the medial side.

6. *Sciatic Stretch Test*

Basis of the test—As suggested by Forst (1981), the basis of this test is to produce tension in the hamstring muscles, which in turn compresses the sciatic nerve. Therefore, the patient experiences acute pain at the level of sciatic notch, and along the course of sciatic nerve.

Method: (a) Ask the patient to lie supine, and support the foot of a fully extended leg in one hand and press over the ipsilateral knee by the other hand. Gradually, flex the lower limb at the hip while lifting the limb above the bed, the patient will feel pain at the level of sciatic notch in cases of sciatic radiculitis. On flexing the knee, the pain instantaneously disappears. In flexed position the hamstrings become lax, so that the sciatic nerve is not compressed (Fig. 8.31).

Sudden Sciatic Stretch Test

Patient sits erect on the table with the legs hanging at the edge from the knees. Then ask the patient to lean back supporting herself with both hands on the table. In the meantime hold the great toe of the suspected side and suddenly lift the bent knee to straight position. In the sciatic root impingement, patient will feel bursting pain at the low back (Fig. 8.32).

7. *Figure of '4' Test*

Ask the patient to lie supine. Flex, abduct and externally rotate the lower limb of the suspected side at the hip and flex the knee to the extent which allows the lower part of the leg to rest on the opposite lower thigh. Now give a jerky pressure over the medial aspect of the knee. In the sciatic root impingement or affections of sciatic nerve, the patient will complain of

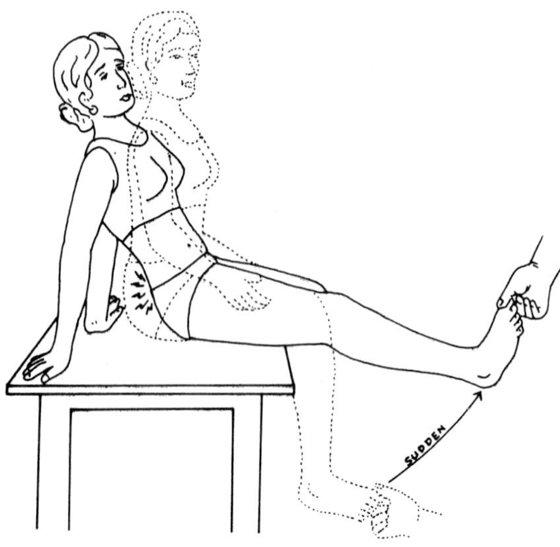

Fig. 8.32: Test to differentiate between a malingerer and a genuine patient of sciatic radiculitis sudden sciatic stretch test

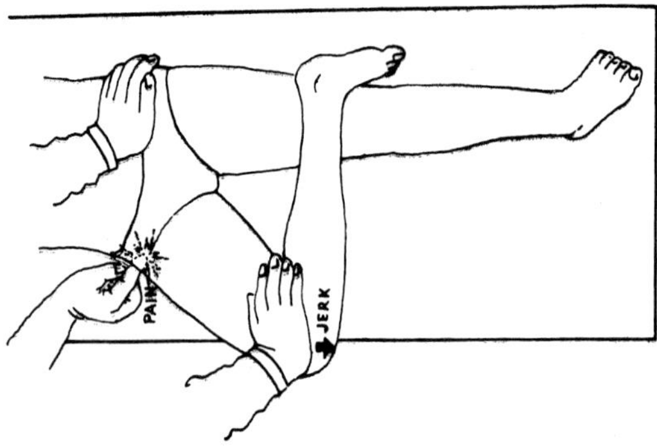

Fig. 8.33: Alternative method of sciatic stretch test (Figure of 4 test)

pain pointing to greater sciatic notch and along the sciatic course (Fig. 8.33).

8. *Bowstring Test*
Patient is asked to lift the straight leg till the pain starts being felt. At this point the knee is flexed, which instantaneously reduces the pain. Pressing the terminal region of the sciatic nerve restarts the painful radicular symptoms.

9. *Sitting Root Test*
Patient sits at the edge of the table with neck bent forward. While the hip remains flexed at 90° the knee is extended. Patient feels pain in the leg which he would like to avoid by attempting to extend the hip.

10. *Femoral Nerve Stretch Test*
Femoral nerve stretch test may be positive if the L2,3,4 roots are affected.

Method (Fig. 8.34): Ask the patient to lie prone. While the other leg is kept extended at the hip and knee, bend the affected side limb to 90° at knee. Hold the leg with one hand just above the ankle. The other forearm and hand should rest on the buttock at hip level, fixing the pelvis on the couch. Lift the bent leg upwards, more by stretching backwards at the hip (as passively testing for extension at hip). The femoral nerve is stretched along with the extension of hip. If the roots are pressed or over stretched, the patient may complain of pain on the front and outerside of thigh even upto knee. This is positive femoral nerve stretch test.

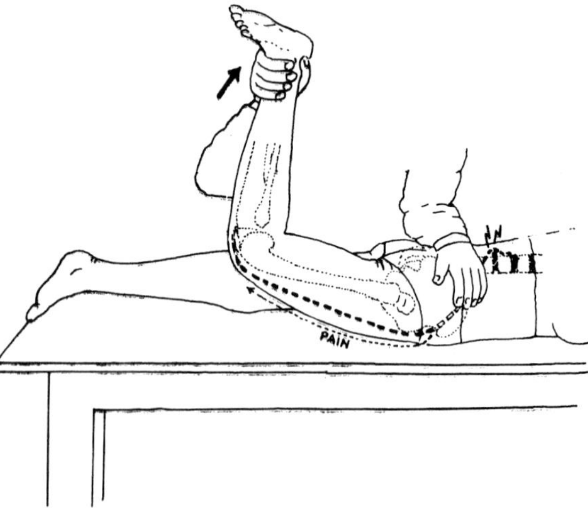

Fig. 8.34: Method of demonstrating the femoral nerve stretch test

Lower lumbar sciatic compressive radiculopathy can be confused with sciatic neuropathy when multiple segments are involved (very rare in disc herniation). Further in straight leg raising just short of discomfort, pain caused by a sciatic neuropathy is increased by internal rotation and relieved by external rotation of the hips, which are not seen in lumbar (sciatic) radiculopathy.

Piriformis Syndrome

This syndrome is the result of entrapment of sciatic nerve (first described in 1928 by Yoeman, and Robinson first used the term 'Piriformis syndrome' in 1947) by the piriformis muscle as it passes through the sciatic notch.

Causes can be hypertrophy of piriformis muscle, trauma, excessive exercises, pseudo-aneurysm of inferior gluteal artery, spasm and inflammation of piriformis muscle, anomalies of muscle, dystonia musculorum deformans, traumatic myositis ossificans.

Clinical findings: There may be history of injury to sacroiliac and/or gluteal region; pain in sacroiliac joint region, greater sciatic notch, and piriformis muscle extending down the lower limb causing difficult in walking; acute exacerbation of the symptoms by lifting the leg or stooping; isolated atrophy of gluteous maximus; dysthesia of posterior aspect of thigh; tenderness over sciatic notch, a palpable sausage shaped mass over the piriformis muscle, which is markedly tender during an exacerbation of symptoms. Tender mass can also be felt laterally during a rectal examination. This feature is pathognomic of the syndrome; a positive straight leg raising test, and Lasegue sign; Freiberg sign (Pain with forced internal rotation of extended thigh; and positive sign of Pace and Nagle (Pain with resistance to abduction and external rotation of the thigh.

The tibial nerve division of sciatic nerve is involved less often than peroneal division, since former is located more medially in the sciatic notch.

Diagnosis can be confirmed by nerve conduction studies demonstrating delayed F waves and H reflexes. CT and MRI show hypertrophy of piriformis muscle. This syndrome is managed by physiotherapy, NSAID, stretching, ultrasound, local hydrocortisone and anaesthetic infiltration. If there is no relief, operative release of piriformis muscle is recommended.

NEUROLOGICAL EXAMINATION

No spinal examination is complete without thorough examination of nervous system. It should be categorically examined under the following headings:

1. A quick assessment of mental state, intelligence, speech, general appearance
2. Cranial nerves
3. Gait
4. Posture
5. Motor functions
6. Sensory assessments
7. Vasomotor functions
8. Reflexes
   —Superficial reflexes
   —Deep reflexes (tendon jerks, clonus)
9. Visceral functions—assessment, specially of the bladder and bowel.

Gait (Fig. 8.35)

The average person takes 8,000 to 10,000 steps in a day, which if added makes about 7,47,000 kilometers in a life time of an average person (on global basis)—enough to take around the planet more than four times.

Usually, gait and posture of the patient, indicates the possible diagnosis of the spinal lesion. Hence, if the patient can walk, notice carefully the type of gait and posture maintained during walking and/or standing. While assessing the gait, the legs should be adequately exposed as feet should be bare. A normal gait must be rhythmic and soundless, having springiness in the feet which work alternatively in a definite cyclic order. This is broadly achieved by alternate effective shortening and lengthening of lower limbs. The gait cycle begins when one foot comes into contact with the ground (initial contact) and ends when the same foot makes

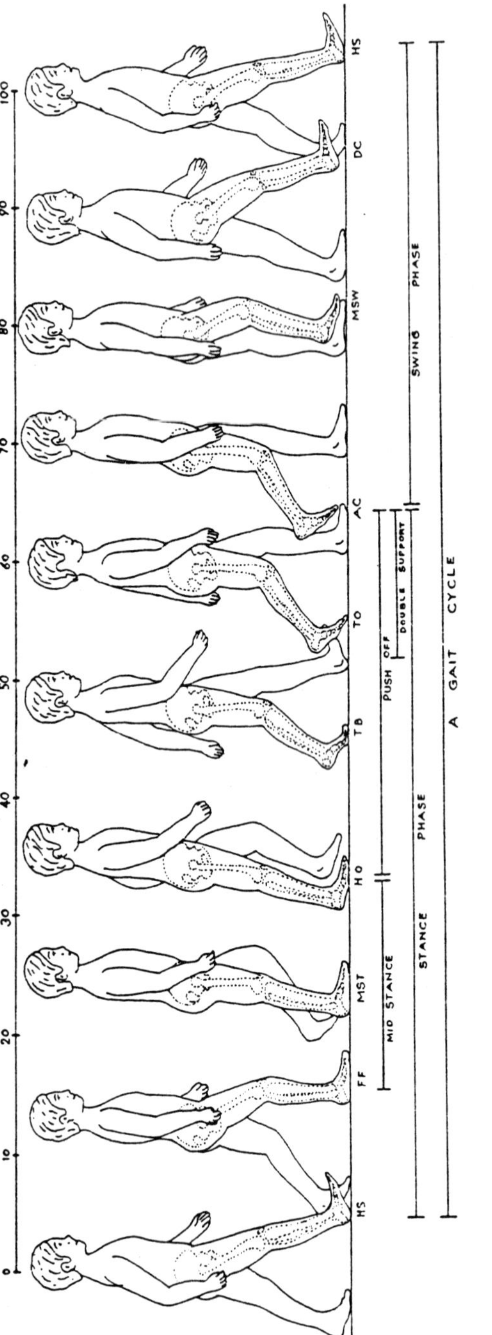

Fig. 8.35: A complete gait cycle. Stance phase 60%; Double support-11% of the gait cycle. HS = heel strike; FF = foot flat; MST = mid stance; HO = heel off; TB = toe break; TO = toe off; AC = acceleration; MSW = mid swing; DC = deceleration

contact with the ground again (subsequent initial contact). The basic unit of measurement in gait analysis is the gait cycle. *A normal gait cycle is divisible into two phases for each extremity: (i) The stance phase, and (ii) The swing phase.*

Stance phase is further subdivisible into-heel strike-foot flat-mid stance-heel off-toe break-push off (toe off). Swing phase is sub-divisible into acceleration, mid-swing and deceleration phases. In a rhythmic gait, while one foot is in the stance phase, the other passes through the swing phase. The stance phase starts with the heel of the leading extremity touching the floor (initial contact) followed by the sole of that foot. When the whole foot is in contact with the ground, this foot is supporting the whole body weight and this is the mid stance phase. Next follows the push off phase. After momentarily stabilising the weight on the whole foot, the heel of the supporting extremity rises from the floor. In succession, the balls of toes prepare to lift-off from the ground. In the meantime, the strong action of gastroc-soleus propels the body forward. With the toes off, the entire foot leaves the ground and enters the swing phase. The leg gets accelerated foward to get in front of the body to be prepared for the next heel strike. This is the acceleration sub-phase of the swing phase. While passing in this direction, at one point the leg has to pass just beneath the body. This is the mid-swing phase. In this phase, the leg is shortened by flexing the hip and knees so that the foot completely clears the ground. Immediately after the leg goes in front of the body, the movement is restrained (deceleration). Now the foot is prepared to go for heel strike.

During normal gait, for a moment, the two lower extremities are in simultaneous contact with the ground. This happens between push-off and toe-off on one side and between heal strike and foot flat on the contralateral side. During this period, both legs support the body weight, and this is known as "double support". The period of this "double support" is inversely proportional to the cadence (number of steps taken per minute) of the gait, i.e. if cadence of gait decreases, the period of double support increases and *vice-versa.*

Walking can be distinguished from running by minimisation of the period of double support in running. Roughly calculated, the relative period of different phases of gait are as follows—stance phase-60%, swing phase 40% and double support 11% of the cycle. With increase in the cadence, gradually the period spent in swing phase increases, and *vice-versa.*

There can be several variations in a normal gait depending upon the weight, the posture, the gymnastic activities, the shape of the foot, and the ground over which the individual walks. Everyone (including a patient) adopts the least energy consuming style of walking. The lay description of abnormal gait can be divided into two patterns—*limping and lurching*. In 'limping' the patient avoids weight bearing on the affected side as far as possible (diminished stance phase). *Limping denotes a painful condition* on the affected side. In lurch, the patient prolongs the stance phase to improve the stability. *Lurching denotes variable failure of abduction mechanism.* However, there are **recognised patterns of gait** which occur in particular clinical conditions:

1. *Scissors gait:* Here one leg crosses directly over the other with each step, like crossing of the blades of a scissor (e.g. cerebral diplegia).
2. *High stepping (steppage) gait (Equine gait):* Here, the patient flexes the hip and knee excessively in order to clear the ground, e.g. foot drop.
3. *Spastis gait:* Here, the spastic muscles do not allow the hip and knee to be flexed enough for the foot to clear the ground. Therefore, the patient partially drags his weight on the spastic leg. In this attempt, there is some circumduction effect on the lower limb (e.g. hemiplegia).
4. *Lathyriatic gait:* In lathyriasis there is a combination of spasticity, hyperabduction and dragging elements in the gait.
5. *Waddling gait or duck gait:* There is increased lordosis. The body sways from side to side on a wide base. Therefore, the patient lurches on both sides while walking, e.g. bilateral congenital dislocation of hip, osteomalacia, pregnancy, myopathy.
6. *Trendelenburg's gait:* It may be unilateral or bilateral. Bilateral trendelenberg's gait is almost like the waddling gait. When unilateral, the patient lurches on the affected side and the pelvis drops on the opposite side of hip. Any condition, in which there is deficit in abduction mechanism of the hip joint, medial deviation of the mechanical axis of the lower limb, and gross costo pelvic impingement (e.g. CDH, fracture of femoral neck, polioparalysis), will cause this.
7. *Drunkards or reeling gait:* Here the patient tends to walk irregularly on a wide base, swinging sideways with tendency of falling with each step (seen in cerebellar incoordination, or in drunken states).
8. *Festinent gait or short shuffling gait:* Here the patient, with stooping body, is propelled forward quickly in successions as if trying to catch up with the centre of gravity, e.g. Parkinsonism. In a few cases of parkinsonism 'RETROPULSION' occurs—i.e. if the patient is pushed backwards, he starts walking backward involuntarily.
9. *Antalgic gait—Painful gait:* Due to pain anywhere from foot to hip, the patient avoids bearing weight on the affected limb (reduced stance phase).
10. *Stamping gait:* Occurs in sensory ataxia, e.g. tabes dorsalis. The patient raises his feet abnormally high and jerks them forward to strike the ground with a 'stamp'.
11. *Knock knee gait:* The gait here is also a typical one, i.e. while walking, the patient flexes the hips slightly, the knees point and appose each other, and the ankles and feet are kept apart with tendency of toe-in.

12. *Short limb gait:* Initially the shortening is made up by equinus. With more shortening (usually more than 5 cms) the patient dips his body on that side.
13. *Short-leg gait (more or less as above no 12):* Mild to moderate shortened lower limb in children is compensated by acquiring 'equinus' position (ending in equinus deformity) of the ankle and foot, when the person walks on the broadened forefoot and toes.
14. *Quadriceps gait or hand to knee gait or five fingers quadriceps (see Figs 11.6A):* In case of very weak quadriceps, the patient stabilizes his knee for weight bearing by little leaning on the affected side and pressing over the lower thigh by his ipsilateral hand or fingers, either openly or through the pocket of the trouser.
15. *Calcaneus gait:* Patient walks on his broadened heel with a tendency of rotating the foot outwards, tendency of genu recurvatum, with no calcaneal pick up, no push off, and is due to weakness of the triceps surae.
16. *Gluteus medius gait* is more or less as Tredelenburg's gait, which is more exemplified in the paralysis of gluteus medius.
17. *Gluteus maximus gait:* Due to weakness in the gluteus maximus muscle, the patient lurches backwards (mostly seen in polio paralysis.
18. *Ataxic gait:* A gait in which the foot is raised higher than is necessary and brought down suddenly in a flapping manner (more or less similar to stamping gait).
19. *Stiff hip gait:* Patient walks without flexing the hip (about 20° of flexing of hip is essential for normal gait).
20. *Stiff knee gait:* During the swing phase, the patient has to raise the affected side pelvis.
21. *Circumduction gait:* If the limb is lengthened, even apparently (e.g. in fixed abduction deformity of hip) the patient has to take the affected limb in round about way to take the forward step.
22. *Hysterical gait:* Patient walks in bizarre fashion as if going to fall on every step, but seldom falls and that too cautiously.
23. *Cerebellar gait:* A staggering gait, often with a tendency to fall to one or other side, forward or backward.
24. *Charcot's gait:* The gait of hereditary ataxia.

Posture

Posture itself is a complex subject and requires clear understanding. The particular posture adopted by the patient while walking and standing should be described clearly. There are certain postures which are very typical of particular conditions, e.g. in parkinsonism the patient has a tendency of stooping forward with the arm adducted, elbow semiflexed, forearm semipronated and 'pill-rolling' movements in between his thumb and fingers. In advanced ankylosing spondylitis, the patient has a typical pokerback appearance, keeping the trunk stooped forward, neck rigidly fixed and thereby has a tendency of looking towards the ground.

Motor Dysfunctions

Main motor dysfunctions are:

i. Loss or less of functions (Lower motor neurone type of paralysis, flaccid paralysis).
ii. Excess of function due to excessive unbriddled neurological stimulation to muscles
 —spastic paraplegia
 —upper motor neurone type of paralysis
iii. Abnormal movements, e.g.
 - Athetosis—writhing type of motion affecting part or whole body.
 - Chorea (the word chorea means a dance)—sudden abnormal discharges along the nerve cause flinging, mostly of one limb. The involuntary movements are brief, fluid and often difficult to discern in the beginning.
 - Dystonia: It expresses an 'abnormally maintained posture', often associated with a plastic rigidity, e.g. flexed posture of Parkinson's disease (flexion dystonia); or the hemiplagic posture (hemiplegic dystonia).

- Dyskinesia: The involuntary movements predominently affect the pharyngeal and facial perioral musculature (e.g. phenothiazene-induced involuntary movements).
- Torticollis: It is a form of dystonia in which a jerky or maintained rotational and abducted posture of neck occurs—spasmodic torticollis.
- Tics: These are normal simple movements which become unnecessarily repeated (producing embarrasing situation). They can be easily imitated, e.g. head-nodding.
- Tetany: It usually occurs in hypocalcaemia or alkalosis in which a peculiar posture of the hand (may be also of toes) develops, in which the fingers and thumbs are held stiffly adducted and partially flexed at the metacarpophalangeal joints. In foot the toes may be similarly effected (carpopedal spasm).

These effects can be reproduced or augmented by producing ischaemia of the affected limb, e.g. by inflating the sphygmomanometer cuff above the arterial pressure for three minutes—Trousseau's sign.

This can also be tested by eliciting Chvostek's sign—tap lightly with patellar hammer at the sternomastoid foramen region through which the facial nerve emerges (3-5 cm in front and below the external auditory meatus)—the facial muscles starts twitching.

Motor Function

Examine under following headings:

i. Bulk of muscle
ii. Tone of muscle
iii. Power of muscle
iv. Reflexes
   - —superficial reflexes (Table 8.4)
   - —deep reflexes (tendon jerks and clonus) (Table 8.5)
v. Co-ordination of movements
vi. Involuntary movements
vii. Contractures.

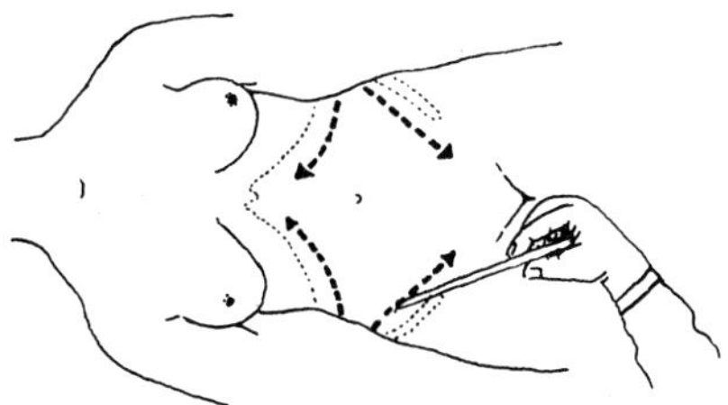

Fig. 8.36: Method of eliciting abdominal reflexes

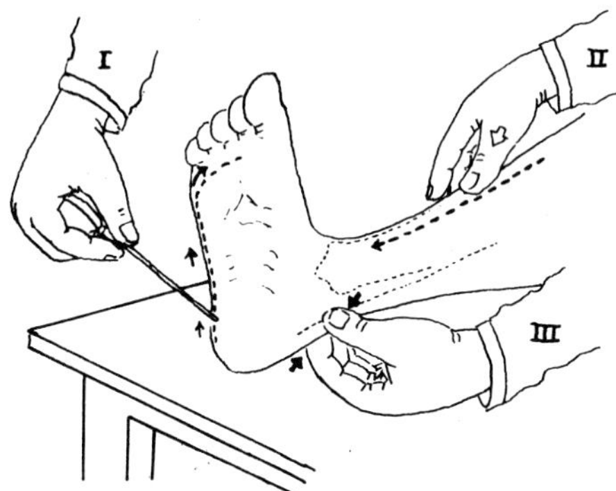

Fig. 8.37A: Different methods of eliciting plantar reflex; I = by stroking the outer sole of the foot; II = by pressing firmly along the medial border of tibia (Oppenheim s sign); III = by squeezing the heel cord (Gordon s sign)

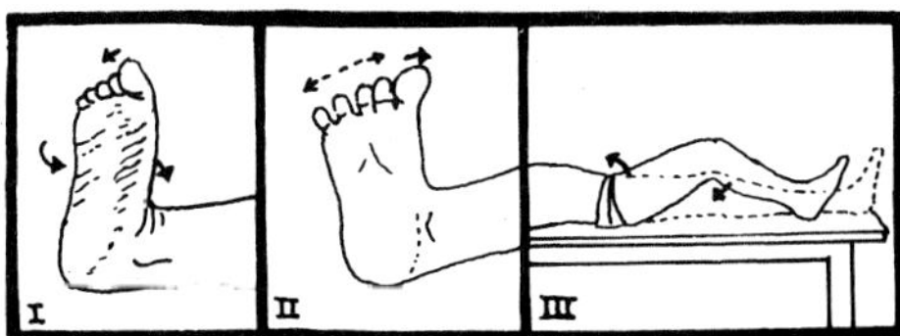

Fig. 8.37B: Showing different responses of plantar reflex. I = flexion of toes; dorsiflexion at ankle and inversion of foot; II = extension of big toe and fanning out of other toes; III = flexion of the hip and knee (In patients with amputated or fallen out toes this response should be looked for. In less severe case hamstrings can be felt and seen contracting)

Bulk of Muscle

i. Look at and feel the bulk of the muscle and assess for any atrophy or hypertrophy. The texture, pliability and flabbiness can also be assessed simultaneously. Confirm by circum-

Table 8.4: Main superficial reflexes

	Reflex	*How to initiate*	*What to observe*	*Inference*	*Cord level*	*Fallacies*
	1	*2*	*3*	*4*	*5*	*6*
1.	Trapezius reflex	— Just proximal to acromion tap the stretched-trapezius	— Contraction of trapezius	Normal (Hyper contraction indicates lesion above C_2 C_1)	C_3-C_4	
2.	Deltoid reflex	— Tap on upper deltoid mass just distal to acromion	— Contraction of deltoid	Normal (Hypercontraction indicates lesion above C_4).	C_5-C_6	
3.	Scapular reflex	— Scratching of skin in inter-scapular region	— Scapular muscle contraction	Normal	C_5-T_1	
4.	Abdominal reflex (Fig. 8.36)	— Scratching of abdominal wall obliquely in all four quadrants, from outer aspect towards midline	— Contraction of abdominal muscles in the testing quadrant.	Normal Absent in UMN lesions above their spinal level	$T_{7\text{-}12}$	Obese, lax abdomen, multipara, anxious and tense patients (diminished or absent)
5.	Cremastric reflex	— With a blunt pointed needle gently scratch over the upper medial side of thigh	— Involuntary contraction of the dartos muscle of scrotum.	Normal	L_1	Huge filarial scrotum. (diminished or absent)
6.	Anal reflex	— Scratch perianal skin or insert one lubricated gloved finger in anus	— Contraction of anal sphincter — No contraction	Normal Caude equina lesion.	S 3-4	Chronic perianal fistula. perianal surgery, patulous anus (diminished or absent)
7.	Bulbocavernosus reflex	— Pinching dorsum of glans penis.	— Contraction of bulbo-cavernosus muscle.	Normal	S 3-4	
8.	Plantar reflex* (Figs 8.37 A and B)	— Stroking the outer part of the sole from heel to base of outer toes (Fig. 8.37A I) — Squeezing the heel cord (Gordon's sign) Fig. 8.37A III — Squeezing the calf — Pressing firmly along the medial surface of tibia (Oppenheim's sign) (Fig. 8.37A II)	1. Flexion of toes, dorsi-flexion of ankle, inversion of foot (Fig. 8.37B I) 2. Extension of great toe, spreading out and extension of other toes. Dorsiflexion of ankle (Fig.8.37B II) 3. Flexion of hip and knee. (withdrawal reflex). (Fig. 8.37B III)	Flexor plantar response (Normal) Extensor plantar responses or Babinski's sign. UMN lesion	L5, S1	Difficult to demonstrate in anaesthetic sole, thick skin of the sole, barefoot walkers. In children below 1 year the extension response is normal. Tense and excited individual may have extensor response.

Contd.

ferential measurements of the bulk, comparing with the normal side. In few cases of muscular dystrophy (Duchenne dystrophy) due to underlying pathology, the muscle bulk increases in size and feels comparatively firm (calf muscles, glutei, infraspinate). Of course, they are weaker in strength.

ii. *Tone of muscle (state of tension found in healthy muscle and contracture)*: Assess the tone of the muscle by palpation. Increase in tone of muscle is *hypertonia*, and decrease *hypotonia*. A hypotonic (flaccid) muscle will be soft and pliable, and provide little or no resistance to passive movements, e.g. lower motor neuron lesions. As the tone increases in the muscle, the muscle becomes less movable from side to side and tighter in feel. Increase and sustenance of tone leads to hypertonia.

Normally, when a particular joint is moved it can be moved freely unless the patient voluntarily resists it. But in presence of hypertonia, the patient does not have much voluntary control over the involuntary resistance offered in moving that joint.

Hypertonia can occur due to lesions of corticospinal systems or extrapyramidal pathways. *Hypertonia due to pyramidal affection is called spasticity*. This spasticity produces rigidity of *clasp-knife type* (when the limb is rapidly flexed or extended, initially there is resistance, after which there is sudden yield).

Hypertonia, following disease of basal ganglion is termed as extrapyramidal rigidity. The rigidity is either *cogwheel type* (the resistance offered is jerky throughout), or *lead pipe type* (uniform rigidity throughout the movement, as in bending a lead pipe)—as in paratonic or catatonic states, e.g. parkinsonism. The physiological basis of this type of rigidity is not clearly known.

In hysteria also the patient offers rigidity. Here, the resistance increases proportionately to the effort applied by the examiner. *Contracture*—here the muscle is wasted, fibrotic and shortened. It feels firm and becomes variably unstretchable. In advanced neglected para-

Table 8.4: Contd.

Reflex	*How to initiate*	*What to observe*	*Inference*	*Cord level*	*Fallacies*
1	2	3	4	5	6
9. Throckmorton's reflex (Thomas-Bentley Throckmorton, American neurologist, (1885)	Percuss the dorsum of foot in metatarscphalangeal joints region	Extension of great toe and flexion of others	Normal		

*In the progressive lesions, the receptive field spreads from outer part of sole over to the whole sole, the leg, knees or even the groin. Hence there also these signs can be elicited

Table 8.5: Deep reflexes (tendon jerks and clonus)

	Reflexes	*How to test*	*What to observe*	*Inference*	*Cord level*	*Fallacies*
	1	2	3	4	5	6
1.	Knee jerk (Figs 8.38 A and C)	1. Patient supine, knees bent 60°, tap the patellar tendon. In the same position of the knee and heel, the forefoot is supported and tapping over the tendo-Achilles from behind elicits ankle jerk. (Figs 8.38A and B) 2. Patient sits with leg hanging at the edge of the table, tap over patellar tendon. In the same position while one hand supports the foot at 90° to leg, tapping over the tendo-Achilles from behind elicits the ankle jerks (Fig. 8.38C) 3. Patient sits on the stool with knee bent 90° and foot planted on the floor. Tap over the patellar tendon to elicit the knee jerk; and tap over the tendo-Achilles to elicit the ankle jerk	Contraction of quadriceps, brief extension of knee Diminished or absent contraction of quadriceps May be brisk contraction of quadriceps Exaggerated contraction of quadriceps. Leg suddenly tends to be thrown off Sustained oscillatory contraction and relaxation of quadriceps (clonus)	Normal LMN Lesion UMN Lesion UMN Lesion UMN Lesion	$L_{2,3,4.}$	Anxious tense individual
2.	Patellar jerk (Fig. 8.39)	Patient supine with extended knee. Tap over your middle finger placed on upper pole of patella	Patella quickly moves upwards	UMN lesion where knee jerk is exaggerated	$L_{2,3,4}$	
3.	Patellar clonus (Fig. 8.40)	Patient supine with extended knee. Hold upper pole of patella between thumb and index finger. Suddenly give a downward jerk and loosen the grip.	Oscillatory up and down movements of patella	-do-	-do-	
4.	Ankle jerk (Figs 8.38B, 8.38C and 8.41)	1. Patient lies supine keeping the leg crossed over opposite leg; slightly dorsiflex the foot with one hand and tap over the stretched tendo-Achilles. 2. As in knee. (Figs 8.38B and C) 3. As in knee 3	A sharp contraction of calf muscle, foot may go in plantar flexion The above response may be brisk/ exaggerated Sustained oscillatory contraction and relaxation of calf muscle (clonus) Diminished or absent contraction of calf muscles	Normal UMN lesion UMN lesion LMN lesion	$S_{1,2}$	

Contd.

Table 8.5: Contd.

	Reflexes	*How to test*	*What to observe*	*Inference*	*Cord level*	*Fallacies*
	1	*2*	*3*	*4*	*5*	*6*
5.	Ankle clonus (Fig. 8.42)	Patient lies supine. Bend the knee 60°. Hold or support the upper leg with one hand. With another hand hold the forefoot and give sudden dorsiflexion jerk and maintain the forefoot support	Oscillatory movements of the foot due to contraction/relaxation of calf muscles	UMN lesion	S1,2	
6.	Triceps jerk (Fig. 8.43)	With one hand support patient's forearm with the elbow bent to 90° and tap over triceps tendon	Diminished/absent Contraction of triceps, brief extension of elbow Brisk exaggerated contraction	LMN lesion Normal UMN lesion	C6,7	
7.	Biceps jerk (Fig. 8.44)	With one hand, support patient's semipronated forearm and elbow bent 90°. Place the supporting hand's thumb on biceps tendon. Tap over the thumb	Diminished/absent Biceps contracts Exaggerated	LMN lesion Normal. UMN lesion	C5,6	
8.	Supinator jerk (Fig. 8.45)	Forearm semipronated, tap over the radial styloid process	Supinator is stretched causing supination of the forearm	Normal.	C5,6	
9.	Inversion of radial jerk	Same as supinator jerk	Brisk flexion of fingers due to hyperexcitability of anterior horn cells at C_{7-8} level	UMN lesion	C5,6	
10.	Jaw jerk (Fig. 8.46).	Patient moderately opens her mouth. Place one finger on the chin, firmly tap over it suddenly	Muscles closing the jaw contract Increased contraction	Normal UMN lesion above fifth cranial nerve		Sometimes absent in health

N.B. (1) When not normally elicited. JENDRASSIK'S manoeuvre, by virtue of its increasing the excitability of anterior horn cells and stretch sensitivity of primary sensory nerve endings, helps in eliciting the deep reflexes (important for lower limbs). Here the patient does some strong voluntary effort with the upper limbs, like forcibly pulling apart the hooked fingers.

(2) Exaggerated tendon reflexes carry pathological significance only when asymmetrical, or when supported by other UMN manifestations, since in tense and anxious persons or tetanus or thyrotoxicosis, there may be hyperreflexia.

(3) The 'ankle clonus reflex' was first described by Dimitrejevic *et al* as a "hyperreflexive state often associated with spasticity and upper motor neuron lesion. It is series of rhythmic contractions of muscle at a frequency of five to seven hertz in response to an abruptly and continuously applied stretch reflex". The clonus reflex requires an intact spinal stretch reflex and sustained hyperexcitability of the lower motor neurones secondary to a loss of central inhibition. In the case of this ankle clonus reflex, the first sacral nerve root mediates the spinal stretch reflex arc

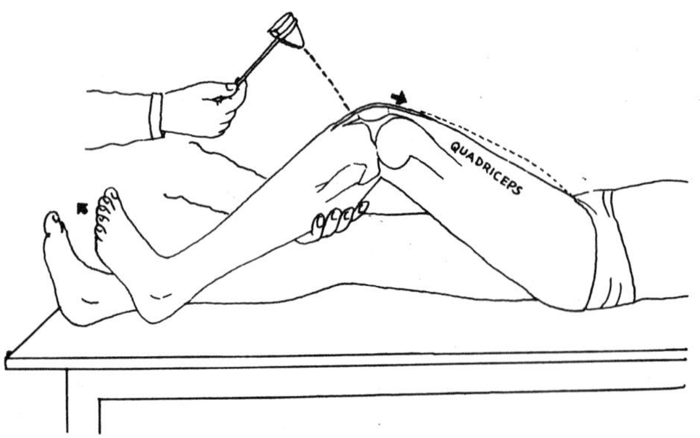

Fig. 8.38A: Method of eliciting the knee jerk while patient is in supine position. Arrow is showing the movement response and the dotted line shows the contraction of quadriceps

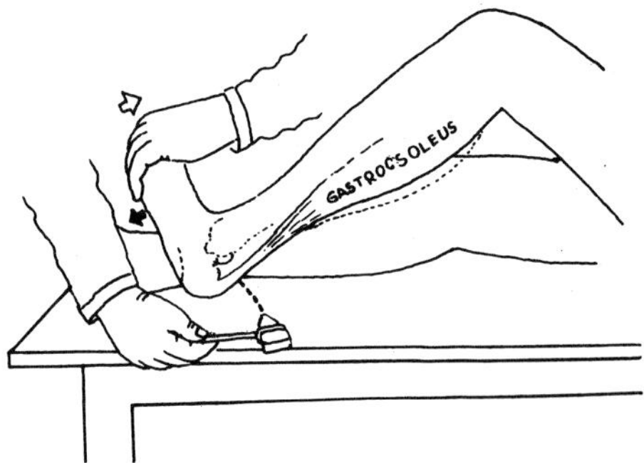

Fig. 8.38B: Method of eliciting ankle jerk while the patient is lying down. Dotted line shows contraction of the gastroc-soleus as a response to ankle jerk. As a consequence a sudden plantar flexion at ankle is shown by dark arrow

plegics, there may be contractures at the joints due to postural negligence or persistent flexor spasms.

iii. *Power of muscle*: To be assessed as given in the chapter on "Introduction".

iv. *Reflexes*
- Superficial reflexes (Table 8.4)
- Deep reflexes (tendon jerks and clonus) (Table 8.5).

The diminution or loss of tendon jerks signifies the presence of a lesion affecting the afferent pathways, anterior horn cells or efferent

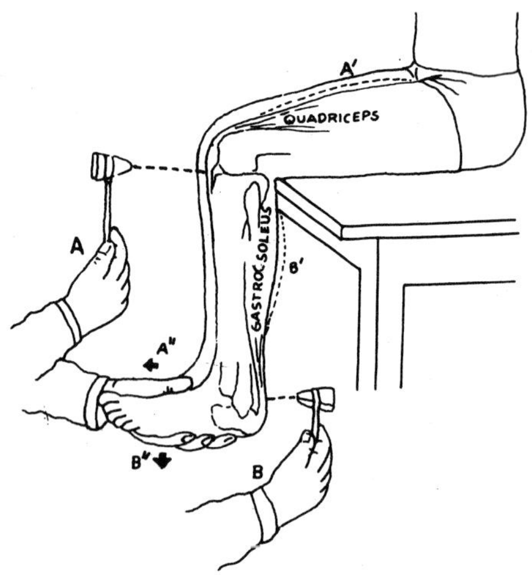

Fig. 8.38C: Eliciting knee (A, A and A*f*) and ankle jerk (B, B and B*f*) while the patient is sitting at the edge of the table

pathways, i.e. the lower motor neuron disease. Assess clearly the diminished or lost jerk. If upper jerks are normal, then the level of cord damage will be lower to the spinal levels which control these jerks, and above the spinal level which controls the immediate lower jerk which is lost.

v. *Coordination of movements*

For a definite motor action, certain separate muscles or group of muscles act in synergism and cooperation, when coordination is intact. For this, perfection in cerebellar control, neuromuscular axis, muscular tone and contractability and sense of joint position (and vision) are essential.

Tests

In upper limbs: Ask the patient to touch his nose tip with his index finger tip, thence with the other index finger, i.e. finger to nose. Similarly, ask him to touch one index finger tip to another index finger tip with arms extended. This should be repeated with his eyes closed, to assess the intactness of the sense of position of the joints of the limb.

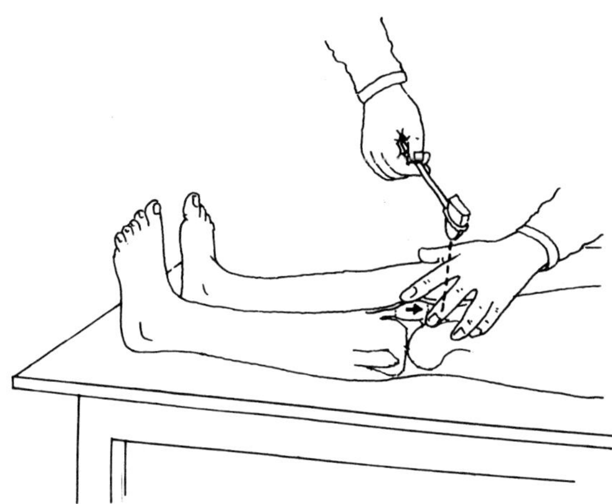

Fig. 8.39: Method of eliciting the patellar jerk. Arrow shows the sudden upward shift of patella after tapping over the upper pole

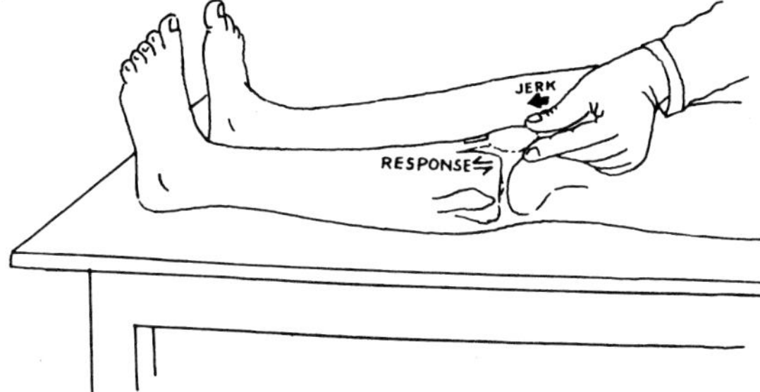

Fig. 8.40: The method of eliciting patellar clonus

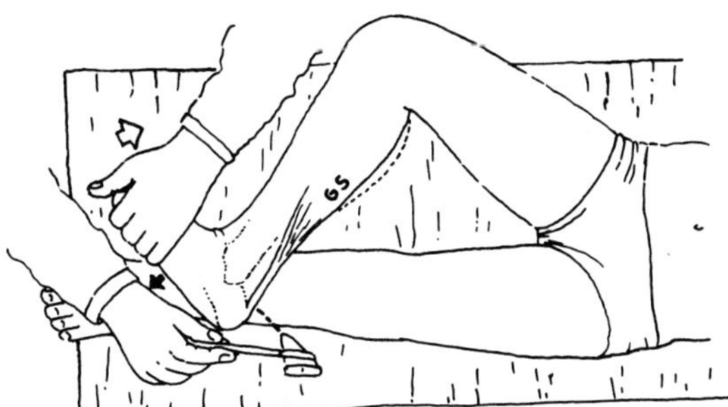

Fig. 8.41: Another method of eliciting the ankle jerk while patient is supine (GS = gastrocsoleus)

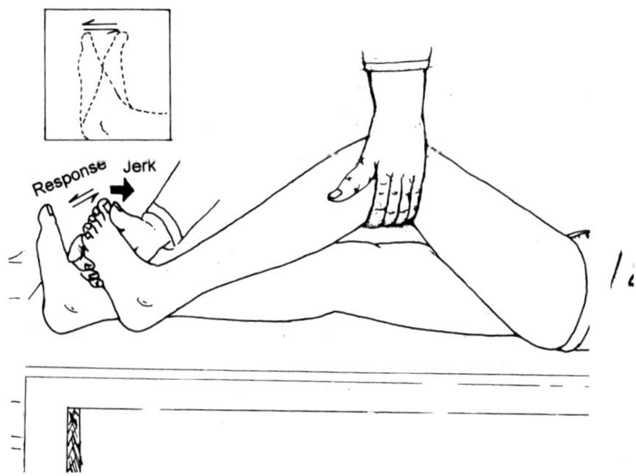

Fig. 8.42: Method of eliciting ankle clonus

In lower limbs: A normal gait indicates perfect coordination. However, in suspected cases, heel to tibial shin coordination can be tested. While lying down and with the eyes open, the patient is aksed to lift one leg in the air, then to bring the heel of that leg over the upper end of the opposite tibial shin and slide it down over the shin towards the ankle.

Romberg's sign: Truely, this sign indicates loss of position sense (sensory ataxia, e.g. tabes dorsalis). However, in advanced vertigo or cerebellar dysfunctions, this test may be positive to a varying extent. Ask the patient to stand with feet approximated and eyes closed. If the test is positive, he starts swaying and may even fall. (cf while in cerebellar ataxia, the patient sways even with the eyes open. This can be further confirmed by observing for dysdiadochokinesia—the patient cannot perform any repeated voluntary movement rapidly).

vi. *Involuntary movement*

Involuntary, undesired movements occur either at rest or during voluntary movements in several diseases, mostly those affecting the extra-pyramidal system, e.g. basal ganglia. Few known varieties are—epilepsy, myoclonus, tremor,

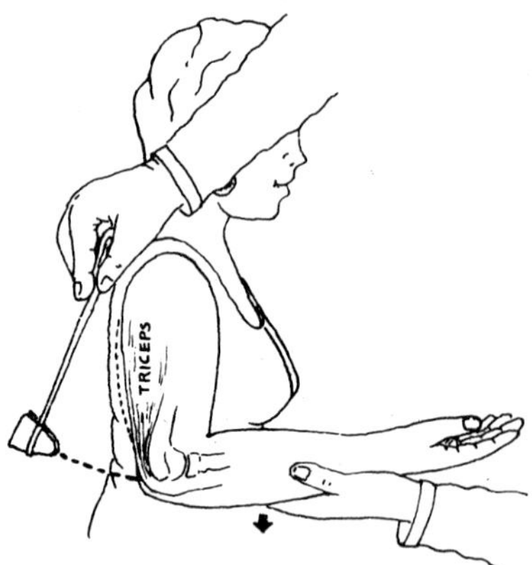

Fig. 8.43: Method of eliciting triceps jerk, dotted line represents contracted triceps after tapping over the tendon. Consequently the elbow shows tendency of extension shown by arrow

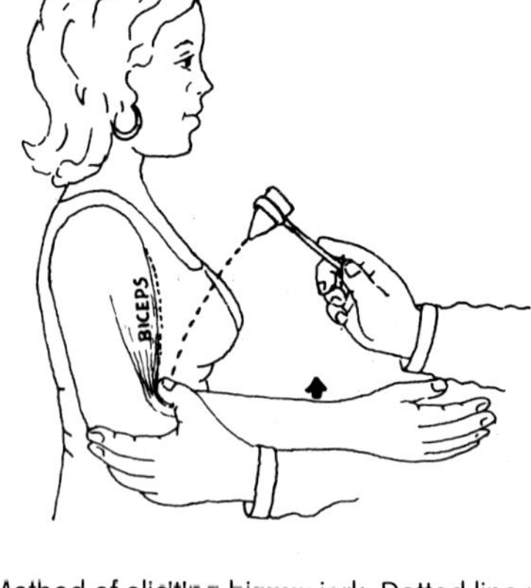

Fig. 8.44: Method of eliciting biceps jerk. Dotted line represents the contracted biceps tendon. Consequently the elbow goes in flexion as shown by arrow

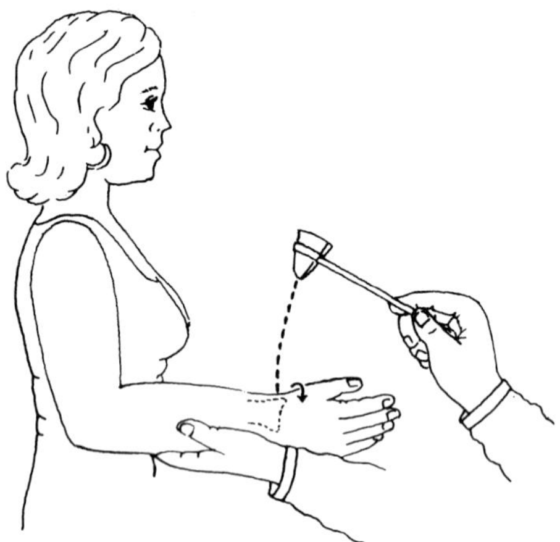

Fig. 8.45: Method of eliciting supinator jerk. Arrow showing the supination of the forearm

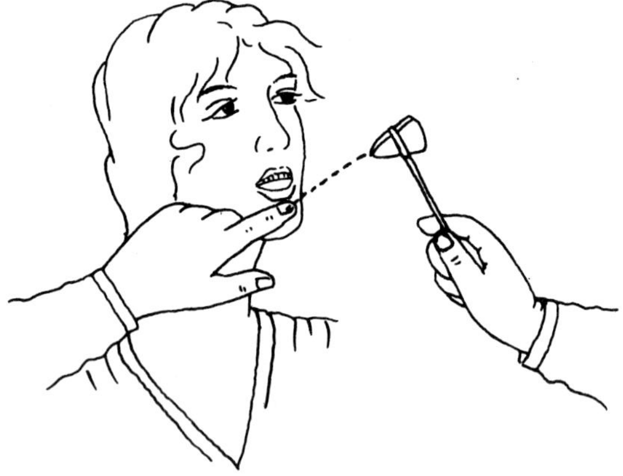

Fig. 8.46: Method of eliciting jaw jerk

athetosis, chorea (meaning a 'dance'), dyskinesia, dystonia, tics, myokymia, hemiballismus, asterixis, tetany, etc.

Sensory Functions

Detailed sensory mapping specially for the limbs should be done for superficial touch, pain, temperature, deep touch, and deep pain, and deficiencies should be noted in terms of root affections.

Superficial Touch

It should be tested with cotton wool after taking the patient fully in confidence. The patient's eyes should be closed or covered with a towel. In spinal lesions specially those in the lumbar region, perianal anaesthesia must be tested along with. In cauda equina lesion—perianal saddle anaesthesia is characteristic.

Temperature

Temperature discrimination can be tested by taking two test tubes, one containing warm and the other cold water. Touch the suspected area, alternately, with the particular test tube and ask for the feeling of the patient. Dissociation of different sensations should be assessed.

Deep Touch

Bathyanaesthesia [Gr. bathos = deep + an = not + aisthesis = perception]—loss of deep sensations should be carefully assessed.

Note the appreciation of deep touch by sharp and blunt objects. Also test for joint sense and sense of position (by asking the patient to close the eyes and to tell about the position of the great toe, while the examiner changes its position from up ♦ neutral ♦ down and *vice versa*), sense of vibration (by tuning fork over bony prominence), sense of discrimination (by divider points), recognition of size, shape, form and weight of known objects (stereognosis).

In *syringomyelia* the pain and temperature sensations are lost while crude touch and postural sensibility is preserved. In *Brown-Sequard syndrome* (hemisection of spinal cord) there is loss of pain, temperature and deep touch sensation of opposite side while there is disturbance of sense of posture, position, movement, loss of recognition of weight, shape, size, vibration and light touch, besides spastic paralysis of same side.

Search for Pressure Sore (Fig. 8.47)

In neurological conditions, (specially in paraplegia or quadriplegia) or following long decubitus or even short decubitus in an unconscious patient, the patient develops pressure sores. When the patient lies supine look the common sites (Fig. 8.47) for pressure sores —the occiput, back of shoulder blades, elbow joint, sacral region, buttock, and heels, over the greater trochanter when he lies on the sides, and over the anterior superior iliac spines when he lies prone.

Vasomotor Changes

Vasomotor changes should be assessed by looking for pallor, cyanosis, redness, atrophy of skin, nailbed and subcutaneous tissues. History of anhidrosis (no sweating) or oligohidrosis (less sweating) or hyperhidrosis (more sweating) should be enquired for. In indeterminate or uncooperative patients this can be found out by certain tests:

i. *Starch iodine test:* Using iodine and starch, this can be done to map out the anaesthetic areas as dry and devoid of sweating.
ii. *Guttman's test:* Sprinkle quinizarine powder on the skin, it will turn purple when it comes in contact with sweat. Hence area of anhidrosis can be clearly mapped out.

Vasomotor swelling, i.e. oedema due to dependant posture, post-plaster, post-surgical, post-infective and post-traumatic conditions should be noted.

Visceral Assessment

Ask for the bladder and bowel control. If there is no voluntary control, enquire regarding retention of urine, retention overflow, incontinence overflow, dribbling or bed wetting. If patient has got voluntary control, ask for any scalding (burning sensation in urethra while passing urine), difficulty in initiation, frequency, precipitancy (unable to control the urge of micturition), etc.

Regarding the bowels—feeling of passage of stools, control of the sphincters, and nature of stool should be asked for.

In females urogenital assessment should be done, while in males the power of penile erection or allied complaints should be asked.

CLINICAL LOCALISATION OF THE LESION IN THE SPINAL CORD (Table 8.6)

Careful assessment should be done at the outset, for any other associated injury (e.g. of head, chest, lung, abdomen, or extremities); extent and depth of paralysis; and for any visceral paralysis (bladder and/or bowel).

The gross idea about the involvement of the motor segment can be obtained with the help of the following anatomicophysiological facts:

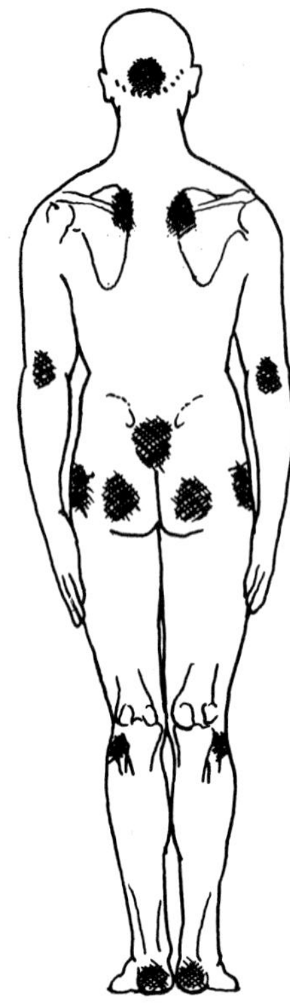

Fig. 8.47: Common sites of pressure sores shown by shaded area

C5 controls flexion of elbow
C6 controls extension of wrist
C7 controls extension of elbow
C8 controls flexion of distal interphalangeal joints of fingers (test the middle finger)
T1 controls abduction of fingers
L2 controls flexion of hip
L3 controls extension of knee
L4 controls dorsiflexion of ankle
L5 controls extension of big toe
S1 controls plantar flexion of ankle.

As the cord proper ends at the upper border of L2 or lower border of L1 vertebra, the actual vertebral level does not correspond to the same spinal cord level. Any neurological damage below the L1 vertebra may affect a few roots of lumbar and sacral outflow. If more roots are affected it will be a cauda equina lesion. The manifestation in this case will be of lower motor neuron type (i.e. weakness, flaccid paralysis, wasting of muscles, fasciculations, less/loss of tone [(hypotonia/atonia), diminished or absent tendon reflexes, plantar reflex absent or down going], perianal saddle anaesthesia, bladder and sexual dysfunction, absent ankle jerk, often accentuation of knee jerk (due to weakness of hamstrings).

Any lesion above the L1 vertebral segment will affect the cord proper. The paraplegia will be of upper motor neuron type, i.e. spastic type of paralysis—increased tone of muscles, spasticity, none or very little wasting of muscles, increased tendon reflexes (may be even clonus), Babinski's sign present, i.e. extensor plantar response, superficial reflexes (like abdominal) absent. In spinal shock stage or in total damage of cord or in terminal stage, the tone may be flaccid.

To assess the actual clinical spinal cord level, the following clinical guidelines should be observed:

1. The surface mark of the vertebral bodies and their relation to that of spinal cord level are as follows in Table 8.6.

Therefore, after localising the vertebral segment, additions must be made accordingly, to assess the cord level. For all practical purposes, the spinous process may be taken as the landmark for the corresponding vertebral body, except in the lower dorsals, where the tip of the spinous process is in level with the body of the vertebra below.

2. If there is sensory loss, the highest level of the sensory loss should be taken as the level of cord damage.

3. Ascertain the hyperaesthetic skin level by passing a key end from below upward. Usually, the irritational zone of the cord affection manifests as the hyperaesthetic zone, i.e. hyperaesthetic zone area will be the lowest level of spared cord above the lesion—this is best demonstrated in viral transverse myelitis.

Table 8.6: Localisation of vertebrae and their relation with spinal cord segments

Surface landmarks of certain vertebrae		*Relation of spine with cord level*	
Spine	*Landmark*	*Vertebral spine*	*Spinal cord segment*
C1	(Transverse process)—below and anterior to the mastoid process	C1-C7	Add 1
C3	At the level of the hyoid bone	T1-T6	Add 2
C4	Opposite the upper border of Thyroid cartilage	T7-T9	Add 3
C6	Opposite the cricoid cartilage	T10	L1, L2
C7	Vertebra prominence	T11	L3, L4
T2	At the level of sternal notch	T12	L5, S1
T2-3	Lies at the level of base of spinous process of scapula		
T4	Against the angle of Louis	L1	Other sacrals and coccygeal segments
T7	Inferior angle of scapula	Below L1	Cauda equina
L4	Highest point of iliac crest		
S1-2	Posterior superior iliac spine		

4. Rough assessment of cord level can be done by correlating with the jerks reflexes. If a particular reflex/jerk is absent, it suggests the damage of the root subserving that reflex jerk.

INVESTIGATIONS FOR SPINAL PATHOLOGY

Besides general investigations, there are certain special investigations which are of value in diagnosing the spinal lesions.

Radiological Investigations

Plain X-ray must be taken in a minimum of two planes:

i. Anteroposterior view
ii. Lateral view.

i. *In anteroposterior view look for*
   a. A general impression of the spinal column and of the particular vertebral segment.
   b. Any pedicular lesion.
   c. Side to side collapse.
   d. Lesions of transverse process.
   e. Paravertebral soft tissue shadows (abscess in caries spine).
   f. Any deviation in the longitudinal axis of the vertebral column (e.g. scoliosis).

ii. *In lateral view look for*
   a. Shape and size of the vertebral body and its relation with vertebrae above and below.
   b. Integrity of anterior and posterior walls.
   c. Wedging or compression of the body.
   d. Texture of the body of the vertebra.
   e. Any localised rarefaction or condensation of the body.
   f. Superior and inferior surfaces of body.
   g. Spinous processes (for its texture and distance from adjacent spinous processes).
   h. Intervertebral space—reduction or increase in the space or any other abnormality in that region.
   i. In the spinal canal—trace the posterior wall of the body of vertebra from above downwards as well as the laminar continuity at the posterior end of the spinal canal. These two lines maintain regular continuity, and in between them is the

space occupied by the spinal cord and soft tissues around it. Note the dimension of the canal from above downwards and the area affected. Take note of any radio-opaque space occupying shadow in the spinal canal.

In cervical region: Lateral view should be taken after fully flexing and fully extending the neck from the neutral position. This not only demonstrates the mobility of the spine, but also helps in delineating degenerative changes in the diarthrodial joints, joint of Luschka and the intervertebral foramen to a great extent.

Oblique Views

These views are essential to delineate the intervertebral foramina and the facet joints, specially in the cervical region. In the lumbar and lumbosacral region, this view has special importance to delineate the integrity of pars interarticularis. In this view this area normally casts a shadow which mimics a Scot terrier's neck. Any defect in pars interarticularis is indicated by a translucent area across the terrier's neck, as if the terrier has been decapitated. This sign is positive in spondylolysis and spondylolisthesis.

Tomography

Tomographic study (measured depth penetration X-ray) is essential to localise certain less obvious lesions in vertebra, e.g. osteoid osteoma, haemangioma.

Screening

Diagnosis and manipulation directly under screening used to be a popular method in managing fractures. But now, its value is more or less restricted to assessments in stress radiography and to observe the flow of contrast medium in myelographic or allied studies.

Cine-Radiography

To know the excursion of the spinal column and flow of contrast medium in the subarachnoid space, cine-radiography is of value.

Scanogram

In the lesions which affect more or less the entire spinal column, or lesions where the relations of the different spinal zones is essential to be assessed, e.g. in scoliosis, it is useful to have a single exposure accommodating the whole of the spinal column. At least lower cervical to lumbosacral regions should be included in the exposure to know the extent of primary and/or secondary curves. This is further important to measure numerically the exact angulation of the scoliotic curves.

Methods of Measuring the Scoliotic Curves

There are several methods of measuring the scoliotic curves, but the following two appear to be of practical use.

i. *Cobb's method* (Fig. 8.48): Locate the upper most vertebral level where the curvature ends (superior end vertebra). This can be delineated by the shape of disc space just above (widening on the concave side), tilt of vertebral bodies (maximum tilt towards the concavity) and the size of pedicular shadows. The pedicular shadows should be symmetrical and horizontally placed.

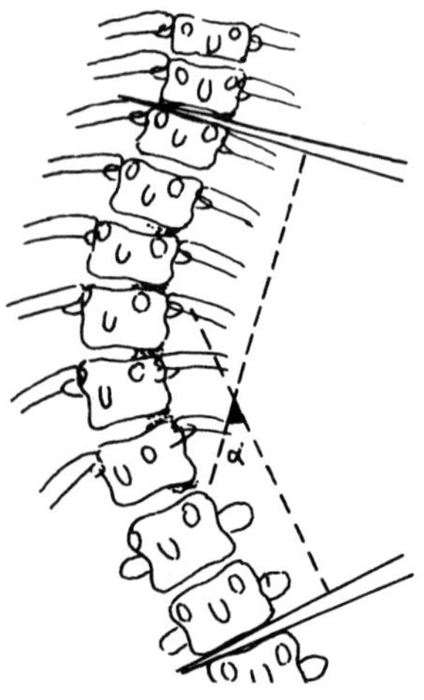

Fig. 8.48: Cobb s method of measuring the angle of scoliosis (α = angle of scoliosis)

Draw a line in continuity with the superior surface of this vertebra. Drop a perpendicular over this line outside the spinal column. Elongate this perpendicular line downwards. Similarly locate the lowest vertebra where the curve ends (inferior end vertebra). At the inferior surface of this vertebra the horizontal line is prolonged to the side in which upper line was projected. Drop the perpendicular on this line outside the spinal column on the same side as above and elongate it upwards. The two perpendicular lines will cut at a point. The angle formed between these lines is Cobb's angle.

ii. *Ferguson's method* (Fig. 8.49): First locate the curve end vertebrae as above. Also locate the vertebra at the apex of the curve. Mark the centres of these vertebrae. Connect the centre of the apex vertebra to that of the centres of the superior and inferior end vertebrae and prolong them to intersect. The superior or inferior angle at the point of intersection of these lines will denote the angle of the curve.

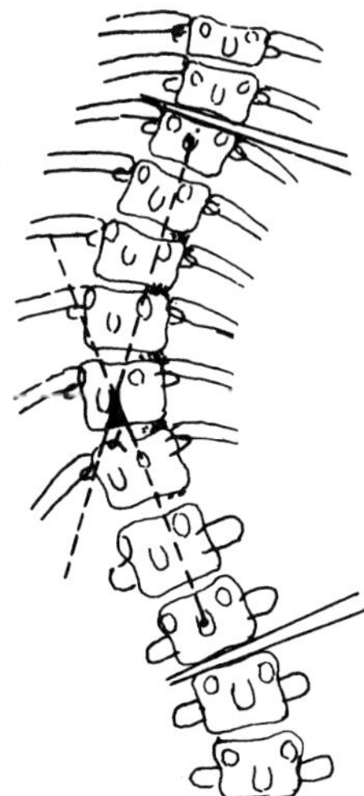

Fig. 8.49: Ferguson s method of measurement of angle of scoliosis (α = angle of the scoliosis)

iii. *Computer-aided assessment of scoliosis:* Patient's spinal column is examined in three dimensions and in colour on a computer screen.To obtain these images two X-rays of the patient (one from the back and other from the side) are placed on luminous digitising table and certain points characteristic of each vertebra are noted. Within seconds the computer shows a 3-D view of the spinal column and pelvis. Numerical and graphical data are also available. By an expert system, all possible corrective measures can be simulated, enabling the surgeon to choose the most suitable option.

Contrast Radiography

To locate any space occupying lesion in the spinal canal, contrast radiographic studies should be done. Four methods are followed:

i. Myelographic studies or contrast-dye-radiography.
ii. Air contrast radiography.
iii. Epidurography.
iv. Epidural venography—to demonstrate impingement upon the epidural plexus.

Myelographic Study

Myelographic delineation is done either through lumbar route (ascending) or through cisternal puncture (descending) after injecting 5 cc of radio-opaque dye into the subarachnoid space. Under fluoroscopy, the movement of the dye column is observed by tilting the X-ray table either way. Any hold up or partial/complete block is noted.

Radioactive Scanning

Radioactive phosphorus or tetracycline, or calcium or strontium are usually used for localising certain osseous growths or other space occupying lesions in the spinal canal.

Discography

Contrast studies of the disc spaces may be helpful in assessing for any prolapse of the disc material. However, the injection into the centre of the biconvex disc space should be done under image intensifier. This is not a popular method of investigation because the method is difficult and the result is not much helpful.

Needle Biopsy

The vertebral body, being deeply situated is not easily accessible for histopathological studies by open biopsy. Therefore, needle biopsy, here, has more importance for:

i. Biochemical studies for osteoporosis.
ii. Cytological studies for assessing the nature of the suspected growth.

A comparatively wide bore aspiration needle is pushed from the posterolateral aspect into the suspected vertebral body.

Modern Imaging Techniques

Modern imaging techniques are revolutionising the process of investigating the spinal problems, e.g.

i. CTS (Computerised tomography scanning).
ii. CTS and intrathecal low osmolality contrast media for assessment of pathology such as tumour and dysraphic condition.
iii. MRI (Magnetic resonance imaging) or NMR (Nuclear magnetic resonance) imaging—This technique has a great future. It is extremely sensitive and affords early detection of avascular necrosis, infection, intraspinal disorders (like disc prolapse, and can also distinguish the disc components), cord compression due to trauma and tumour. It delineates various bony and soft tissue growths without the use of contrast media, differentiation of muscular dysfunction (atrophy, paresis, and myopathy).
iv. Spinal cord monitoring technique to record somatosensory evoked potentials SEP's—mainly being used during surgery on spine and spinal cord to simultaneously observe any dysfunction of spinal cord, especially while performing corrective surgery for spinal deformity.

Key Diagnostic Points of Common Spinal Pathology

1. *Cervical Spondylosis*
   - Middle age, males dominate.
   - Usual complaints—pain, tingling, numbness and even pin-prick sensations manifest along the irritated roots, more in the night.
   - In acute root irritation, the patient usually presents with keeping his hand over the head on the affected side. Any attempt to bring the hand downwards, aggravates the symptoms. In upper root affections, the features of vertebral artery syndrome, like tinnitus, giddiness, occipital headache and transitory fainting attack may occur.
   - Rest in lying down position (by avoiding the weight of head) usually relieves pain to a variable extent.
   - Strained walking, overactivity, jerky drive, moist humid weather aggravates the symptoms.
   - Movements of cervical spine variably restricted, usually at the extremes.
   - Cervical compression test usually positive.
   - Paraesthesia in periscapular region, deltoid region and in lower cervical root affections, even in the fingers.
   - Local tenderness in the cervical region in acute and subacute manifestation.
   - Rarely motor power weakness in the fingers and thumb and other muscles according to affection.
   - X-ray—especially the lateral and oblique views are confirmatory.
   - Congenital malformations may be a confusing factor (Figs 8.50A and B).

2. *Klippel-Feil Syndrome (1912) (Congenital Webbed Neck; Congenital Short Neck, Brevi Collis) (Figs 8.51A to C)*
   - Short or absent neck due to congenital malformation (fusion of several vertebrae) of C2 to C7 in multiple or single level of cervical vertebrae.

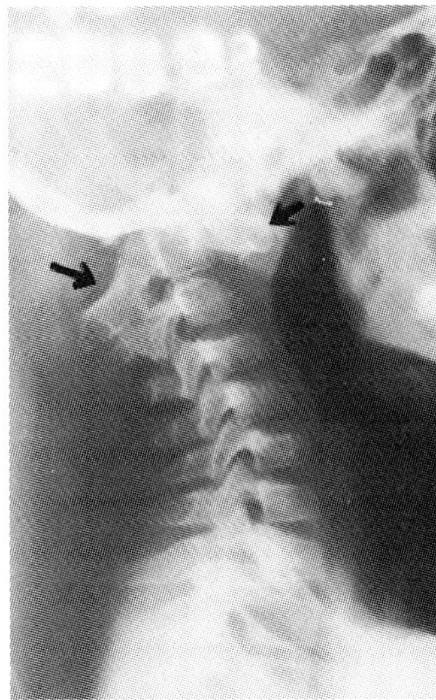

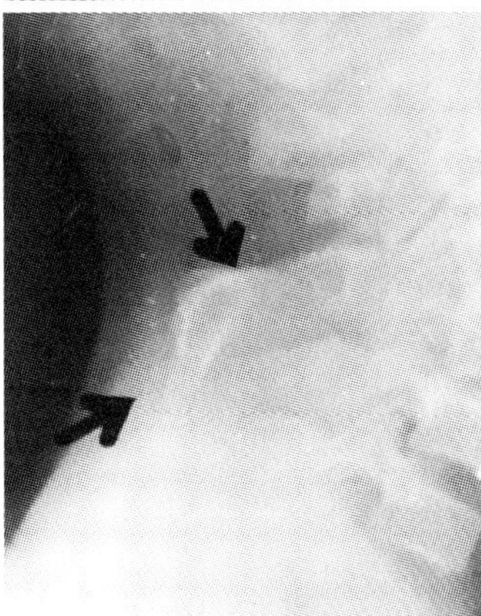

Figs 8.50A and B: Congenital fusion of the spinal processes of in cervical vertebrae

— Hair margin quite lowered, sometimes even on shoulder level.
— Marked limitation in mobility (specially lateral bending and rotation) of cervical spine.
— May be associated with congenitally high-placed scapula (Sprengel's shoulder), and/or cervical spina bifida.
— May be associated with mongoloid type of face.
— Symptoms manifest in young adults.
— Deafness may be associated in about 30% of cases.
— Scoliosis (alone or with kyphosis) is commonly associated spinal deformity in about 50% of cases.

3. *Spina Bifida*

Any environmental or other effect may interfere with the fusion of neural tube and encasing mesenchyme, which starts from the cephalic end on the 25th intrauterine day and ends at the caudal end on the 29th intrauterine day.

Varieties: (a) Posterior (due to defect in the posterior bony arch: (i) occulta (ii) manifesta. (b) Anterior (due to defect in the development of bodies)—very very rare.

i. *Spina Bifida Occulta (Fig. 8.52)*
— Usually in lumbosacral region.
— Manifested by the presence of—naevus, or tuft of hair or fibro fatty mass or dimpling of skin.
— Usually symptomless, and discovered accidently in X-ray.
— May be associated with—deformity of the foot (usually bilateral equinocavovarus), bladder disturbance, sensory deficits in foot.
— Dissociated growth between cord and canal and tugging of the filum terminale with the surrounding and subcutaneous tissue lead to decreased ascent of the spinal cord; which may manifest as cord-traction or filum terminale or Arnold-Chiari syndrome. Clinically, symptoms like peculiar gait, features of increased intracranial pressure, spastic paralysis and cervical root pain start manifesting between 4 and 6 years of age.

ii. *Spina Bifida Manifesta (Cystica) (Figs 8.53A to C)*
— Midline tense, cystic saccular protrusion in lumbar, dorsal, occipitocervical region, present since birth.
— Depending on level and type of lesion—variable neurological manifestations.

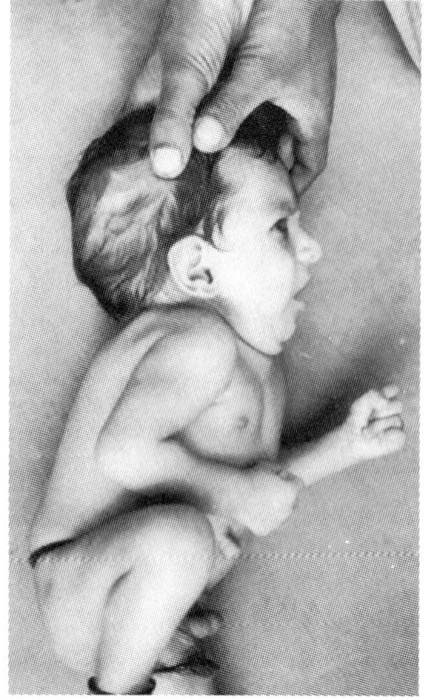

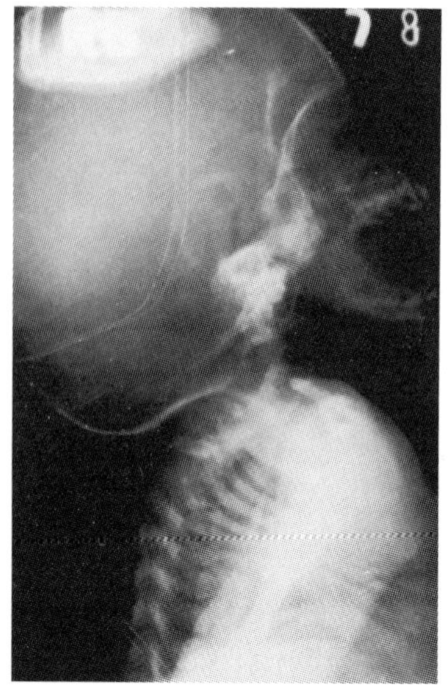

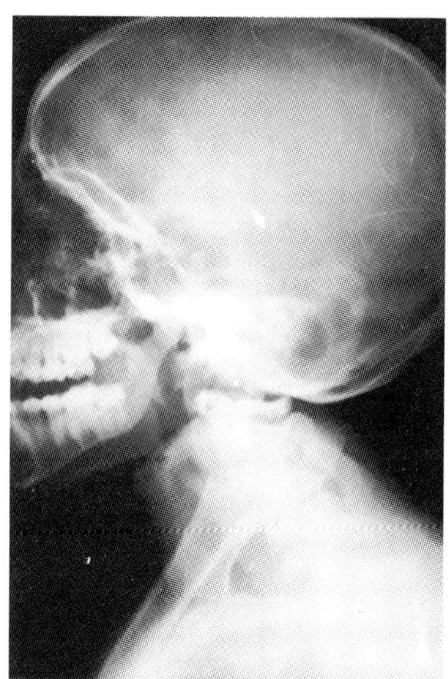

Figs 8.51A to C: Klippel-Feil syndrome

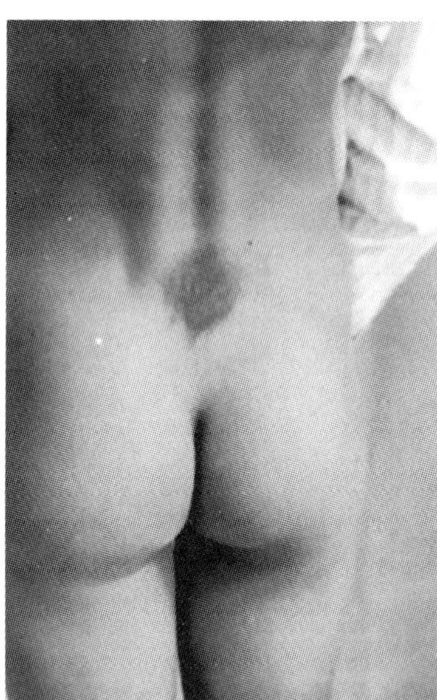

Fig. 8.52: Spina bifida occulta to be suspected by seeing the tuft of hair

— May be impulse on coughing.
— Transillumination may be obtained delineating the darker shadow of the cord and nerves from the bright fluid portion.

Types

i. Meningocele (Figs 8.53A to C)—protrusion of meninges only.
ii. Myelomeningocele (commonest of the three)—protrusion of a plaque of neural tissue surrounded by meninges.

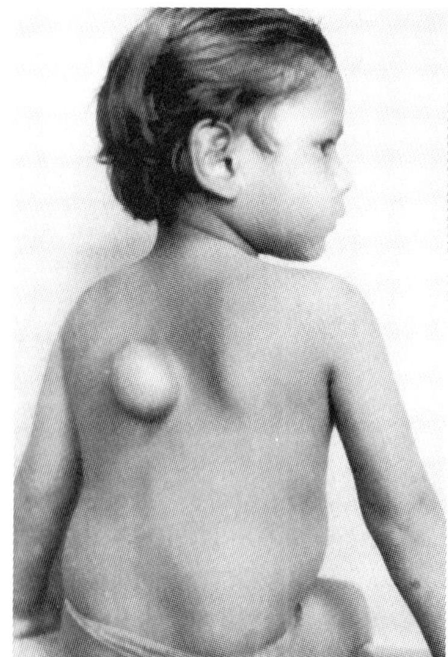

Fig. 8.53A: Spina bifida manifesta (cystica)

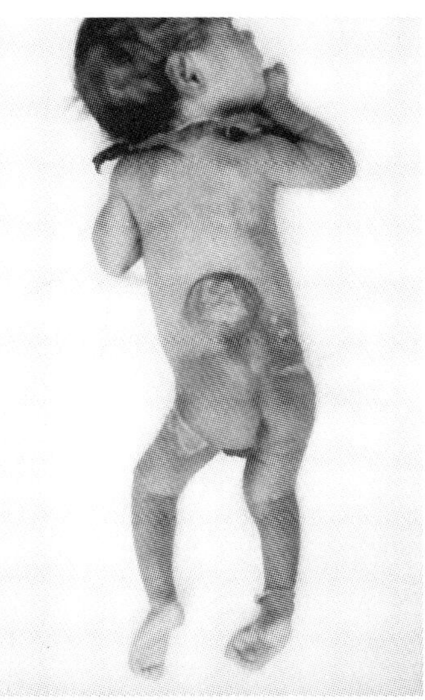

Fig. 8.53B: Spina bifida manifesta (cystica)

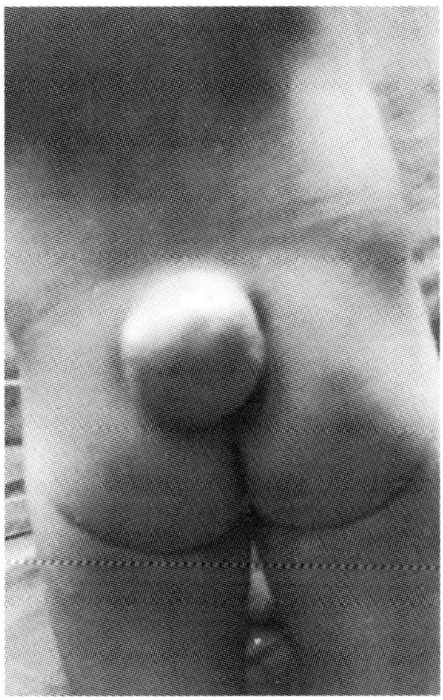

Fig. 8.53C: Spina bifida manifesta (cystica)

iii. Syringomyelocele—central spinal canal is dilated and the spinal cord is expanded to form the lining of sac.
iv. Myelocele—gross spinal cord deformity, an elongated fissure surrounded by hair or telangiectasis which is in direct contact with the central canal.
v. Rachocele—roots spread in the walls of protrusion.

4. *Caries Spine—(Pott's disease—Percival Pott 1779/Tuberculosis Spine)*
   — Pain in the back or referred pain which aggravates with activities and spinal stress test.
   — Common sites: Lower dorsal, mid dorsal, lumbar, cervical, upper dorsal, lumbo-sacral.
   — Persistent local tenderness in the affected spine.
   — Spasm of muscles in early case, muscular wasting later on.
   — Limitation of spinal movements, especially flexion.
   — Presence of kyphosis, usually angular kyphosis.
   — Presence of cold abscess, usually distant from the primary focus.
   — May be associated with complications, like paraplegia (Table 8.7)
   — Raised ESR.
   — Primary focus (e.g. in lungs, lymph node). In spite of advanced technology such as gas liquid chromatography and polymerase chain reaction, smear microscopy (for AFB) remains the most reliable diagnostic test (of pulmonary tuberculosis).
   — In chronic, late deformed dorsal caries cases—features of cor pulmonale, due to reduced thoracic capacity.
   — X-ray—reduced intervertebral disc space, rarefaction/destruction/collapse of vertebrae, paravertebral abscess shadow (Figs 8.18A to C).
   — Possible sites of cold abscess in caries spine—vide Table 8.2, page 163.

5. *Ankylosing Spondylitis*
   — Age and sex predilection—males in the age group of 18-30 years.
   — Pain and stiffness, in the dorsolumbar and both sacroiliac regions, which are

variably relieved by spinal stress test (cf. tuberculosis and septic arthritis where pain is increased).
— More in the morning after getting up from the bed or after getting up from prolonged rest.
— Patients get comparative relief after daily routine activities, walking around or after certain exercise.
— Progressive limitation of chest expansion (if less than 2.5 cm, it is highly suggestive).
— Rest aggravates, and activity relieves the pain and stiffness.
— Sometimes bizarre manifestation occur, e.g. pain occurs locally or is generalised all over the body and may be over calf muscles, both heels, shoulder regions, back, and cervical spine.
— Earlier, boarding of back, specially in lower region; later on poker back in advanced cases (Figs 8.13A to C).
— Restricted spinal movements, especially flexion.
— Later on, hip, and still later, shoulder, knee, cervical region, rather all bigger joints to smaller joints, (even temporomandibular joint), become stiff.
— May be history of urethritis, uveitis, ulcerative colitis.
— Predilection for positive HLA-B 27 individuals and their family members.
— X-ray—sacroiliac joints fusion; in AP view (mainly in the lower dorsal and lumbar region) bamboo spine due to calcification of collateral ligaments (Figs 8.54A to C). In cervical spine after fusion, it gives an appearance of CANE-STICK in lateral view.

6. *Intervertebral Disc Prolapse (mainly occurs in the lumbosacral and lumbar region)*
— There is usually a history of low back pain, which may have had moderate to severe intensity, with radiation to the lower limb (usually in sciatic distribution). The onset is usually acute/subacute, following some exertive work or lifting of heavy weights. Usually symptoms are intermittent.

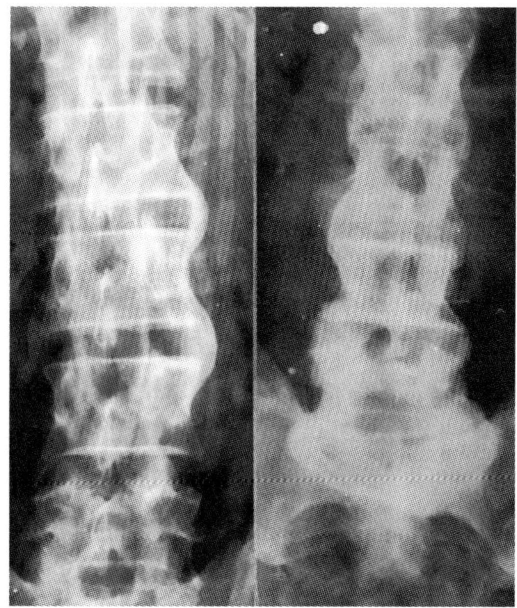

Fig. 8.54A: Ankylosing spondylitis to note the bambooing of the 1,2,3 and 4 lumbars

— The symptoms increase on exertion, coughing, sneezing, changing of posture, (from standing to sitting to lying down or *vice-versa*) and on spinal stress test.
— Rest relieves and activity aggravates the symptoms.
— Neural complications may be presenting feature: variable sensory disturbances; motor weakness (extensor hallucis longus, dorsiflexors of ankle, tendo-Achilles), and even cauda equina syndrome.
— Lower back muscles are usually in spasm, thus restricting the movements (mainly flexion).
— Sciatic scoliosis (antalgic or functional scoliosis) is usually present (this scoliosis gradually disappears when the patient gradually bends forward). The protruded disc usually presses the root from the lateral sides. Hence, in order to keep the root away from the disc, the spine bends

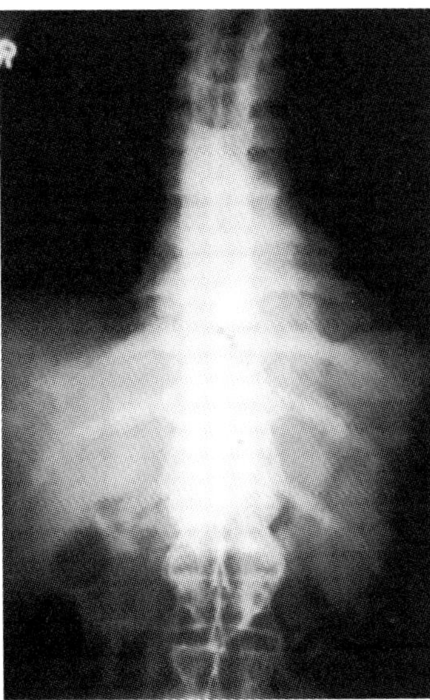

Fig. 8.54B: Ankylosing spondylitis bambooing getting more marked in L_2-L_1 upwards

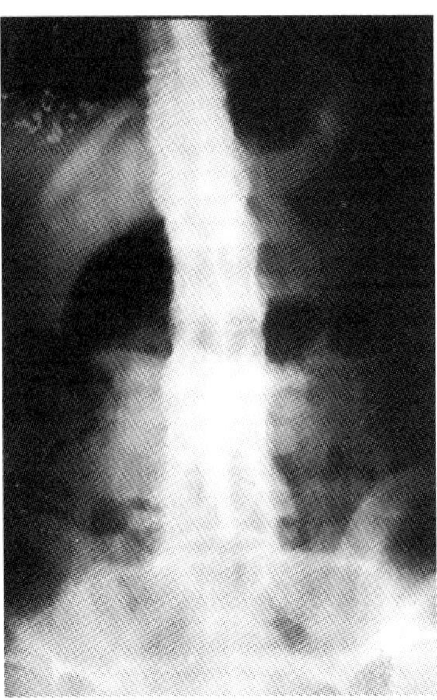

Fig. 8.54C: Ankylosing spondylitis all ligaments and intervertebral spaces calcified in advanced stage of ankylosing spondylitis

to the opposite side. However, the less common pressure on the root from the medial side by disc protrusion, may produce a list on the same side.

— Deep thrust tenderness is present usually over the L4-5 or L5-S1 region.
— Straight leg raising less than normal. Lasegue's test positive.
— Femoral nerve stretch test may be positive.
— Ask the patient to walk on the heels (not possible in L5 weakness) and the toes (not possible in S1 weakness) alternately. In case of sciatic root stretch, the patient will complain of pain in the sciatic distribution while walking on the heel. In case of femoral root stretch, patient may complain of pain in front of and on the medial aspect of the thigh.
— In more common S1 root compression in intervertebral disc prolapse, the ankle jerk is depressed (more easily detected and assessed when patient is in prone or sitting position) or even absent.

7. *Spondylolisthesis (see Figs 8.15 and 8.16)*
— Mostly, middle aged or even elderly ladies are the subjects.
— Complaints of persistent pain in low back with/or without radiation in lower limbs. No definite relation with rest or activities. In advanced cases there may be a waddling gait.
— Clinically, feeling of a step in the central furrow, in the lower lumbar region, reduction of distance between last rib and highest point of iliac crests (common sites L4-L5, L5-S1, L3-L4).
— Transverse furrows in the loin region.
— Comparative limitation of movements of spine in that region, in these subjects.
— Palpation through the pelvis may reveal the step because of the slipped vertebral body.
— The pain along the sciatic root may be only presenting clinical symptoms, and in that case, the features of prolapse intervertebral disc will also be present.

Table 8.7: Pott's paraplegia (caries spine) (Percival Pott 1779)
Compression paraplegia of upper motor neuron type; very rarely cauda equina lesion

	Paraplegia of early onset	*Paraplegia of late onset*	*Paraplegia of sudden onset*
1	*2*	*3*	*4*
1. Definition	Paraplegia setting in during active stage of disease	Paraplegia setting after the disease has been cured/or remained quiescent for a pretty long time	Any time coming suddenly with or without earlier diagnosed caries spine
2. Time factor (no hard and fast rule)	Usually within 2 years of the onset of the disease	Usually after 7-10 years of the earlier diagnosed disease	-do-
3. Age	Children/adults	Adults	Any age (usually adults)
4. Common site of spinal lesion	Lower dorsal, mid dorsal upper dorsal, lower cervical	Mid dorsal, lower dorsal	Dorsal lesion
5. Affections	—Motor: Staggering gait, spasticity with spastic gait Gradually increasing muscular weakness Paraplegia in extension Paraplegia in flexion Flexor spasm Mass reflexes —Sensory affection —Visceral affection —Contractures —Decubitus ulcers, chest infections —Urinary complication —Cachexia —Death	Motor and/or sensory (partly sensory) Staggering gait, very slowly increasing muscular weakness	Sudden presentation—total paralysis or variable paresis

Contd.

Table 8.7: Contd.

	Paraplegia of early onset	*Paraplegia of late onset*	*Paraplegia of sudden onset*
1	*2*	*3*	*4*
6. Cause	Pressure over spinal cord —Tuberculous pus (paravertebral abscess ♦ intervertebral foramen ♦ spinal canal) —Caseous material —Tubercular sequestra —Sequestrated intervertebral disc —Pathological subluxation —Dislocation of body backward	—Recrudescence of the disease —Due to constant rubbing of spinal cord against internal gibbus	Usually vascular, i.e. tuberculous embolism or thrombotic phenomena of segmental spinal artery
7. Depth of paraplegia	Incomplete/complete	Always incomplete	Usually complete may be incomplete
8. Pathology in the cord	Cord is spared till very late stage	Gliosis where cord rubs against internal gibbus	Immediate no change. May suffer necrosis if collaterals do not develop quite early
9. Prognosis	Variable—usually good if treated promptly	Never good—some legacy always remains	Usually recovers
10. Treatment	Chemotherapy Conservative: rest preferably on plaster bed/ spinal frame; Traction Operative— —Costotransversectomy —anterolateral decompression —anterior excision with or without bone graft	Conservative Rarely operation indicated Chemotherapy only in recurred cases	Chemotherapy Conservative

— Classical X-ray pictures—slipping of vertebra in lateral view.
— Decapitated 'terrier' neck in oblique view (in isthmic, commonest type) (Fig. 8.55).

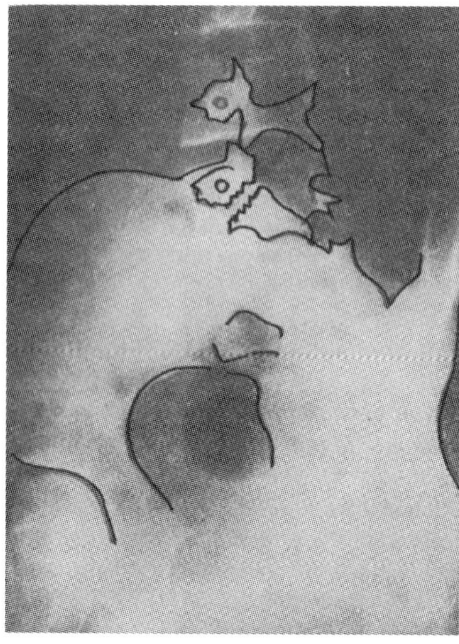

Fig. 8.55: Spondylolysis to note the decapitated terrier sign

8. *Spinal Tumours (Table 8.8)*

It is very difficult to clinically diagnose authentically the benign tumours of the spine. Of the malignant conditions, secondaries are the most common, which may present with/or without compression of the cord. Common features of secondaries:

- Elderly persons, without any history of injury, run-down conditions.
- Localised or spread over tenderness, angular or no kyphosis—suspect secondaries.
- Search for all possible primary sites (prostate, breast, bronchus, thyroid, GI tract, kidney, etc).

— Multiple myeloma—spine is a common site of affection. Spinal presentation may be minimal or even the patient may present with compression paraplegia.

- Suspect multiple myeloma when:
  - In elderly subjects with disseminated pain in the bones, increasing weakness, anaemia, bony tenderness, (specially over the flat bones)
  - Spinal tenderness at affected zone.
  - Usually no deformity in spine.
- No pulmonary symptom (no pulmonary metastasis).
- Bence Jones protein in urine (in 30% of the patients).
- X-ray—multiple punched-out osteolytic lesions.

— Rare tumours of spine like osteosarcoma. Ewing's sarcoma, osteoclastoma and haemangioma, etc. are more or less diagnosed after histopathological investigations.

Compression Paraplegia of the Spinal Cord

Upper motor neuron (UMN) type of paraplegia resulting from compression of the dorsal segments of the spinal cord due to various causes:

1. Congenital malformations (very rare)
   —Severe scoliosis.
2. Inflammatory (infective)—caries spine, arachnoiditis, meningitis, serosa circumscripta, epidural abscess.
3. Traumatic
   —Fracture, fracture-subluxation/dislocation; foreign body (bullet injury).
4. Vascular
   —Vascular malformations.
   —Spinal artery embolism/thrombosis.
   —Aortic aneurysm.
5. Miscellaneous
   —Paget's disease.
   —Cysts in spinal canal, e.g. *Echynococcus granulosus*
   —Spinal cord cyst, which can be extraspinal or intraspinal, e.g. cysticercosis (infection by the larval (cysticercus) stage of the tapeworm *T. solium*).

Compression of cord in cervical region should produce compression quadriplegia/triplegia or even monoplegia of UMN type. Besides the

Table 8.8: Spinal tumours

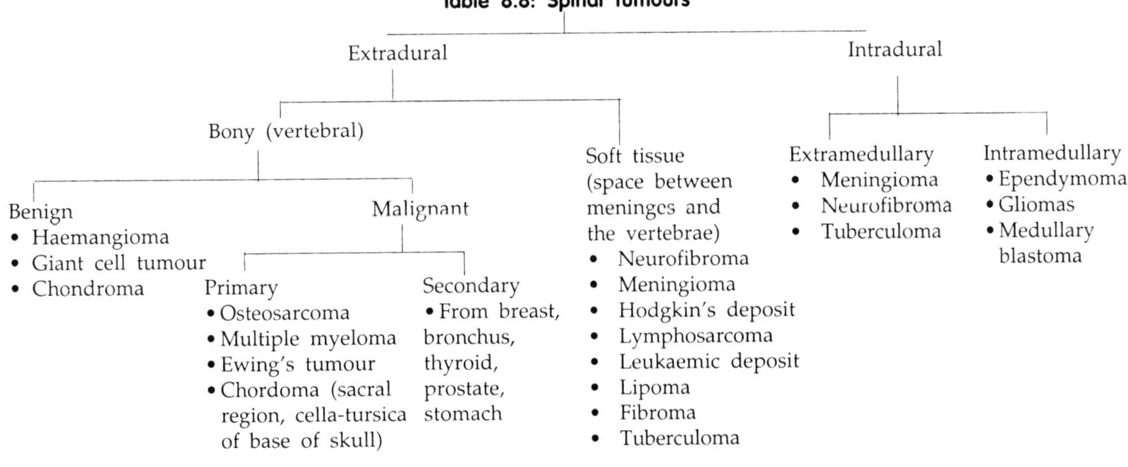

aforesaid causes, following can also produce compression—

i. Prolapsed intervertebral disc.
ii. Cervical spondylosis.
iii. Atlantoaxial subluxation in collagen arthropathy (e.g. rheumatoid arthritis, ankylosing spondylitis).

Cauda Equina Syndrome

It occurs due to pressure on the roots of the cauda equina due to various causes (mostly the herniated disc of central type).

Lower motor neuron (LMN) type of paraplegia produced due to compression on the cauda equina (distal to L1 vertebra) with following features:

Complains of backache, sciatica (unilateral or bilateral), sensory disturbances in feet and leg, foot drop.

Signs:

i. Motor—varying (seldom complete) LMN type of weakness (usually below the knee).
ii. Sensory—Usually perianal saddle-shaped hyperaesthesia, hypoaesthesia or anaesthesia.
iii. Visceral—Bladder (usually retention overflow) and bowel involvement. In males impairment of sexual functions.
iv. Reflexes
   —Ankle jerk—sluggish or absent.
   —Knee jerk—normal or brisk (due to weaker hamstrings).
   —Anal reflexes—sluggish or absent.

Causes of Cauda Equina Syndrome

A. *Acute:*
   —Trauma (fracture/fracture dislocation of lumbar vertebrae).
   —Intervertebral disc prolapse (usually central).
B. *Chronic:* Spinal canal stenosis—common causes are:
   —Congenital
   —Vascular malformations
   —Degenerative
   —Iatrogenic (following fenestration or hemilaminectomy, spinal fusion).
   —Caries spine
   —Neoplastic (secondary deposits)
   —Spinal tumours (space occupying lesions in the vertebral canal—e.g. neurofibroma, meningioma, Hodgkin's deposits, lymphosarcoma, haemangioma).
   —Spondylolisthesis.

Prompt surgical decompression is rewarding in most of the cases.

BIBLIOGRAPHY

1. Bradford FK, Sprurling RG: *The Intervertebral Disc* (2nd ed). Springfield II: Charles. C. Thomas, 1945.
2. Schmorl G, Junghanns H: *The Human Spine in Health and Disease* (2nd ed). New York: Grunn Stratton 1971.
3. Dimitrejevic M, Sherwood A, Nathan P: Clonus, peripheral and central mechanisms. In Desmedt JF (Ed) *Neurology*. New York: Karger 173-182, 1978.
4. Brown MD, Hornicek FJ, Lebwohl NH: Phantom Sciatica. *J Bone Joint Surg* **79A**: 252-53, 1977.
5. Beachesne RP, Schutzer SF: Myositis ossificans of the piriformis muscle: an unusual cause of piriformis syndrome. *J Bone Joint Surg* **79A**: 906-10, 1997.
6. Novacheck TF: Running injuries—a biomechanical approach. *J Bone Joint Surg* **80A**: 1220-33, 1998.

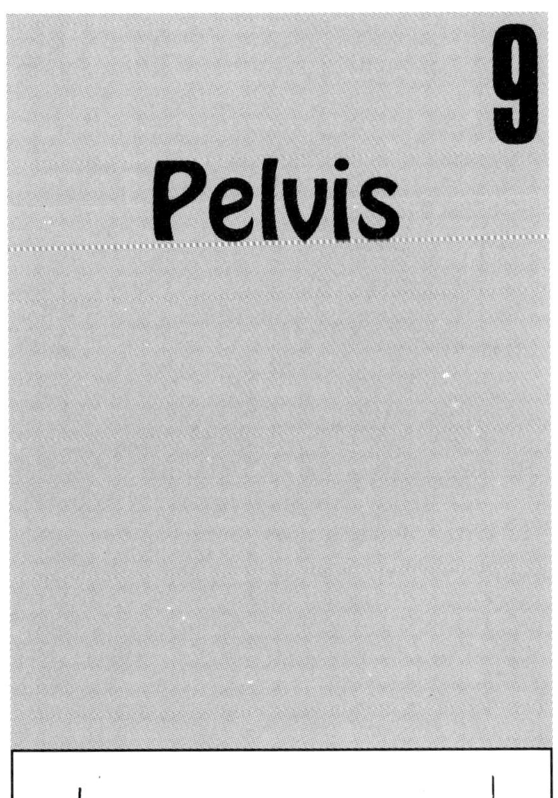

9 Pelvis

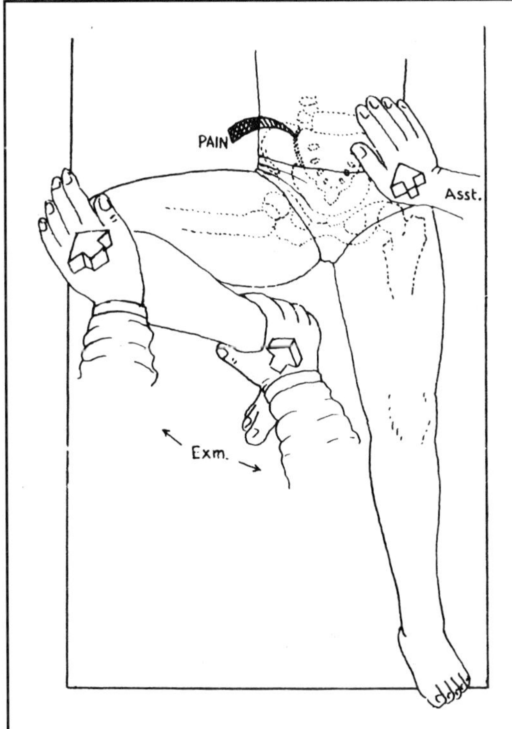

INTRODUCTION

Pelvic injuries basically comprise two sets of involvements: (i) skeletal framework of pelvis and (ii) soft tissues and visceral contents in the pelvis and around it.

Many a time, simple fractures of the pelvic bone may be insignificant from the treatment point of view. However, on the other hand, even without obvious fracture of the pelvis, visceral injuries may be so serious as to have lethal consequences, unless promptly and adequately attended to. Unfortunately, pelvic peritonitis is often severe in its manifestation.

ANATOMICAL CONSIDERATIONS

1. The pelvis is more or less in a ring form. Its inlet is broad and shallow, and the outlet is constricted and deep.
2. The ring comprises of two hemi-pelvises, with intervention of the sacrum posteriorly and a fibrocartilaginous disc anteriorly.
3. The joints in between the sacrum and posterior ends of ilial plates are either amphiarthrodial (fibrocartilaginous bridging) or dia-arthrodial. Articular surfaces having irregular elevations contribute to the restricted movements and strength of the joint. The tough interosseous ligaments spread from the postero-superior rough area of the articular surface on the ilial plates to the lateral mass of sacrum. Anteriorly, the anterior sacro-iliac ligaments are thin, and thus get easily distended by any intra-articular pathology and can be felt by rectal examination. The lumbosacral nerve trunk lies anterior to it, hence any sacroiliac joint pathology can lead to inflammatory neuritis. The posterior sacro-iliac ligaments are quite tough and can withstand violent trauma. These joints allow very slight antero-posterior rotational movements, occurring around a transverse axis about 7.5 cm vertically below the promontory of the sacrum. In most of the activities during locomotion, these joints have an insignificant role. Anteriorly, the two pubic bodies

more or less adhere together with the intervention of a fibro-cartilaginous disc, forming the pubic symphysis.

4. The normal shape of the pelvis is more or less that of a signet ring. In conditions where the bone gets softened (e.g. osteomalacia, rickets), under influence of the body weight and thrust of the two femora upwards during locomotion, the sacral promontory protrudes antero-inferiorly and the two acetabular floors project superomedially, giving a trefoil shape to the pelvis.
5. When the hips are normal, the pelvis has almost negligible involvement, except for transmitting the weight through the acetabulofemoral head axis, but in altered situations, the pelvis accommodates disabilities, deformities, and disparities in the length of the lower limbs to a very significant extent. This postural adjustment of the pelvis leads to pelvic obliquity. Pelvic obliquity may be in anteroposterior axis (to accommodate the aforesaid effects in anteroposterior direction) or in lateral axis (to compensate the effects in the side to side axis).
6. In pelvic injuries, following viscera and important soft tissues are affected (in order of frequency)
   a. Urethra and bladder
   b. Vagina and uterus
   c. Sciatic nerve
   d. Rectum and anal canal
   e. Pelvic peritoneum
   f. Iliac vessels
7. If one of the bones of the hemi-pelvis is fractured, it is not going to affect the integrity of the pelvis in any significant way. This is because the muscles are firmly adapted to the inner and outer pelvic bone plates and act as firm splintage from both sides of the bone.
8. Pelvis is a common site for inflammatory pathology. Besides the complications following any abdominal and gynaecological pathology, infections in the form of iliac abscess and psoas abscess are quite common. Being a container with a dependent position, pus and other infected materials accumulate at the bottom to present as abscesses (e.g. psoas and iliopsoas abscess in caries spine, infected collection in pouch of Douglas).
9. Even major injuries affecting the pelvis may not be of much significance in males, if the viscera and neurovascular bundles are intact. However, in females of child bearing age, any disruption of the normal anatomy or overall shape of pelvis may affect the pregnancy and delivery.
10. The disposition and attachment of the deeper layer of superficial fascia in the lower abdomen determines the extent of extravasation of urine due to rupture of the urethra. The deeper condensed membranous layer of the superficial fascia of abdomen (Scarpa's fascia) continues as the Collie's fascia investing the penis and the scrotum. Then it continues as the superficial fascia covering the superficial perineal muscles.

    The attachments of Collie's fascia are as follows:

    Above-continuous as Scarpa's fascia.

    Medially—continuous with the Collie's fascia of the opposite side.

    Laterally—attaches on the conjoint ischio-pubic ramus.

    Inferiorly—fuses with the posterior border of urogenital diaphragm.

    The spread of any extravasated urine following rupture of the urethra in the perineum is limited below the attachment of Collie's fascia with the urogenital diaphragm. Laterally it can go upto the conjoint ischio-pubic rami. Upwards, it may spread over the penis and scrotum. Further, it may extend over the abdominal wall passing along the spermatic cord. From the lower abdominal wall, urine may track down below the inguinal ligament upto the attachment of the Scarpa's fascia to fascia lata.

Table 9.1: Innominate bone or hip bone

Primary centres	*Secondary centres*
Primary centres—One for ilium—8th weeks IUL One for ischium—4th month One for pubis—4-5th months At birth, acetabulum is a cartilaginous cup with a triradiate stem appearing on the pelvic surface as a 'Y' shaped epiphyseal plate between the ilium, ischium and pubis	Secondary centres appear about puberty and join with rest of the bone between 15-25 years. Iliac crest—two secondary centres. Acetabular cartilage ossifies by two centres. Anterior inferior iliac spine, ischial tuberosity, pubic crest, symphyseal surfaces may have separate centres

Ossification (Table 9.1)

METHODOLOGY

History taking—As in chapter on Introduction.

General and systemic examinations—As in chapter on 'Introduction'.

If there is history or suspicion of pelvic injury, the features of shock and haemorrhage must be carefully looked for. Unstable fractures of the pelvis are the third commonest cause of death following road traffic accident.

Regional Examination

If the patient can walk, note the gait. Note the obvious pelvic tilt, the posture of lower back (lordosis, scoliosis, kyphosis) and any obvious deformity while standing. Perform the Trendelenberg test (see Fig. 12.21). The trauma and chronic pathology of the pelvis closely mimic the hip, sacroiliac, lumbosacral and lower lumbar involvements. Therefore, one should examine these regions separately. The corresponding lower limb should be assessed as a whole.

Most of the patients suffering from traumatic conditions are initially unable to stand due to pain. On the other hand, in most of the diseases of pelvis, except for acutely manifesting ones, the patient can stand, and walk about with a limp and deformities of varying extent.

Local Examination

Inspection

Besides looking at the surface and condition of skin, the following points must be given due attention while patient is lying supine. Note the symmetry and level of anterior superior iliac spines, iliac crests, iliac plate flares, symphysis pubis, groin folds, Scarpa's triangle, contour and bulge of abdomen, the level of umbilicus and genitalia. Usually, it is painful for the patient to turn to the lateral or to a prone position. But if possible, it should be done. While on side, note the symmetry, any bulge, prominence of iliac crest and the gluteal region, dimples of Venus, symmetrical prominences of posterior superior iliac spines, gluteal bulge, internatal cleft, gluteal folds, and back of thighs. In case of injury, look for any bruising particularly in perineum, any swelling or sinus or scar in perineum (Figs 9.1 to 9.3) and any bleeding from urethra/anus/vagina.

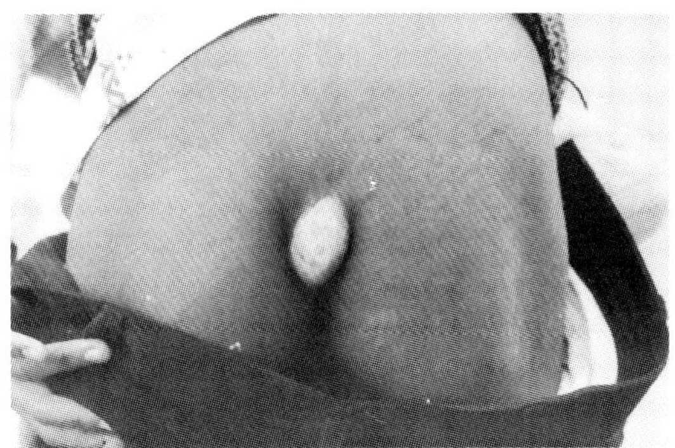

Fig. 9.1: Condylomata (syphilitic) in internatal cloft

Palpation

Palpation should be done systematically, as in inspection. Significant points to be noted in palpation:

Superficial palpation (Touch): Besides noting the findings of touch (e.g. skin sensation, temperature, tenderness, etc.) in case of any suspected pelvic injury, palpate the lower abdomen thoroughly. Note any rigidity of abdominal

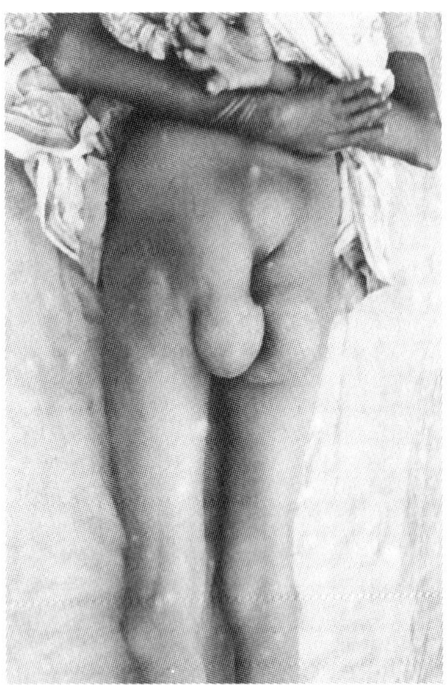

Fig. 9.2: Atypical neurofibromatous swelling

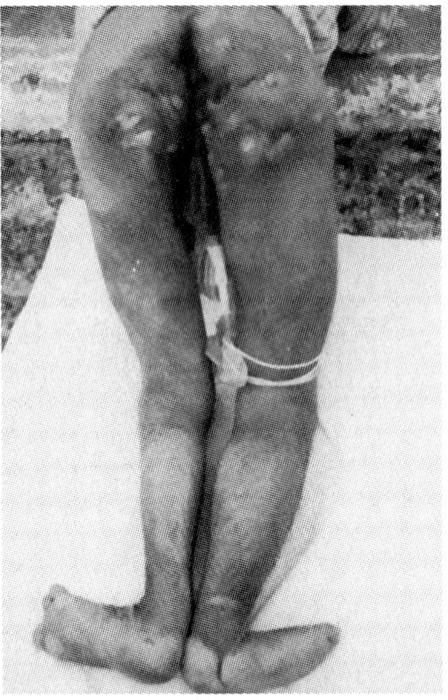

Fig. 9.3: Multiple sinuses in perineum (draining) in a patient of spina bifida

muscle, generalised/localised tenderness, hollowness/fullness of iliac fossae and pelvis.

Deep palpation (Feel): It should also include the cave of Retzius region, i.e. behind pubic symphysis. Palpate pubic symphysis for symmetry, regularity of surfaces or any gap in between the two halves. In disruption and any fracture dislocation of the pubic symphysis, one can insinuate a finger/fingers or even the fist if there is wide separation. In subluxation, a regular step may be felt. Palpate the inlet and outlet of pelvic margins systematically. The outer side and back of pelvis should be palpated on routine lines. The alignment and tenderness of sacral spines, sacroiliac joints, ischial tuberosities and coccygeal regions should be noted. Tenderness just beneath the posterior superior iliac spine and down to about 3-5 cm denotes sacroiliac joint tenderness. In very early pathology, tenderness of sacroiliac joints can be elicited by firmly tapping or guarded deep thrust applied over that region. At the bottom of the pelvis, any bulge and tenderness should be noted in the region of ischiorectal fossa.

Rectal Examination

No pelvic examination is complete without per rectal and per vaginal digital examinations. During this examination, palpate the ischiopubic rami, coccyx and inferior part of sacroiliac joints on the sides. Acetabular tenderness can also be elicited in acute pathology. In males, the condition of prostate, and, in both sexes any abnormal soft tissue bulge should be noted.

In pelvic fractures if the patient has not passed urine smoothly, do not ask him to strain and pass urine. Check up for any extravasation of urine in the scrotum, labial region, groin and in the lower abdominal wall.

Palpation of urethra is difficult. However, gradually palpate backwards from penile urethra towards the membranous part. It is always safe to pass a sterilised rubber catheter cautiously for testing the integrity of the urethra.

Auscultation

Quadrants of abdomen must be auscultated, especially in traumatic cases. Silent abdomen (along with rigidity) should be a definite sign of peritonitis.

MOVEMENTS

In connection with pelvic examination, movements at lumbar spine, lumbosacral region, hip and sacroiliac region must be tested separately, as described in corresponding chapter. The movements of the sacroiliac joints can be tested only by indirect methods, i.e. stress tests.

Stress Tests

These are of four types:

1. Straight leg raising test.
2. Compression stress test.
3. Distraction stress test.
4. Axial rotation stress tests.
   a. Pump handle test.
   b. Gaenslen's test.
   c. Laquer's sign.
   d. Goldthwaite's sign.

1. *Straight Leg Raising Test (See also Fig. 8.30)*

(Also done to test sciatic radiculitis and hip-stability)

In most of the affections of the hemipelvis and corresponding sacroiliac joint, patient has difficulty or even inability in raising ipsilateral straight leg.

Method: While the patient lies supine, ask him to elevate the ipsilateral lower limb with the knee fully extended. He is asked to stop as soon as he feels pain. The angle between the back of the thigh and the bed is measured. Normally, one can lift the straight leg to about 90° without tilting the pelvis. Beyond that, it will not be possible, unless the knee is bent. Even with a normal lower limb, straight leg raising may be deficient in affections and cause pain in the pelvis and sacroiliac joint.

2. *Compression Stress Test (Fig. 9.4)*

The patient lies supine on a flat bed and with the legs approximated together as far as possible. The examiner leans forwards, and compresses both anterior superior iliac spines, towards each other. Forceful compression often elicites pain in the affected sacroiliac joint, but will have no effect on lumbosacral affections. Of course, in fractures/dislocations of pelvis, this manoeuvre will elicit pain at the affected site.

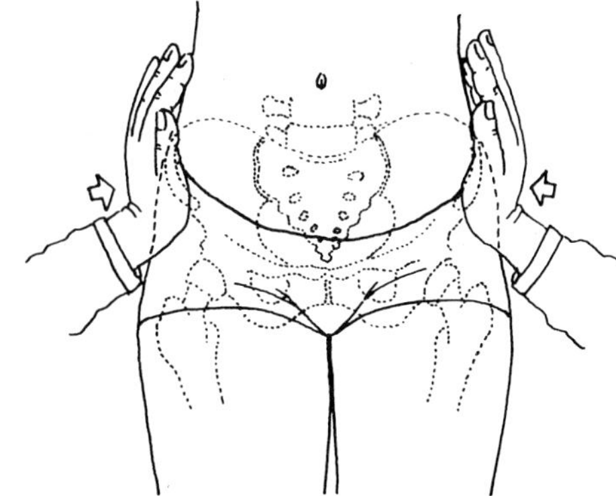

Fig. 9.4: Method of eliciting compression stress test of pelvis to elicit pain at sacroiliac joints

3. *Distraction Stress Test (Fig. 9.5)*

The patient lies supine with legs extended and approximated together. The examiner leans forwards and presses on both anterior superior iliac spines from the inner aspect with a tendency of distracting them away from each other. The inferences will be similar, as in 'compression stress test'.

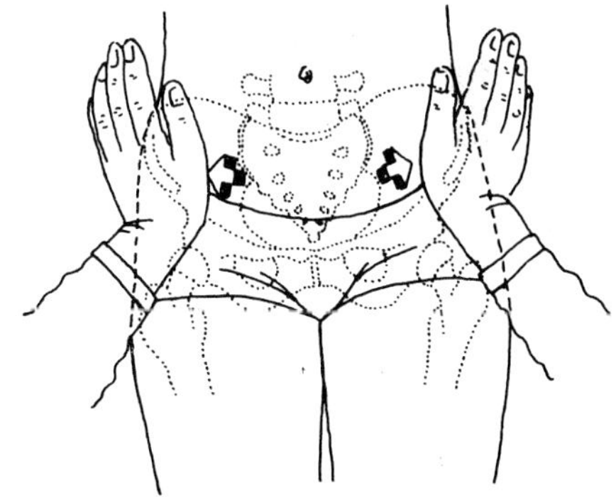

Fig. 9.5: Method of eliciting distraction stress test for pelvis to elicit pain at sacroiliac joints

4. *Axial Rotation Stress Test*
   a. *Pump handle test* (Fig. 9.6): The patient lies supine. Press with your left hand over patient's left shoulder. While the patient keeps her right lower limb extended, hold

her left upper leg and fully flex the knee and the hip (left) with a tendency to bring her left-knee towards her right shoulder. If right sacroiliac is diseased, the patient will feel pain on the right side in this manoeuvre (Reverse the position of the hand and test for opposite sacroiliac joint).

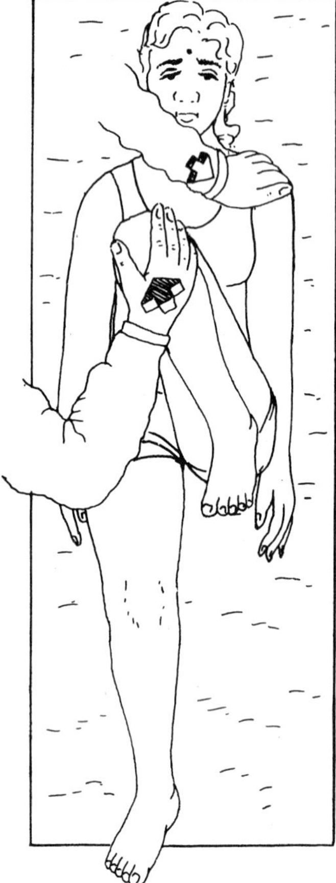

Fig. 9.6: Method of demonstration of pump handle test

Patho-mechanics of the test—By fully flexing the knee and hip, that side of hemipelvis is more or less locked with the sacrum. Attempts to forcibly flex the knee and hip (flexed across the abdomen) produces rotational stress at the opposite sacroiliac joint. In this manoeuvre, even in early pathology, pain will be felt at the sacro-iliac joint.

b. *Gaenslen's Test* (Fig. 9.7)—The patient lies supine, with the pelvis preferably lying on the edge of examination table. On the unaffected side, hip and knee are fully flexed and pressed over the abdomen. The affected side of hip is hyperextended. While doing so, the patient feels pain in the affected sacroiliac joint due to rotational strain.

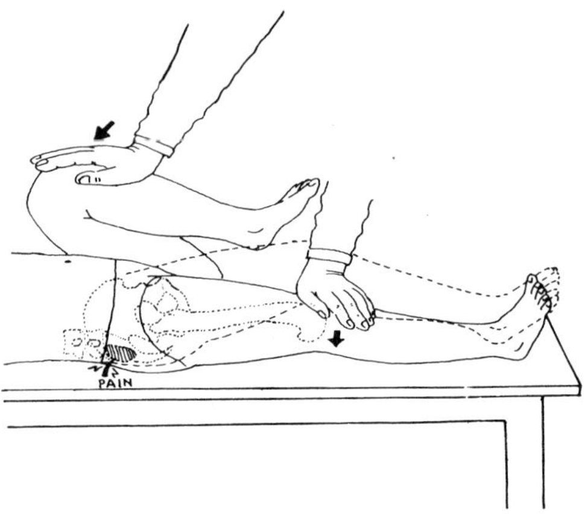

Fig. 9.7: Method of demonstration of Gaenslen's test

c. *Laquer's sign* (Fig. 9.8): If the ipsilateral lower limb is forced into flexion, abduction and external rotation at the hip, the patient experiences pain in the affected sacroiliac region.
d. *Goldthwaite's sign* (Fig. 9.9): The patient lies supine. While the knee is fully extended, the thigh is strongly flexed. The tense hamstring muscles produce rotatory strain upon the sacroiliac joint of ipsilateral side. Therefore, in sacroiliac affections, the patient feels pain on the same side on doing this manoeuvre.

MEASUREMENTS

In pelvic examination, it has not much significance. The girth of the pelvis at different levels, specially at the highest points of iliac crests and

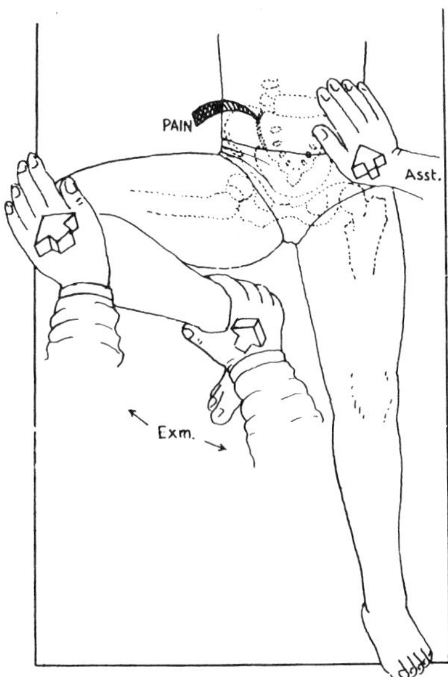

Fig. 9.8: Method of demonstration of Laquer s sign

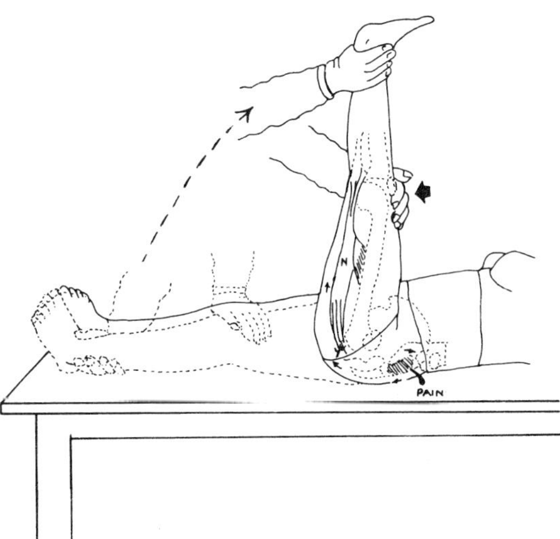

Fig. 9.9: Method of demonstration of Goldthwaite's sign. H = hamstrings; T = ischaial tuberosity

supra-trochanteric regions, should be noted. The linear measurements of the lower limbs should be done as described in the chapter on 'Hip Joint'.

Neurovascular examination of the lower limb should also be done routinely.

INVESTIGATIONS FOR PELVIC PATHOLOGY

Besides specific investigations indicated for particular pathological conditions, X-ray (in different planes) is an essential investigation for pelvic injuries and pathology.

In taking the X-ray for pelvis, the following points must be taken into account:

i. Bowel must be cleared of gases and faecal matter.
ii. Pelvis must be centred on the X-ray table, i.e. symphysis pubis and umbilicus should be in the same vertical line.
iii. The whole pelvis must be included in the exposure, rather, inclusion of lower three lumbars and lower down upto subtrochanteric level is very much helpful in considering the symmetry of the two hemipelvises.
iv. In ordering for an X-ray of the pelvis, the clinician must be clear in his mind as to which part he wants to delineate. Anteroposterior X-rays of pelvic inlet, pelvic outlet, and sacrum—all require different positioning. One must remember that the pelvis is not placed in a plane horizontal to the long axis of the body, rather, even the fully squared up pelvis is set at an anterior inclination. Therefore, if one wants to have a true anteroposterior exposure for the pelvis, the plate should be placed in contact beneath the pelvis supported on a sandbag and the X-ray beam should be focussed at the centre of the pelvic inlet.

For Sacroiliac Joints

Place the patient on the X-ray table with a wide sandbag supporting the upper pelvis, i.e. just below the lumbosacral areas. The lower limbs will be in lithotomy position. The X-ray beam is to be centred on the third sacral body. In this position, the longest zone of the auricle shaped sacroiliac joints is traversed by the X-ray beam. Confirmation of correct exposure of the sacroiliac joints can be had from the fact that the pelvic outlet will project a constricted bean shaped impression. For exposing the full length of sacrum, place a wider pillow beneath lower lumbar region transversely. Put the patient in wider lithotomy position. The beam is centred to imaginary S3 body.

Since the sacroiliac joint is placed obliquely, oblique anteroposterior and posteroanterior views are essential to visualise the joint clearly in its major extent. For oblique posteroanterior view, the patient lies prone. Then the unaffected side of the pelvis is elevated by 30°. The film is centred on the level of the anterior superior iliac spines and the beam is projected centering the mid point of the film. For oblique antero-posterior, the patient lies supine, and the affected side is elevated by 30°.

For delineating ilial plates, ischial and pubic rami, a plain anteroposterior X-ray exposure is good enough.

Key Diagnostic Points of Common Pelvic Affections

Classification of pelvic fractures (Table 9.2 and Fig. 9.12).

An extremely rare injury—ipsilateral triple dislocation of pelvis, produces gross instability (Fig. 9.10).

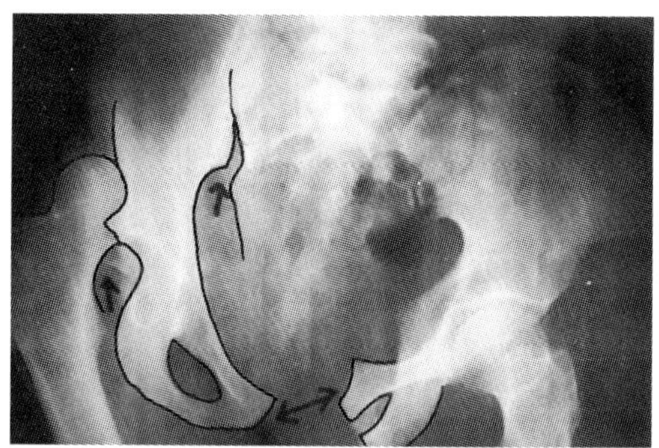

Fig. 9.10: Ipsilateral triple dislocation of pelvis: dislocations of hip, sacroiliac joint and pubic symphysis

DISEASES

I. Congenital Anomalies

Important are:

i. Undeveloped/Underdeveloped pelvis/congenital abscence of any segment/zone/part of pelvis (Figs 9.11A, and B).
ii. Trefoil pelvis.
iii. Protrusio acetabuli.
iv. Ectopia vesicae with deficient pubic symphysis.
v. Morphological alterations according to associated congenital conditions, e.g. in CDH.

Table 9.2: Injuries of pelvis

	Skeletal (Figs 9.15 and 9.16)			*Visceral (usually in severe injury)*
	Stable (usually due to minor injury)		*Unstable* (due to severe injury)	
(i)	Avulsion fracture, e.g. Anterior superior iliac spine (by sartorius), Anterior inferior iliac spine (by rectus femoris), Ischial tuberosity (by hamstrings)	(i)	Vertical—fracture Ilium, Pubis, Ischium	Urethra (membranous most common) Bladder
		(ii)	Bilateral fracture of—Ilium, Pubis, Ischium with various combinations	Vagina/Uterus Sciatic nerve
(ii)	Fracture individual components of pelvis Fracture ilial plates Fracture pubic ramus/body Fracture sacrum Fracture coccyx	(ii)	Fracture dislocation of pelvis.	Rectum and anal canal Pelvic peritoneum with its reflections Iliac vessels
(iii)	Subluxation of the joints, e.g. Pubic symphysis Sacroiliac joints Sacrococcygeal joint			

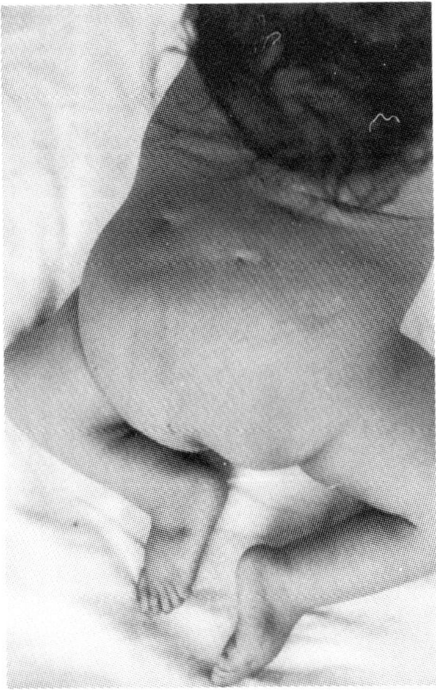

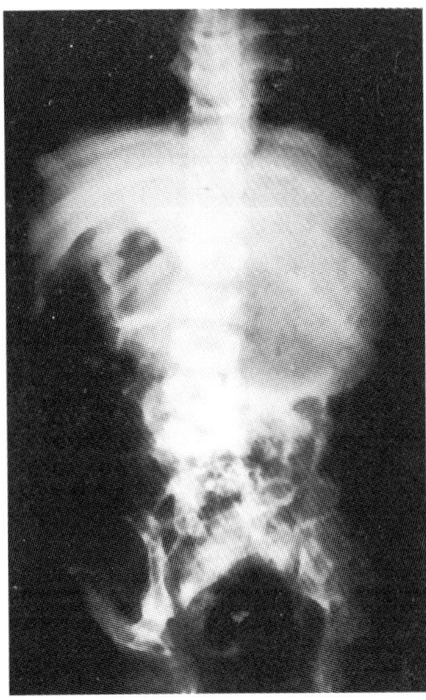

Figs 9.11A and B: Congenital abscense of sacrum

II. Inflammatory Conditions

i. Tuberculous focus in acetabulum and sacroiliac joints.
ii. Pyogenic inflammation of iliac plates, specially near about supraacetabular zone.
iii. Secondary involvement of pelvic bones following infective conditions of pelvic viscera, iliac abscess, compound injuries and injection abscess.

III. Metabolic and Deficiency States

— Rickets
— Osteomalacia:
  — Looser's zone (pseudofractures at ribs, axillary border of scapula, pubic rami, medial cortex of femur)
  — Trefoil pelvis
  — Protrusio acetabuli (Fig. 9.12)
  — Paget's disease.

IV. Collagen Arthropathy

— Ankylosing spondylitis
— Rheumatoid arthritis

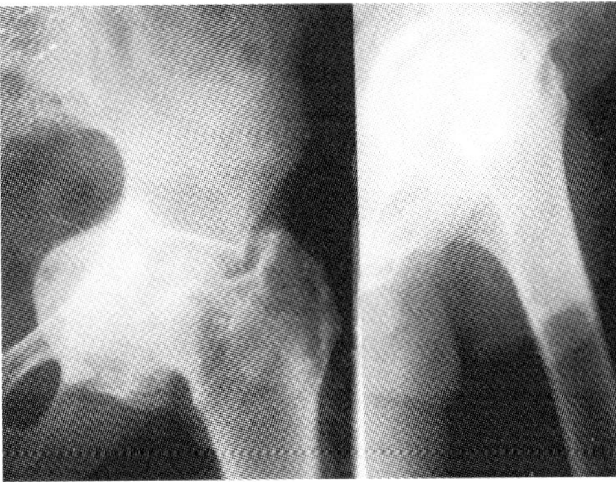

Fig. 9.12: Protrusio acetabuli

V. Degenerative Conditions

— Degenerative arthrosis of sacroiliac joint and acetabular margin (hip joint).

VI. Neoplasm

Benign: —Osteochondroma
—Haemangioma
—Osteoid osteoma

Malignant: —Chondrosarcoma
—Multiple myelomatosis
—Secondary carcinomatosis
—Others (rare)

Tuberculosis of Sacrolliac Joint

The patient is usually young female, with chronic history of low backache and pain in buttock region, specially on changing posture while sleeping, getting up from sitting and *vice-versa.* Sitting on the buttock of affected side is painful, whereas sitting on the opposite buttock relieves the pain. Bending forward with the knee extended is painful (tight hamstrings pulling the sacrotuberous ligament), whereas bending with the knee flexed (relaxed hamstrings) is painless.

—Little or no relief by analgesics.
—Localised tenderness, fullness (?) in sacro-iliac region.
—May be cold abscess—intra-pelvic/gluteal region/posterior part of iliac crest.
—Stress tests positive.
—Rectal examination demonstrates swelling and tenderness.
—ESR usually not much raised.
—X-ray—initially may be noncontributory, later on shows usual changes of tuberculosis.

Pyogenic Infection of Iliac Plate

In young children, pyogenic osteomyelitis of lower part of ilium with secondary septic arthritis of hip (and *vice-versa*) is not uncommon.

—Constitutional and local inflammatory features as in any pyogenic infection.
—May be local abscess.
—Hip movements affected.
—Pus culture and X-ray—confirmatory.

Ankylosing Spondylitis

—Young adults (male:female = 9:1) complaining of low backache and morning stiffness, which are relieved after exercise or activity and aggravated after prolonged rest.
—Deep thrust tenderness over sacroiliac regions.
—Other associated clinical findings (as in chapter on Spine).
—X-ray—periarticular rarefaction, fuzzines across sacroiliac joint, sclerosis of articular margins (Fig. 9.13), obliteration of joint line. As pathology advances, trabeculations across the joint (Fig. 12.51).

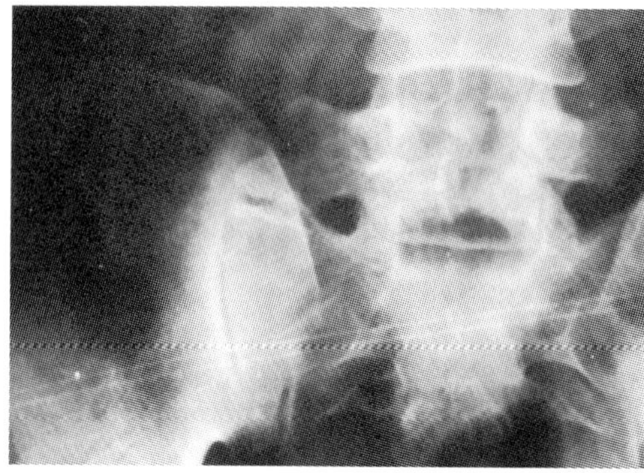

Fig. 9.13: Ankylosing spondylitis. Note the sclerosis of articular margins

Osteochondroma

—Pelvic bones are common sites.
—Variable knob like irregular, hard swelling arising from bone.
—Symptoms are usually due to pressure effects, cosmetic effect, or when it turns malignant, e.g. chondrosarcoma.
—X-ray is highly suggestive.

Coccydodynia (Coccydynia)

—Usually, overweight ladies in their forties.
—May or may not be a history of fall on buttock (on the edge of a hard object).
—Pain complained of on sitting on a hard object, or after walking a long distance, in advanced cases even when passing hard stools.
—Local tenderness at sacrococcygeal junction, coccyx, coccygeal tip.
—Per rectum examination elicits pain while finger tip presses posteriorly towards coccyx.

Osteitis Pubis

—Painful condition about the pubic symphysis with tendency to spontaneous cure.

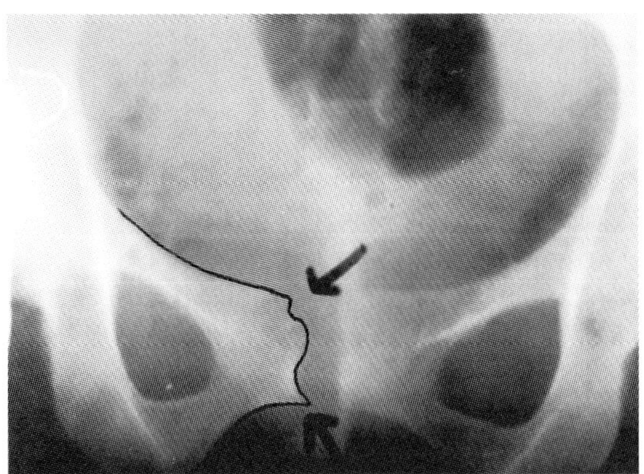

Fig. 9.14: Osteitis pubis

— Exact cause unknown but may follow trauma, usually surgical procedure about the pelvic region, and in women during pregnancy.
— Waddling gait.
— Lateral compression/distraction tests are positive.
— Cross leg test positive.
— Direct pressure elicits tenderness over pubic symphysis and origin of adductor muscles.
— Pain more on abduction of lower limb.
— No local or general signs of inflammation.
— X-ray—Early stage—no change. Late stage—pubic bodies look moth-eaten, rarefied and gaping (Fig. 9.14), which gradually reossify as normal, bony architecture is restored.

Classification of Fracture Pelvis

See Figs 9.15 and 9.16.

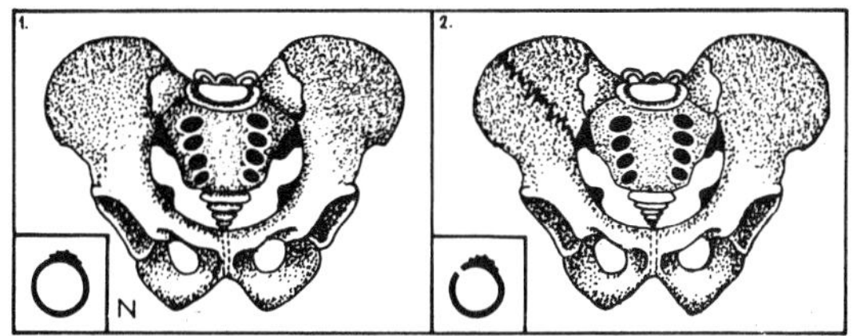

Fig. 9.15: (1) Normal pelvic ring; (2) stable fracture of pelvic ring

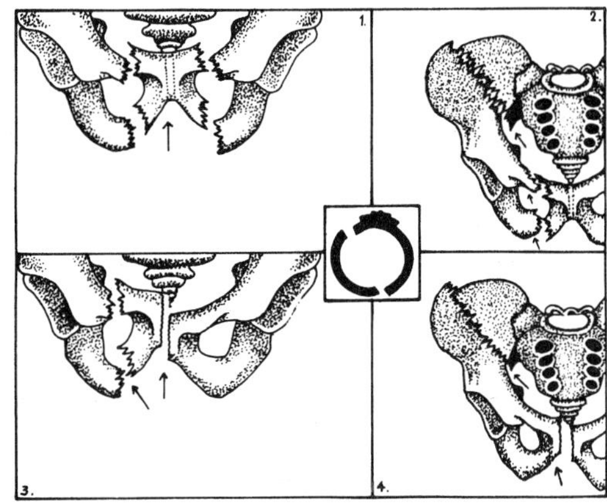

Fig. 9.16: (1 to 4) Unstable fracture of pelvic ring

10 Backache

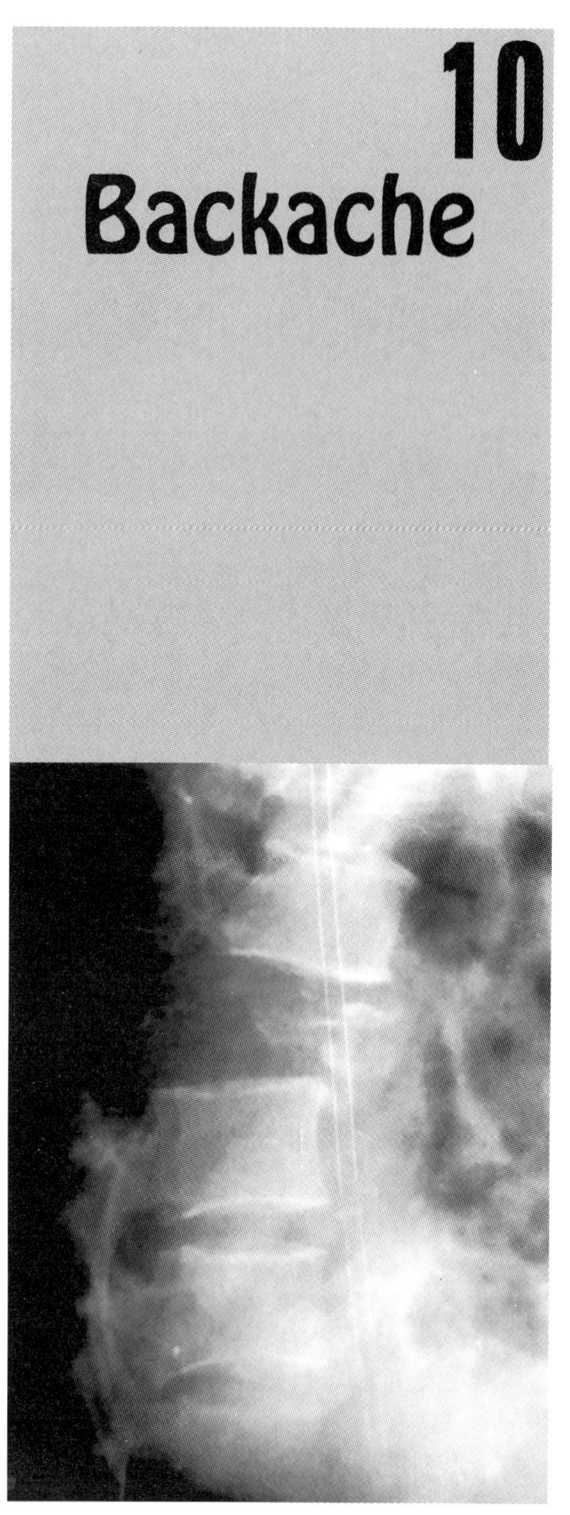

200,000 years ago the Neanderthal man did not suffer from low back pain, because he was not yet fully vertical. However, as the human being assumed upright posture, the manifestations of backache grew almost proportionately to the progress in civilization.

Examining a patient with backache can itself cause both backache (because one must examine again and again from top to bottom performing different clinical tests) and headache to a clinician (because the cause can be numerous and intricate and malingerers are not easy to identify).

On no subject in orthopaedics can more controversies arise than on the problem of backache. Backache is one of the most common orthopaedic problems, and manifests as society's most expensive disease in the productive years. It is a common problem almost all over the globe. Any part of the back may ache, but the commonest site is the lower back, i.e. lumbar and lumbosacral regions, followed by dorsolumbar and dorsal regions. The commonest age group affected are adults and elderlies, with the incidence more among females. With the march of civilisation and the consequent increasingly stressful life, the list of the causes of backache has also increased, as such that it has now assumed nearly epidemic proportions. However, increasing automation and robotisation, by helping to reduce 'backbreaking' stresses, hold promise in reducing the incidence of backache.

Anatomically and functionally, the lower lumbar spine forms a more or less transitional zone from the more mobile trunk to the more static pelvic region. Thus, the lower lumbar region is the site for rotatory and shearing strains. Mechanically also, it is not suitably designed for biped weight bearing. Further this region is often a site for structural abnormalities (e.g. canal stenosis, pars inter-articularis defects). These reasons may explain the predilection of this region for backache.

The disabilities, length disparities and deformities of the lower limbs are accommodated to maximum possible extent by tilting of the pelvis either side ways or anteroposteriorly. This inherently puts the lower back to strain and gradually, patients start complaining of low backache.

Deformities, like scoliosis, kyphoscoliosis or even kyphosis of the spine (dorsal and/or lumbar), by changing the physiomechanics of posture and weight transmission also ultimately lead to strain at the low back.

USUAL CAUSES OF BACKACHE

As such, the list of causes of backache can be a very long one, but the common causative factors are:

1. *Posture:* Certain postural defects while sitting, standing, sleeping, heavy weight lifting, prolonged standing, prolonged walking, working on heavy machines, working in stooping posture with legs close together, riding on fast and jerky vehicles (horse riding, jeep riding, motor-bike riding) may lead to backache. Explore this possibility if no other organic cause is evident. Persons with protuberant abdomen, by virtue of constant dragging strain on the spinal ligaments, are liable to have backache, specially when they sit or stand for prolonged periods.

   Individuals with tall slender physique, may develop postural defects, like gradual kyphosis in dorsolumbar region (usually in a young tall girl) or lumbar lordosis, both of which can cause dull backache.

2. *Congenital defects:* Defects in the vertebrae and their soft tissue allies (e.g. spina bifida, sacralisation of 5th lumbar vertebra (Fig. 10.2) scoliosis, spondylolysis, spondylolisthesis, transitional vertebra can be potent causes of chronic backache—X-ray usually helps in the diagnosis.

3. *Injury:* Strain, sprain, ligamentous (e.g. sprung back—occurs due to tearing of all posterior supportive ligaments of lumbosacral region) and muscular injuries, fractures, dislocations, fracture-dislocation of vertebrae are common causes of backache. History of trauma and X-ray findings suggest the diagnosis.

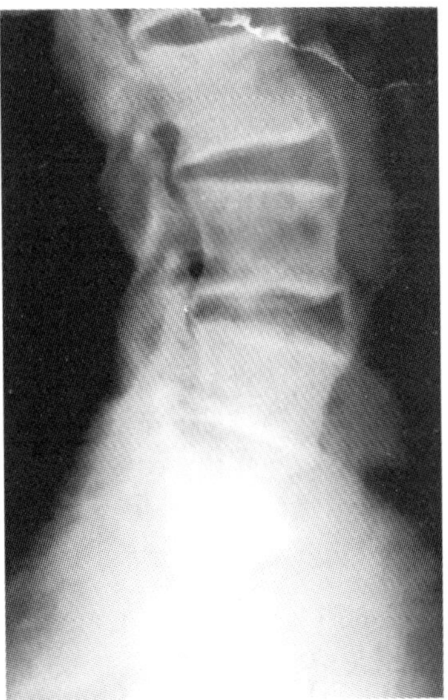

Fig. 10.1: Lumbar spondylosis

   Sometimes the history of injury is completely forgotten but the patient may suffer chronic backache due to a very old injury (Kummell's disease).

4. *Intervertebral disc pathology:* In 1934 Mixter and Barr were the first to identify herniation of lumbar disc as a cause of low-back pain and sciatica.

   Either due to increased turgidity or herniation (prolapse) of the nucleus pulposus, the intervertebral disc can become a potent cause for low backache. The subject is usually a young male complaining of low backache mostly of sudden onset, with or without radiating pain in the lower limb and perhaps with some numbness and tingling.

   In acute disc herniation (prolapse)—At the lower back, board like muscular rigidity and/or sciatic scoliosis are seen; coughing, sneezing, stooping, increased intra-abdominal pressure augment the symptoms; straight leg raising upto or below 60°, positive sciatic stretch test and myelography confirm the pathology.

Allied conditions which may lead to backache are:

Lumbar spondylosis (degenerative changes in the lumbar region) (Fig. 10.1).

Spondylolysis (weakness in pars interarticularis).

Spondylolisthesis (slipping of the vertebra along with the spinal column above, over the vertebra below).

5. *Spinal stenotic syndrome*
It can be defined as the narrowing of the osteoligamentous vertebral canal and/or the intervertebral foramina causing compression of the thecal sac and/or the caudal nerve roots; at a single vertebral level, narrowing may affect the whole canal or part of it (Postacchini 1983).

Spinal canal stenosis can be of three forms:

i. Primary stenosis
   — Congenital
   — Developmental—postnatal defective development of vertebrae; achondroplastic and constitutional stenosis.
ii. Secondary stenosis—Compression is due to acquired causes, e.g. spondylotic changes, Paget's disease, old vertebral fracture.
iii. Combined stenosis—Combined causes of primary and secondary stenosis.

Causes: Congenital narrowing of vertebral canal.

Acquired—Traumatic, degenerative, neoplastic, iatrogenic. Clinical features are low backache, intermittent claudications and there may be deep tenderness in the affected zone.

Lumbar spinal stenosis remains one or the most frequently seen and clinically important degenerative spinal disorders in the aging population.

6. *Ankylosing spondylitis and rheumatoid spondylitis (Sacroiliatis)* (Fig. 10.2): Ankylosing spondylitis is a common condition affecting young males below 40 and usually diagnosed by complaints of morning stiffness, pain in the back (dorsolumbar or lumbar region) which gets relieved after exercises (spinal stress tests). On examination, limited chest expansion (limitation below 2.5 cm expansion at the 4th intercostal space) is diagnostic. X-ray shows fuzziness and later on fusion of sacroiliac joints, and bamboo spine.

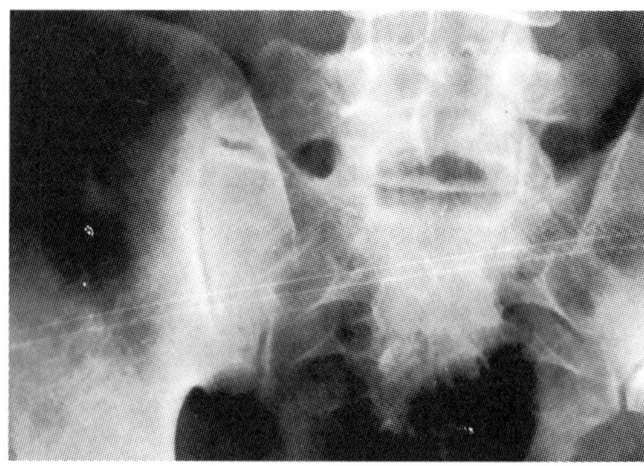

Fig. 10.2: Sacralisation of lumbar vertebrae can also cause low backache. Also note the features of sacroiliatis

Rheumatoid arthritis can also affect the sacroiliac joints, causing low backache.

7. *Infective conditions:* Acute infection presents apparently and is not a common cause. Among the chronic infections, tuberculosis of the spine is the commonest cause. Other causes may be pyogenic osteomyelitis, syphilitic back, or *B.coli* infection.

8. *Neoplastic conditions*
   In the benign group
   — Osteoid osteoma, aneurysmal bone cyst, haemangioma, neuro-fibroma and meningioma (Fig. 10.3)
   In the malignant group
   — Secondary carcinomatosis, multiple myeloma, Hodgkins deposit, lymphosarcoma, giant cell tumour, osteogenic sarcoma.

Apart from these, malformations (angiomatous) and neoplasms of the spinal cord may also be responsible for backache.

9. *Degenerative arthrosis of spine:* In elderly subjects, low backache, usually variably relieved after some activities and massage, may be due to degenerative changes in the spine, with or without primary healed pathology and/or deformity.

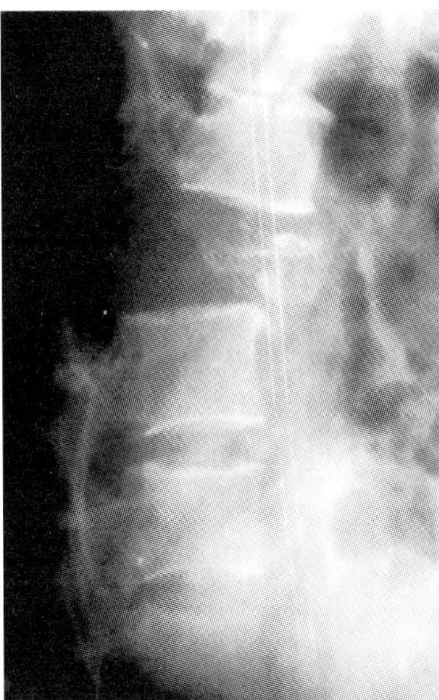

Fig. 10.3: Meningioma of L3 leading to chronic backache

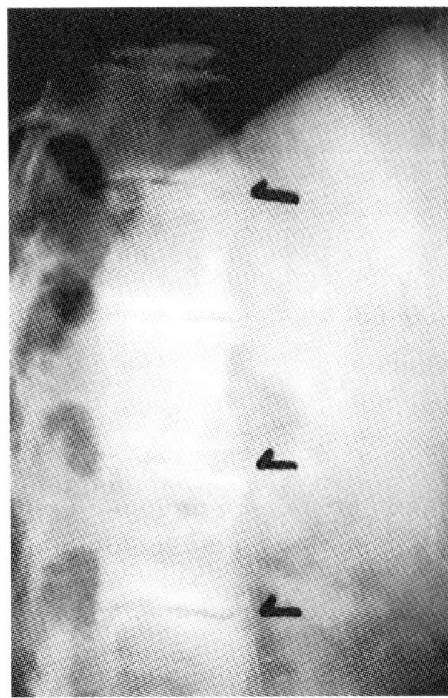

Fig. 10.4: Alkaptonuria (Ochronosis, Onchronotic arthritis). Note the degenerative calcification of the intervertebral discs.It is a congenital and inherited as Mendelian recessive trait mostly occurring in offsprings of consanguineous mairrages. Homogentisic acid is deposited in tissues like sclerae, ligaments, tendons, cartilage, intervertebral disc which turn black due to the pigment. Bluish green colouration of urine with the addition of a drop of dilute ferric chloride solution is diagnostic

10. *Senile osteoporosis:* Elderly subjects, usually ladies complain of constant mild backache. With typical rounded kyphosis X-ray is confirmatory.

11. *Other causes in ladies:* Leucorrhoea, pelvic inflammatory diseases, repeated pregnancy, uterine disorders (prolapse, growths), and intrauterine contraceptive devices.

12. *Metabolic:* Osteomalacia, alkaptonuria (Fig. 10.4)

Osteomalacia (analogue of rickets occurring in the adult skeleton)—Usually child bearing mother with multiple quick succession of pregnancies complains of constant dull boring pain. Flat bones are tender. Pelvis may be deformed (trefoil pelvis), classical Looser's zone in X-rays (especially of femur and tibia), which are transverse radiolucent lines surrounded by a small amount of sclerotic bone.

13. *Malingerer's backache:* This is a usual problem in industrial workers, which can be suspected in lack of any organic pathology, and confirmed by their bizarre manifestations (mostly unrelated), and watching the patients activities at home and in society.

14. *Compensation backache:* With a view to exploit the employer and/or insurance company for undue compensation, several workers keep on complaining about backache with no definite and discernible organic pathology.

15. *Abdominal and pelvic causes:* Backache may be a manifestation of abdominal visceral or pelvic (genitourinary) pathologies. Upper abdominal conditions can cause pain in the dorsolumbar region; lower abdominal conditions in lumbar region; and pelvic pathologies in lumbosacral, sacral and sacroiliac regions. Nowhere in the spine can any accountable pathology be delineated.

16. *General (miscellaneous) causes:* Exposure to cold, viral infections (e.g. influenza virus), fibrositis, myositis, chronic constipation, febrile illness, depressive psychosis.

17. *Idiopathic:* In examining a patient with low backache one should follow the method of examination of the spine. However, as seen in the above mentioned causes of low backache, one will be obliged to examine the lower limbs, abdomen and pelvic region. Diagnosis by 'exclusion' is markedly helpful in coming to a conclusion. Of course, corroboratory investigations should also be done in order to clinch the diagnosis.

If no obvious cause (e.g. caries spine, spondylolisthesis, or advanced ankylosing spondylitis) is detected on routine examinations, it is worth while to put the lower back to stress and recommended postural exercies and note the results. In backache, due to postural defects, spondylotic changes and in early ankylosing spondylitis, patient definitely feels better after doing the exercises.

REFERENCES

1. Postacchine F: Lumbar stenosis and pseudostenosis: Defination and classification of pathology. *Inl J Orhop Traumatol* **9**: 939-50, 1983.
2. Mixter WJ, Barr JS: Rupture of the intervertebral disc with involvement of the spinal canal. *New England J Med* **211**: 210-15, 1934.
3. Spivak JM: Degenerative lumbar spinal stenosis. *J Bone Joint Surg* **80A**: 1053-66, 1998.
4. Harrold AJ: Alkaptonuric arthritis. *J Bone Joint Surg* **38**: 532, 1956.

11 Examination of a Paralytic Patient*

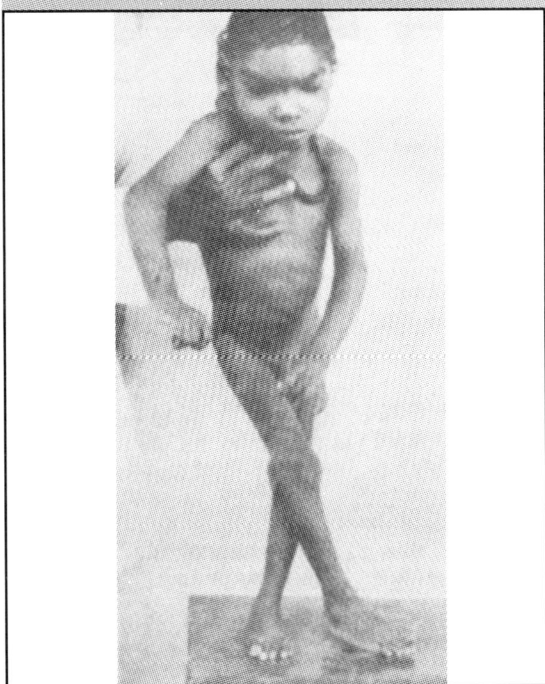

* Besides the considerations in the chapter on examination of the Spine

INTRODUCTION

The examination of a paralytic patient must be rehabilitation-oriented from the very beginning.

Most of the paralytic conditions do not recover fully. Assessment should be psychologically, socially, economically and rehabilitation oriented. The assessment must aim not only at finding out the disability of the patient, rather, the functional capabilities with which the patient has been left, and the potentiality of improvement must be fully explored.

In examining such a patient hitherto, the main aim has been to find out the cause of paralysis by assessing as discussed in the chapter on spine. This chapter mainly aims at assessing the extent of residual disabilities and the potential for improvement.

Syzygiology (the study of interrelationships or interdependencies especially of the whole, as opposed to the study of seperate parts or isolated functions)—is of great importance in these paralytic patients (Figs 11.1A to C).

ANATOMICAL CONSIDERATION

1. Muscles Commonly Affected in Polio-Paralysis (Figs 1 and 2, Coloured Plate 1)

Poliomyelitis is a viral infection causing degeneration of the anterior horn cells and ventral nerve roots leading to the lower motor neuron type of paralysis of the affected muscles.

A. *In lower limb* (in order of frequency and severity of affection)
   - Tibialis anterior
   - Quadriceps femoris
   - Gluteus medius
   - Gastroc-soleus
   - Gluteus maximus
   - Tibialis posterior
   - Peroneus tertius
   - Hamstrings
   - Peroneus longus and brevis.

B. *In upper limb* (in order of frequency and severity of affection)
   - Deltoid
   - Biceps brachii

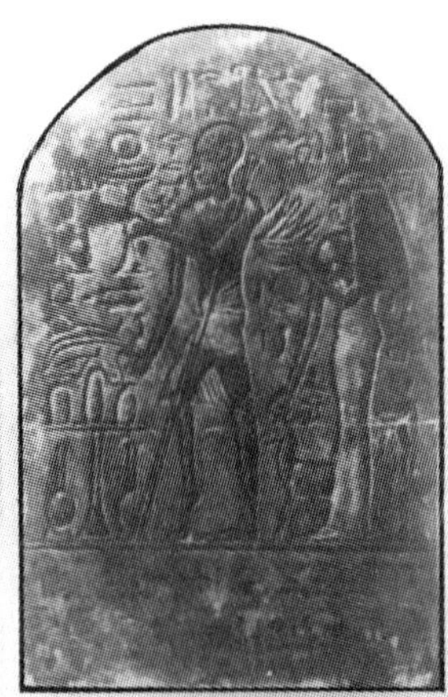

Fig. 11.1A: Roma (eighteeth dynasty), door-keeper and priest of the temple of Astarte at Memphis, who suffered from poliomyelitis of the right lower limb (still kept at the Ny Carlsberg Museum, Copenhagen)

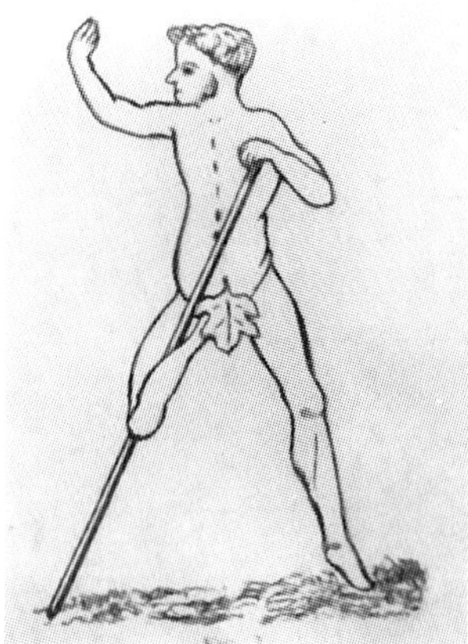

Fig. 11.1B: Poliomyelitic deformities of the lower limbs drawn on an antiquc Italian jar dating from thc fourth century BC. (Musée du Louvre, Paris)

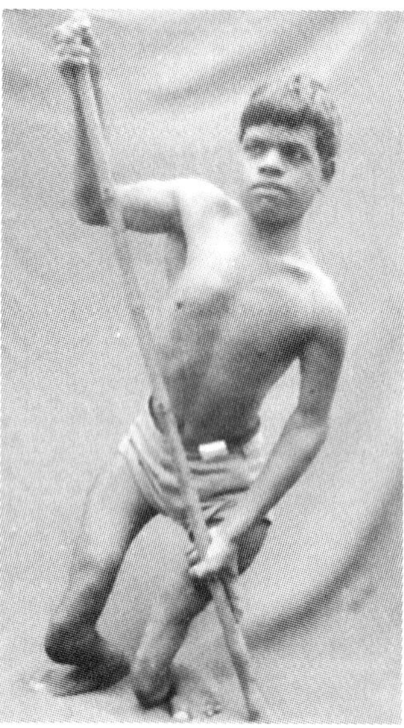

Fig. 11.1C: Judge ability more than disability of a handicapped person. In spite of gross deformities he is in job

— Short rotators of shoulder
— Extensor carpi ulnaris
— Extensor pollicis longus
— Extensor digitorum
— Supinator
— Flexor digitorum profundus
— Flexor digitorum sublimis.

C. *Trunk* (in order of frequency and severity of affection)
— Sacrospinalis
— Pectoralis major
— Latissimus dorsi
— External oblique abdominis
— Internal oblique.

2. Muscles Commonly Escaping Polio-Paralysis

— Tensor fascia femoris
— Ilio psoas
— Pronator teres
— Trapezius
— Subscapularis
— Intrinsics of foot and hand.

3. The Muscles Having Wider Representation at the Neural Level Usually Escape unless the Affection is of Very Severe Magnitude

History Taking

Besides the general considerations, the main stress should be given to:

1. Complaints—Congenital (e.g. for spina bifida)/acquired (in case of trauma—mode of injury).
2. Any familial tendency (may be positive history in myopathy).

3. Social and economic background:
   — Geographical topography.
   — Place of residence and its surroundings.
   — Structural barriers around residence.
4. Any constitutional features (e.g. for febrile onset in poliomyelitis).
5. Immunization status.
6. Chronological history of milestones of development.
7. Pregnancy and delivery:
   — Antenatal period.
   — Mode of delivery.
   — Any problem during or after delivery.
   — Drugs taken during pregnancy

General Examination

(Besides general and systemic examination as written in 'Introductory chapter'). Most of the paralytic patients are carried to the clinician by attendants. However, if they can walk, note the following:

1. The effect of the disability on the general posture of the patient.
2. The apparent mode of compensation for the residual disabilities, deformities and limb length discrepancy.
3. Mode of stabilisation while standing.
4. Mode of walking.
5. Aids required for walking.
6. Mode of clearing hurdles and negotiating steps.

The examiner must look for and note the expression, mental alertness, approximate IQ, any change in facial appearance, salivation, tongue position.

Regional Examination

Usually the disabilities are initially localised to a particular region, but with the passage of time the patient develops associated deformities and disabilities of the adjoining joints or even the contralateral limb and trunk. Therefore, general assessment of the patient as a whole is necessary. Try to identify the primary site of lesion and then assess the deformities which chronologically developed as a mechanism of compensation to achieve functional gain. In longstanding paralysis, natural compensatory mechanisms may be present and give a grotesque, ugly look, but they may be of immense functional value to the patient in helping to meet his bare minimum needs (Fig. 11.1C). This can be very well exemplified while assessing a neglected patient.

Local Examination

This should be done at the different sites of deformities and residual disabilities.

Prerequisites

1. Expose the affected regional zone and the contralateral limb fully.
2. The patient should be examined in the compensated position which he assumes for his daily activities.

Attitude and Gait

In such patients, attitude depends upon:

1. The type and extent of paralysis.
2. The period of paralysis.
3. Compensatory mechanisms developed by the patient to combat the disabilities, deformities and limb length disparities.

CERTAIN COMMON ATTITUDES

[Especially in neglected polio and cerebral palsy (a group of disorders resulting in nonprogressive brain damage) patients].

THE TENSOR FASCIA FEMORIS DEFORMITIES COMPLEX

This is the commonest deformity complex of the lower limb in neglected polio (Figs 11.2 and 11.3) and myopathy patients (Fig. 11.4).

This develops due to contracture of tensor fascia femoris muscle-ilio-tibial tract axis. By virtue of its alignment on the anterolateral aspect of hip and posterolateral aspect of knee, it primarily produces flexion, external rotation and abduction at the hip and flexion at the knee. Further assisted by contracture of outer hamstring and gravity, posterolateral subluxation of

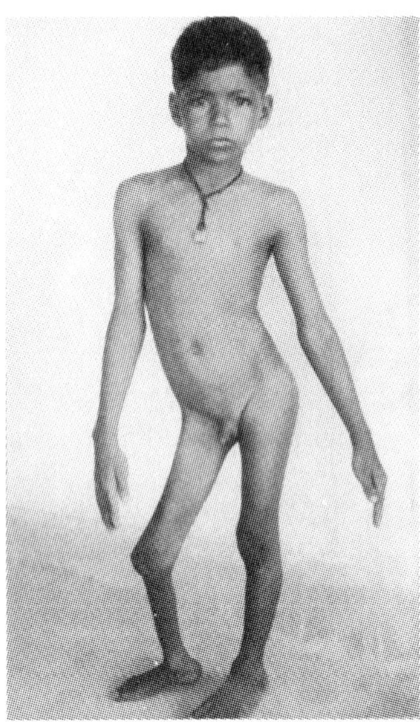

Fig. 11.2: Boy with mild tensor fascia femoris deformity note flexion, abduction and external rotation deformity at hip, mild flexion at knee, secondary equinus tendency at ankle, secondary scoliosis tendency at spine to compensate the pelvic tilt

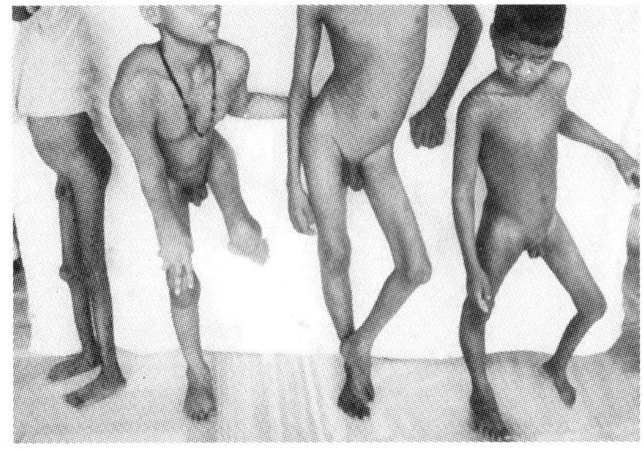

Fig. 11.3: Various stages of tensor fascia femoris contracture (TFF complex deformities) due to polio paralysis

knee develops. If further neglected, posterolateral rotation and genu valgum of leg develop. Secondarily, equinovarus deformity develops at ankle and foot.

In severely neglected cases, pelvic obliquity, lordosis, fixed lower lumbar scoliosis and varying shortening of the affected limb develop.

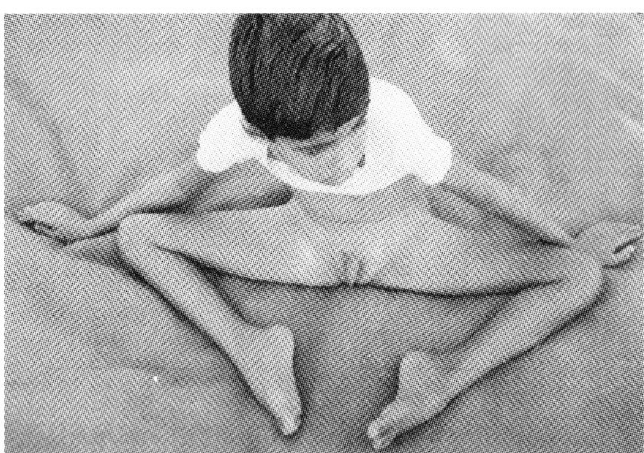

Fig. 11.4: Boy of myopathy developed bilateral tensor fascia femoris deformities complex due to neglected posture. Upper limbs and trunks are also weak

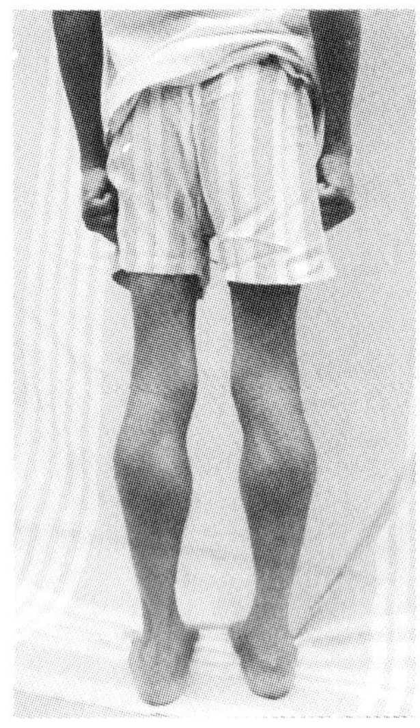

Fig. 11.5: Pseudomuscular hypertrophy in myopathy. Note the wasted thigh muscles but hypertrophy of calf muscles

Five Finger Quadriceps (in Hand to Knee Gait) (Fig. 11.6A)

It is usually to be seen while the patient is walking. The affected limb is always put forward in stepping, with the body leaning towards it anteriorly. With weak quadriceps, the patient gradually learns to stabilise his knee by directly transferring his body weight over the lower thigh, through his ipsilateral hand, usually by keeping the knee in variably flexed position.

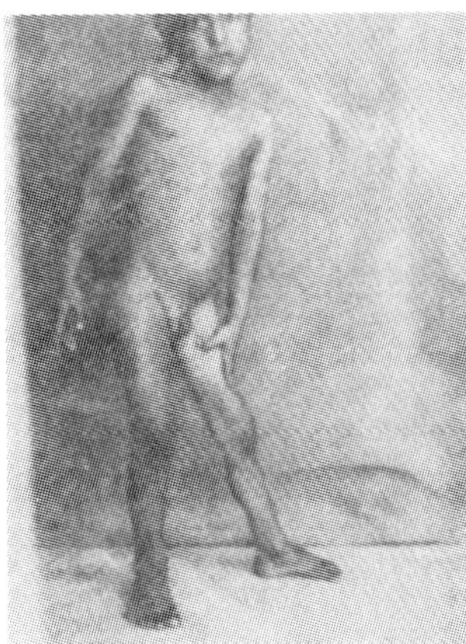

Fig. 11.6A: Hand to knee gait (five finger quadriceps) in children of polio-paralysis with weak quadriceps, managing to walk

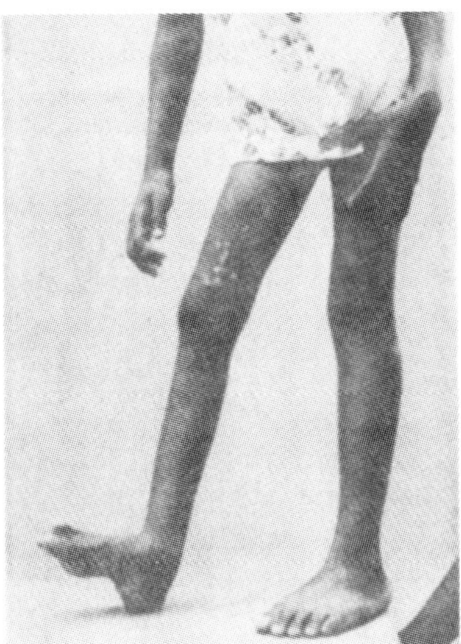

Fig. 11.6B: Note the hyperkeratotic, tough and warty skin in front of lower right thigh of a polio-paralysis patient walking for years with five finger quadriceps. He has also calcaneo-cavo-valgus deformity of right foot

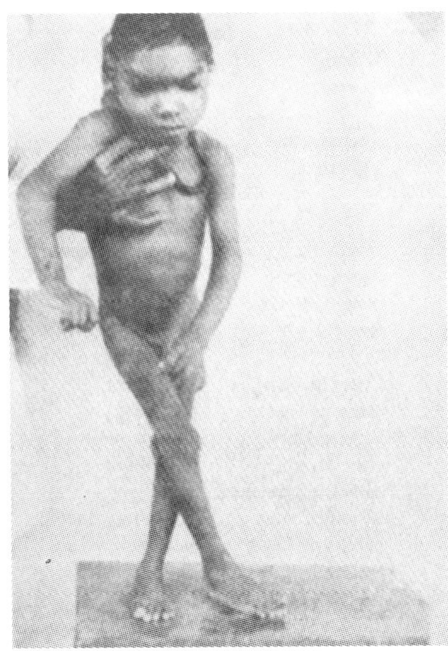

Fig. 11.7: Typical cerebral palsy child, note the scissoring of the legs in attempt of standing/walking; microcephaly; thumb in palm deformity

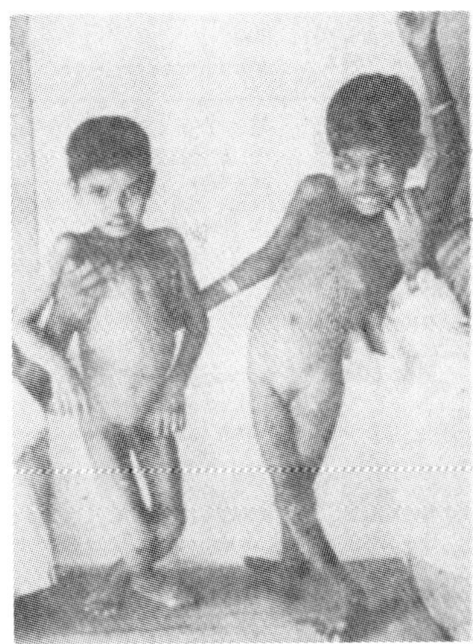

Fig. 11.8: Cerebral palsy in brother and sister

With markedly weak quadriceps, especially when it is associated with shortening of the limb, the foot is in equinus, the knee flexed and the fingers and thumb of the ipsilateral hand are firmly anchored on the front of the lower thigh. The skin of that region of thigh may become hyperkeratotic, even warty, tough and hyperpigmented (Fig. 11.6B) while the underlying quadriceps mass is markedly atrophied. In moderately weak quadriceps even two finger support over the region helps the patient in stabilising the knee joint. The intelligent patient adopts this function by keeping his hand in ipsilateral pant-pocket and pressing over the thigh through it.

Gluteal Lurch

Gluteus medius or gluteus maximus or both paralysis lead to an unstable hip and unsightly and flinging lurch. In isolated paralysis of gluteus medius, the trunk sways towards the affected side and the pelvis sags on the opposite side. When gluteus maximus is paralysed alone, the body lurches backwards. Trendelenburg test will be positive in gluteal paralysis. However, when the gluteal paralysis is severe, the test cannot be performed, as it will become impossible to balance on the affected side.

TYPICAL ATTITUDES OF FOOT DEFORMITIES (vide chapter on the Foot)

Cerebral Palsy

Cerebral palsy is a group of disorders resulting in nonprogressive brain damage. Basically, it is a neuromuscular disorder of cerebral origin occurring due to injury or insult to the developing brain in prenatal, natal or neonatal (postnatal) period and is nonprogressive. Neurologically cerebral palsy patients are mostly of six types:

1. Spastic (about 60%)
2. Ataxia
3. Athetoid
4. Rigid
5. Mixed types (about 10%)
6. Atonic

Clinically cerebral palsy may be monoplegic (rare) diplegic (most common), hemiplegic, triplegic (more theoretically) or quadriplegic.

— The cerebral palsy patients (Figs 11.7 to 11.9) with mental retardation are usually microcephalic with or without dribbling of saliva.

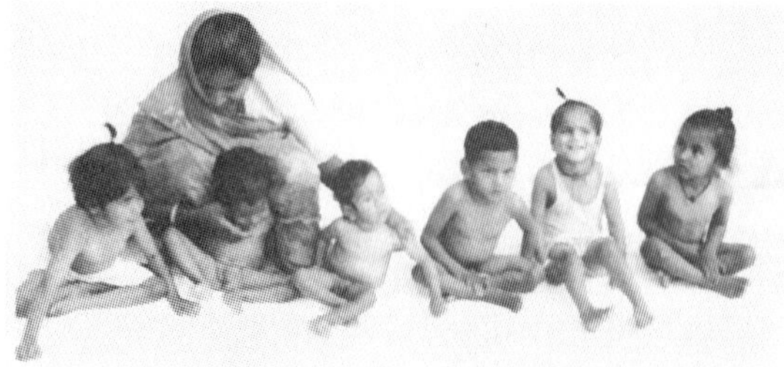

Fig. 11.9: Cerebral palsy patients in group—in various stages of exercises, rehabilitation and training

In a few cases, there may be squint or nystagmus. Typically, they show flexion, adduction and internal rotation at the hip, flexion at the knee, mild tendo-Achilles tightness and valgus of the foot with or without toe-in.

— In the upper limb, the shoulder is adducted and internally rotated; the elbow is kept variably flexed; the forearm is in pronation; flexion and ulnar deviation develop at the wrist with fanning tendency of the fingers. In hand the fingers also have the tendency for hyperextension at the metacarpophalangeal joints (usually affecting the index and ring fingers) and thumb in palm deformity. However, presentations may be mild to severe.

— In cerebral diplegia, the lower limbs assume a typical "scissor-gait" on attempts at stepping, mainly due to spasticity of the adductors of the thigh (Fig. 11.7).

— In hemiplegics, the foot develops equinovarus deformity and the shoulder may be adducted and internally rotated with or without other aforesaid deformities of upper limb. The patient walks with spastic gait.

Before the typical features of cerebral palsy develop, even the early cases can be clinically diagnosed by carefully assessing the response to certain primitive reflexes, as charted in Table 11.1.

For prognostising about the sitting and walking abilities of a CP child, the following observations may be of help (After Paine, 1966):

— If the child starts sitting even by the age of 2 years, it should be a favourable sign for his walking.

— If sitting of its own comes between 2 to 4 years, the chances of standing and walking independently are about 50%.

— If independent sitting is not learnt before 4 years, independent standing or walking will hardly be possible.

— If a CP child, without severe contracture, can not walk by the age of 8 years, there is hardly any chance of his ever walking in future.

Table 11.1: Reflexes of neonates

	Name of reflex	*When to appear/disappear*	*How to elicit*	*What to observe*	*Inference*
1.	Tonic neck reflex	Appears at 2 months and disappears at 6 months	Neck flexion	Arms flex and legs extend	Presence of this reflex is incompatible with independent standing and walking
2.	Asymmetric tonic neck reflex		Head is turned to one side	Arm and knee of opposite side flex	Absent reflex indicates poor prognostic signs for walking
3.	Moro's reflex	Appears at birth, disappears at 3 months	Neck is suddenly extended	Upper limbs extend away from body and then come together in embracing pattern	Persistence indicates bad prognosis for walking
4.	Neck righting reflex	Appears at 4 to 6 months, disappears at 24 months	Head is turned to one side	Shoulder, trunk pelvis and lower limb follow the the turned head	Persistence, indicates bad prognosis for walking
5.	Parachute reaction	Appears at 9 months and persists forever	Child is lifted horizontally by the waist and suddenly lowered on the table	Arms and hands fan out towards the table as though to protect from fall	Absence, indicates bad prognosis for walking
6.	Palmar grasp reflex	Appears at birth and disappears at 6 months	A pencil is passed along the medial side of palm	Tries to grasp the pencil	Persistence indicates bad prognosis for walking

A cerebral palsy patient should be assessed for functional abilities, e.g.:

1. Sitting ability: Can sit independently/can sit only when propped/cannot sit.
2. Walking ability: (a) Community walker—can move about independently in society, (b) can walk about inside the house only independently, (c) can walk with some assistance or aids/cannot walk.
3. Eating ability: (a) Can eat with his hand independently, (b) can eat only with the help of some aids and/or appliances, (c) can not eat of his own even with aids and/or appliances and has to be fed.
4. ADL (Activities of daily living): (a) Can manage ADL independently, (b) can manage ADL with some assistance, (c) cannot carry out ADL and has to be helped by others.

Inspection

Besides the apparent position due to unbalanced contracture of opposite groups of muscles of the limb, a rough idea of the extent of involvement of the muscles can be obtained by inspection. In the abdominal wall, a definite ballooning of the particular sector in which the muscle is paralysed, can be noted.

Palpation

Besides general consideration, palpation should particularly ascertain:

1. The bulk of the muscles.
2. The tone of muscles.

3. Any affection of contralateral muscles and tendons.
4. The extent and thickness of callosities at the joints due to abnormal weight bearing.

In acute cases (mainly in polio), muscle tenderness should be elicited, since this will give a guideline to the depth of involvement.

MEASUREMENTS

This must be a routine procedure even in the early follow up of a paralytic patient, especially in polio patients in growing age. It has been found that:

a. The earlier the age of affection—the more is the limb length discrepancy.
b. The more extensive is the affection (especially if it has been neglected) the more is the disparity—unless a balance between the paralysed and unaffected opposing group of muscles has been maintained (by physiotherapy-stretching, splintage and/or operation). The presence of severe deformities in paralytic patients, especially bilateral affections, sometimes presents a real problem in measuring the true limb length discrepancy. However, in such circumstances the nearest possible value should be worked out in as far identical position as possible.

Mode of Measurement (see relevant chapter)

In poliotics, with the involvement of hip region, it is difficult to do exact true measurement mainly because of ill-developed hemipelvis. Even without any fixed deformity anterior-superior iliac spines are not at the same level, and further, it is not possible to levelise them. However, the measurement can be done in the following manner.

The patient lies comfortably supine, stretching both his lower limbs in as much neutral a position as possible. Identify the fixed deformity on the affected side. Keep the opposite limb in identical position. In bilateral affections keep both lower limbs in as much identical position as possible. Measure the total and segmental distances on one side (which appears to be normal or nearly normal). From the anterior-superior iliac spine of other side (which is lower), draw a horizontal line towards the opposite anterior-superior iliac spine. Draw another horizontal line from other anterior-superior iliac spine up to the midline. The difference between the two lines at the midline will indicate the structural deficiency in developing the anterior-superior iliac spine. This difference is substracted from the measurement done on the side in which the anterior-superior iliac spine is high up. For all practical purposes, the remaining length will indicate the total length of that limb.

Circumferential Measurement

A paralysed limb is invariably wasted. Hence, circumferential measurement is mostly for compilation of records.

Linear Measurement

This measurement has its main importance for lower limb. However, measurement should be done as described in concerned chapters.

MOVEMENTS (see the relevant joint chapter)

Since in a limb, several joints may be affected due to paralysis of the controlling muscles, the movements at each individual joint must be charted separately.

Flail joints are hypermobile and mostly subluxated. Paralytic dislocation usually occurs in hip and shoulder.

Muscle Assessment Chart

While assessing muscle power, a rough estimation of the group action should be done (e.g. the dorsiflexion and palmar flexion at the wrist, the flexion and extension at the elbow, and so on). Thence individual muscles should be tested and its power charted in proper proforma (page 235 to 239). For testing the power of individual muscle, one should proceed as follows:

Ask the patient to perform the normal actions which can be done by that functioning muscle

Table 11.2: Depending upon the given criteria, contractures can be graded as mild, moderate or severe

	Mild	*Moderate*	*Severe*
Skin	Normal	Callosity on convex surface starts appearing	Callosities almost always present
Pain on stretching	None or very mild	Pain on stretching beyond 25%	Pain almost from the beginning of stretching
Stretchability	Full or almost full	25-50%	0-25%
Effect of stretching on vascularity	No blanching on full stretching	Blanching beyond 50% stretching	Blanching in range of 0-25% stretching
Effect on the underlying joint	No effect	It starts subluxating after stretching beyond 50%	Underlying joint mostly remains subluxated and/or presents tendency of subluxation on attempts of stretching

against standard resistance and gravity. If this is not possible, then he should be asked to complete the functional action of that muscle against only gravity, which if not possible should be done with gravity eliminated. In all these procedures, note the extent of action (movement) achieved. If initiation of movement is not possible, look at and feel the contracting muscle as it attempts to perform its function. After testing as above power should accordingly be graded from 5-1. If even flickering of the muscle is not appreciated then it is graded as '0'. Power between grades 5-4, 4-3, 3-2 can be subgrouped as indicated in the chapter on 'Introduction'.

Grading of Muscle Power

(As in the chapter on Introduction).

Assessment of Contractures (Table 11.2)

This examination is essential to:

1. Reveal the degree of contractures.
2. Assess whether the contracture is stretchable or not.
3. Know the effect of the contractures on the underlying joint.
4. Know the effect of the contracture on the vascularity of distal joints.

Special Test for Particular Joint (see the relevant joint chapter).

ASSESSMENT OF EARLY POLIO CASES

Any paralysed patient, but especially the polio cases, must be assessed thoroughly to form a base line. Of course, this will be a specialised job for the physiotherapist, but as a clinician, one should have an overall picture of the regions affected, along with the extent and complications of the affection. Problems in assessment arise in very young children, i.e. below the age of 2 years. In such cases, proceed as follows:

Ask the attendant of the child to hold the baby's upper chest from the sides and keep the child away from him so that the limbs hang in the air. Observe from the front and do mild continuous pinching over the lower quadrants of the abdomen and observe the movements at each joint and the working of the muscle groups/important individual muscles. If only one limb is affected it provides a good comparison. However, even if both limbs are affected the overall functions of the limbs, movement at the joints, group actions of the muscles and individual action of important muscles can be assessed while the child screams. Weakness of the abdominal muscle becomes apparent by ballooning of a sector of the abdominal wall when the child cries.

Now the child is held from the front and observed from the back. Give a mild continuous pinch on both sides of the lower back and assess as above. Besides the movements and power in the lower limbs, the power of the spinal muscles can be assessed while the child is wriggling the back.

For the upper limbs—the child is held at the lower chest from the sides, while the upper limbs are hanging by the side of the chest. Pinch at the upper medial aspect of the arm and observe, as for the lower limbs.

In extensive and very early affections the child should not be examined as above, rather, observe the movements while the patient is lying comfortably on the bed. Muscle tenderness should be elicited gently in the suspected areas. If power is markedly weak (grade 2 or less) assess while the patient is lying in such a way as to eliminate the effect of gravity.

ASSESSMENT OF THE TENSOR FASCIA FEMORIS COMPLEX DEFORMITIES (TFF)

By and large, this is the commonest deformity complex affecting the lower limbs in poliomyelitis and in myopathy. It also starts appearing quite early in neglected convalescent cases (even by 3-4 weeks). If detected early, guarded stretching usually corrects it.

Method of Detecting Early Deformity

Ask the attendant to hold the child at the chest from the sides with the legs hanging in the air. The deformed limb will not hang straight. If the other lower limb is normal even the earliest deformity of the affected side will be obvious. Hold the opposite buttock with one hand and with the other hand hold the suspected limb at the knee level (thumb over the knee, index and middle fingers above the popliteal fossa, and ring and little fingers below the popliteal fossa). While the knee is kept in maximum extension, the lower limb is moved medially and backwards. Resistance will be felt. Simultaneously, palpate along the iliotibial band for any tightness (compare with other side). In advanced cases, a subluxating tendency of the head of the femur can be felt during manoeuvre.

Second method—The child is laid on the bed on his side with the side to be tested kept up. The trunk is held straight with one hand fixing the buttock. With the other hand holding the knee as above, the lower limb is taken medially and backwards. Observations are made as above by comparing with the opposite side.

To confirm that abduction contracture is only due to iliotibial tightness, the following observation is useful when the patient lies supine with extended hip and knee, the abduction contracture is present, but it disappears with flexion of hip and knee. Iliotibial band contracture can be assessed quantitatively by the following test.

The patient lies prone. The examiner, standing on the opposite side of the limb to be tested, holds with one hand the affected limb just above the ankle with the knee in 90° flexion, hip in maximum abduction and the limb in neutral rotation, while his other hand presses over the buttock to keep pelvis fixed on the table. The limb is then gradually adducted till the firm resistance is encountered. The angle sustained between the vertical axis of the body and the limb is the angle of abduction.

Testing for Tightness of Tendo-Achilles

Individually, this is the commonest deformity of the lower limb, especially in polio-paralysis. Even in flail ankle and foot (with 0 to 2 powers of the tendo-Achilles) tightness due to gravity occurs.

Method of Testing

The child is held and the knee fixed as in testing for TFF deformity. Hold the foot in the other hand in neutral position (midpatella, mid ankle and second web in one line) and try to dorsiflex it at the ankle. In case of tightness, resistance will be felt. In further advanced cases, rocking of the foot at the ankle to one side can be felt while performing the above manoeuvre. Once rocking is felt, the foot should not be subjected to forceful stretching lest the developing talus will be compressed and damaged.

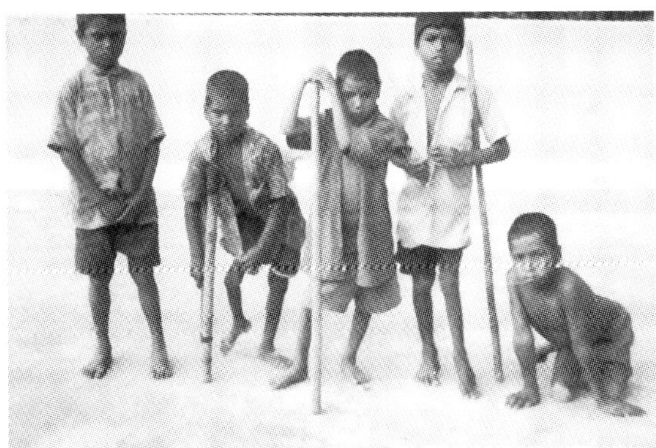

Fig. 11.10: A group of polio-paralysis patients waiting for operating management

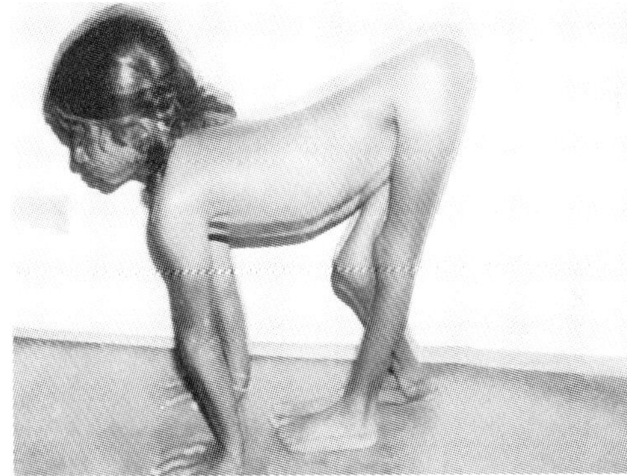

Fig. 11.11: Due to polio-paralysis with gross weakness in hip, pelvic girdle and lumbar regions, the child is walking like quadruped

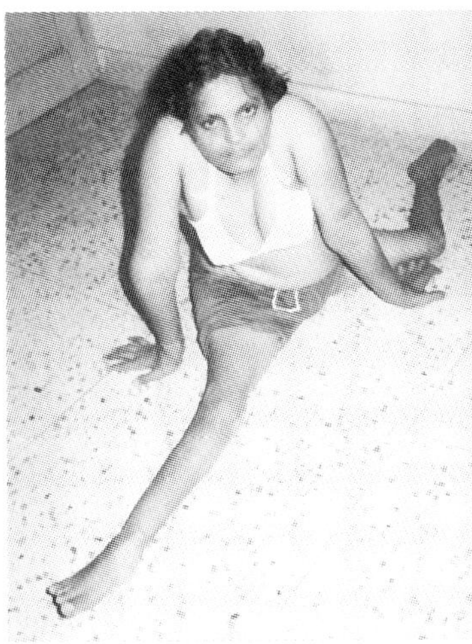

Fig. 11.12: Due to polio-paralysis with gross weakness in both lower limbs and lumbar region, the girl is managing to sit and also to glide on wider base and supporting herself on her both upper limbs (note the hypertrophy of upper limb muscles)

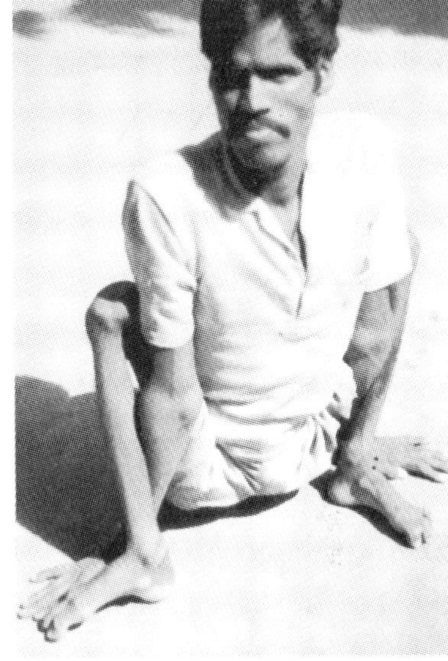

Fig. 11.13: Neglected flail lower limbs with various contractures. The man is walking on his hands

In neglected cases of mild tendo-Achilles tightness the child is brought with the following complaints—inability to squat, pain in the calf, pain in the heel, thinning of the calf and small size of the foot. Observe the patient while walking—he will walk with a tendency of high stepping and later on with an equinus tendency of the foot. On asking him to walk on his heels, he will not be able to do so on the affected side. On asking him to squat, he will do so by keeping his affected foot in front and away from the other foot. If he is then asked to bring the affected foot to the level of the normal foot, he will either lose his balance and tend to fall backwards and therefore support himself with his hand kept on the ground behind his body, or he will balance himself by raising the heel, thereby transferring the weight onto just the forefoot.

The calf is comparatively thin and firm, the heel is small and comparatively clean looking than the other as it does not touch the ground.

Severe cases of tightness of tendo-Achilles result in equinus deformity of the foot.

Assessment of Instability

The main problem in a paralytic patient is instability at different joints, which should be assessed individually. The sum total of instabilities at different joints of a limb may result in the grotesque unstable disabilities for that patient. Hence, the degree of instability of that limb in carrying out the different grades of function should be assessed.

Grades of function are basically:

- —ADL (Activity of daily living)—Mainly consist of eating, attending the natural calls and bare minimum dressing.
- —Critical functions: At every joint, certain range of movements are critically needed for basic functions, e.g. at wrist 0° to 20° dorsiflexion to hold and grasp; at right elbow 30° to 100° of movement for eating; at left elbow 20° to 40° of movement for cleaning the private parts; at the knee 0° to 30° of movement for walking, etc.
- —Job oriented function.
- —Full function.

Neurological Examination

(As in chapter on the Spine)

Investigation

The principal investigation in a paralysed patient is to keep a proper photographic record and prepare a detailed neuromuscular-sensory charting, which not only helps in diagnosis but also forms a base line for comparison in future.

Radiology

This is the other important investigation. In case of lower limb, radiograph should be done of both sides in as much symmetrical a position as possible.

For practical assessment of any trunk deformity, radiograph should be taken in standing weight bearing position—specially to assess paralytic scoliosis and pelvic obliquity. For the hips, weight bearing position is much useful, to know its exact position under the stress of body weight and the ground reaction against it.

For the knees, lateral view is more useful, in which flexion deformity and any subluxation of upper tibia will be clear.

For the ankle and foot, it is also beneficial to expose the film while weight bearing, keeping the ankle-foot relation at right angles (or as much as possible towards right angle). Both feet should be simultaneously exposed in superoinferior projection. In lateral view, lower half of the leg, ankle and the foot should be exposed in the same film for charting the different angles and measurements.

To assess exact lower limb discrepancy, radiologically both the lower limbs should be exposed together in standing position right from hips to ankles, if possible, in one film or in two films, after keeping a common metallic marker to be included in both films.

Serum enzyme: Serum creatine phosphokinase estimation in early myopathy is more specific and is 200 to 300 times the normal value.

Blood and urine chemistry: In muscular dystrophy, serum creatinine and urinary creatinine estimation is an important aid to the diagnosis, which is increased.

Key Diagnostic Points of Certain Paralytic Diseases

1. *Poliomyelitis (Figs 11.10 to 11.18)*

- —History of fever, gastrointestinal upset or respiratory tract infection.
- —Onset—acute and mostly in early childhood.
- —Lower motor neuron type of asymmetrical paralysis.
- —Non-progressive muscle weakness.
- —Practically no sensory loss.

2. *Cerebral Palsy*

- —Delayed disappearance of congenital reflexes (few may even persist much longer).
- —Usually spastic bilateral and almost symmetrical deformities, affecting all four or any three or any two or even one limb.
- —Upper motor neuron type of paralysis.

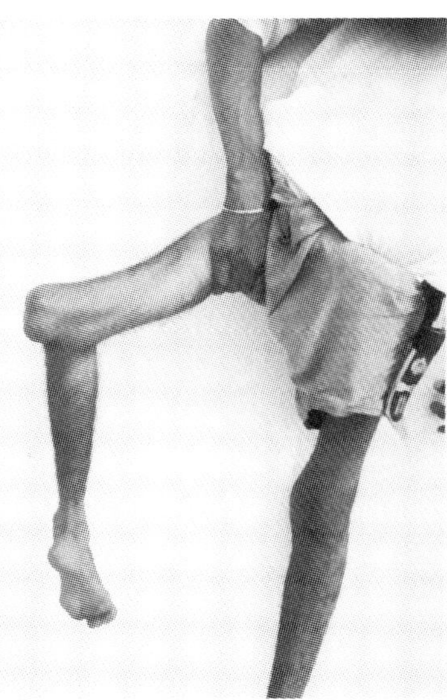

Fig. 11.14: Flail right lower limb (due to polio-paralysis) with bizarre deformities. He is managing to walk with one crutch and supporting his flail lower limb with other hand

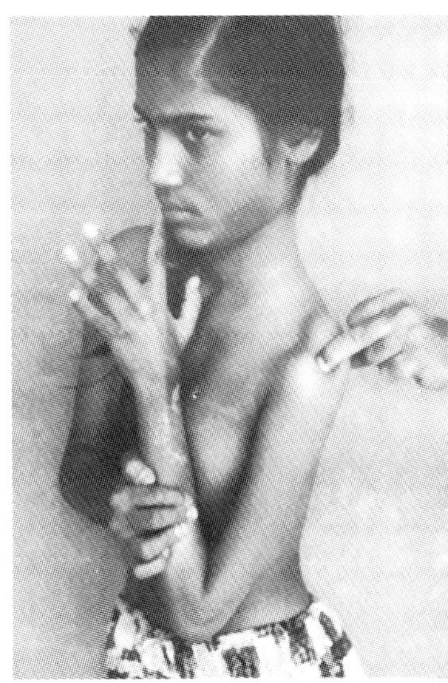

Fig. 11.15: Polio-paralysis of left upper limb.Note the wasting of paralysed deltoid and the humeral head can be subluxed out with a finger pressure

Left wrist has been arthrosed for the gross weakness, after which the latent functions of the fingers and thumb have markedly improved

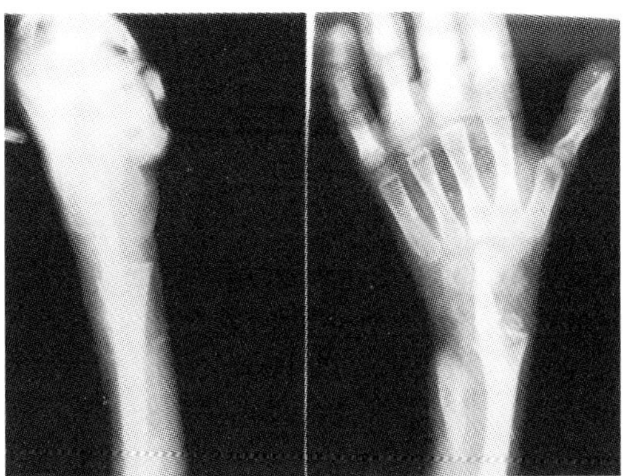

Fig. 11.16: X-ray showing arthrodesed wrist using ipsilateral ulnar graft

— Varying mental retardation (about 25% of cases).
— May be associated microcephaly, squint and dribbling of saliva.

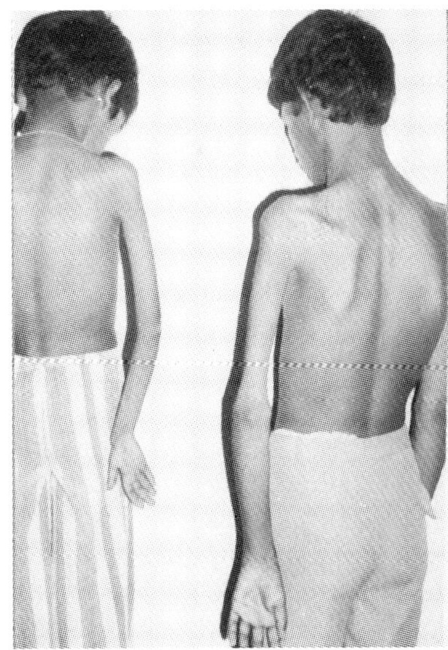

Fig. 11.17: In polio-paralysis of upper limb the shoulder is the commonest site of paralysis

3. Myopathy (Figs 11.19 to 11.21)
— May be familial history of disease.
— Manifestation usually after 5 years of age.
— Lower motor neuron type of mostly bilateral symmetrical lesion (in fascioscapular-humeral or Landouzy-Dejerine myopathy only one side is affected).

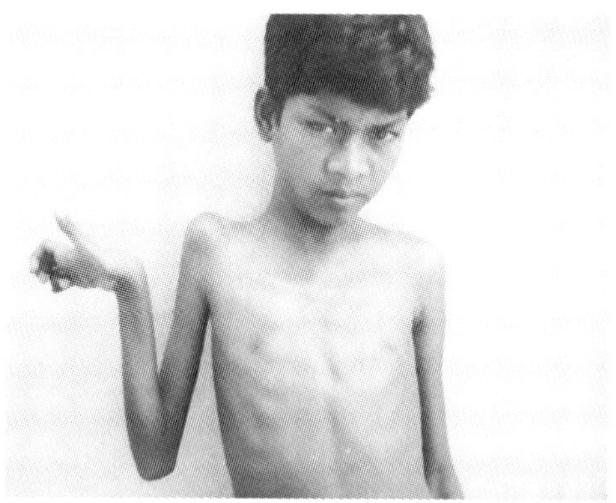

Fig. 11.18: In polio-paralysis affecting the upper limb, the common combination of affected regions (with magnitude of affection in that order) is the shoulder, wrist, hand, elbow

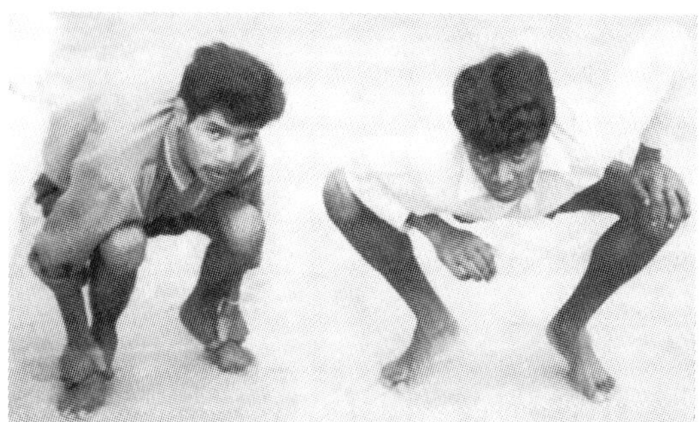

Fig. 11.20: The boys are climbing up on their own knees to get up from the sitting posture (G sign)

—No sensory loss.
—Pseudohypertrophy of muscle may be present.
—Increased blood creatinine and urine creatinine levels. Decreased creatinine level in urine is characteristic of the disease.
—Much increase of serum creatinine phosphokinase is diagnostic of myopathy.
—Tongue sign—In advanced cases, the child keeps the tongue semiprotruded, with mouth partially opened.

4. *Motor Neuron Disease*
—Usually young adults presenting with gradual weakness, atrophy and fibrillation in the shoulder girdle muscles.
—May be lower motor neuron type of lesion in the upper limbs and associated upper motor neuron type of lesion in lower limbs.
—No sensory loss.

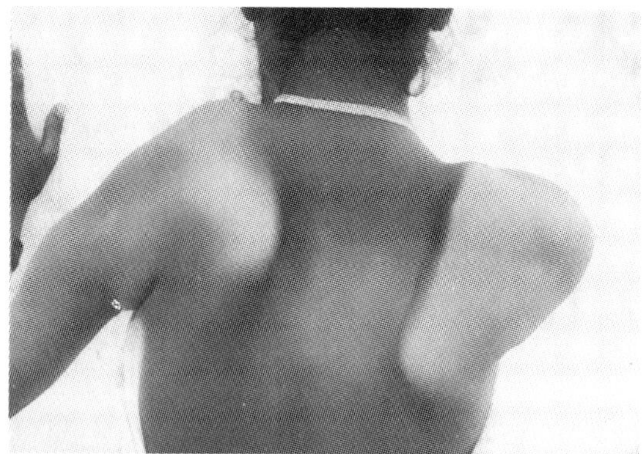

Fig. 11.19: Gross wasting of scapulae muscles in myopathy

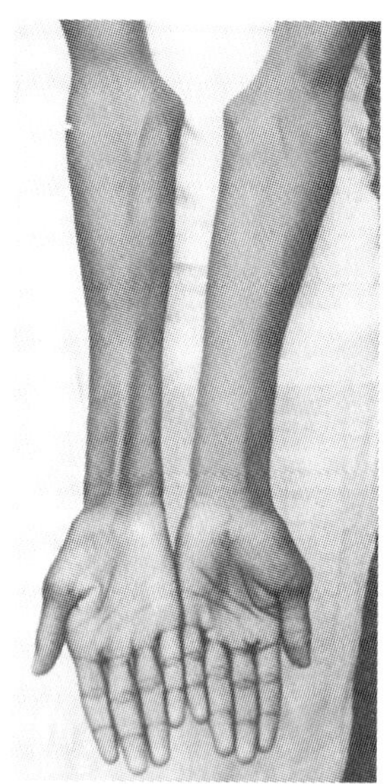

Fig. 11.21: Myopathy: note the wasting of muscles in both distal forearm and hands (right more than the left)

5. *Polyneuritis*
—Usually adult female complaining of sensory disturbances which may be bilateral or unilateral.
—Lower motor neuron type of lesion.
—Variable muscular weakness and sensory disturbances affecting more than one site.

RECORD OF MUSCLE POWER

Po/Sp—(I/D)/PN—(I/D)/My/MND/Others. . . . . No

Group 0,1,2,3,4

Prophylactic Vaccines- Po/Wh. cgh/Dep/Tet/Meas/any other

Name of Patient________________ Age________ Sex________ Ward________ Hospital No.
Complete Address ________________ Tel: ________ Fax: ________

LEFT							RIGHT			
					Therapist's signature					
					Dates					
					HEAD, NECK and TRUNK					
					Facial muscles	Cr. VII				
				Flex.	Sternocleidomastoid	Cr. IX				
				Ext.	Neck extensors	C1-T1				
				Flex.	Rectus abdominis	T7-L1				
				Ext.	Dorsal spinal muscles	Segmental supply, Post div. of spinal nerves				
					Lumbar spinal muscles					
				Rot	To the right					
					To the left ≠					
				El. Pel.	Quad lumb	T12,L1,2,3				
					Scoliosis					
					Lordosis					
					General posture					
					Spine flat or flexed					
					LOWER LIMBS					
					HIP					
					Iliopsoas	L1,2,3,4				
				Flex.	Sartorius	L2-4				
					Rectus femoris	L2,3,4				
				Ext.	Gluteus maximus	L5, S1,2				
				Abd.	Gluteus medius minimus	L4,5 S1				
					Tensors, fascia lata L4,5 S1					
				Add	Adductor longus, brevis, magnus	L2,3,4				

Po = Poliomyelitis
Sp = Spinal Injury
Dep = Diptheria
I = Injury
D = Diseases
Tet = Tetanus
PN = Peripheral Nerve
My = Myopathy
Meas = Measles
ND = Motor Neuron Disease
Wh Cgh = Whooping Cough

Contd.

LEFT							RIGHT			
				Rot	Ext rotators	L2-5, S1,2				
					Int rotators	L4,5, S1,2				
					KNEE					
				Flex	In-hamstring	L4,5, S1,2				
					Out-hamstring	L5, S1,2,3				
					Gracilis	L2-4				
				Ext	Quadriceps	L2,3,4				
					ANKLE					
				Plant Flex	Gastroc and Soleus	S1,2				
					Soleus	L5, S1,2				
				Dorsi Flex	Tibialis anterior	L4,5 S1				
					Peroneus tertius	L4,5 S1				
				Inversion in dorsiflexion	Tibialis anterior	L4,5, S1				
				Inversion in plantar flexion	Tibialis posterior	L4,5 S1,2				
				Everters	Peroneals— longus, brevis, and tertius	L4,5, S1 L5, S1				
				Eversion in dorsiflexion	Poroneus tertius	L4,5 S1				
				Eversion in plantar flexion	Peroneus longus Peroneus brevis	L4,5, S1 L5,S1,S2				
					TOES					
				Flex	Lumbricals	L4,5, S1				
					Fl dig Longus	S2 S3				
					Fl dig brevis	S2 S3				
				Ext	Ext. digit longus	L5 S1				
					Ext. digit brevis					
					HALLUX					
				Flex	Fl hall brevis	S2 S3				
					Fl hall longus	S2 S3				
				Ext.	Ext hall longus	L5 S1				
					Ext hall brevis (a part of Ext digit brevis)					

Contd.

LEFT							RIGHT			
					MEASUREMENTS IN LOWER LIMBS					
					Ant Sup iliac spine to med malleolus					
					Ant Sup iliac spine to knee jt line					
					Knee jt line to Med malleolus					
					Apparent shortening/lengthening					
					Mid thigh circumference					
					Mid calf circumference					
					UPPER LIMB					
					SCAPULA					
				Abd	Serrat, anterior	C5-7				
				Elev	Upper trapezius	C2-4				
				Add	Mid trapezius	C2-4				
					Rhomboids	C4-5				
				Depr	Lower trapezius	C2-4				
					SHOULDER					
				Flex	Coracobrachialis & ant deltoid	C5-6				
				Ext	Latissimus dorsi	C6-8				
					Teres major and post deltoid	C5-7				
				Abd	Deltoid and Supraspinatus	C4-6				
				H ABD	Post deltoid	C5-6				
				H ADD	Pect major	C5-8, T1				
				Rot	Ext rotator					
					Int rotator					
					ELBOW					
				Flex	Biceps brachii	C5,6				
					Brachioradialis	C5,6				
				Ext	Triceps	C6-8				
					FOREARM					
				Sup	Biceps	C5,6				
					Supinator	C6				
				Pron	Pronators	C6				
					WRIST					
				Flex	Fl carp rad	C8				
					Fl carp uln	C8				
				Ext	Ext carp rad	C6,7				
					Ext carp uln	C7				
					FINGERS					
					Lumbricals	C7,8 T1				
				Flex	Fle dig subl	C7,8 T1				
					Fle dig prof	C8, T1				

Contd.

LEFT							RIGHT			
				Ext	Finger Exten	C7				
				Abd	Dorsal Int & Abd digiti minimi	C8, T1				
				Add	Palm Inteross	C8				
					THUMB					
				Flex	Fl pol brev	C6-8				
					Fl pol long	C8, T1				
				Ext	Ext pol brev	C7				
					Ext pol long	C7				
				Abd	Abductor Poll	C7				
				Add	Adductor Poll	C6,7				
				Oppos	Thumb & tip of lit fing	C6-8, T1				
					RESPIRATION					
					Intercostals					
					Diaphragm	C4,5,6				

Remarks: Including gait and deformities.

ADDITIONAL DATA: Eyes__________Hearing__________Face__________Tongue__________Speech
__________Mastication__________Swallowing__________Diaphragm__________Intercostals__________

WALKING STATUS:

Cannot stand	Date__________	Walks in parallel bar	Date__________
Stands with support	Date__________	Walks with invalid walker	Date__________
Stands without support	Date__________	Walks with crutches	Date__________
Cannot walk	Date__________	Walks with canes	Date__________
Walks with braces	Date__________	Walks unaided	Date__________
Walks with corset	Date__________	Climbs stairs with support	Date__________
		Climbs stairs without support	Date__________

Contractures and Deformities Upper limb: Rt__________ Lt__________
Lower limb Rt__________ Lt__________

Scoliosis and trunk deformities:

Key to grouping of the extent of paresis/paralysis

Group 0 Cases which have a general residual weakness with functional value just below normal.

Groud 1 Cases with involvements of face or neck or trunk or one limb only.

Group 2 Cases where two limbs are affected either wholly or partially. The paralysed limbs may be both upper limbs or both lower limbs or one upper limb and one lower limb or one limb and the trunk.

Group 3 Cases where three limbs are affected either wholly or partially or it may be two limbs with trunk or neck or face and so on.

Group 4 Cases where all four limbs are affected wholly or partially, or it may be three limbs with trunk or face or neck and so on.

Scaling of Muscle Power
0. No contraction 1. Flicker 2. Joint motion with gravity eliminated
3. Joint movement—antigravity 4. Joint movement—antigravity with resistance
5. Normal.

Any *sensory disturbance* should be depicted in diagrammatic dermatomal distribution.

CEREBRAL PALSY—CASE RECORD

Patient's name. . . . . Hosp No. . . . . CP No. . . . . Age. . . . . . . Sex. . . . . . .

Complete address. . . . . Telephone No. . . . .

Prophylactic vaccinations with dates . . . .

Whooping cough and Diphtheria. . . . . .Tetanus toxoid. . . . .

Any other sera or protective vaccines . . . .

Complaint . . . .

History
1. Mother's health during pregnancy
2. Length of pregnancy
3. Special features of labour and presentation
4. Delivery at hospital or home. Mode of delivery
5. Age and any blood relation in between the parents at time of birth of child: Father Mother
6. Condition of baby at birth:
   a. Cried b. Blue baby
   c. Suck when weak/strong
   d. Temperature e. Jaundice
   f. Transfusion given or not
   g. Twitchings
   h. Convulsions
   i. Rh Factor.-Mother Father Child
   j. WR, Kahn or allied tests
   h. Weight at birth

7. *MILESTONES*

i. *Gross:*	Normal within	Delayed		Normal within	Delayed
Neck holding	4 months		Crawling	7–° months	
Rolling over	6 months		Standing	15 months	
Sitting	7 months		Walking	18 months	

ii. *Details*

MENTAL	Age	*MOTOR*	Age
Smiles		Turns on sides.	
Recognise familiar faces.		Raises head prone.	
Grasp.		Raises head supine.	
Waves bye bye		Rolls over.	
Throws		Crawls	
Monosyllables.		Sits up	
Speaks in sentences.		Stands up	
Articulation.		Walks without support.	
Drools.		Teething.	
Control over bladder and bowel		When achieved.	
Handedness (right/left)			
Hearing.		Vision.	
Behaviour.		IQ	

8. PRIMITIVE REFLEXES (as on next pages 241 and 242)
9. *Habits:*
   a. Sleep
   b. Appetite: Good — fair — Poor
   c. Feeding habits: Breast fed — Weaned when / Weaned how / any difficulty
   d. Diet: Liquid — Solids — Chewing
      Swallowing
   e. Eating: With hand — Spoon
   f. Dressing
10. PREVIOUS ILLNESS
11. PREVIOUS TREATMENT
12. Schooling: Ordinary School — Special School — Home Education
13. Family history of Congenital deformities. . . . .
    a. Abortions
    b. Still birth
    c. Premature birth
    d. Brothers and sisters with ages
    e. Casualties among children and cause of death
    f. Epilepsy in family
    g. MD in family
    h. CP in family
14. When and how did the parents become aware of the child's condition
15. Clinical Examination:
    a. General examination
    b. Type of CP
    c. Motor system
    d. Degree of muscle tone
    e. Voluntary control
    f. Involuntary movements
    g. Abnormal reflex postures
    h. Contractures
    i. Deformities
    j. Coordination
    k. Gait
    l. Sensations

16. Urine test for phenyl pyruvic acid

17. *Management plan:*

Therapy	Physical
	Occupational
	Speech
	Vocational
Drugs	Any other
Aids/orthosis	
Surgery	
Follow ups	

PRIMITIVE REFLEXES

Reflex	*Present*	*Absent*	*Age*				
	months	*months*	*Date*				*Comments*
Spinal level:							
(Apedal stage)							
(Primitive reflexes)							
1. Flexor withdrawal	Upto 2	After 2					
2. Extensor thrust	Upto 2	After 2					
3. Crossed extension	Upto 2	After 2					
Brainstem Level (Apedal stage)							
(Primitive reflexes)							
1. ATNR	Upto 4-6	After 4-6					
2. STNR	Upto 4-6	After 4-6					
3. Tonic Labrynthine	Upto 4	After 4					
4. Associated reaction	Absent	Absent					
5. Positive supporting reaction	Upto 4	After 4					
6. Negative supporting reaction	Upto 4	After 4					
Midbrain Level							
(Quadripedal stage)							
(Rightning reaction)							
1. Neck rightning	Upto 6	After 6					
2. Body rightning	6 on wards	From 6					
3. Labyrinthine on head prone	1-2 onwards	From 0-1-2					
4. Labyrinthine on head supine	6 onwards	From 0-6					
5. Labyrinthine on head lateral	6-8 onwards	From 0-8					
6. Optical rightning	1-2 onwards	From 0-1-2					
Automatic reaction:							
1. Moro	Upto 4-6	After 4-6					
2. Landau	From 6-30	After 0-6-30					
3. Protective extensor thrust	6 onwards	From 0-6					
Cortical level							
Equilibrium reaction							
(Bipedal stage)							
1. Supine	6 onwards	From 0-6					
2. Prone	6 onwards	From 0-6					
3. All fours	8 onwards	From 0-8					

Contd.

Reflex	*Present*	*Absent*	*Age*				
	months	*months*	*Date*				*Comments*
4. Sitting	10-12 onwards	From 0-10-12					
5. Kneeling-standing	15 onwards	From 0-15					
6. Hopping	15-18 onwards	From 0-18					
7. Sea saw	15-18 onwards	From 0-18					
8. Squatting	15-18 onwards	From 0-18					
9. Walking	18 onwards	From 0-18					

REFERENCE

1. Gautam VK, Anand S: A new test for estimating iliotibial band contracture. *J Bone Joint Surg* (B) **80-B**: 474-75, 1998.

12 Hip

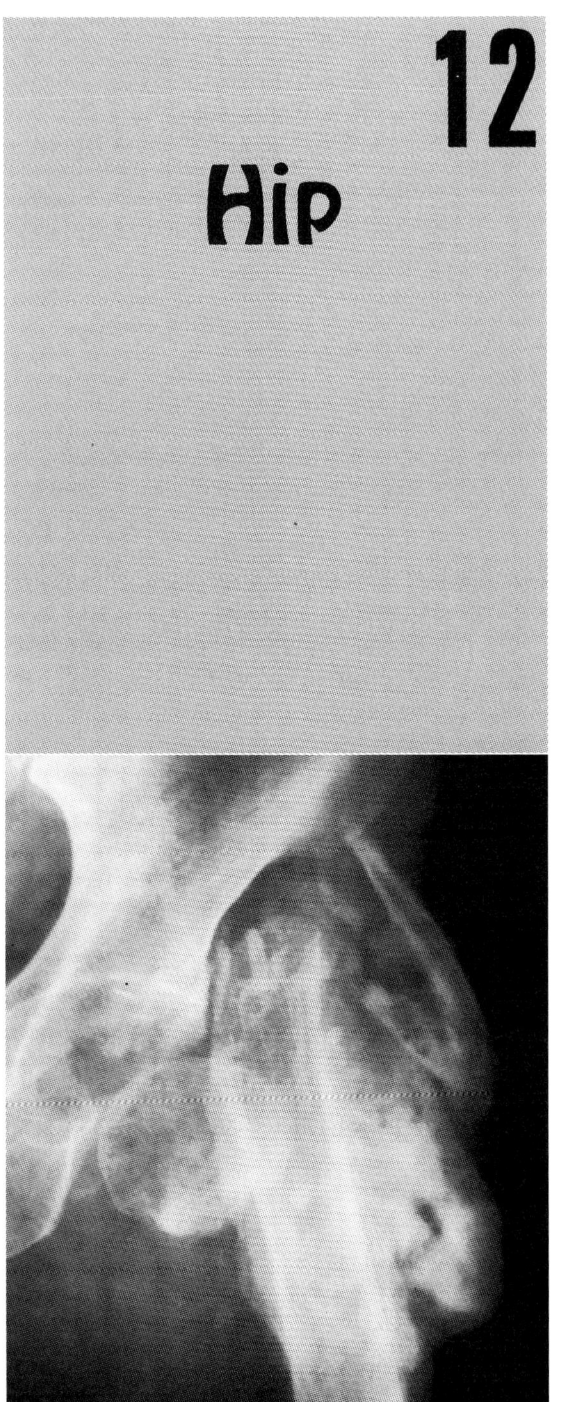

INTRODUCTION

In bipeds, the hips have the great responsibility of transmitting the ground reaction against the body weight while at the same time preserving mobility. To mechanically accommodate this postural change, the head and neck of femur undergo angulation and rotation at the base. Any affection of the hip is of much concern to the patient since it affects locomotion from the very beginning. The patient mostly tries to accommodate the disabilities following such pathology, as far as practicable, by various compensatory mechanisms.

ANATOMICAL CONSIDERATIONS

1. Compensations for deficits at the hip are usually made by various tiltings at the (i) pelvis, (ii) lower spine, (iii) ankle and foot, and (iv) knee.
2. Early pathology at the hip may manifest as pain on the anteromedial aspect of the knee (being referred along the anterior division of the obturator nerve). Hence, it is imperative to examine the hip fully for any unexplained pain in the knee.
3. Development of neck-shaft angle (upward inclination: 120°-130°) and anteversion of the neck (forward inclination of the neck relative to the shaft 15°-20°), gained in morphological evolution, has to pay its price by making the neck very much susceptible to rotational shearing stress.
4. The arterial supply (retinacular, metaphyseal and that through ligamentum teres) of the head and neck of the femur is such as to make it very vulnerable in intracapsular injuries of the hip.
5. Calcar femorale (an oblique longitudinal condensation of the compact trabeculae on inferomedial aspect of the neck, trochanteric region and upper shaft) provides an internal support for the mechanically disadvantageously placed head and neck of the femur. It also determines to a great extent the displacement of subcapital and trochanteric fractures.

6. Capsular reflections of the hip encases the whole of the neck anteriorly. Posteriorly it is deficient by about 1.5 cm from intertrochanteric crest, thereby encasing most part of the upper metaphyseal end of the femur. Hence, infective pathology (e.g. pyogenic infections) are very much likely to affect the hip joint quite early.

   The capsule is reinforced by the ligaments almost all around, strongest of which is anteriorly placed as the ileo-femoral ligament ('Y' ligament of Biglow).
7. The hip is a ball and socket joint. Since the femoral head has to transmit the ground reactions against the body weight, it becomes vulnerable to dislocation. However, the watershed created by the reinforced margins of deep acetabulum (except for the posteroinferior region) mostly prevents this.
8. Fortunately, the hip is surrounded by thick layers of stout muscles, which can take the greater load of hip functions even when there is deficit in the intracapsular bony lever.
9. The hip is commonly vulnerable for the congenital deformities—i.e. dysplasia/ subluxation/dislocations; infective pathology—pyogenic/tuberculosis; fractures—fracture neck of femur (intracapsular)/ trochanteric fracture (extracapsular); dislocations and degenerative arthrosis, besides a host of other pathologies. Hence, at almost all ages, detailed assessment of the hip is essential.

   In hip involvement, the first movement to be lost is extension, the hip gradually assuming a varying flexion attitude with progress of the underlying pathology. With erosion of the articular cartilage, rotational movements, besides extension, are lost early.
10. The hip joint space becomes most accommodative in the posture of flexion, abduction and external rotation. Hence, this is the most common postural attitude in case of pathologies where there is a collection in the joint.
11. The protective natural splint for the painful conditions of hip is by spasm of the powerful flexors (ilio-psoas) and adductors. Therefore, in any erosive pathology, these deformities are commonly seen. However, the effect of prolonged decubitus in a particular posture and compensatory mechanisms by the patient, do affect the ultimate posture of the limb.

Certain Important Anatomical Landmarks

i. *Pubic tubercle*: In adults pubic tubercles are about 2.5 cm on either side of pubic symphysis. A line joining them and prolonged on either side crosses the normal femoral head in the normal pelvis.

ii. Anterior landmark of femoral head is about 1 cm below and out to the mid inguinal point.

iii. From a central point at the base of the greater trochanter, a line drawn to the ipsilateral mid inguinal point (or to opposite anterior superior iliac spine) represents the femoral neck.

iv. A line joining the posterior superior iliac spines in normal pelvis crosses at the second sacral segment (where spinal dura ends) and if prolonged on either side, this line transects the sacro-iliac joint almost in the middle.

v. A line joining the most prominent point of ischial tuberosities lies almost at the level of the base of greater trochanter.

METHODOLOGY

History taking: Besides as given in the Chapter on 'Introduction', certain leading questions are essential to elicit certain points, specially in early pathology and that too in children. The main complaints in a hip disease are pain, limp (may be after some activity), stiffness, deformities, limb length disparity, swelling and paralytic disabilities.

Most of the pathologies affecting the hip (traumatic or non-traumatic) can be roughly guessed by seeing the attitude of the patient and taking his age into consideration.

Common Pathologies (according to different age groups)

A. *Traumatic*

- Up to 5 years of age, fracture or dislocation involving the hip joint is very rare
- In 5 to 20 years of age—fracture neck of femur (intracapsular) is seen
- In sportsmen, there is a possibility of avulsion of the lesser/greater trochanter
- In young adults, the injuries around hip are dislocations; fracture of neck of femur (intracapsular); fracture pelvis; fracture of trochanteric region (extracapsular)
- In the middle age the usual incidence is of fracture of neck of femur (intracapsular), fracture of trochanteric region (extracapsular), dislocation, fracture pelvis
- In the elderly fracture of trochanteric region (extracapsular), fracture of neck of femur (intracapsular), pathological fractures and fracture pelvis commonly occur.

B. *Non-traumatic*

- 0-5 years of age—congenital hip dysplasias/ dislocations; Tom Smith arthritis (transient synovitis), pyogenic infections, tuberculous infection
- 5-10 years—Perthes' disease, tuberculous infection, pyogenic infection
- 10-15 years—Adolescent coxa vara, Perthes' disease, tuberculous infection, pyogenic infection and bone cysts
- 15-35 years—Ankylosing spondylitis, rheumatoid arthritis, tuberculous infection, idiopathic osteonecrosis, secondary osteoarthrosis and bone cysts
- Elderly—Degenerative osteoarthrosis (primary or secondary), secondaries, tuberculous infection.

In case of trauma, hip is usually involved in indirect violence (e.g. slip in the bath room, missing of step, etc.), which mostly results in the unsolved problems of fracture of the neck of femur. The immediate status of the patient, especially as regards standing, weight bearing and using the affected limb in locomotion, should be enquired into.

General and Systemic Examination

It is done as usual, with a special emphasis on the type of gait (refer to the Chapter on 'Spine' pages 177 and 180), if the patient can walk; and mode of weight bearing, if the patient can stand.

An overall assessment of the patient and the hip condition should be noted while the patient is walking, standing and sitting on a stool. Any particular attitude or abnormal finding should be noted, such as scoliosis of the lower back (See Fig. 8.9), elevation of the buttock region and prominence of trochanters. Five fingers quadriceps purchase (See Fig. 11.6A) in polio patient can only be marked while the patient is standing and walking.

Regional Examination

Since various compensatory mechanisms right from the lower lumbar spine to the ankle and foot can occur to accommodate the hip pathology, these regions must be examined in any hip involvement.

Local Examination

Prerequisites of hip examination:

1. Patient should be supine on a flat bed or couch.
2. Both lower limbs, hips and abdomen must be exposed (a narrow strip to be placed over private parts, specially in females). A female attendant must be by the side while examining a female patient.
3. To note the attitude, patient should be asked to lie comfortably in as far neutral a position as possible.

Attitude

Although attitude of the limb varies in various stages of different pathological and traumatic

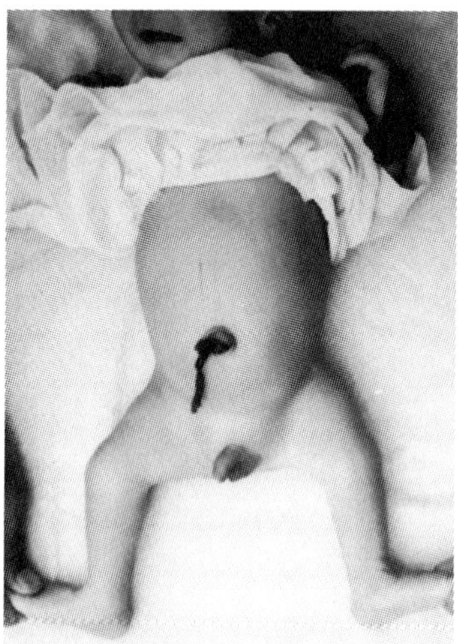

Fig. 12.1A: Photograph of the child. CDH showing widening of perineum, duplication and asymmetry of gluteal fold and shortening

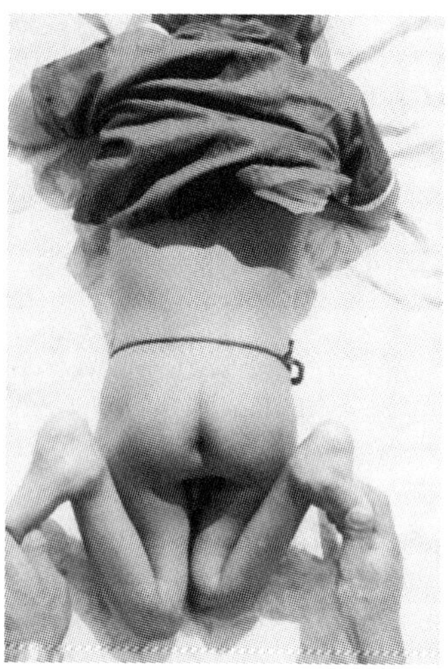

Fig. 12.1B: Marked dissociation in gluteal fold in CDH

conditions, certain attitudes may be considered as typical.

In congenital dislocation of the hip—broadening at trochanteric level, widening of the perineum, asymmetry and/or duplication of gluteal fold (Figs 12.1A and B).

In synovitis of hip joint—mild flexion, abduction and external rotation, with apparent lengthening of the limb.

In true arthritis of hip joint—flexion, adduction and internal rotation with or without true shortening of the limb.

In pure posterior dislocation—flexion, marked adduction and internal rotation with apparent and true shortening.

In anterior dislocation—flexion, abduction, and external rotation, with apparent lengthening of the limb in low type, whereas in the high type there is marked external rotation in full extension and some abduction.

In trochanteric fracture, marked external rotation (outer part of foot mostly touching the bed) of the lower limb, is characteristic. In fracture neck of femur also, there is external rotation but not so marked (due to catch in the capsule); in late cases variable flexion and adduction may be superadded (except where patient has managed to walk).

Inspection (Table 12.1)

It should be done from the front, side and the back (Figs 12.2A to C).

Palpation

As in the Chapter on Introduction, confirm the findings of inspection from different sides. While palpating, mark with a skin pencil the bony points (anterior superior iliac spine, tip of greater trochanter, pubic tubercle, ischial tuberosity) required for assessing measurements and movements. It is more convenient and accurate to localise the sharp bony points by the metal end of the measuring tape.

If the presentations of the hip pathology are vague, *percussion on the heel pad* in the extended position of leg, and over the trochanter usually induces discomfort and/or pain in the groin region if there is any disease or injury in the hip.

Superficial Palpation (Touch)

Touch and assess the temperature, skin surface (smooth/rough), any hyperaesthesia/anaesthesia, venous prominence, sharp bony points.

Table 12.1: Inspection of the hip joint

	Fixed bony points	*Soft tissue region*	*Abnormal findings*
From front (Fig. 12.2A)	Anterior superior iliac spine, pubic symphysis and pubic tubercle	Iliac fossae, inguinal ligament, groin fold, femoral triangle (Scarpa's), front of the thigh	Muscular wasting, any swelling, sinuses, scar marks, ulcers, obvious pulsations, abnormal skin conditions, level of anterior superior iliac spine
From the side (Fig. 12.2B)	Iliac crest and trochanteric region	Gluteal bulge, supratrochanteric depression, infratrochanteric depression, lateral thigh muscle mass	Same as above and level of tip of trochanter in relation to the anterior superior iliac spine
From the back (Fig. 12.2C)	Back of iliac crest, posterior superior iliac spine represented by dimple of Venus, ischial tuberosity region	Gluteal bulges, gluteal folds, back of the thigh	Muscular wasting, any swelling, sinuses, ulcers, obvious pulsations, abnormal skin condition, contracture (Figs 12.3A to C)

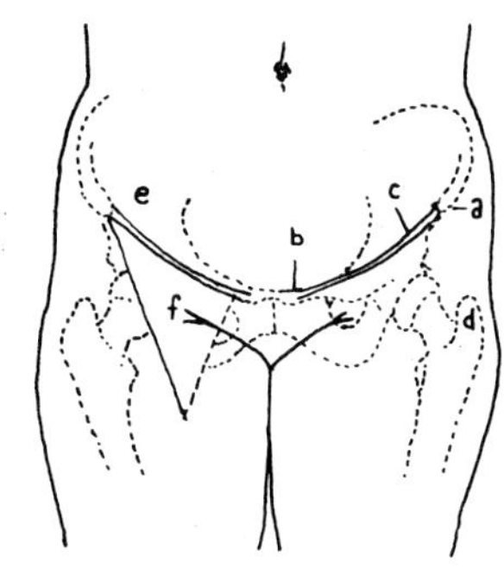

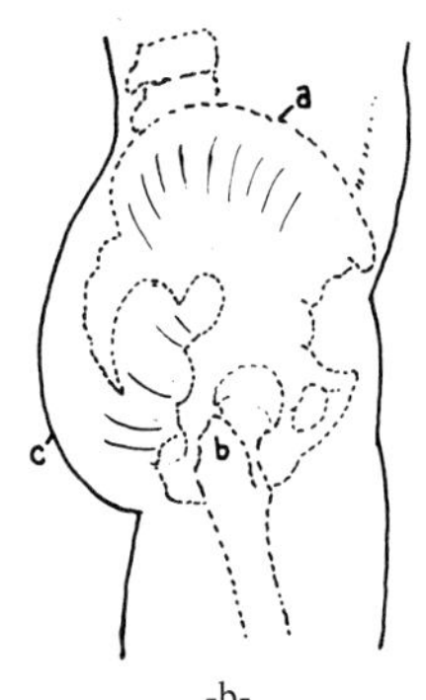

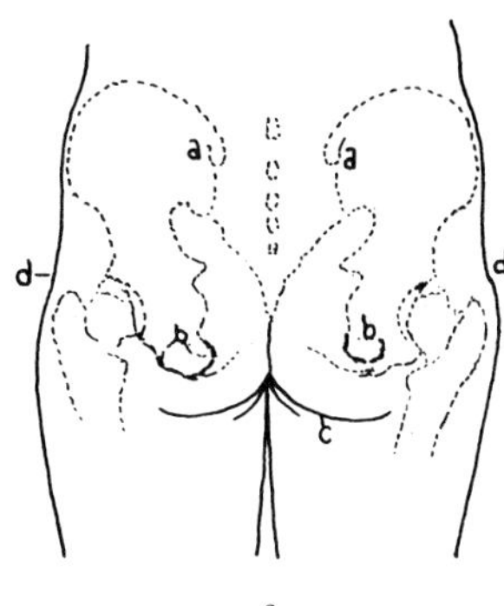

Figs 12.2A to C: (A) Inspection from front. Note the following: a = anterior superior iliac spine; b = pubic tubercle; c = inguinal ligament; d = greater trochanter; e = iliac fossae; f = Scarpa's triangle, (B and C) Inspection from sides and back. Note the following: a = posterior superior iliac spine; b = ischial tuberosity; c = gluteal fold; d = supratrochanteric depression

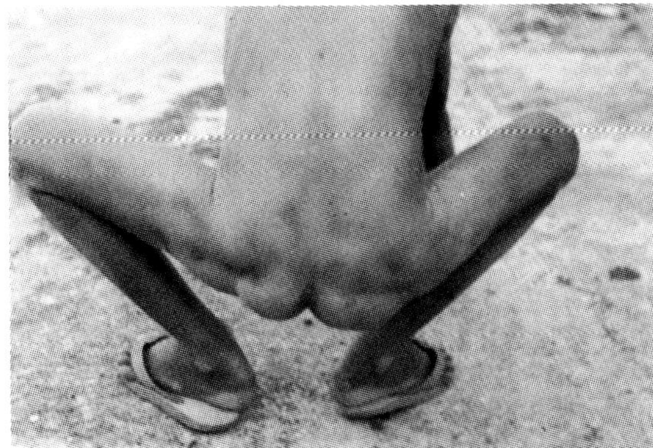

Fig. 12.3A: Photograph showing puckering in the buttock and thigh due to fibrosis along the line of gluteus maximus, especially when the patient attempts to squat or stoop forewards

Deep Palpation

Besides that in Chapter on Introduction, note the hollowness/fullness/tenderness of the iliac fossae and site and volume of femoral pulsation at the base of the Scarpa's triangle. In conditions like posterior dislocation of hip, excised or dissolved head and neck of femur, Buerger's disease the femoral arterial pulsation is weak, or sometimes not palpable (Positive Narath's sign).

Points to be palpated (by applying deep finger pressure) to locate tenderness of the hip joint (Figs 12.4A to C):

1. *Anteriorly*: Just below and lateral to the mid inguinal point at the base of the Scarpa's triangle.

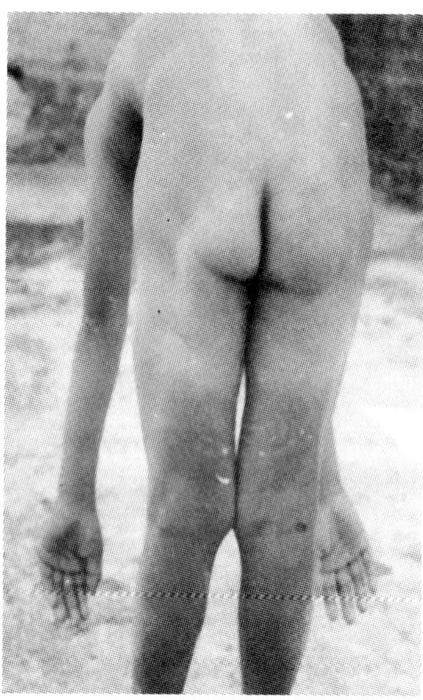

Fig. 12.3B: Due to gluteus maximus contracture the patient is not able to stoop fully

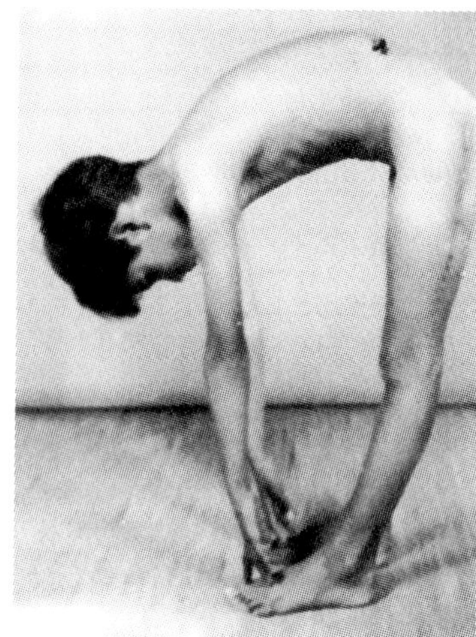

Fig. 12.3C: Same patient, after operative release of the fibrotic contracture, he is able to stoop fully and there is no puckering

2. *Laterally*: Just above the tip of the greater trochanter by giving direct pressure or thrust over the trochanter. The patient points towards the hip joint, if it is tender. Intensities of trochanteric tenderness can hint towards underlying pathology, e.g.:
   i. Touch tenderness—fresh trochanteric fracture, acute inflammatory lesion in that area.
   ii. Deep pressure tenderness—healing trochanteric fracture, trochanteric bursitis, trochanteric cyst, fracture neck femur.
   iii. Thrust tenderness—transmitted tenderness in fracture neck femur, fracture acetabulum, tuberculosis hip and other inflammatory hip involvements.
3. *Posteriorly*
   i. About the centre of a line joining the trochanteric tip to the ischial tuberosity.
   ii. About the centre of a line joining the ischial tuberosity and posterior superior iliac spine.
4. *Iliac fossa:* In the base of iliac fossae more inferiorly.
5. *Medially:* At the junction of the groin with the medial aspect of the thigh.

Sites to be inspected and palpated for cold abscess or for any collection from the hip joint (Figs 12.4A to C)

1. Base of Scarpa's triangle.
2. Gluteal region.
3. Supratrochanteric region.
4. Iliac fossa.
5. Anteromedial aspect of mid thigh even up to knee joint, in that direction.

Lymph Nodes

Inguinal and external iliac groups of lymph nodes should be examined.

MOVEMENTS (Table 12.2)

In examining the hip joint, two aspects which present maximum difficulties to young clinicians and students are:

1. Eliciting the range of different movements of the hip joint.
2. Measurement of the limb for limb length disparity.

It is essential to know the normal range of movements in the different directions.

For measuring opposing movements (e.g. flexion-extension; abduction-adduction; internal

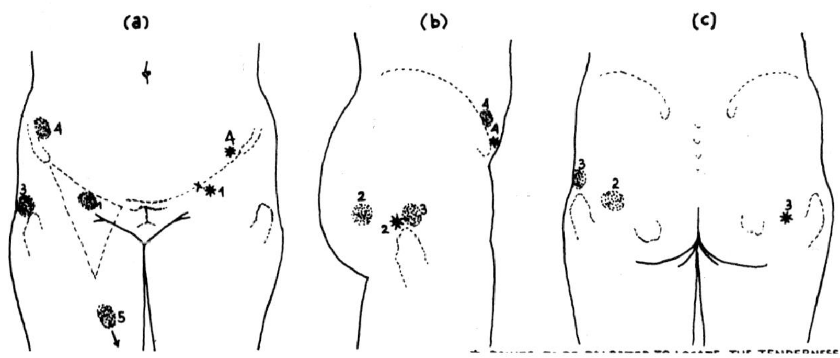

Figs 12.4A to C: Points to be palpated to locate the tenderness of hip joint, and sites to be suspected/palpated for cold abscess

rotation-external rotation) there must be a zero position of the joint for that group from where it will be convenient and accurate to measure the range of motion in that particular direction.

Normal Range of Movements

For flexion-extension: The back of the thigh, calf and heel points must touch the bed (zero position). The limb going above, or in front, will be flexion (to be measured from zero position onwards). While lying prone or on the side, limb going posteriorly is extension. While lying on the sides, the long axis of the limb as a whole should be in line with the trunk and parallel to the bed (zero position).

For abduction-adduction: The long axis of the limb must be parallel to each other and to the axis of the trunk (the line joining the mid inguinal point (practically anterior superior iliac spine may also be taken), mid patellar point, midpoint on anterior aspect of ankle joint and second web of the foot, is the long axis of the limb). From this zero position, abduction, i.e. the limb moving outwards and adduction, i.e. the limb moving towards the opposite limb or inwards without moving the pelvis, are measured.

For Internal Rotation-External Rotation

For this, the zero position is that in which the patella is almost horizontal and the great toe is pointing vertically upwards (except in toe-out and toe-in deformities). From this zero position, the rotational movement in either direction are measured.

FIXED DEFORMITIES

Persistent muscular spasm; persistent posture assumed to avoid pain or to conceal any obvious deformity/disparity of the limb-lengths; destructive changes in the joint; fibrotic contractures in periarticular soft tissues and surgical interventions may lead to particular fixed positions of a joint, from where limb cannot be brought back to neutral position, but further movement in the same axis may be possible—"fixed deformity."

The hip joint commonly gets fixed in flexion, adduction or abduction, internal rotation or external rotations, either singly or in various combinations. Common fixed deformities are flexion, abduction, external rotation, in that order. The combination of fixed deformities are flexion, adduction and internal rotation; flexion, abduction and external rotation; adduction and external rotation in that order.

For understanding the pathomechanics of these deformities, one must clearly understand the following points:

1. The hip, being a ball and socket joint, allows a certain range of motion in all directions. Beyond that normal range, if one tries, either actively or passively, to move the hip, it is not that the femoral

head is moving in the acetabular socket, rather the head is fixed in the acetabulum and the opposite ligaments get tighter and thereby both the head and acetabulum move as one unit moving the hemipelvis. Thus, beyond the normal range movements are achieved by moving the pelvis. In case of limitation of the terminal movements, this situation will come early, i.e. short of the normal range. In presence of any fixed deformity in that direction, if we attempt to bring the limb to zero position, the pelvis will start moving from the very point of fixity.

2. Beyond the position of fixed deformity, it may be possible to have some free range of the same motion.
3. If the joint is fixed in a particular direction, the opposite motion is automatically not possible.
4. In measuring this fixed range, one should measure from the zero position.
5. The pelvis must be fixed to the bed while testing for the range of motion. The moment the pelvis starts moving (manifested by movement of the anterior superior iliac spine), one must stop and bring the limb back to just short of this situation. Then measure the range from the zero position.
6. Even though a patient may have a fixed deformity, he usually adopts some compensatory measure in order to:
   a. conceal the deformities.
   b. maintain the equilibrium by shifting the centre of gravity.
   c. apparently make up the disparity of the limb length.
   d. stabilise the unstable hip.

Therefore, in most of the fixed deformities, there are compensatory, secondary functional (postural) deformities, e.g. in fixed flexion deformity—lordosis at the lumbar spine (Fig. 12.5); fixed abduction deformity—lowering of the pelvis on that side and scoliosis with convexity towards the affected side; fixed adduction deformity—raising of the pelvis on that side and scoliosis with convexity towards the unaffected side.

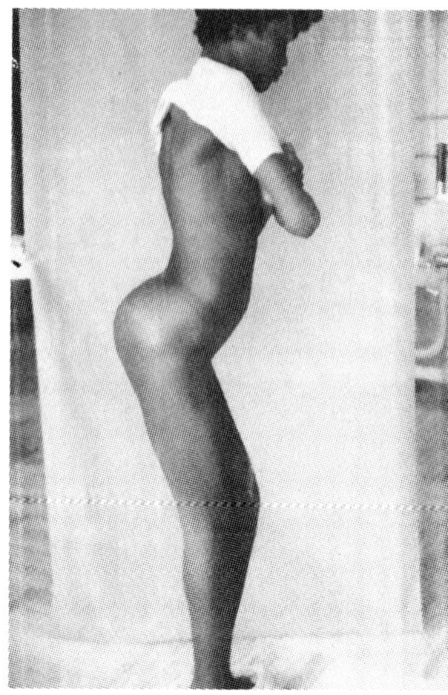

Fig. 12.5: Photograph showing lumbar lordosis due to fixed flexion deformity at hip

Fixed external/internal rotation deformities remain more or less revealed because of lack of proper compensation. Any attempt to properly compensate these deformities produces stress at the lumbar and lumbosacral region, as well as on the knee, ankle and foot.

Hence, in assessing the fixed deformities first of all it is essential to neutralise the postural compensatory deformities.

Fixed Flexion Deformity

In most of the pathological conditions of the hip, the first movement to be lost in extension, i.e. the backward movement from the zero position. Thereafter, the hip goes in for increasing flexion deformity with progress of the disease. If there is fixed flexion deformity at the hip, there will be compensatory lumbar lordosis to conceal it. This must be obliterated to see the actual fixed flexion deformity.

For assessing the fixed flexion deformity, the whole credit goes to Hugh Owen Thomas who described his test in the year 1876.

Methods (Fig. 12.6A)—The patient lies supine on a firm flat surface. The examiner gradually flexes the normal hip, holding the bent knee till the compensatory lordosis is obliterated. This should be judged by insinuating the hand between back and the bed. When the finger can no longer be insinuated, flexion of the normal hip is stopped. In this manoeuvre, the affected hip, if in fixed flexion deformity, will automatically be lifted anteriorly upto a certain angle. While the normal hip is kept in the flexed position, the affected hip is actively or passively extended as far as possible keeping the limb in neutral longitudinal alignment (i.e. '0' position in between abduction and adduction, and '0' position in rotation)—which can not be extended beyond the angle of fixed flexion. Now the angle subtended between the back of the thigh and the bed, will be the angle of fixed flexion deformity.

Severity of the flexion contracture at the hip will not be appreciated if the hip is allowed to abduct while the Thomas test is performed.

Criticism of Thomas Test

1. The patient is hurt further in a painful hip.
2. In obese or heavily built individuals, it is not easy to perform this test, because of improper appreciation of obliteration of lumbar lordosis.
3. In bilateral fixed flexion deformity of the hip it is difficult to perform this test. Since the unaffected side is manoeuvred to elicit this test it would never facilitate comparative evaluation in bilateral cases.
4. Quite often, inappropriate amount of force is applied in flexing the thigh over the abdomen, which leads to anterior tilting of the pelvis. Then the actual measurement would be of the angle made in the long axis of the distal part of the pelvis and the bed, rather than the long axis of the thigh and the bed, leading to fallacious measurement.
5. In presence of ankylosed knee (in extension), it is difficult to perform this test.

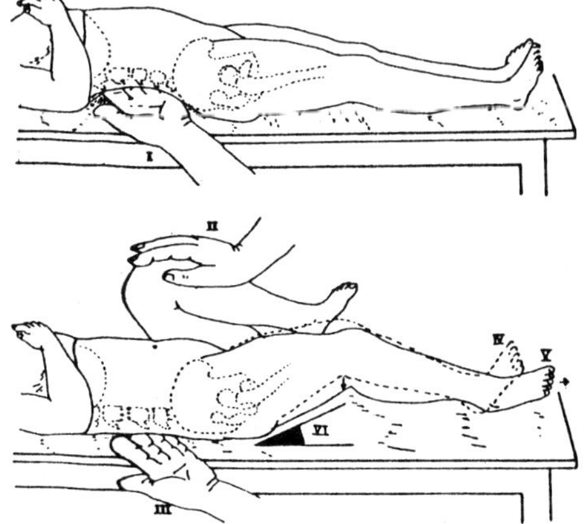

Fig. 12.6A: Method of eliciting Thomas test for fixed flexion deformity at hip

Alternative Methods (Fig. 12.6B)

This method is more useful in bilateral fixed flexion deformities of hip. Put the patient prone on the couch in such a fashion that the trunk lies fully supported on the couch and the hip region is at the edge of the couch. Support both the knees with your hands to avoid hurting the patient. Then, passively, extend the hips till resistance is felt. No force should be used. Keeping the thigh in this position the angle made between the long axis of the trunk (easily manifested, by putting the forearm on the back with hand projected beyond the buttock) and the thigh would be the angle of fixed flexion deformity. In the same attempt, flexion deformities of both the hips can be evaluated.

If there is superadded cause for lordosis, like spondylolisthesis, this can be evaluated more easily in a prone position than a supine. If there is simultaneous fixed flexion deformity of the knee, that also can be measured easily in this position. While the knees are kept supported, the legs are allowed to fall towards '0' position (i.e. fully extended position) of the knee. If the fixed flexion deformity is more than 90°, gently take the leg passively towards zero position. In presence of fixed flexion deformity, the knee can not be extended beyond the angle of fixity.

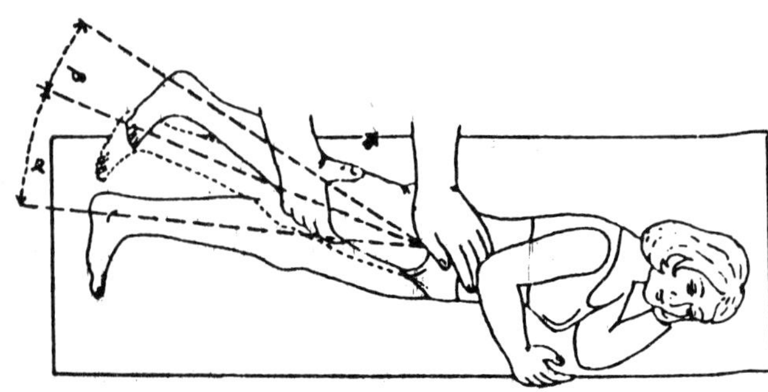

Fig. 12.8A: Showing the active extension at hip while the patient is lying on side; further extension will be possible by passive backward pressure with examiner's other hand. α = range of active extension; β = possible passive extension

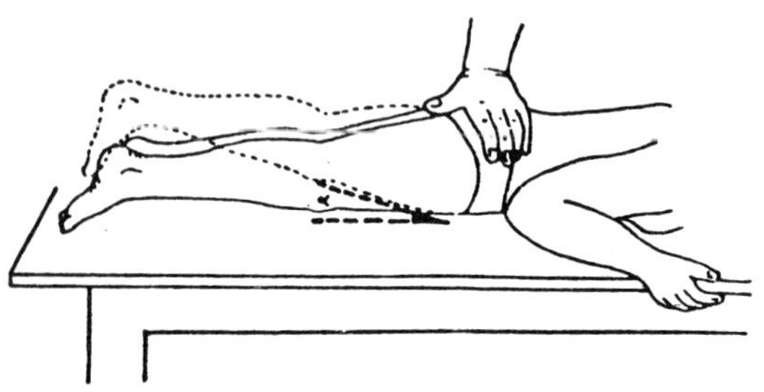

Fig. 12.8B: Showing the active extension at the hip while patient is lying prone. Note the fixation of pelvis by examiner's hand during movement. α = range of active extension at hip. Further few degree of passive extension can be achieved when the examiner assists by lifting up the extended thigh

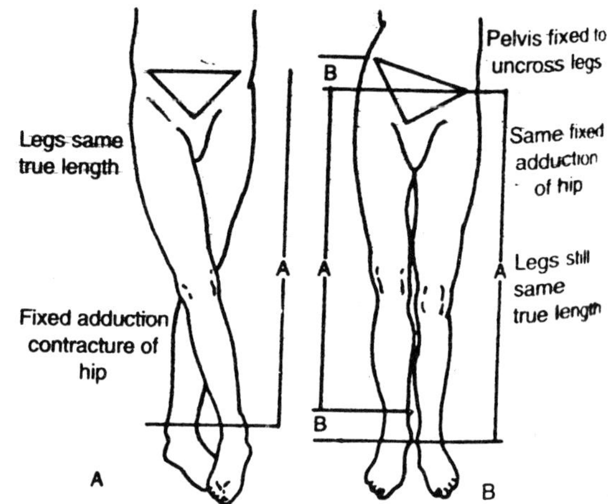

Fig. 12.8C: Functional shortening

additional degree of extension may be elicited (passive range) by passively extending his hip beyond the active range.

Flexion (Fig. 12.9)

Keeping the one lower limb extended, the patient is asked to flex his other lower limb at the hip with knee fully flexed till the front of the upper thigh touches the front of the abdomen, or the pelvis just starts moving. With the knee extended normally one can flex up to 90°

Abduction (Fig. 12.10)

Hold the ipsilateral iliac crest by the spread out hand so that thumb is on anterior superior iliac spine (in children the same hand can hold both anterior superior iliac spines, i.e. the pelvis). Ask the patient to move out his extended limb in the horizontal plane till the thumb just appreciates movement of the anterior superior iliac spine (limit of normal abduction). If patient cannot reach this point (end of active movement), hold the lower part of the leg with the other hand and gradually move it out till the thumb just appreciate any movement of the anterior superior iliac spine.

Abduction in Flexion (Fig. 12.11)

Ask the patient to flex both the hips as far as possible up to 90° (optimum). In this position, with the soles of his feet approximated together, the patient is asked to touch the couch with the outer aspect of his knees. Note the deficit. Normal range in children is 80°-90°, which gradually decreases to 60°-70° in adults.

Table 12.2: Movements of hip

Movements	*Axis*	*Range of movement*	*Prime mover*	*Nerve supply*	*Assisted by*	*Limiting factor*
Flexion	—	0°-110° to 130°	Psoas major	L 2-3	Rectus femoris, Sartorius, Pectineus, Tensor fascia lata Adductor longus Adductor brevis Adductor magnus (Oblique fibres)	With extended knee—tension on hamstrings With flexed knee—contact of thigh with abdomen
Extension (Extension beyond zero position)	—	0°-20°	Gluteus maximus Semitendinosus Semimembranosus Biceps femoris	Inferior gluteal (L5, S1-2) Sciatic nerve (L4, 5, S1, 2, 3)		Tension of anterior capsule is re-enforced by iliofemoral ligament Tension of hip flexors
Abduction	Anteroposterior axis passing through head of femur	0° to 45°-55°	Gluteus medius	Superior Gluteal nerve (L4, 5, S1)	Gluteus minimus Gluteus maximus (Upper fibres) Tensor fascia lata	Tension of hip adductors, Tension of medial band of iliofemoral ligament and adjoining capsule
Adduction	Do	0° to 35°-45°	Adductor longus Adductor magnus Adductor brevis Pectineus Gracilis	Obturator nerve (L3, 4) Femoral nerve (L2, 3, 4)		With extended knee—contact of upper part of thigh with the opposite one With flexed knee—tension of abductors and tension of lateral band of ilio-femoral ligament
External rotation	Vertical axis, passing through centres of head and mid-patellar point	0° to 40°-50° (except in persons not used to Budha position) (eg Europeans, Americans etc) in whom the terminal 10° to 20° are limited on either side	Obturator externus Obturator internus Quadratus femoris Piriformis Gemelli superior Gemelli inferior	S3, 4 S1, 2, 3 L5, S1 S1, 2 S1, 2, 3 L5, S1	Sartorius, Long head of biceps femoris	Tension of internal rotators of hip Tension of ilio-femoral ligament
Internal rotation	-do-	0° to 30°-40°	Gluteus minimus Tensor fascia lata	Superior gluteal nerve (L4, 5, S1)	Gluteus medius (anterior fibres) Semimembranosus Semitendinosus	With flexed hip, tension of ischio-femoral ligament Tension of hip external rotators With extended hip, tension of ilio-femoral ligament
Flexion, abduction and external rotation of hip, while knee is flexed			Sartorius (Tailor's muscle)	L2, 3, 4	Hip flexors Knee flexors Hip abductors	
Abduction of hip in flexion			Tensor fascia lata	L4, 5, S1	Hip external rotators Gluteus medius Gluteus minimus	

Circumduction:
Limitation of any movement will not allow free range of circumduction

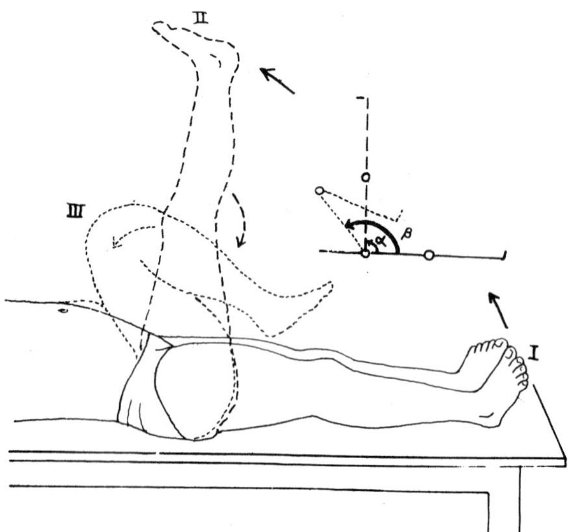

Fig. 12.9: Showing the method of active flexion at hip; α = with knee extension (II); β = with the knee flexed (III)

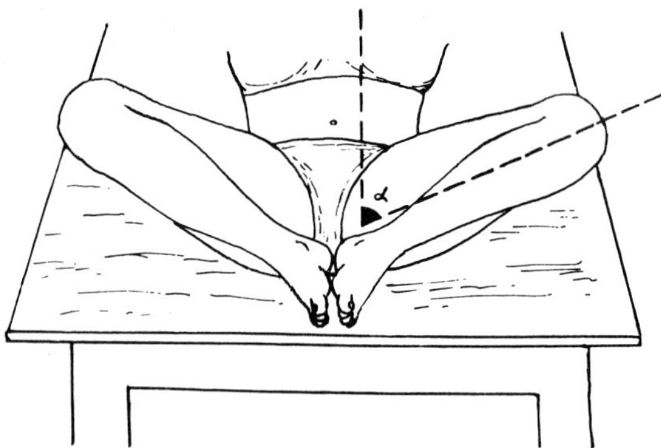

Fig. 12.11: Showing the active abduction at hip with hip and knee flexed; α = range of active abduction at hip

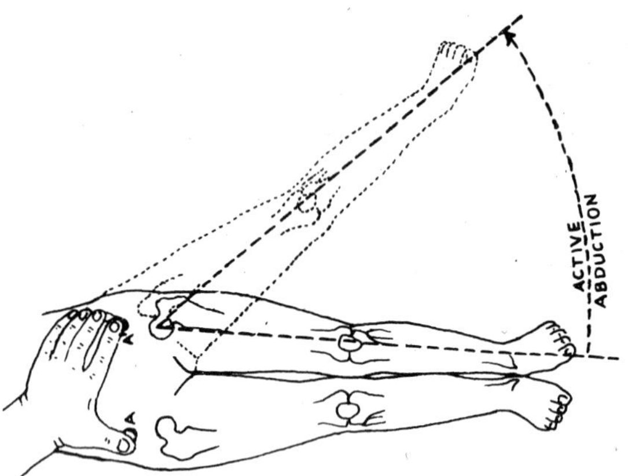

Fig. 12.10: Showing the active abduction at hip with hip and knee extended range of active abduction at hip. A and A = anterior superior iliac spines

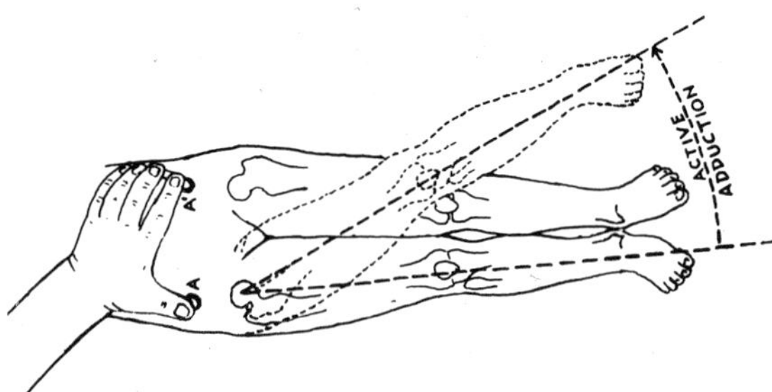

Fig. 12.12: Showing the active adduction at hip = range of active adduction at hip

Restriction of this movement occurs in congenital dislocation of the hip, Perthes' disease, tuberculosis of hip.

Adduction (Fig. 12.12)
Holding the pelvis, as in testing for abduction, ask the patient to cross his opposite neutrally placed extended limb till the pelvis just starts moving (normally the middle third of the opposite thigh is crossed before the pelvis moves).

External/Internal Rotation (Figs 12.13A and B)
For clarity, rotational movements should be tested passively. To get an approximate idea, the extended limb is rolled in and out holding the junction of the middle and lower third of the thigh by the palm (Fig. 12.13A). However, to measure these, the hip and knee are flexed to about 90°. Fixing the knee by the left hand, and securing the heel by the right, with the hip as fulcrum, the leg is taken in and out to elicit the external and internal rotations of the hip correspondingly. The range through which

the foot moves in, will be the angle of external rotation and the range through which the foot moves out, will be the range of internal rotation (Fig. 12.13B). After a certain range the rotational movements are limited by feeling of a terminal catch and then if force is applied in the same direction, patient lifts his buttocks simultaneously. Therefore, one should stop just short of this.

The rotational deformities can also be assessed by similar manoeuvres in prone position of the patient (position as in alternative method of measuring fixed flexion deformity of hip).

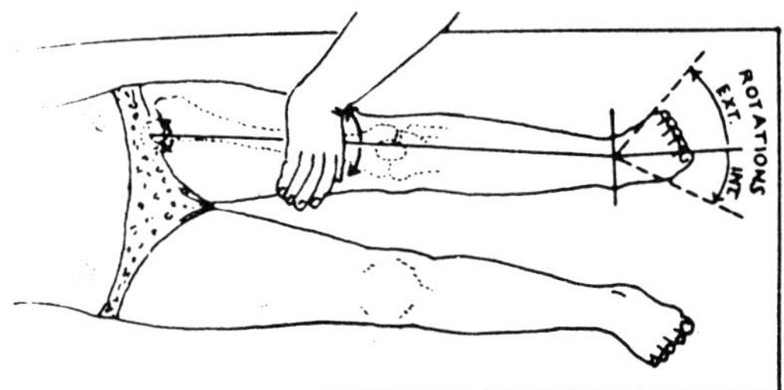

Fig. 12.13A: Quick method of eliciting rotations at hip

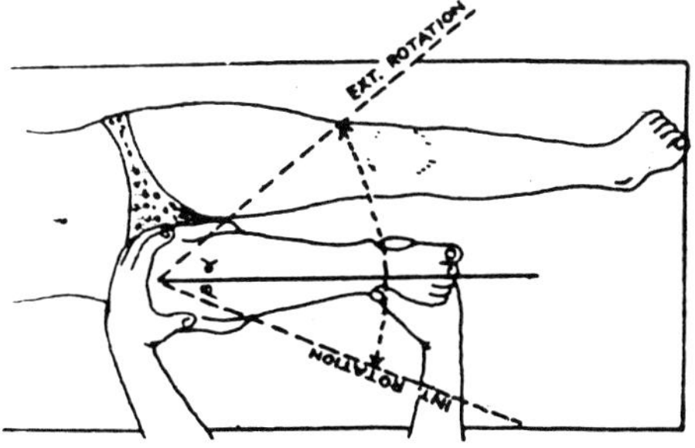

Fig. 12.13B: Method of exact assessment of rotational movement at hip; α = angle of external rotation at hip; β = angle of internal rotation at hip

Circumduction

This can only be possible when all movements are free, hence, as a corollary it may be taken that a hip having full circumduction is almost a normal hip. For getting a rough idea about hip pathology, if the hip can be extended and rotational movements are free, in most of the cases this should be taken as a normal hip.

Snapping hip syndrome: This is mostly of extra-articular type, in which a snap is heard and felt when the knee is flexed and the hip is rotated medially.

MEASUREMENTS

Linear Measurements

Shortening in one lower limb is usually compensated (while walking) by:

i. tilting the pelvis down (i.e. anterior superior iliac spine dips at lower level)
ii. gradual acquiring of equinus position of foot
iii. flexing the opposite lower limb at hip and knee when shortening is beyond the compensatory capacity of pelvic tilt and equinus posture.

a. Apparent measurement
b. True measurement

a. *Apparent measurement:* This measurement helps in assessing the extent of natural compensation developed for concealing the actual deformity/disability/disparity at the hip joint, specially by tilting the pelvis sidewards (fixed abduction and fixed adduction deformity).

While standing, the patient with a hip or hips involvement unawarily tries to assume a posture, by developing natural compensations, which would broadly aim at:

i. Concealment of the deformities.
ii. Bringing the centre of gravity towards the median plane.
iii. Postural equalisation of the limbs.
iv. Stabilizing the unstable hip.

Method

Prerequisites

1. Apparent measurement should be done while the patient is lying supine in a comfortable posture with the affected limb in the line of the trunk (Fig. 12.14A).
2. The lower limbs should be in parallel position. To achieve this handle the unaffected limb to make the limbs parallel. In bilateral affections apparent measurement is not of much significance.

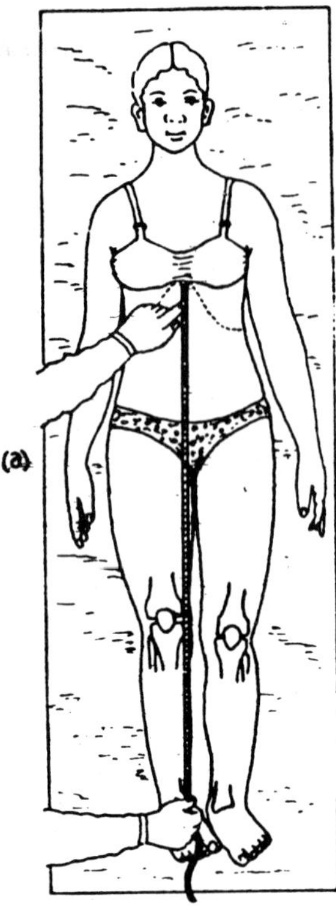

Fig. 12.14A: Method of apparent measurement of lower limb. Note that the limbs are in parallel position and body is aligned to the limbs

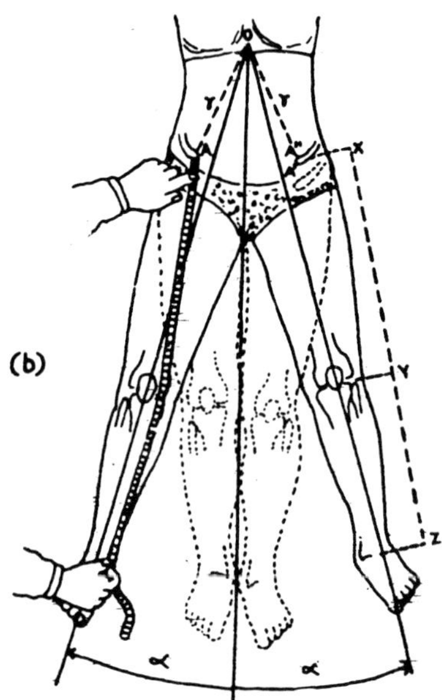

Fig. 12.14B: Method of true measurement of lower limb. XZ= Total length of the lower limb; XY = length of thigh component; YZ = length of the leg component; α = angle of abduction required for squaring the pelvis, the normal limb has also to be taken out by α angle to make it identical

The measurement should be taken from any central fixed point on the trunk (e.g. central point of suprasternal notch, xiphisternum, umbilicus) distally to the sharp bony point of the medial malleolus.

Significance of Apparent Measurement

1. Assessment of the compensations that the patient has developed to conceal any fixed deformity of hip and/or disparity of the limb lengths.
2. On many occasions, this natural compensation also improves the cosmetic aspect.

True Measurement (Fig. 12.14B)

It is the measurement taken from anterior superior iliac spine to the medial malleolar tip while both lower limbs are kept in identical position and pelvis is squared. This can be done either in standing or in lying down position.

In a suspected case of limb length disparity, its effective assessment should be done in ambulatory patients by block adjustment method (Fig. 2.6A) in standing weight bearing position.

Method of measuring limb length disparity while patient is standing.

Usually the patient compensates shortening by abducting the limb, thereby making the pelvis on that side tilt downward. This is represented by lower level of anterior superior iliac spine on that side. Ask the patient to bring the abducted lower limb to as far as the zero position, while the trunk is erect. He is able to do so by gradually lifting the heel, in the process of which the anterior superior iliac spine starts moving upwards. As soon as it comes in the horizontal plane, insert the measured wooden block beneath the foot so as to keep up that level. The height of the wooden block required, is the limb length disparity.

Similarly, if there is lengthening of the limbs, anterior superior iliac spine remains higher up. Insert the measured wooden block beneath the opposite foot to the extent that it brings anterior superior iliac spines in horizontal level. The height of wooden block required will be the amount of lengthening of the opposite affected limb.

Measurement in Lying Down Position

a. *Prerequisites:*
   1. Patient must be fully exposed.
   2. The bony points must be distinctly marked with a skin pencil. The bony points are the anterior superior iliac spines, medial central or lateral central point of the knee joint line (or tibial flare), distal sharp bony point on the inferoposterior aspects of the medial malleolus, sharp point on the posterosuperior aspect of the greater trochanter, sharpest point on the ischial tuberosity, which can be marked conveniently by flexing the hip joint and knee at 90°.
   3. The concealed fixed abduction or adduction deformity must be accurately revealed by squaring up the pelvis, i.e. where the line joining the tips of the two anterior superior iliac spines is horizontal, i.e. it should cut the central line at right angles or the anterior superior iliac spines should be equidistant from the umbilicus or any other central fixed point.
   4. The limbs must be kept in identical position.
   5. The affected limb should be handled to square up the pelvis (level the pelvis) by exaggerating the noted abduction/adduction deformity. The normal limb should then be handled to make it in identical position to the affected limb.
   6. For localising any bony point or joint line, palpation by finger tip may be misleading and may cause some false recording due to stretching of the skin. The metal end of the measuring tape is best utilised for this purpose, e.g.:
      - For the anterior superior iliac spine, the metal end of the measuring tape should be gently slided over the inguinal ligament towards the anterior superior iliac spine and the first bony resistance catching the metal tip should be marked without squeezing or stretching the skin.
      - For the trochanteric tip, the metal end of the tape is passed down and laterally over the gluteus medius till it is obstructed by a sharp bony resistance. This point is marked.
      - At the knee, the adductor tubercle may be difficult to mark, specially in a fatty or a heavily muscular limb. Hence, mark the joint line which can be very easily located by sliding the metal tip of the tape upwards over the medial surface of medial tibial condyle, till it engages into a transverse slit, i.e. the joint line. The central point of the joint line, on the medial surface of the joint, should be taken as the fixed point at the knee.
      - For the medial malleolus, the metal tip should be slided up vertically towards the medial malleolus, and the first bony point catch should be taken as the point and marked.

Total Length

A quick assessment of limb length disparity can be done by eliciting Allis or Galeazzi sign (Figs 12.28 and 12.29). Here the hips are flexed, as much as possible, upto about 60 degrees and the knees are bent at 90 degrees with feet planted over the bed. Both the closetted knees should normally be in same horizontal level. Any disparity in level indicates limb length disparity.

Actual measurement should be done first on the normal side. Total length is measured from the anterior superior iliac spine to the tip of medial malleolus. If the true shortening is equal to earlier done apparent shortening, it indicates that there is no compensation. If the true shortening is more than the apparent one, it indicates that part of the shortening has been compensated by tilting the pelvis downwards (fixed abduction deformity). If the true shortening is less than the apparent shortening, it indicates fixed adduction deformity besides shortening without any compensation.

Any disparity in the limb lengths can be localised by taking the segmental measurement.

a. *Leg length*: Central point on medial knee joint line to tip of medial malleolus.
b. *Thigh length*: It is divisible into two segments:
   i. Infra-trochanteric (from the tip of the greater trochanter to the knee joint line).
   ii. Supra-trochanteric (measurement for the length of the neck and head of femur).

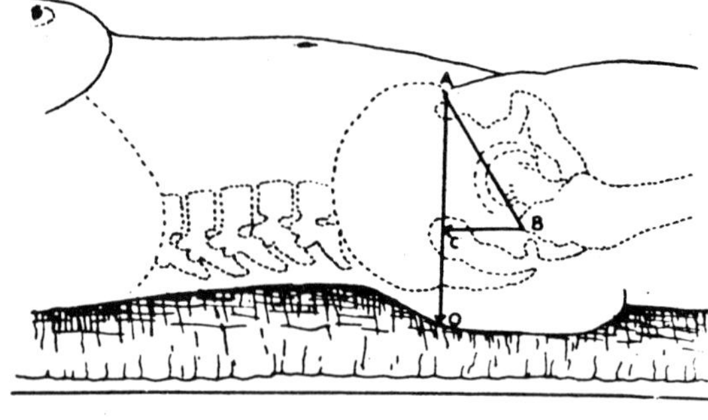

Fig. 12.15: Method of drawing the Bryant's triangle (ABC); AD = perpendicular on the bed from ASIS; BC = perpendicular from the tip of greater trochanter to the first line; AB = line joining the anterior superior iliac spine to tip of the greater trochanter

Supratrochanteric Measurement

A quick approximate assessment of the supratrochanteric disparity can be done by comparing the limbs by 'digital Bryant's triangle'. Here the tip of the thumbs are placed on anterior superior iliac spines, the tips of the middle fingers over the trochanteric tips and the tips of the index fingers over the imaginary points of intersection of the perpendiculars dropped from anterior superior iliac spines over the bed and from the trochanteric tips over the first line.

By drawing the geometrical Bryant's triangles on both the sides, the quantitative supratrochanteric disparity can be assessed.

Method (Fig. 12.15): In already squared up pelvis, from the anterior superior iliac spine, a perpendicular line is drawn down to the bed/ couch. From the tip of the greater trochanter, draw a perpendicular line over the first line (base of the triangle). Join the tip of the greater trochanter to the anterior superior iliac spine (hypotenuse). Each side of this right angled triangle is compared with its counterpart on the normal side.

Interpretation

Any shortening of the base (i.e. more or less femoral axis continuation line) indicates riding up of the trochanter, which may be due to the shortening in the neck, head, joint proper or dislocation of the joint. In gross overriding of the trochanter, the trochanteric tip may lie above the perpendicular drawn from the anterior superior iliac spine over the bed. Here, Bryant's triangle will be drawn above the perpendicular (reversed Bryant's triangle), and the shortening will be the sum total of base of reverse Bryant's triangle and the base of Bryant's triangle on the normal side.

Any shortening of the perpendicular line drawn from the anterior superior iliac spine over the bed indicates anterior sliding or tilting, internal rotation of the trochanter/or head of the femur (e.g. posterior and central dislocation of the hip joint); in flexion contractures of the hip, following old fractures or destructive lesion of the joint, and in trochanteric fractures, the length of this line will increase.

Any shortening of the hypotenuse indicates approximation of the trochanter towards the central point of the body, e.g. in central dislocation of the hip, old fracture neck femur with neck absorption, absence of head due to disease or surgery, protrussio acetabulii.

Fallacies of Bryant's triangle: In bilateral affection of the hip; excision of anterior superior iliac spine, e.g. for bone graft; a limb disarticulated at the hip.

The quantitative measurement of the Bryant's triangle can be confirmed by the qualitative assessment done by following drawing:

—Nelaton's line.
—Schoemaker's line.
—Chiene's test.
—Morris's bitrochanteric test.

Nelaton's Line (Fig. 12.16)

Turn the patient on the normal/opposite side, the limb preferably bent 90° at the hip and knee. A line is drawn from the sharpest bony point on the ischial tuberosity to the anterior superior iliac spine. Normally, this line should pass through the tip of the greater trochanter. In the case of supratrochanteric shortening, the trochanter will be above this line. This line is to be drawn on the affected side only.

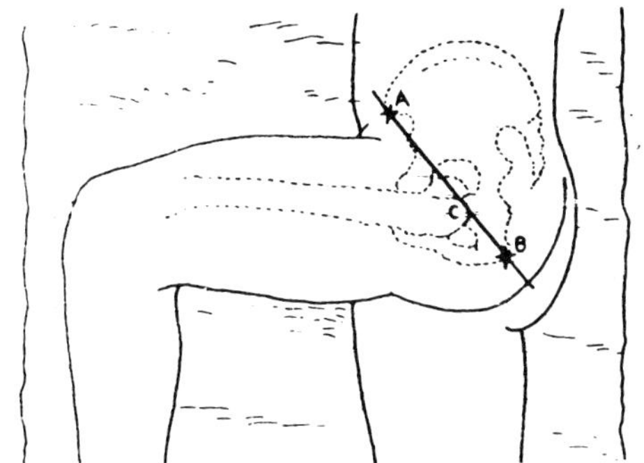

Fig. 12.16: Method of drawing the Nelaton's line; note that line joining anterior superior iliac spine (A) to ischial tuberosity (B) is just touching the tip of the greater trochanter (C)

Schoemaker's Line (Fig. 12.17)

The patient lies supine. A line joining the trochanteric tip and anterior superior iliac spine is prolonged in its direction on the abdomen on each side. Normally, this should meet in the central line at, or above the umbilicus. In case of riding up of the trochanter the line on that side will meet its counterpart below the umbilicus and on the opposite side. In a bilateral coxavara or congenital dislocation of the hip, both lines will meet in the centre, but below the umbilicus.

Chiene's test (Fig. 12.17): The lines joining the two anterior superior iliac spines and tips of greater trochanter should be parallel. If the tip of the trochanter is upridden, then the lines will converge on that side.

Morris's bitrochanteric test (Fig. 12.17): The distance from the tip of the trochanter to the pubic symphysis should be equal. If the trochanter is externally rotated or displaced back, on that side distance will be increased, and *vice-versa*. These distances should be measured by using graduated callipers.

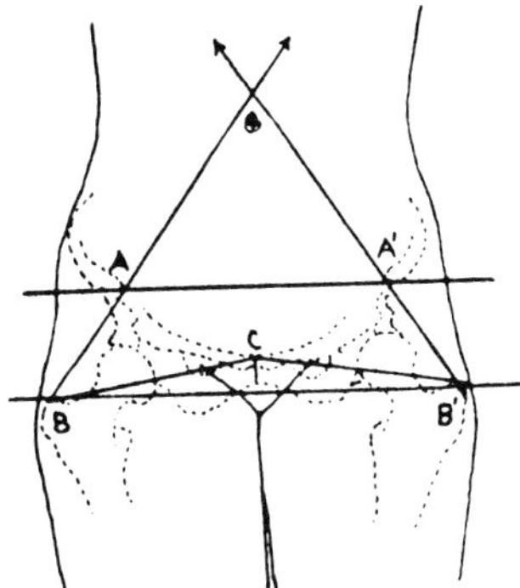

Fig. 12.17: Method of drawing Schoemaker's line (BA and B'A'); Chiene's test (AA' and BB' are parallel); Morris's bitrochanteric test (CB and CB' are equidistant).

In bilateral hip affections, true measurement is inconclusive. In such cases do segmental measurement (supra and infratrochanteric thigh components, and leg component). Add them and compare with the other side measurement. Then corroborate with indirect evidences about the shortened side (e.g., if trochanter is ridden up—that will be the shorter side).

Circumferential Measurements (Fig. 12.18)

i. At the affected sites—to indicate swelling or widening or collections or wasting.
ii. Ideally at the mid thigh on both sides to indicate any muscular wasting or hypertrophy, however it can be taken at equidistant points.

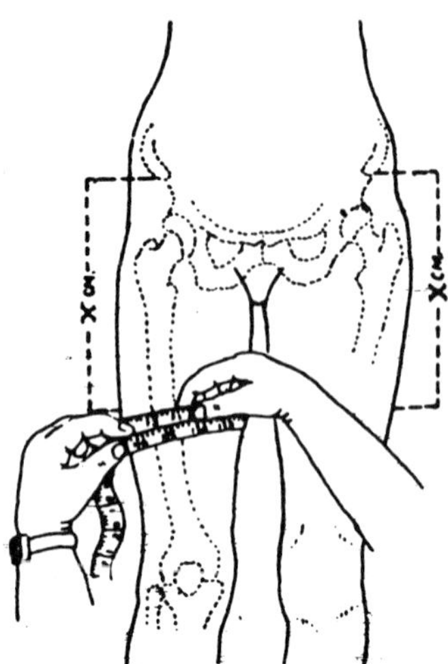

Fig. 12.18: Method of circumferential measurement of thigh

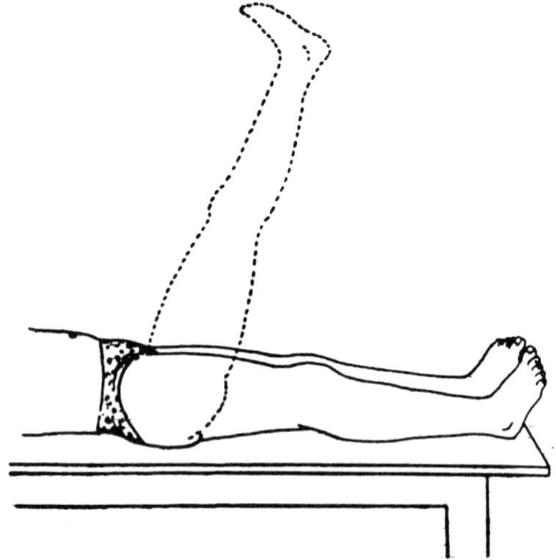

Fig. 12.19: Showing the straight leg raising test

SPECIAL TESTS

Tests for Stability of Hip

1. *Straight Leg Raising Test* (Fig. 12.19)

If the acetabulum, joint space, head, neck and rest of the lower limb are normal, the patient can easily raise his straightened leg up to about 80°-90°. Any affection of the aforesaid regions or even the sacroiliac and adjoining areas or sciatic root irritation, or acute, painful lumbar pathology may affect straight leg raising. The method will be the same as given in the Chapter on Spine.

2. *Telescopic Test* (Fig. 12.20)

By this method, the intactness and adaptation of the head and acetabulum are assessed.

Method: Patient lies supine. Flex the knee and hip as much towards 90° position as possible. For the patient's right hip, put your opened up left hand closely adapted to the trochanter and outer part of the buttock. The right hand, while firmly holding the lower end of femur, pulls up and pushes down the thigh away from and towards the bed. Even in normal condition, a slight amount of excursion of trochanter can be felt underneath the palpating hand. If the excursion is more, then this indicates instability of the hip joint (e.g. old unreduced posterior dislocation, paralytic hip, loss of neck and/or head).

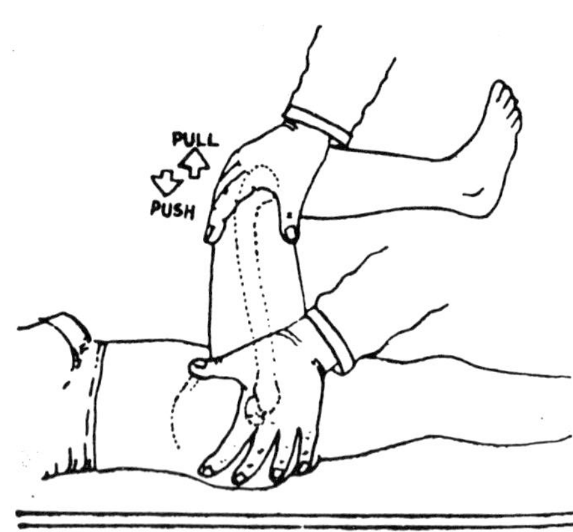

Fig. 12.20: Showing the method of demonstration of telescopic test

3. *Trendelenburg's Test*

Friedrich Trendelenburg described this test in the year 1895 for assessment of congenital dislocation of hip. This test is done while the patient is standing.

Principle of the test: It is done to assess the integrity of the abductor mechanism of the hip, which constitutes of the fulcrum, lever arm and power. Intact abduction mechanism ensures stability of the hip joint. With the fulcrum at the hip joint, normal lever arm of the head, neck and shaft of femur intact, and good power in the controlling group of muscles, especially in the gluteus medius, one can have a normal rhythmic gait with alternate measured and controlled steps and load bearing on the hips. With affection of any of the aforesaid, the normal mechanism of weight bearing is disturbed and a gluteal or Trendelenburg lurch develops.

Method (Fig. 12.21): While one stands on one leg, the opposite part of the body, pelvis [represented on the surface by anterior superior iliac spine (ASIS)] and the lower limb are lifted up to clear the ground. This is effected by the force of contraction of the ipsilateral gluteus medius, an intact lever arm and fulcrum, working from below and pulling the upper part of the pelvis down. Therefore, the opposite pelvis is lifted up. This is indicated on the surface by elevation of the gluteal fold, the iliac crest, the level of the scapula and the shoulder top on the other side. This should be better observed by standing behind the patient. While doing Trendelenburg's test, ask the patient to stand on one leg, and keep your thumbs on the iliac crests, by which it will be easy to assess the dipping down of the pelvis. 5° drop of pelvis or gluteal fold may be taken to be that within normal limits. More than 5° is definitely abnormal.

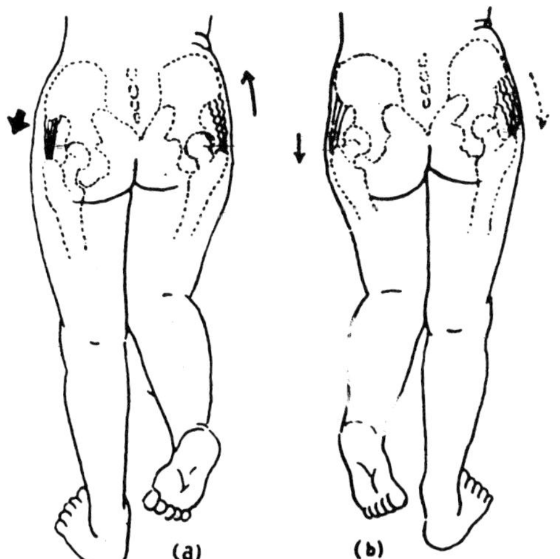

Fig. 12.21: Demonstration of Trendelenburg's test: a = patient is standing on the normal limb; b = patient is standing on the affected limb

If this gluteal mechanism does not work, the opposite pelvis sags down which is indicated by lowering down of the gluteal fold (illiac crest, scapula/shoulder top), on that side. This is Trendelenburg's positive test. This test is positive in the conditions in which any of the above three (fulcrum, lever and power) is affected, e.g. congenital dislocation of hip, fracture neck femur, abductor paralysis due to poliomyelitis, etc.

Fallacies:

a. The intact quadratus lumborum muscle plays its role in effecting the normal gluteal mechanism. The ipsilateral quadratus lumborum working from below pulls down that side of the trunk, while the opposite quadratus lumborum working from above lifts up iliac crest, i.e. pelvis. Hence, affection of the quadratus lumborum can also give a positive Trendelenburg's test.
b. In certain congenital conditions, where there is dissociation of coordination of different groups of controlling muscles of joints (even other than the hip), there may be affection of these mechanism, e.g. cerebral palsy, congenital displacia of hip.
c. Affections of sacroiliacs by virtue of producing pain may produce a pseudo-positive Trendelenburg's test.
d. The medial shift of the mechanical axis of leg below the hip (e.g. in bow knee, bow leg, malunited fracture of femur or tibia) the test may be pseudo-positive.
e. In obese and bulky persons, the test may be pseudo-positive.

4. *Ortolani's Sign*

Ortolani's sign was described by Marino Ortolani in the year 1937 to diagnose congenital dislocation of hip even in the neonates.

Principle: Almost similar in principle and manoeuvre as that of Barlow's test (1962). Here, when attempt is made to reduce the dislocated hip, the head enters the original acetabulum after jumping over the acetabular labrum, giving a sensation of snapping.

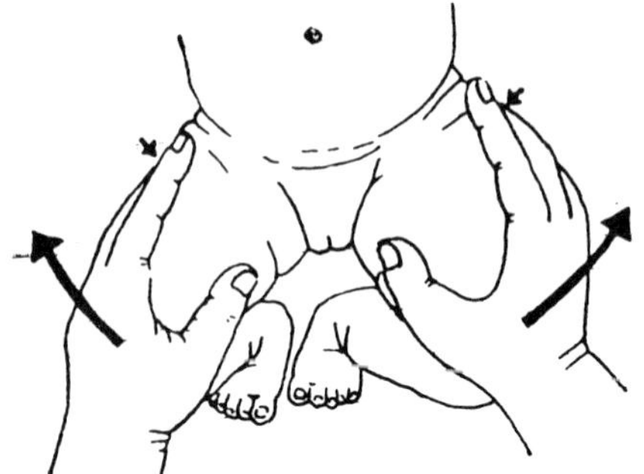

Fig. 12.22: Demonstration of Ortolani's sign

Method (Fig. 12.22): The child lies supine in as much relaxed a position as possible. Flex both hips to right angles, slightly internally rotate and hold the bent knees by both palms, with the thumb placed over the upper inner side of the knees. Both thighs are abducted and externally rotated, while the spread up fingers press inwards and medially over the greater trochanter. As the head jumps over the labrum, snapping is felt and/or heard.

5. *Barlow's Test* (Fig. 12.23)

Patient lies supine, the flexed hips are abducted as much as possible. Hold the upper femur with the middle finger on the greater trochanter and the thumb in the groin. Using alternate pressure from both sides the head can be levered in and out of the acetabulum.

6. *A Test for Diagnosing Dysplasia/Subluxation/ Dislocation of the Hip Joint Early* (Figs 12.1B, 12.24A to D)

The child lies supine. Both thighs are approximated together in the midline. Holding the lower leg, flex the knees symmetrically as far as possible beyond 90°. Now internally rotate and extend the thigh as much as possible. In this position, note for:

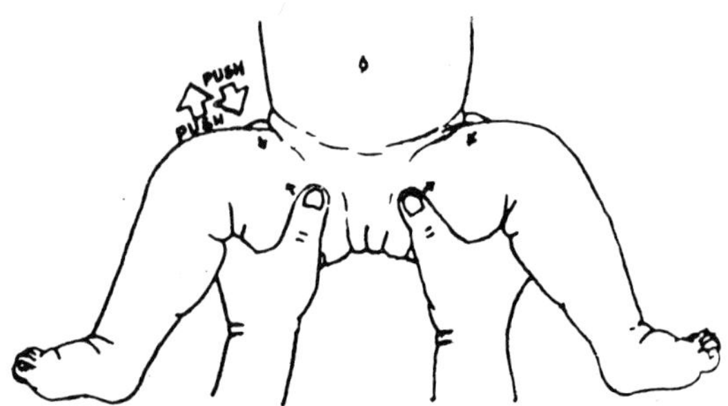

Fig. 12.23: Demonstration of Barlow's test

a. any resistance felt in terminal internal rotation, on the affected side of the hip.
b. any widening of the perineum (Fig. 12.1A).
c. any abnormal crease in the groin (may be seen on the affected side).
d. the level of the groin folds/labial folds (may be raised on the affected side).
e. the trochanteric prominences (obviously prominent and up on the affected side).
f. the level of the bent knees—a flat sheet placed tangentially over the normal knee will not touch the affected knee and the deficient distance will give a rough measurement of the shortening of the affected thigh.

The same test can be done by putting the child in prone position (Figs 12.24C and D). Put the child in prone position. Approximate the extended thigh in the midline. Holding at the lower leg, bend the knees symmetrically as far as possible beyond 90°. Now, internally rotate the hips to the maximum possible extent. In this position, note for:

a. The level of the gluteal folds—on the affected side, the gluteal fold may be higher.
b. Widening of perineum if present.
c. Presence of abnormal gluteal folds, which may appear on the affected side.
d. Level of the knees—on the affected side the knee may fall short of the tangential (horizontal) level of the normal knee. The deficient distance gives the rough estimate of the shortening of thigh component.

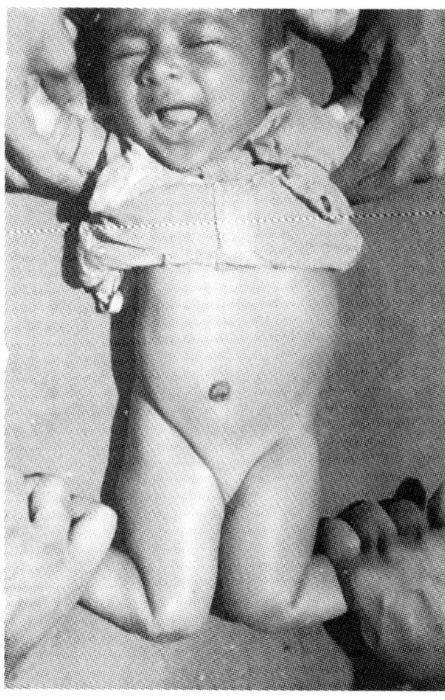

Fig. 12.24A: In supine position

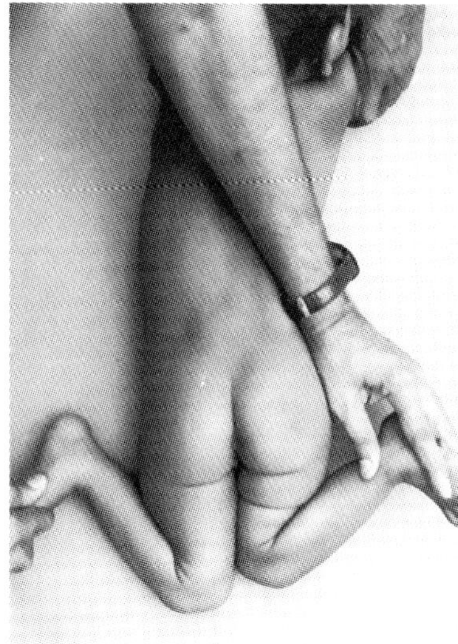

Fig. 12.24C: Test in prone position of the patient

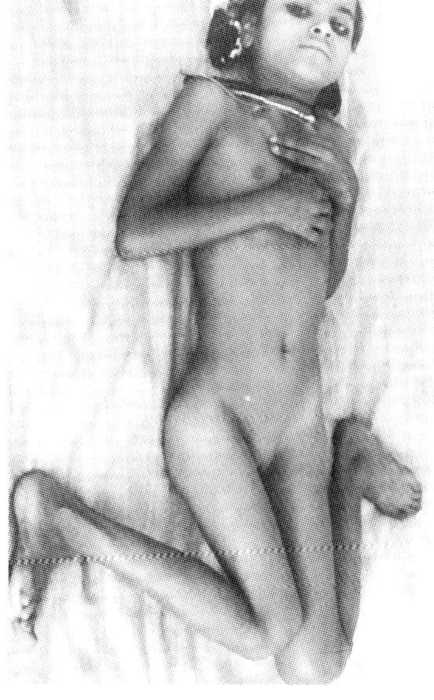

Fig. 12.24B: In older children this test can be demonstrated even without assistance

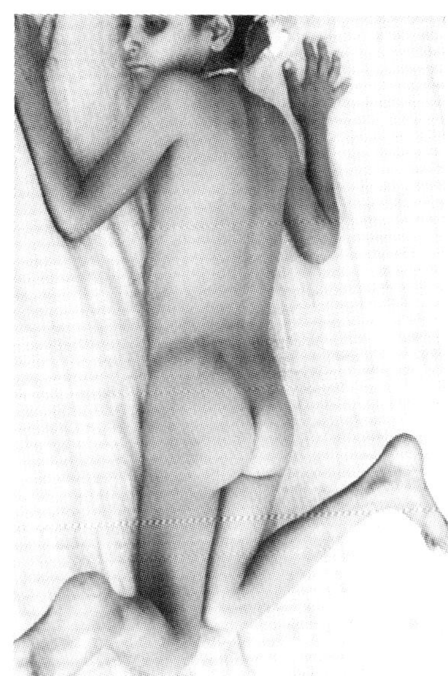

Fig. 12.24D: Same test can be demonstrated even without assistance

Other Tests

1. *Gauvain's Sign*

Sir Henry Gauvain described it in the year 1910. This is of value in early doubtful cases of tuberculosis hip.

Principle: In active tuberculosis of the hip, on initiating its rotatory movements, the muscles around the hip and lower abdomen go into spasm.

Method: Holding the lower end of femur, the thigh is rotated at the joint inwards and outwards. After the movement is checked, any further slight sharp rotation is followed by spasmodic contraction of the muscles of the joint as well as those of the lower abdomen. The reason of abdominal muscles going into spasm is that in this manoeuvre, the rotational movements of the femur is transmitted to the ipsilateral iliac spine.

2. *Sciatic Stretch Test*: (See the Chapter on 'Spine') Though it is important for eliciting the sciatic stretch, it will also be positive where external rotation of the hip is limited.

3. *Narath's Sign*
Normally, femoral arterial pulsation can be felt quite appreciably on both sides. But when the head is not in the socket, e.g. posterior dislocation of the hip joint, the vessels fall back unsupported so femoral arterial pulsation, which is felt against the head of the femur, will be feeble or even may not be palpable—positive Narath's sign.

Patrick's test (Faber test) The patient lies supine, and the examiner places the patient's test leg so that the foot of the test leg is on top of the knee of the opposite leg. The examiner then slowly lowers the test leg in abduction towards the examining table. A negative test is indicated by the test leg's falling to the table or at least being parallel with the opposite leg. A positive test is indicated by the test leg's remaining above the opposite straight leg. If positive, the test indicates that the hip joint may be affected (Fig. 12.25).

Craig's test: In Craig's test, the patient lies prone with the knee flexed to 90°. The examiner palpates the posterior aspect of the greater trochanter of the femur. The hip is then passively rotated medially and laterally until the greater trochanter is parallel with the examining table or reaches its most lateral position. The degree of anteversion can then be estimated, based on the angle of the lower leg with the vertical. The test is also called the Ryder method for measuring anteversion or retroversion (Figs 12.26 and 12.27).

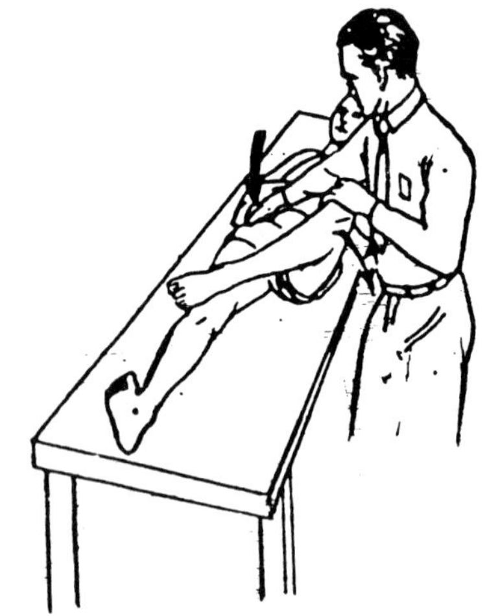

Fig. 12.25: Detection of limitation of motion in the hip

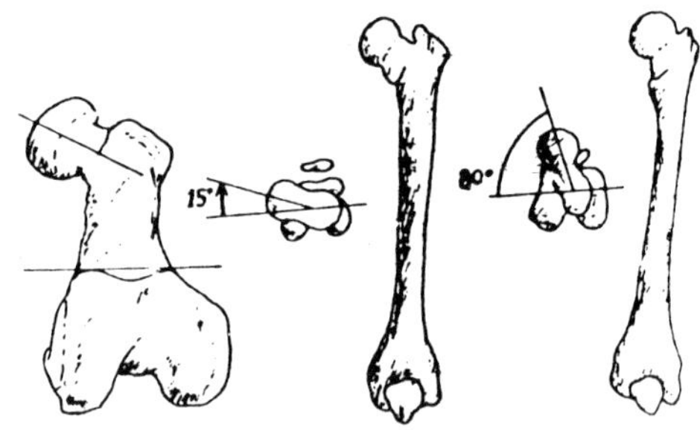

Fig. 12.26: Anteversion of the hip

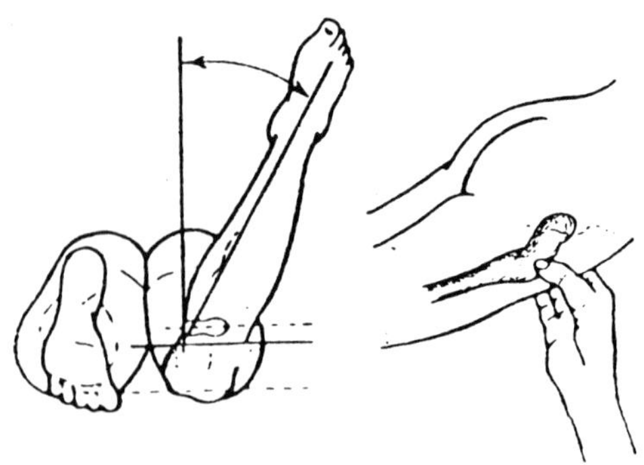

Fig. 12.27: Degree of anteversion and palpate greater trochanter parallel to table

Galeazzi's sign: The Galeazzi's test is good only for assessing unilateral congenital dislocation of the hip and may be used in children from 3 to 18 months of age. The child lies supine with the knees flexed and the hips flexed to 90°. A positive test is indicated by one knee being higher than the other (Figs 12.28 and 12.29).

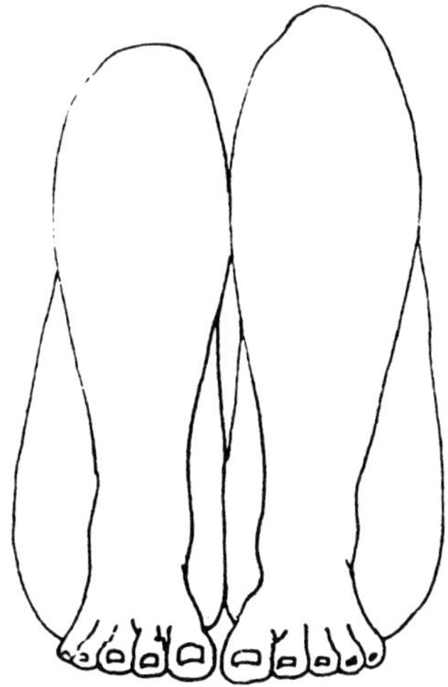

Fig. 12.28: Galeazzi's sign (Allis' test)

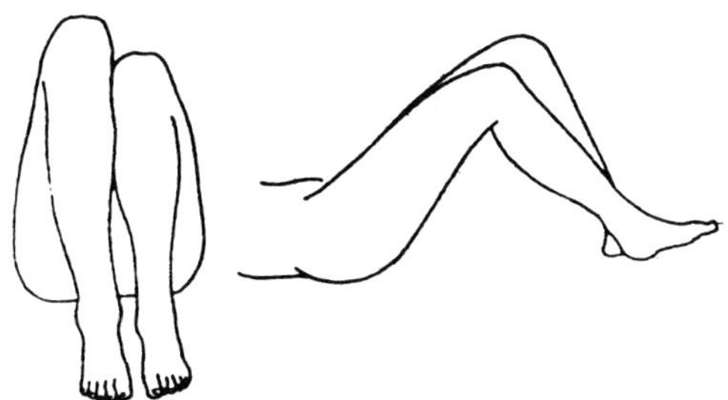

Fig. 12.29: Left shortened tibia and right shortened femur

Rectus femoris contracture test (Ely's test): The patient lies prone and the examiner passively flexes the patient's knee. On flexion of the knee, the patient's hip on the same side will spontaneously flex, indicating that the rectus femoris muscle is tight on that side and that the test is positive. The two sides should be tested and compared.

Noble compression test: This test is used to determine whether iliotibial band friction syndrome exists near the knee. The patient lies supine, and the knee is flexed to 90° accompanied by hip flexion. The examiner then applies pressure with the thumb to the lateral femoral epicondyle or 1 to 2 cm proximal to it. While the pressure is maintained, the patient slowly extends the knee. At approximately 30° of flexion (zero degree being a straight leg), if the patient complains of severe pain over the lateral femoral condyle, a positive test is indicated. The patient will say it is the same pain that accompanies the patient's activity (e.g. running).

Testing for normal flexibility in hamstrings: The patient flexes the hip to 90° while the knee is bent. The patient then grasps behind the knee with both hands to stabilise the hips at 90° of flexion. The patient actively extends each knee in turn as much as possible. For normal flexibility in the hamstrings, knee extension should be within 20° of full extension.

Erichson's sign: When the iliac bones are sharply pressed toward each other, pain is felt in sacro-iliac disease, but not in hip disease.

Hart's sign: Hart's sign is the limitation of abduction of the hips seen in congenital dislocation of the hip.

Per Rectal Examination

In suspected central fracture dislocation, fracture floor of acetabulum, pathological affection of acetabular floor, protrusioacetabuli (Otto pelvis), per rectal examination will elicit tenderness with or without abnormal bulge in that region.

Examination of related peripheral nerves and vessels: The sciatic nerve can be involved in several pathologies of the hip, e.g. dislocation of the hip, fracture of acetabular margin, or in surgery on the hip, etc. Hence, it is imperative to examine for integrity of this nerve.

Ask the patient to dorsiflex and plantarflex the ankle. If he can do so properly, the sciatic nerve, for all practical purposes is intact.

Fortunately, affections of the hip are less likely to affect the main blood vessels of the lower limb, i.e. femoral blood vessels.

However, peripheral vascular diseases sometimes present with baffling symptoms, even mimicking a hip pathology. Exclude them by palpating the dorsalis pedis, anterior tibial, posterior tibial and popliteal arteries.

INVESTIGATIONS

A. General investigations—as in Chapter on Introduction.
B. Special investigations.

I. X-ray is most important

Both anteroposterior, and lateral projections are essential to know the exact femoroacetabular relations; conditions of the head, neck and acetabulum; neck-shaft angulation; axial rotations of the head, and length of the neck.

a. While taking anteroposterior view, the following points must be kept in mind:

i. Keeping the pelvis in as much symmetrical a position as possible, comparative view of both the hips must be taken.
ii. Both lower limbs should be kept in zero position in as far as rotation, adduction and abduction are concerned (i.e. hips extended, legs parallel, and patellae in neutral positions).
iii. Contrast radiography will be helpful in delineating early infective pathology of the hip and its surrounding structures.

Special Points to be Noted in AP Projections

i. Continuity of Shenton's arc—The lower margins of the neck of femur and superior pubic ramus make up parts of the same arc. Any breakage of continuity suggests dislocation of hip or disruption of neck of femur.
ii. The relation of capital epiphysis to the femoral neck.
iii. Relations of capital epiphysis/femoral neck to the acetabular cup.

Lateral view of the hip is often a difficult task for projection, though it is mandatory (e.g. to diagnose and also to assess for perfect reduction after the femoral capital epiphysis slip; to assess perfect reduction, positioning and fixation of fracture neck of the femur).

Method: The extended limb is abducted to about 20°. The X-ray tube is focussed on the groin at mid point of anteroposterior plane. The plate is placed almost adapted to the outer aspect of the hip region.

Alternative method: Patient is put in lithotomy position (hip flexed abducted and externally rotated). X-ray tube is centred on the mid-inguinal point, while the cassette is kept behind the hip.

b. Oblique projection of the hip: Three quarters internally and externally rotated views—essential for detailed assessment of fracture and displacement in central fracture dislocation.

c. In comparatively old fracture neck of femur, X-ray should be taken in 15° abduction and 15° internal rotations to neutralise the anteversion of femoral neck (to assess the length of neck).

d. In coxa plana or Legg-Calves-Perthes disease, anteroposterior projection, keeping the hip maximally abducted and internally rotated gives an assessment about containment of the flattened head in the acetabulum.

II. Arthrography

It is of special importance in conditions like congenital dislocation of hip, Perthes' disease.

III. Arthroscopy

It is not of much value for hip.

IV. Aspiration and Aspiration Biopsy (anterior or lateral route)

Except where the capsule is distended due to collection of fluid, it is difficult to aspirate the contents of the hip joint.

Table 12.3: Harris hip function scale

(Circle one in each group)

Pain (44 points maximum)	
None, ignores	44
Slight, occasional, on compromise in activity	40
Mild, no effect on ordinary activity, pain after unusual activity, uses aspirin	30
Moderate tolerable, makes concessions, occasional codeine	20
Marked, serious limitations	10
Totally disabled	0
Function (47 points maximum)	
Gait (walking maximum distance) (33 points maximum)	
1. Limp:	
None	11
Slight	8
Moderate	5
Unable to walk	0
2. Support:	
None	11
Cane for long walks	7
Cane—full time	5
Crutch	4
Two canes	2
Two crutches	0
Unable to walk	0
3. Distance walked:	
Unlimited	11
Six blocks	8
Two to three blocks	5
Indoors only	2
Bed and chair	0
(Functional Activities 14 points maximum)	
1. Starts:	
Normally	4
Normally with banister	2
Any method	1
Not able	0
2. Socks and tie shoes:	
With ease	4
With difficulty	2
Unable	0
3. Sitting:	
Any chair, 1 hour	5
High chair, 1/2 hour	3
Unable to sit 1/2 hour any chair	0
4. Enter public transport	
Able to use public transportation	1
Not able to use public transportation	0
Absence of Deformity (requires all four) (4 points maximum)	
1. Fixed adduction <10°	4
2. Fixed internal rotation in extension <10°	0
3. Leg length discrepancy 11/4"	
4. Pelvic flexion contracture <30°	

Range of Motion (5 points maximum)

Instructions

Record 10° of fixed adduction as "–10° abduction, adduction to 10°"

Similarly, 10° of fixed external rotation as "–10° internal rotation, external rotation to 10°"

Similarly, 10° of fixed external rotation with 10° further external rotation as "–10° internal rotation, external rotation to 20°"

Permanent flexion (1) ______ °	Range	Index Factor	Index Value*
A. Flexion to	______°		
(0-45°)		1.0	
(45-90°)		0.6	
(90-120°)		0.3	
(120-140°)		0.0	
B. Abduction to	______°		
(0-15°)		0.8	
(15-30°)		0.3	
(30-60°)		0.0	
C. Adduction to	______°		
(0-15°)		0.2	
15-60°)		0.0	
D. External rotation in extension to	______°		
(0-30°)		0.4	
(30-60°)		0.0	
E. Internal rotation in extension to	______°		
(0-60°)		0.0	

*Index Value = Range × Index Factor

Total index value (A + B + C + D + E) ______

Total range of motion points (multiply total index value × 0.05) ______

0 Pain points: ______
Function points: ______
1 Absence of Deformity points: ______
0 Range of Motion points: ______
Total points (100 points maximum)

Comments:

Modified from Harris WH: *JBJS* 51: 737-55, 1969.

Table 12.4: Traumatic hip differential diagnosis

	Capsular tear haematoma	*Fracture neck*	*Fracture trochanter*	*Anterior dislocation*	*Posterior dislocation*	*Central fracture dislocation*	*Fracture pelvis*
1	*2*	*3*	*4*	*5*	*6*	*7*	*8*
Age (more common)	Adults/elderly	Elderly -> 50 years	> 65 years	Young 20-40 years	30-50 years	20-45 years	20-50 years
Sex (more common)	Male	Female	Male	Male	Male	Male	Male
Violence	Indirect twist	Indirect twist	Direct/indirect	Forced external rotation and abduction in flexion—low type; forced external rotation and abduction in extension—high type	Internal rotation adduction strain on flexed hip	Internal rotational, abduction Direct fall on the heels. Indirect violence along the shaft of femur with direct violence from the trochanteric region (eg thrown from dashboard injury) Produce type I. Main violence transmitted along the femur while hip in slight internal rotation and some abduction in extended limb (fall from height produces type II)	Fall from height or direct run over by automobile
Presentation	Pain on walking and standing	Walking/standing—not possible. Sometimes in abduction type or impacted type can do guarded walking	Bed ridden, Swelling ++ Ecchymosis + Trochanteric region	Initially in bed; later on, even if not treated, may walk about with deformity and limp	Initially in bed. Later on, even if not treated, may walk about with deformity and limp	Not able to stand/or walk for pretty long time Swelling and bruises/abrasion over trochanteric region and knee	Varying presentation, depending upon planes and severity of fracture May not be able to walk
Pain	Pain ± (in certain movements +)	Pain ++	Pain +++	Pain +	Pain +	Pain ++	Pain ±
Attitude	Not particular	Spasmodic adduction with slight external rotation. In old neglected fracture—mild flexion, adduction and even internal rotation	Limb lies extended and externally rotated almost till the outer side of the foot touches the bed	Low type—marked abduction and external rotation with some flexion High type—some abduction and external rotation with full extension	Hip flexion, adduction, internal rotation	Internal rotation with adduction	Nothing particular
Limb length	Not affected	Shortening (in fresh cases usually 1 cm and to usually 3 cm in late cases)	Shortening usually 1-2 cm; in unstable type or neglected cases, may be even 5 cm or more	Lengthening of limb	True shortening may be about 5 cm	True shortening 05 to 2 cm	None except in displaced vertical fracture of ipsilateral ilium, pubis and ischium

Contd.

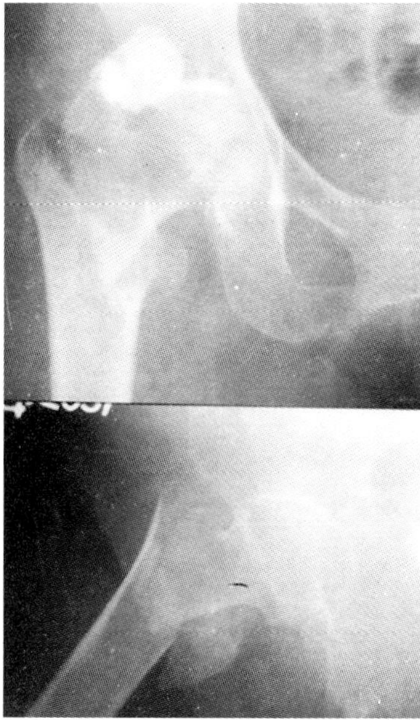

Fig. 12.34: Fracture trochanter—fracture line running from upper outer to inferomedial direction. All such fractures are stable, except the grossly comminuted ones

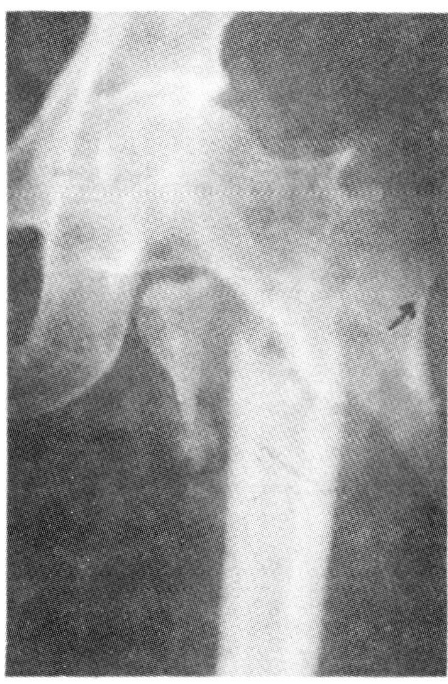

Fig. 12.36: Fracture trochanter with fracture line running from superomedial to infero-lateral direction (all are unstable fractures)

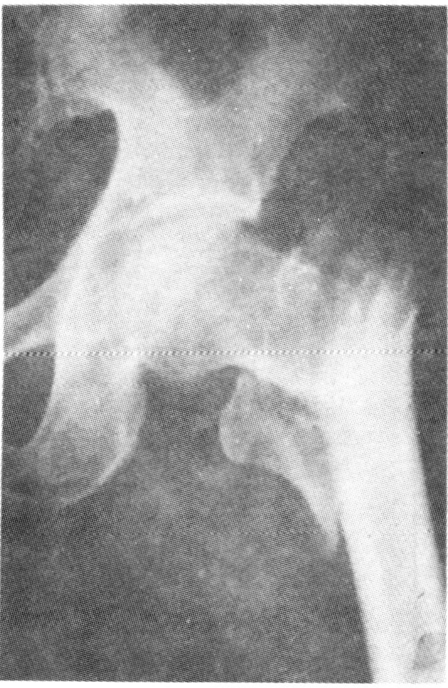

Fig. 12.35: Fracture trochanter with fracture line running from upper outer to inferomedial direction with comminution (mostly stable fracture)

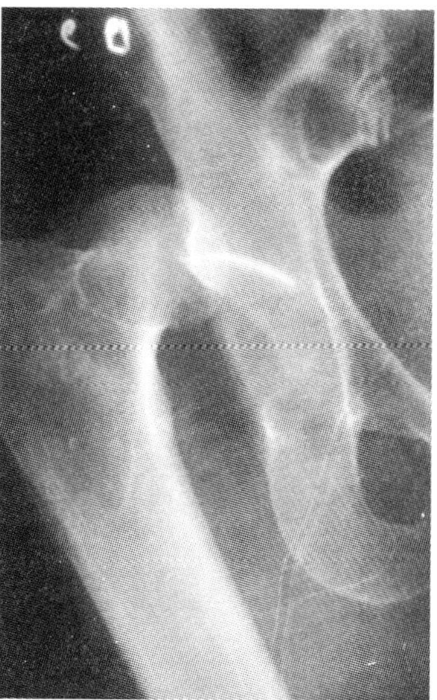

Fig. 12.37A: Posterior dislocation of hip joint (typical high type;ilial type) in adult

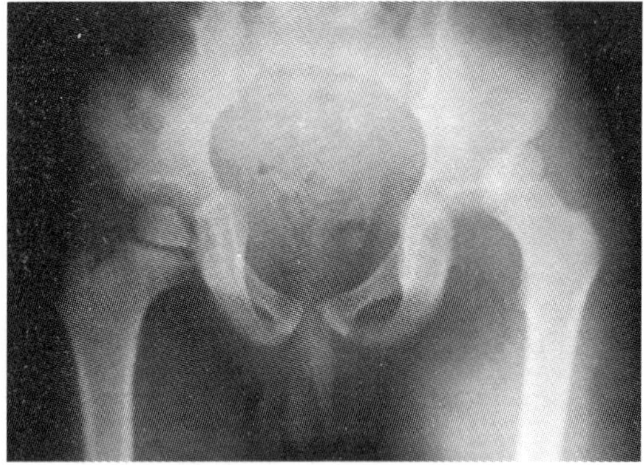

Fig. 12.37B: Neglected posterior dislocation of hip in a boy aged 11 years

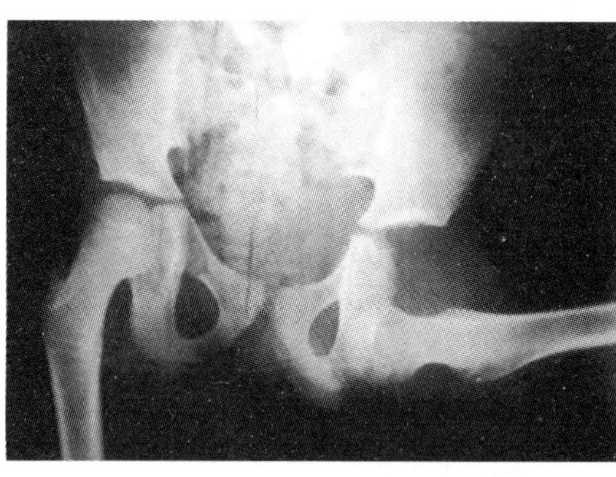

Fig. 12.39A: Anterior dislocation of hip joint (obturator type)

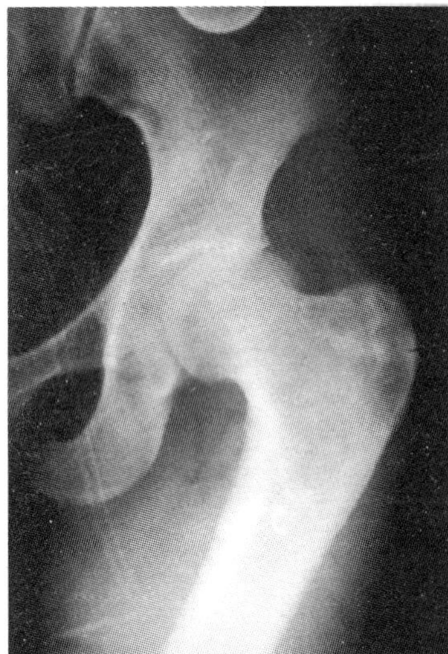

Fig. 12.38: Posterior dislocation of hip joint (low type; sciatic type)

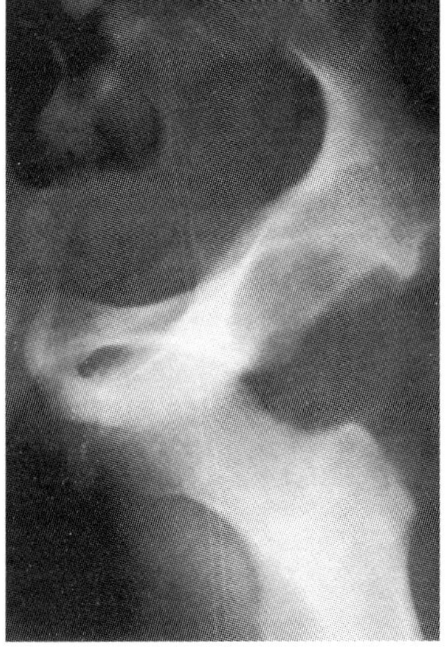

Fig. 12.39B: Anterior dislocation of hip joint (obturator type)

Table 12.6: Classification of fractures in trochanteric region (Based on Evan's classification)

- Type I
  - Fracture line running from superolateral to inferomedial direction
    - Undisplaced (always stable-
      (Treatment: Conservative;
      internal fixation may be done)
    - Displaced (Figs 12.34 and 12.35)
      - Reducible
        (Stable—treatment: fixation preferable; conservative also satisfactory)
      - Non-reducible
        (Not stable—treatment: possible reduction and internal fixation; or osteotomy + internal fixation)
- Type II (Fig. 12.36)
  - Fracture line running from superomedial to inferolateral direction—always unstable.
    (Treatment: Possible reduction and internal fixation)

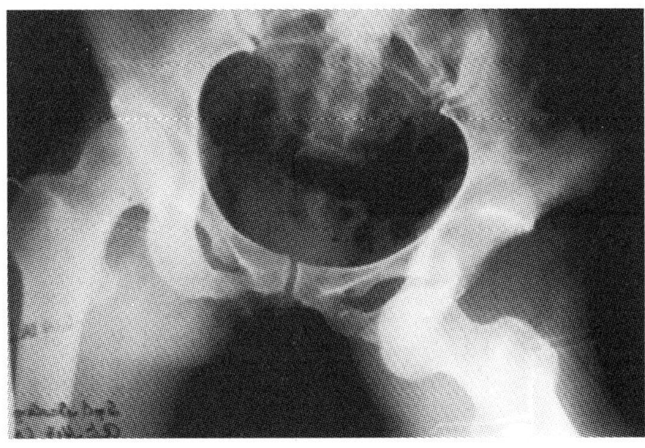

Fig. 12.40: Anterior dislocation of hip joint in adult (pubic type)

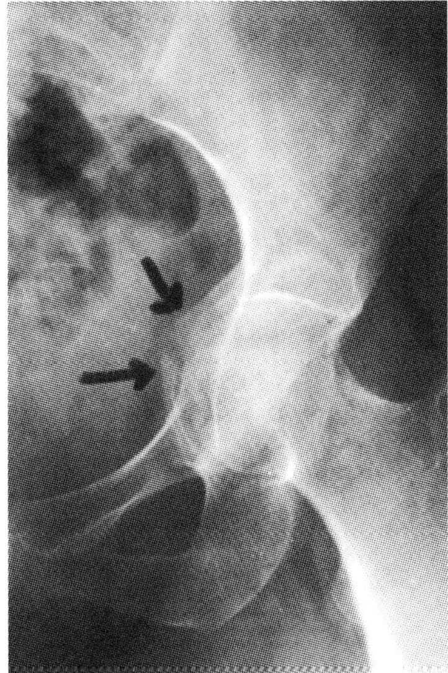

Fig. 12.41: Central-fracture dislocation of hip joint (Grade I)

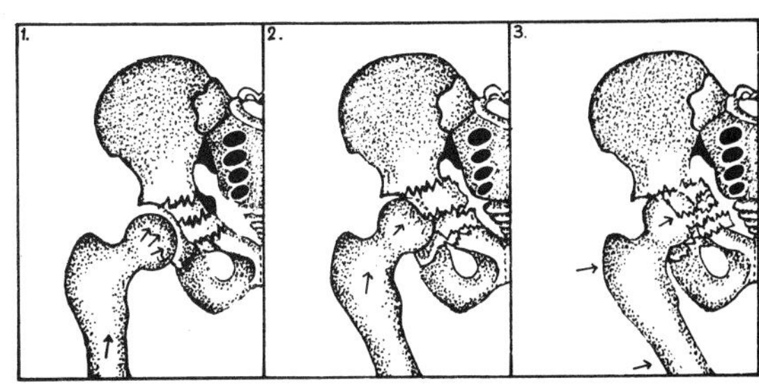

Grade I representing Fig.12.41

Grade II representing Fig. 12.42

Grade III representing Fig.12.43

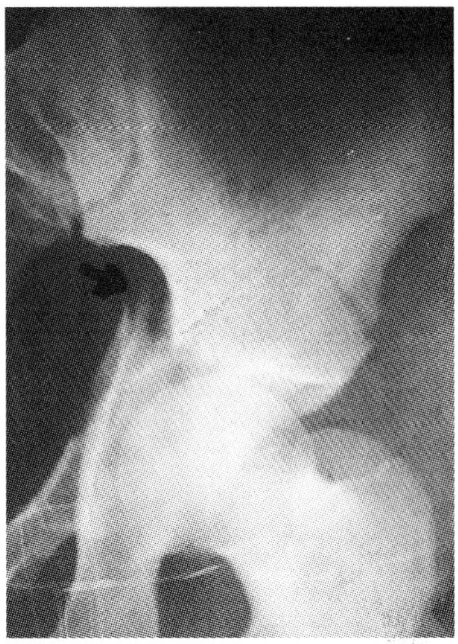

Fig. 12.42: Central-fracture dislocation of hip joint (Grade II)

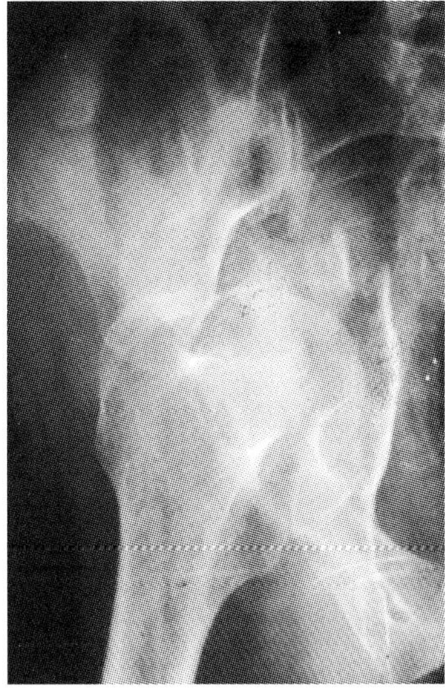

Fig. 12.43: Central-fracture dislocation of hip joint (Grade III)

Line drawing representation of central fracture dislocation of hip joint (Figs 12.41, 12.42 and 12.43)

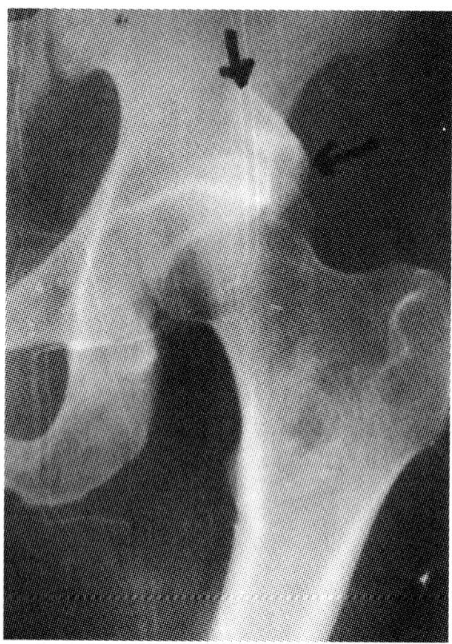

Fig. 12.44: Fracture-dislocation(Fracture of posterosuperior rim of acetabulum) of hip joint

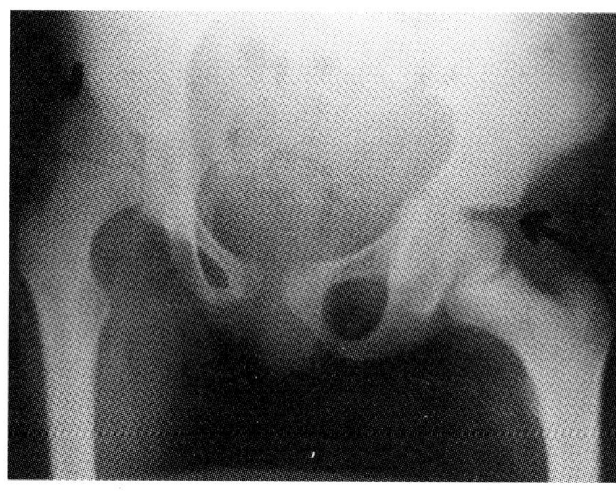

Fig. 12.46: Paralytic subluxation of hip joint (unilateral)

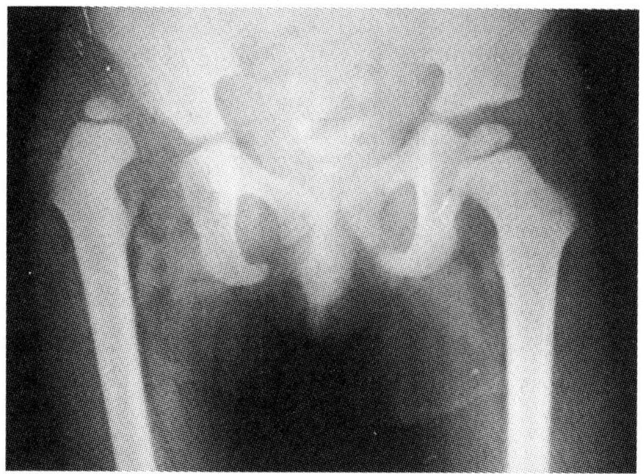

Fig. 12.45: Congenital dislocation of right hip joint

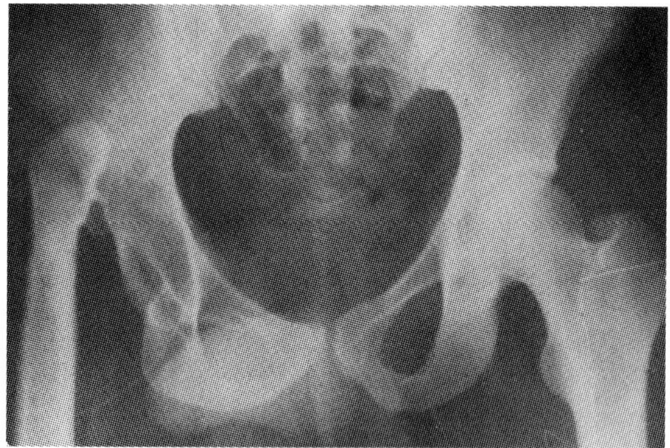

Fig. 12.47A: Pathological dislocation of hip joint following old septic arthritis

Table 12.7: Classification of dislocation of hip joint

A	Traumatic	—Posterior	Ilial type (Figs 12.37A and B)
			Sciatic type (Fig. 12.38)
		—Anterior	Low type (Figs 12.39A and B) (Obturator type)
			High type (Fig. 12.40) (Pubic type)
		—Central	Type I— Where weight bearing articular area intact (Fig. 12.41)
			Type II— When weight bearing area is fractured, but not grossly displaced (Fig. 12.42)
			Type III—Where acetabulum is grossly comminuted (Fig. 12.43)
		—Fracture dislocation	With fracture of posterosuperior rim of acetabulum (Fig. 12.44)
			With chip fracture of head
			With fracture neck of femur
B	Non-traumatic		—Congenital dislocation of hip (Fig. 12.45)
			—Paralytic (Poliomyelitis) (Fig. 12.46)
			—Pathological (septic arthritis) (Fig. 12.47A)
			—Spastic (cerebral palsy)

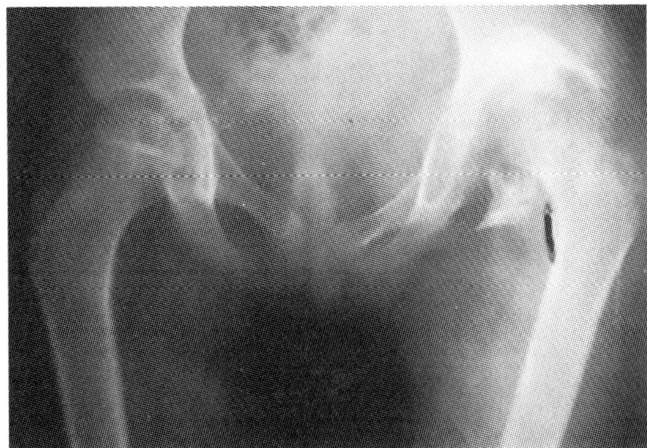

Fig. 12.47B: Myositic mass around hip in a neglected posterior dislocation

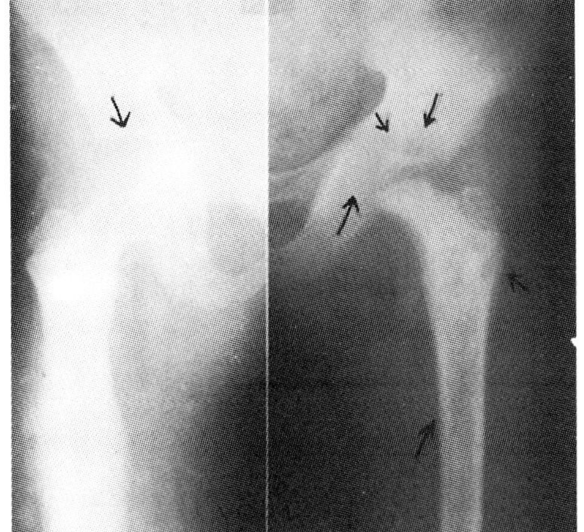

Fig. 12.47C: Septic arthritis hip sequestrating capital epiphysis

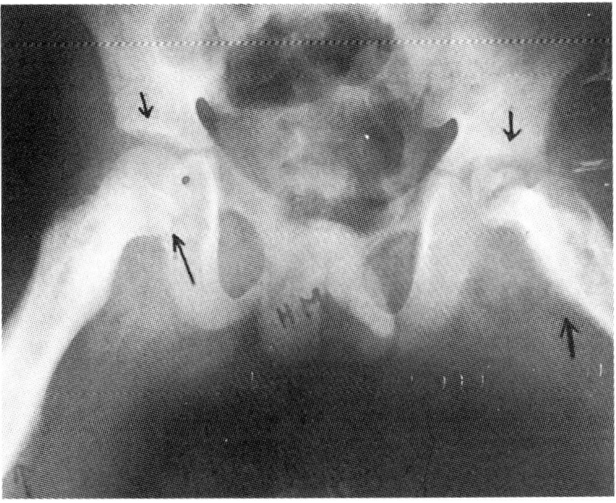

Fig. 12.47E: Septic arthritis hip bilateral septic arthritis of hip (left more affected)

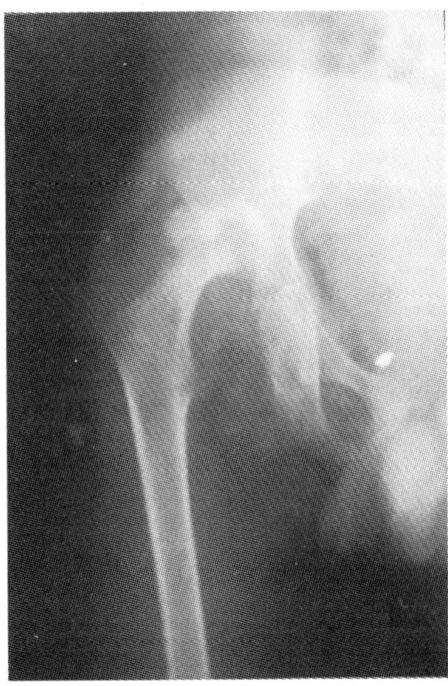

Fig. 12.47D: Septic arthritis hip sequestrated capital epiphysis dislocating out

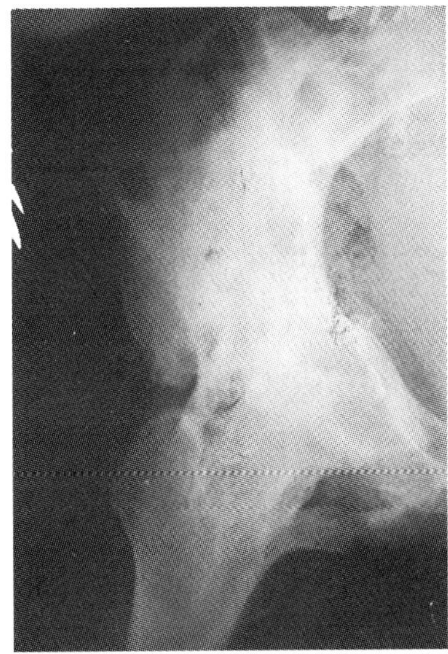

Fig. 12.47F: Septic arthritis hip bony ankylosis

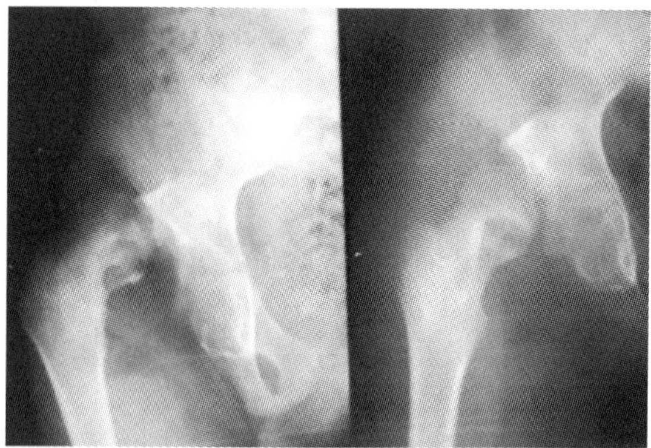

Fig. 12.48A: Tuberculous arthritis of right hip joint with encysted lesion in cervicol area

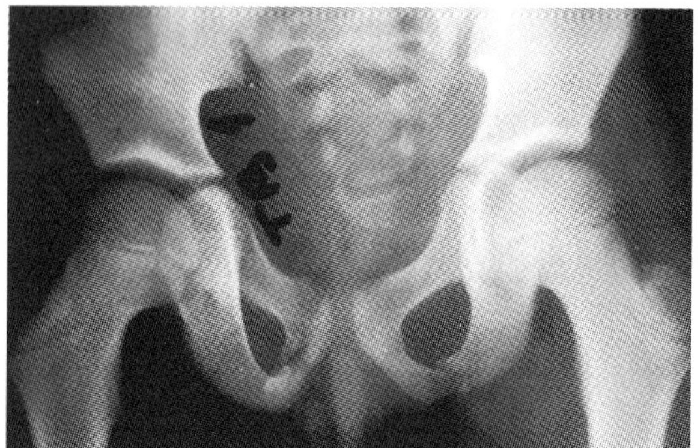

Fig. 12.48B: Tuberculous synovitis of right hip. Note the increase in joint space and rarefaction of adjoining bones

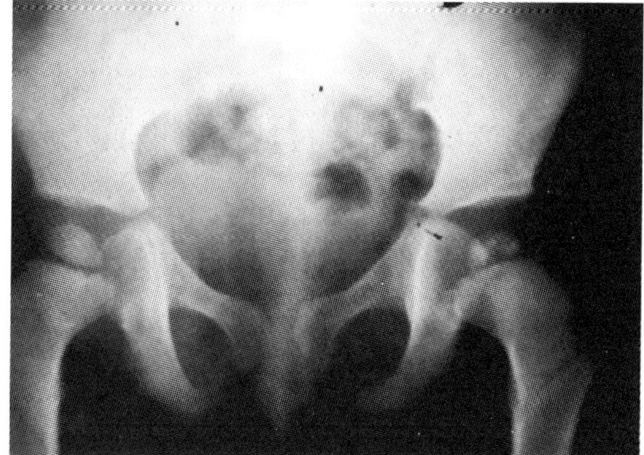

Fig. 12.50A: Perthes disease early stage

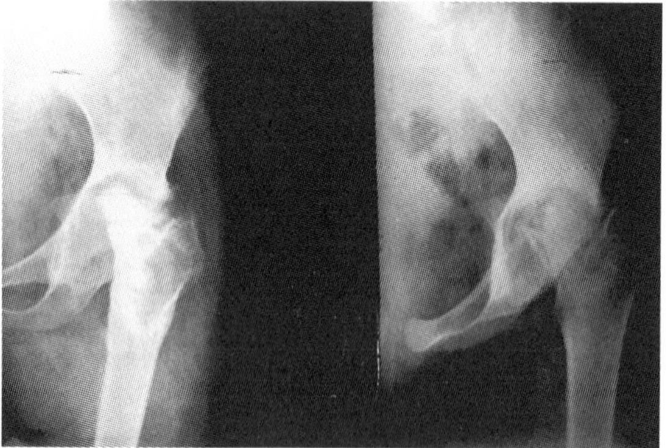

Fig. 12.49: Advanced tuberculous arthritis of hip joint, with a destruction of head and wandering acetabulum

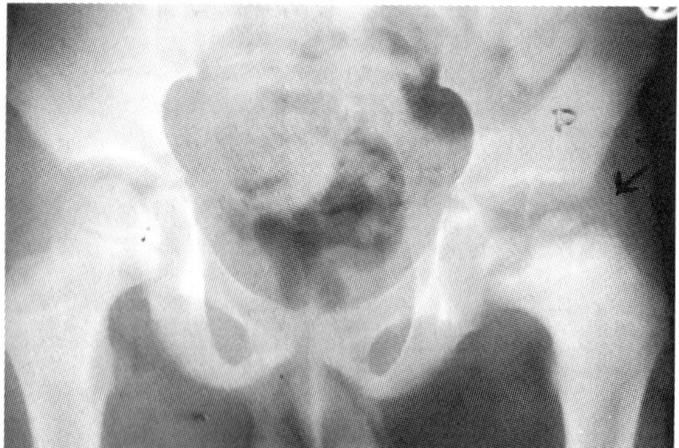

Fig. 12.50B: Perthes disease advanced stage

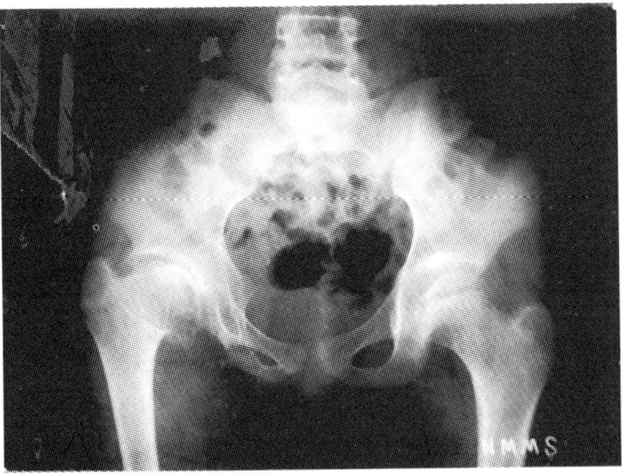

Fig. 12.50C: Slipped capital epiphysis of right hip

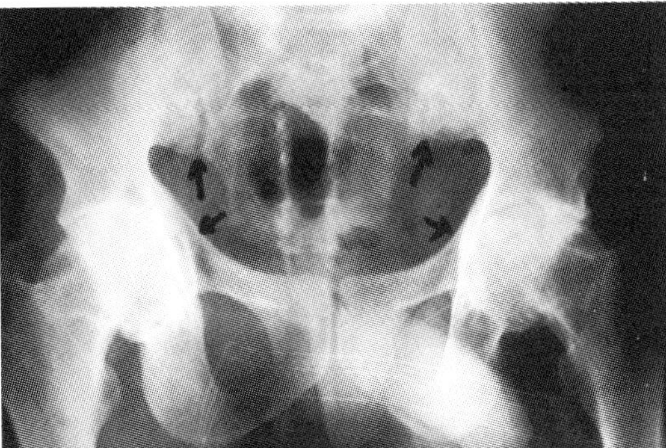

Fig. 12.51A: Prebony ankylosis stage of ankylosing spondylitis

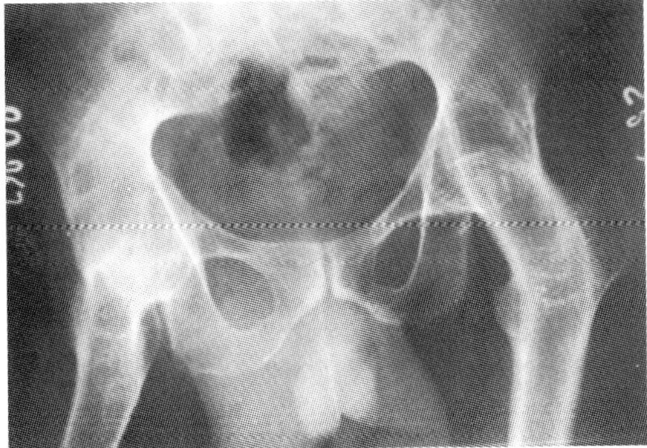

Fig. 12.51B: Ankylosing spondylitis with markedly advanced totally fused hips and sacroiliac joints

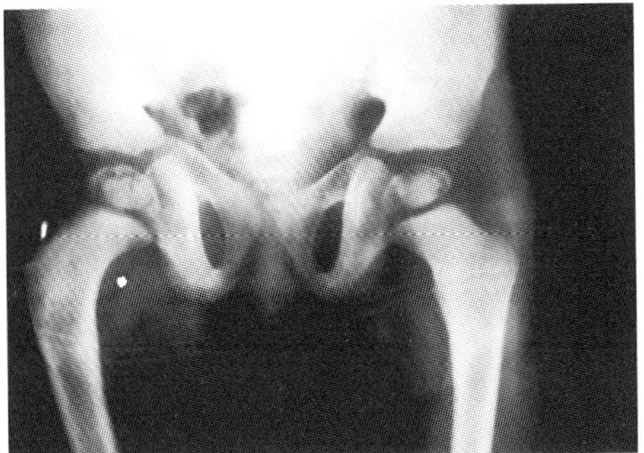

Fig. 12.52: A typical affection of hip in cretinism (note fragmentation of capital epiphysis)

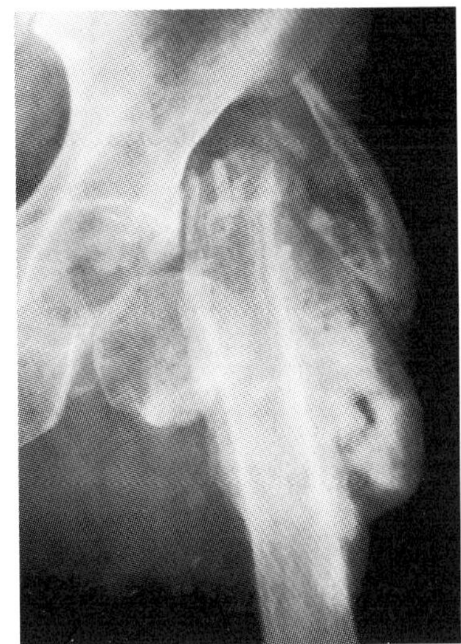

Fig. 12.53: Charcot s disease of hip

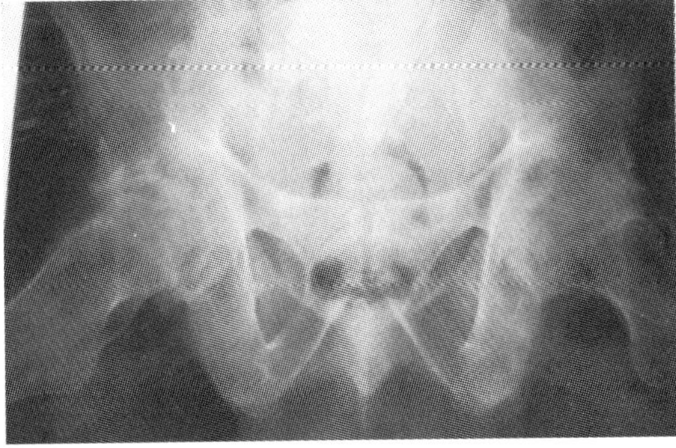

Fig. 12.54A Bilateral idiopathic avascular necrosis of hip joint (right more than left)

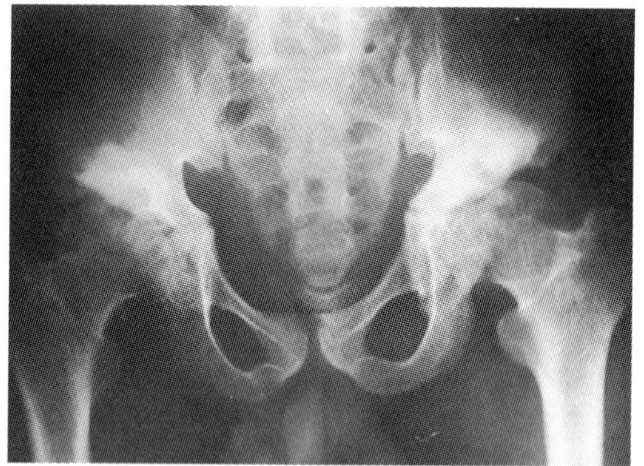

Fig. 12.54B: Bilateral avascular necrosis of femoral head in a chronic alcoholic

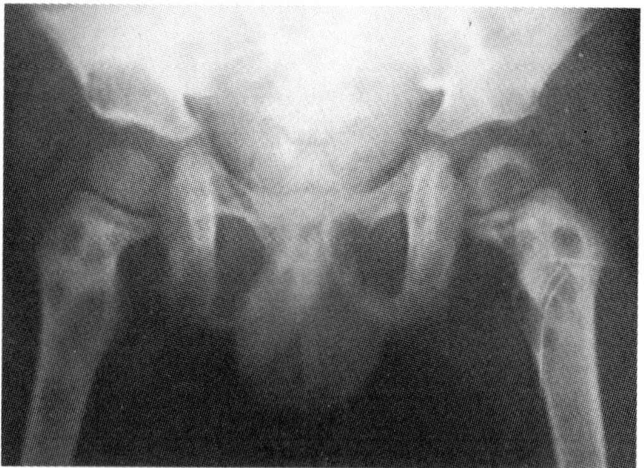

Fig. 12.54C: Sickle cell anaemia

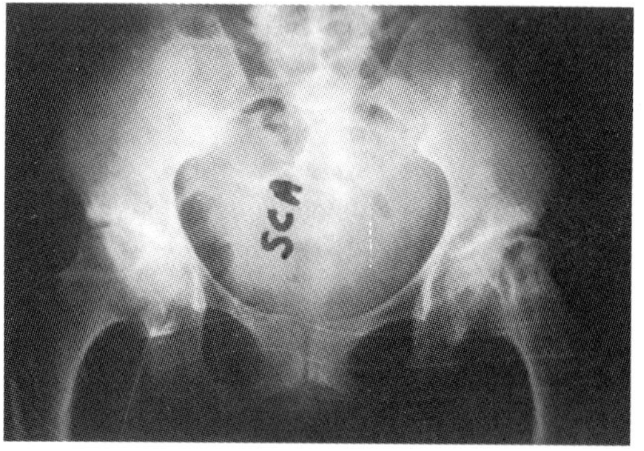

Fig. 12.54D: Sickle cell anaemia

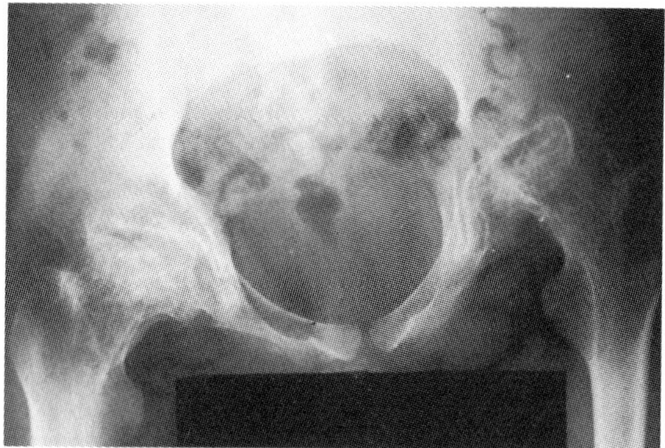

Fig. 12.54E: Bilateral avascular necrosis of femoral head with collapse (left more than right)

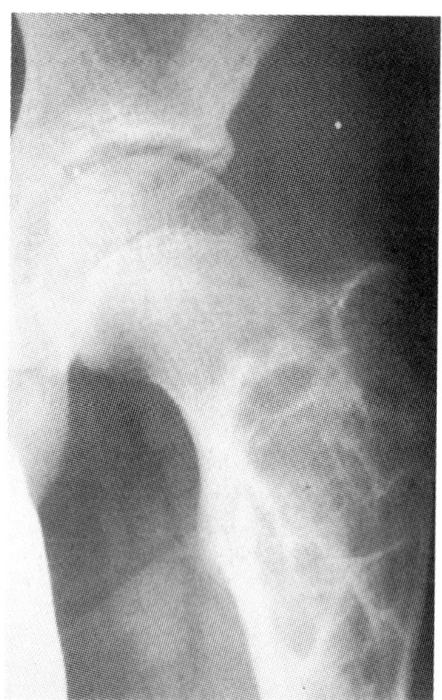

Fig. 12.55: Fibrous dysplasia of trochanter

V. Ultrasound

Presence of fluid inside the joint and unossified articular cartilage can be evaluated. It is important in case of septic arthritis in children.

Assessment of overall functions of the hip is essential in every case, and much more of the hip, which has been operated upon, especially

Table 12.8: Non-traumatic—differential diagnosis

	Congenital dislocation of hip (Fig. 12.45)	*Tuberculous hip (Figs 12.43A to 12.49)*	*Septic arthritis hip (Figs 12.47A to F)*	*Perthe's hip (Figs 12.50A to C)*	*Adolescent coxa vara (Fig. 12.50C)*	*Ankylosing spondylitis (Figs 12.51A and B)*	*Rheumatoid hip*	*Degenerative arthrosis*	*Paralytic hip (Fig. 12.46)*
1	2	3	4	5	6	7	8	9	10
Age	Newborn	3-10 yrs age	Newborn to 5 ++ 5 to 15 +	5 to 10 yrs	10-16 yrs	18-30 yrs	25-35 yrs	Primary > 40 yrs Secondary > 20 yrs	1-4 or more yrs
Sex	Female > male	Male	Male = Female	Male > Female	Male > Female	Male > Female	Female > Male	Male > Female	Female > Male
Geographical distribution.	More in cold countries (Caucasions)	Third wo:ld	Third world	More in white race.	—	—	More in cold climate.	More in cold climate.	Third world
Presenting symptoms	Initially detected by doctor. May be other associated congenital deformities. Later on, waddling gait, still later on, pain in hip on exertion.	Limp, pain, deformity, abscess, sinus, constitutional features, stiffness limb length disparity (LLD) +	Constitutional features, pain, swelling, spasm, local inflammatory features, deformity, stiffness LLD ++	Limp after exertion, vague pain, stiffness. LLD ±	Pain, limp, LLD ±	Pain, stiffness, limp	Pain, limp.	Pain after rest, stiffness gradual limp.	Weakness, deformity, LLD
Salient features	Trendelenburg's test +, gluteal fold asymmetry, Ortolani's and Barlow's +, painless movements, abduction in flexion limited to varying extent, adduction excessive, telescopic test positive, Galeazzi's test positive	Spasm + all movements restricted. Typical attitude— *Synovitis stage— flexion, abduction, external rotation, *Arthritis stage — flexion, adduction, internal rotation. Later on flexion, adduction, internal rotation +, pseudo—dislocation. (if patient has been walking— abduction instead of adduction)	In collection stage, initially-flexion, abduction, external rotation. Later on flexion, adduction, internal rotation. All movements restricted. Thickening and tenderness in trochanteric or ileal region	85% unilateral. Abduction and internal rotation limited. Abduction in flexion limited, antalgic gait	Abduction and internal rotation limited. External rotation and adduction may be excessive. Gradually, fixed adduction and external rotation deformities. Trendelenburg's test/gait.	Mostly bilateral affection, marked stiffness. Ankylosis develops in flexion, external rotation and abduction (mostly due to posture)	Flexion, adduction and internal rotation limited.	Initially limited extension, abduction and external rotation, later on, all movements may be restricted	Hypermobility, gross wasting
Investigations: a. X-ray: Both hips must be X-rayed in as much comparative position as possible	Up to 6 months—no diagnostic X-rays picture. Dysplastic feature, shallow acetabulum, capital epiphysis up and out, Shenton's arc broken (Fig. 12.45)	General rarefaction. Localised destruction, reduction in joint space, wandering acetabulum, sequestration. (Figs 12.43 and 12.49)	Soft tissues shadow, osteomyelitic changes in adjacent ileum or trochanter, bone formation, bone destruction, sequestrum, pathological dislocation, damage of capital epiphysis (Fig. 12.47).	In early stage, head-socket distance increased. Flattening, fragmentation and mushrooming of femoral head. Broadening of neck. Areas of avascular necrosis in denser areas. X-ray must be taken in full abduction and internal rotation to see the containment (Fig. 12.50)	Posteroinferior slipping of capital epiphysis, neck shaft angle reduced	Reduced joint space, condensation at joint margin, tendency of cross trabeculation, associated sacroiliac ankylosis (Fig. 12.51)	Marked osteoporosis, thinning of cortex, later on—joint space reduction, subchondral cysts, tendency of ankylosis	Reduction in joint, space, subchondral osteophytes, subarticular sclerosis	Osteoporotic and thin bone, dislocation/subluxation, push-pull films can detect abnormal excursion of head

Contd.

Table 12.8: Contd.

	Congenital dislocation of hip (Fig. 12.45)	*Tuberculous hip (Fig. 12.48A to 12.49)*	*Septic arthritis hip (Fig. 12.47A to E)*	*Perthes hip (Figs 12.50A to C)*	*Adolescent coxa vara (Fig. 12.50C)*	*Ankylosing spondylitis (Fig. 12.51)*	*Rheumatoid hip*	*Degenerative arthrosis*	*Paralytic hip (Fig. 12.46)*
1	2	3	4	5	6	7	8	9	10
b. Blood and others	Nothing particular	ESR raised lymphocytosis	Total WBC count increased, polymorph count markedly raised Aspiration of pus from joint	Nothing particular	Nothing particular	ESR raised, Rose-Waaler negative HLA B 27 antigen present	Rose-Waaler positive.	Nothing particular	Nothing particular
Classification	1. Dysplasia 2. Congenital subluxation 3. Congenital dislocation	Earlier classification of staging of tuberculosis hip is more academic rather than practical. —Stage of synovitis —Stage of arthritis —Arthritis with gross destruction and pathological dislocation	Stage of —Collection in joint (exudate + pus) —Sequestration of capital epiphysis. —Pathological dislocation —Ankylosis	Catterall's radiological classification based on area of epiphyseal involvement, its collapse and metaphyseal reaction—into four grades—is most popular	— —	— —	— —	—Primary (Idiopathic) —Secondary to • trauma • infection • Perthes' disease • coxa vara • osteonecrosis in adults • Obesity	—Subluxation —Dislocation
Management—	Conservative 1. —Splints (Harnesses, e.g. von-Rosen's splint), 2. Reduction and plaster in 60° abduction Operation on pelvis—acetabuloplasty, pelvic osteotomy —On upper shaft-osteotomy, total hip replacement.	Conservative: General rest, local rest by POP, splint, traction. Chemotherapy. Operative: Excision, excision-arthrodesis. Later on may go for total hip replacement after 5 to 10 years of complete quiescence.	Conservative: Rest, antibiotics, aspiration Operative: Drainage, excision	Conservative: Splint, POP (Broom stick type), physiotherapy, traction, Operative; Adduction osteotomy of femur/pelvic osteotomy. Later on abduction osteotomy of femur, total hip replacement (THR)	Conservative: closed reduction and POP. Operative: open reduction + internal fixation; later on abduction osteotomy THR	Conservative: Physiotherapy, analgesics, corticosteroids, deep X-ray Operative: Girdlestone arthroplasty, total hip replacement (THR) Corrective high femoral osteotomy	Conservative: Analgesic, (NSAID), Corticosteroid, goldsalts, heat therapy, physiotherapy, rest by traction Operative: Synovectomy, cup arthroplasty, THR	Conservative: Stick support, Physiotherapy, analgesics, postural adjustments. Operative: Abduction displacement type osteotomy of femur, THR, Girdlestone arthroplasty	Conservative: Physiotherapy, Orthotics Operative: Tendon transfer to improve stability, osteotomy, arthrodesis

NB. In children the criteria for treatment should be based on measurements on both ultrasound and radiography; both should show abnormality before intervention is considered necessary.

* Neoplasms in and around hip region manifest in bizzare fashion, depending upon the site of onset, nature of neoplasm and aggressiveness of the growth. Presenting features are mainly pain and limp. Later on, pathological fractures, swelling, deformities,.

• Certain rare but typical photographs: Figs 12.52, 12.53 and 12.54) after total hip replacement. For this purpose Table 12.3 (based on Harris hip function scale) is useful.

BIBLIOGRAPHY

1. Chung SMK: The arterial supply of developing proximal end of the human femur. *J Bone Joint Surg* **58A**: 1961, 1976.
2. Fahey JJ, O Brien, ET: Acute slipped femoral epiphysis. *J Bone Joint Surg* **47A**: 1105, 1965.
3. Green WB: Treatment of hip and knee problems in myelomeningocele. *J Bone Joint Surg* **80-A**: 1068-82, 1998.
4. Handerson RS: Traumatic anterior dislocation of the hip. *J Bone Joint Surg* 338-602.
5. Harris WH: *J Bone Joint Surg* **51**: 737-55, 1969.
6. Harty M: Anatomy of the hip joint. In Tronzo RG (Ed): *Surgery of the Hip Joint* Lea Febrger: Philadelphia, 1973.
7. Trendelenburg F: *Dtsh Med Wochenscher* **21**: 21, 1895.
8. Trueta J: Normal anatomy of human femoral head and its clinical importance. *J Bone Joint Surg* **318**: 82, 1965.
9. Vasudevan PN, Vaidyalingam KV, Bhaskaran Nair: Can Trendelenburg's sign be positive if the hip is normal? *J Bone Joint Surg* (Br) **79B**: 462-66, 1997.

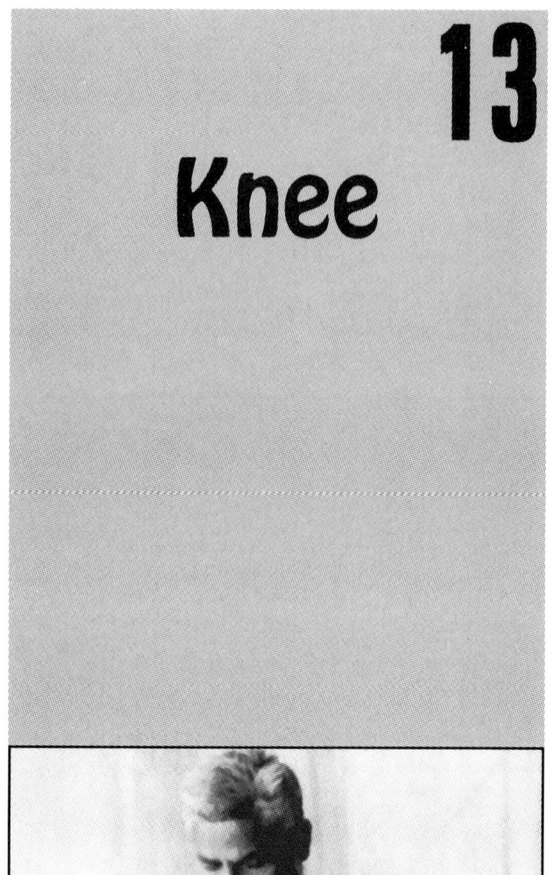

13 Knee

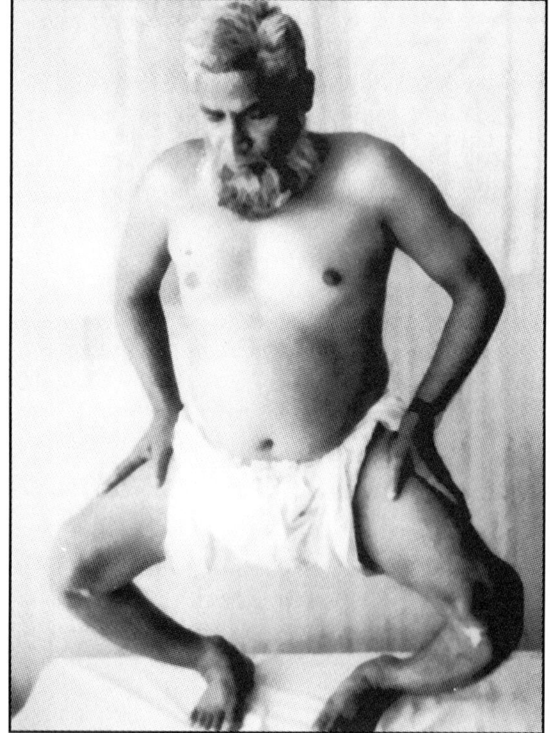

INTRODUCTION

Evolutionwise the basic characteristics of the human knee were present almost 300 million years ago. Broadly the knee is a triaxial joint having three sets of interrelated articulations, i.e. tibiofemoral , patellofemoral and upper tibio-fibular.

The knee, being one of the most exposed joints, is much more vulnerable to trauma and disease, specially in sports activities. With the advancements in the sports medicine, the knees are becoming more and more important. Accurate clinical diagnosis is essential to provide an adequate base for arthroscopic surgery, which plays a major role in the management of the lesions of the knee.

ANATOMICAL CONSIDERATIONS

1. It is a complex synovial joint, in which fibro-cartilaginous menisci are present. It is mainly comprised of: (i) femorotibial compartments (lateral and medial which are separated by vertical fibroligamentous structures attached to the intercondylar eminence of the tibia and the intercondylar notch of the femur), and (ii) patellofemoral compartment.

2. The synovial reflections of the joint are quite extensive and complicated. Therefore, (i) any synovial affection can remain synovial for a pretty long time before invading the articular components, (ii) most of the pathologies of the knee joint first manifest either as synovial swelling or as a swelling produced from synovial secretions, (iii) diseases which have more predilection for synovial affection are much more common in this joint.

3. The articular surfaces are so oriented that their adaptations are vulnerable in any horizontal and/or rotatory stress, i.e. abduction, adduction, anteroposterior or rotatory stresses.

4. Except posteriorly, the joint is quite superficial in its other aspects.

5. The integrity of the joint is dependent mainly on the ligaments and muscles in and around the knee joint.

6. There is no other joint in the body which contains so much of intra-articular ligaments or cartilaginous structures and bony prominences as the knee joint. Therefore, internal derangements of the knee joint are quite common.

7. There is no other joint which is associated with such a big sesamoid bone, i.e. patella, which subserves several important functions—(i) it acts as a natural knee cap protecting the joint proper from direct external violence, (ii) it acts as a buffer to the violent quadriceps contractions, (iii) acting on a pulley like mechanism, it augments the action of the quadriceps apparatus, transmitting the forceful quadriceps contractions to tibial tuberosity through the ligamentum patellae, (iv) It prevents unwarranted friction of the quadriceps tendon over the femoral condyle thereby mechanically easing the quadriceps mechanism, (v) It aids in the nourishment of the articular surface of the femur, (vi) Patients after total patellectomy feel difficulty in suddenly getting up from a fully crouched position, perhaps due to comparative diminution in the power of extension (from a fully flexed position). This indicates the importance of the patella.

The blood supply of patella is from patellar plexus formed by the branches of superior, medial and inferior geniculate arteries.

8. The vestigial synovial folds can be a cause of internal derangement of the knee joint, like impingement of the infrapatellar pad of fat even with a trivial injury.

9. Being superficial, even any insignificant prick can lead to severe infective arthritis of the joint.

10. *Movements:* From the stability point of view, the knee joint has been allowed only one axial movement, i.e. flexion and extension. Rather, it should be taken as only one movement, i.e. flexion from zero degree anatomical position of full extension. However the kinematics in the human knee encompass much more than flexion and extension, the important one being medial pivoting kinematics. Therefore, from trauma point of view, rotational stresses on the knee joint produce more damage. The anatomically provided checks do not allow the leg component to go beyond the zero position and are probably not strong enough to withstand moderate to severe rotational strains (e.g. in missing a step or while running or playing).

11. The main neurovascular bundle of the leg and foot lies in close vicinity of the posterior capsule of the knee joint. Hence, it is quite vulnerable to certain types of injuries around the knee (specially dislocations of the knee joint and displaced supracondylar fractures). However, extensive collateral network around the knee may make it possible to obliterate the popliteal artery without jeopardising the circulation of distal portion of the extremity. Therefore, it is imperative to assess the integrity of these vital structures in affections of the knee joint.

12. Whatever may be the pathology, traumatic or cold, the methodology of examination remains the same. However, in traumatic cases, more importance should be given to stress-integrity of the knee joint, while in cold cases, the condition of the articular components is more important.

13. *Consideration of Bursae Around the Joint*: These are situated in between the tendons and the coverings of the joints. They are quite often affected by pathologies, varying right from non-specific to malignant neoplastic conditions. In these conditions, the patient presents with knee complaints.

14. Menisci: Menisci, the wedge shaped fibrocartilaginous structures lie in the outer region of the tibiofemoral component of the knee joint. They are anchored at their ends firmly to the slopes of the tibial spine, attached to the upper end of tibia by the coronary ligaments, and have their inner margins free. The range of excursion of medial meniscus is less than that of the lateral, hence it is more vulnerable to rotational strains.

The internal structure of both menisci is primarily collagen with a small amount of proteoglycan.

The blood supply of the medial and lateral menisci is from the medial and lateral genicular arteries.

Earlier, when the functions of the menisci were not fully studied, they were considered by the anatomists as fillers of the vacant joint space, and as working for spreading of the synovial fluid in between the articular surfaces. With these considerations in mind, the treatment of meniscus tear was excision at the earliest. Therefore, even on clinical suspicion, meniscectomy was done as a routine. Now, the functions of menisci in human being have been very well studied. Besides the aforesaid functions, other functions are:

i. by virtue of its location, it prevents synovial and capsular impingement during flexion extension movement,
ii. helps in stabilising the joint in all planes, especially during rotatory strains,
iii. about 50% of the insignificant weight bearing or load transmitting forces are carried by the menisci.
iv. mechanically, it deepens the tibial condylar surface.
v. acts as shock absorber.

Thus, based on better understanding of functions of the menisci, and supported by the arthrographic and arthroscopic findings, now the aim is to save and repair the torn menisci than to excise it.

15. The long axis of the thigh and leg (i.e. femorotibial angle) are not in the same line, rather, the leg axis is placed at 7° ± 3° valgus to the thigh axis. The thigh axis is placed at an angle of 81° on the outer side over the horizontal line, whereas the leg axis makes an angle of 87° over the horizontal knee axis on the inner side (Fig. 13.1).

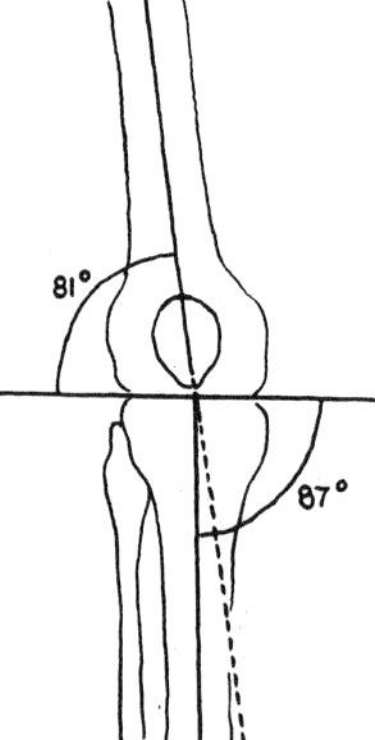

Fig. 13.1: Showing normal longitudinal axis of femur and tibia (femorotibial angle)

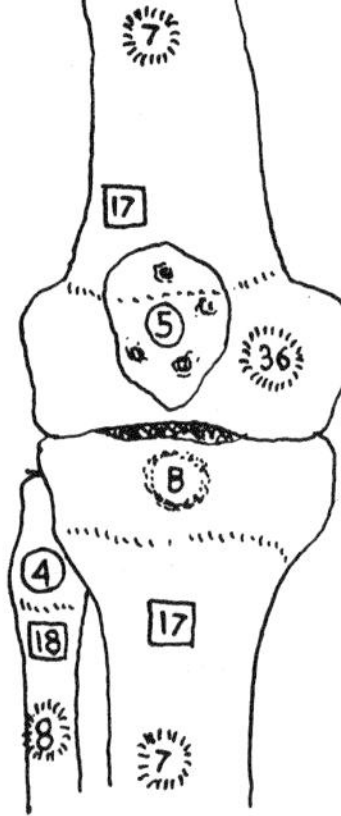

Fig. 13.2: Ossification around the knee. Dotted circle primary centre in weeks IUL. Complete circle secondary centres in year. Square fusion in years. B at birth

Ossification around knee joint (Fig. 13.2) (Table 13.1)

METHODOLOGY

1. History Taking

Usual complaints in case of knee pathologies are pain, swelling, limitation of movements (usually painful) and deformity. Though history taking will be as usual, however, certain factors should be particularly ascertained. In recurrent swellings of the knee in a child, history of bleeding from gums and any increase in duration

Table 13.1: Ossification around the knee

Bone	*Primary for shaft*	*Secondary*	*Unites with shaft*
Tibia	7th week IUL	1. For the lower end, early in 1st year 2. For upper end, usually present at birth	15th year-female 16th year-male 16-18 years
Fibula	8th week IUL	1. For lower end 1st year 2. For upper end 3-4 years	17th year-male 15th year-female 19th year-male 17th year-female
Patella	Ossifies from several centres which appear at 3-6 years and quickly coalesce. Accessory marginal centres appear later and fuse with the central mass		
Femur	7th week IUL	Secondary centres -one each for head 3-6 months, greater trochanter-4th year, lesser trochanter-12-14th year. For the lower end at 9th months IUL	14-17th year 16th year-female 18th year-male

of bleeding due to any cut, if present, must be noted. In case of injury to the knee, the nature of violence, immediate effect of injury on the patient as a whole and the knee in particular should be noted. In older knee injuries, history of locking of joint, sense of 'giving way' at the knee on walking or running should be ascertained. Any other relevant point should be categorically noted.

2. General and Systemic Examinations

These should be done as in the chapter of Introduction. In case of pain or swelling of the knee joint, one must enquire about involvement of other joints, especially the smaller joints, because the knee is a common site for collagen arthropathy. Besides, any obvious generalised pathology and clinical manifestation must be noted.

3. Regional Examination

In regional examination, at least the hip and the ankle are to be examined, since the involvement of either can have an impact on the knee, thus confusing the clinical examination. However, it will be much informative and desirable if lumbosacral to foot region is examined in the purview of regional examination.

ANALYSIS OF KNEE COMPLAINTS DUE TO REGIONAL PATHOLOGY

Occasionally, the patient complains of pain in the knee, specially on the anteromedial aspect, though there is no pathology in the knee joint itself. This is the referred pain from the hip joint (especially where the superomedial aspect of femoral head is affected) through the anterior division of the obturator nerve which also supplies a twig to the hip joint.

In the sacroiliac affections, pain referred along the sciatic nerve, either due to sciatic radiculitis or fibro fatty nodules over the sacroiliac region, may be felt mainly at the back of the knee.

In ankle pathology or painful hindfoot syndrome, sometimes the patient complains of pain in the knee, specially in the anteromedial compartment. This is because, in these conditions, the patient wants to avoid weight on hindfoot, so the ankle and foot are put in equinus position, which automatically has an external rotational tendency of the knee joint. With continued effort in this posture, the knee is strained more and more, resulting in stretch pain sensation.

In spastics, spasm of the hamstrings gets an upper hand over the quadriceps. This sustained spasm leads to pain in the back of the knee joint. In the long run, degenerative changes manifest quite early in such a knee, leading to actual pain in the knee proper.

4. Local Examination

Prerequisites

1. Both the knees must be examined simultaneously for comparative study.
2. Pelvis to toes must be exposed.
3. Patient must be examined on a hard couch.
4. Examine the patient in walking, standing, sitting, squatting and lying down position (if possible). Observe gait from the side. Watch the attitude of the knee in full weight bearing and in the relaxed position.
5. While patient is sitting, attitude should be noted in as far as extended and flexed positions of the affected knee. The normal knee should be kept in identical position for comparison.

Attitude

While examining in lying down posture, supine position should be adopted. Back should be relaxed by resting it on the couch. Mark the attitude of the affected knee from the front and the side. Normal limb must be kept in identical position for comparison. In most of the cases with recent pathology or trauma, the joint is swollen all around, more so anteriorly, and assumes an attitude of about 30° flexion. In most of the chronic diseases, the knee goes for a peculiar deformity complex, i.e. triple deformity. Here in flexed position of the knee, the tibia subluxates posteriorly and laterally and also rotates laterally over the femoral condyle. Gradually, leg also goes in valgus. Thus, though it has been identified as "triple subluxation deformity," in its full form, actually it is a *"quadruple deformity complex"*. It is common in advanced tuberculosis and rheumatoid arthritis, but even postural contractures can produce such deformity and subluxation.

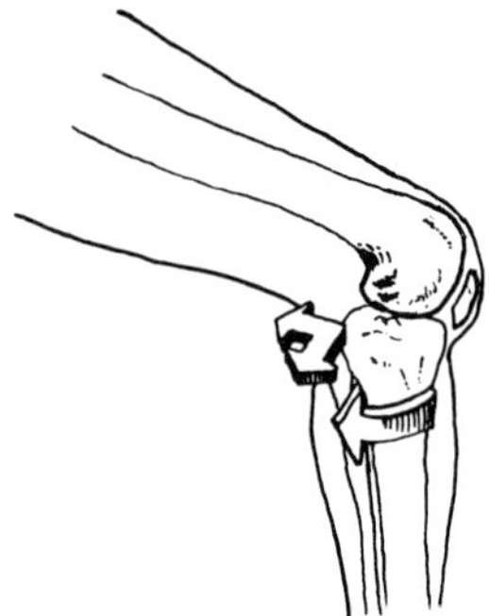

Fig. 13.3: Diagrammatic representation of the mechanism of triple deformity of the knee

Patho-dynamics of Triple Deformity
(Figs 13.3 and 13.4A and B)

The flexed attitude of the knee joint is a protective position and position of rest. Therefore, following any painful condition there is early tendency of spasm of the hamstring group of muscles. This position allows enough of posterior space in the knee joint for collection of blood or exudates. With constant flexed attitude of varying extent, the posterior capsule starts contracting. This flexion provides further mechanical advantage to the hamstrings, specially the biceps femoris and iliotibial band which now become important flexors of the joint. While lying down, the patient tries to keep the hip in external rotation, till the outer part of the knee rests on a support or the couch. In this position, gravity assisted contraction of the iliotibial band helps in outer subluxation of the tibiofibular component. Taking further mechanical advantage, the biceps femoris and iliotibial band further keep on contracting, the fibulotibial component therefore rotates laterally. These three conjoint and successive deformities are grouped together as triple deformity of the knee joint. Besides, the above deforming forces also pull the leg outwards, i.e. in valgus.

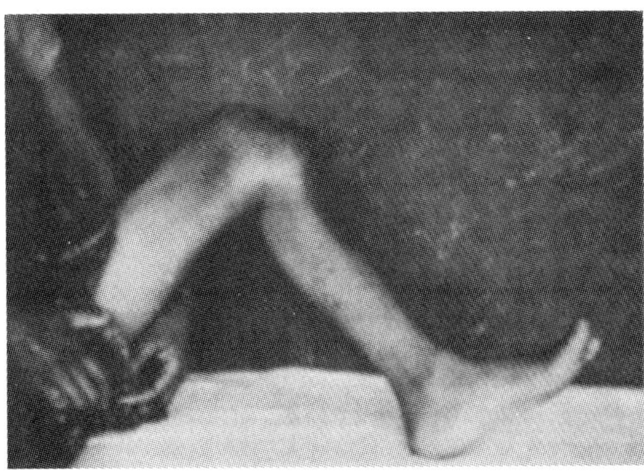

Fig. 13.4A: Triple deformity of knee joint showing flexion contracture of knee, in which tibia has subluxated posteriorly and rotated laterally

Clinical Assessment of Triple Deformity of Knee

In observing from the outer side, the flexion of knee will be obvious. Simultaneously comparing with the equally flexed normal knee, depression of the upper tibial end denotes posterior subluxation, which can be further confirmed by palpating the subluxated posterior upper end of the tibia through the popliteal fossa. In this position, the distal end of the condyles of femur are more prominent and more palpable anteriorly as compared to the other side (specially the medial one).

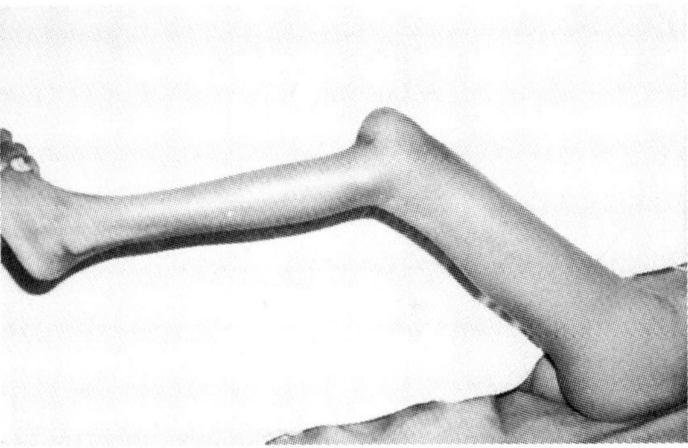

Fig. 13.4B: Triple deformity of knee joint showing flexion contracture of knee, in which tibia has subluxated posteriorly and rotated laterally with genu valgum

In case of outward subluxation of the upper end of tibia, observing from the front, the tibial tubercle will be placed more outward, the tibial shin will be aligned more outwards and the fibular head will be placed more posterolateraly. Valgus of the leg can be confirmed by measuring the outward drift of the medial malleolar tip from the midline.

Genu Valgum/Varum

Observe the alignment of the leg component to the thigh component. Normally, the mid inguinal point, centre of patella and mid ankle joint are in one line. If this line is prolonged

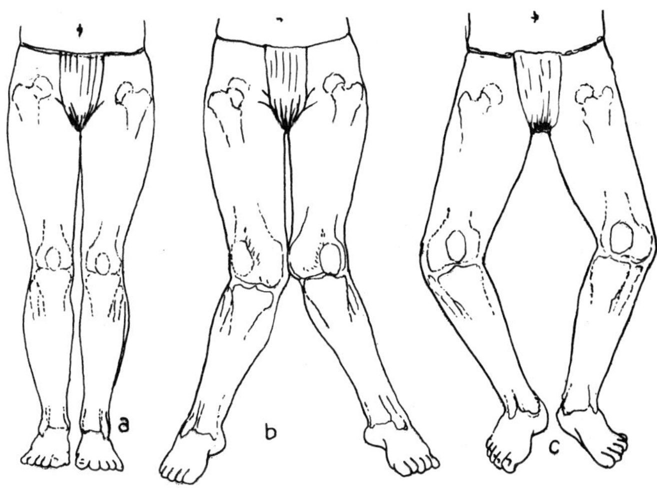

Fig. 13.5: (a) Normal alignment of thigh and leg; (b) Genu valgum; (c) Genu varum

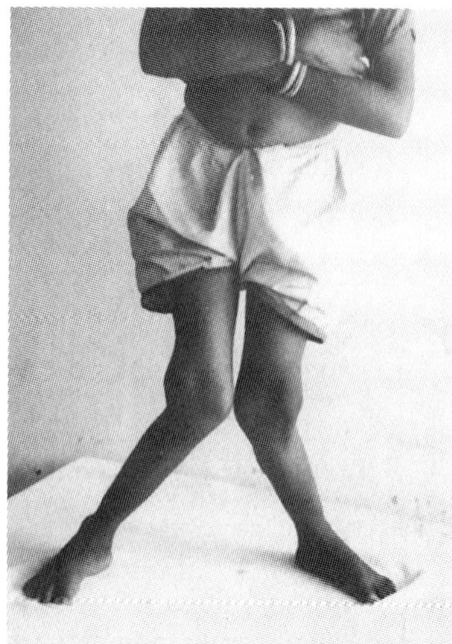

Fig. 13.6A: Photograph of rachitic bilateral marked genu valgum

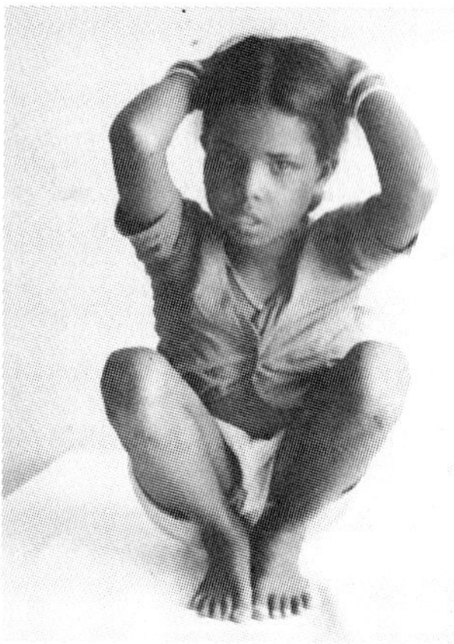

Fig. 13.6B: Same patient in squatting position. Note disappearance of genu valgum which indicates the seat of deformity at the lower femur

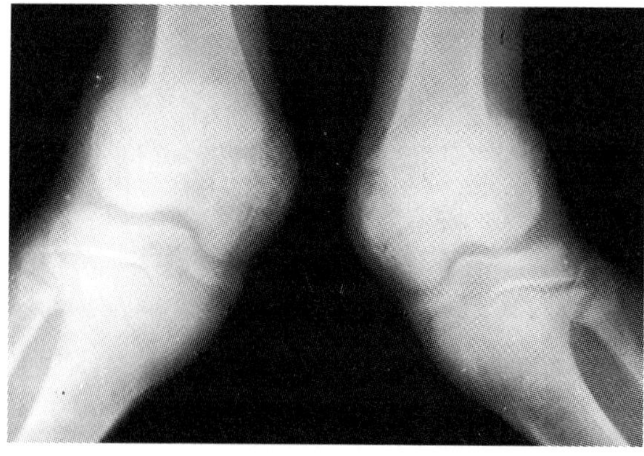

Fig. 13.6C: X-ray of both knees of same patient (Fig. 13.6A)

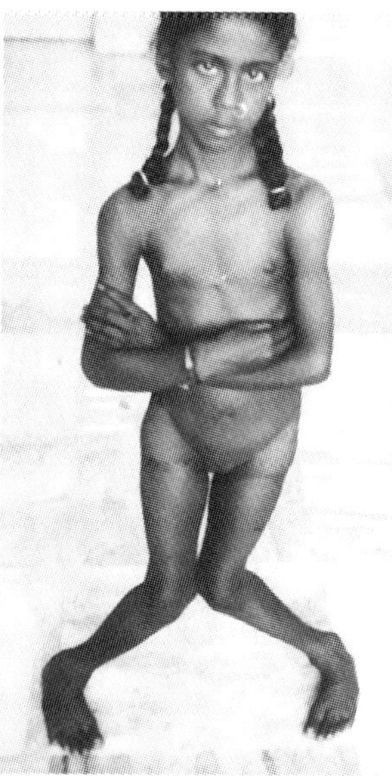

Fig. 13.6D: Rachitic bilateral genu valgum (advanced) with varus and toe in deformities of the feet (developed to catch the centre of gravity while standing and walking

to the foot, it should pass through the second web (Fig. 13.5a). Deviation of the leg axis (for all practical purposes from centre of the knee, i.e. centre of the patella) outwards is called valgus (Figs 13.5b, 13.6A to F) and inwards as varus (Figs 13.5c, 13.7A to G). This must be tested for in both lower limbs.

In the first 2 years of life some lateral bowing of tibia and some genu varum should be taken as normal. After the age of 2 years, genu valgum becomes apparent, which may even increase upto the age of 4 years. After that age genu valgum improves and should come to normal of about 7° at about the age of 8 years.

The physiological genu varum or valgum are bilateral.

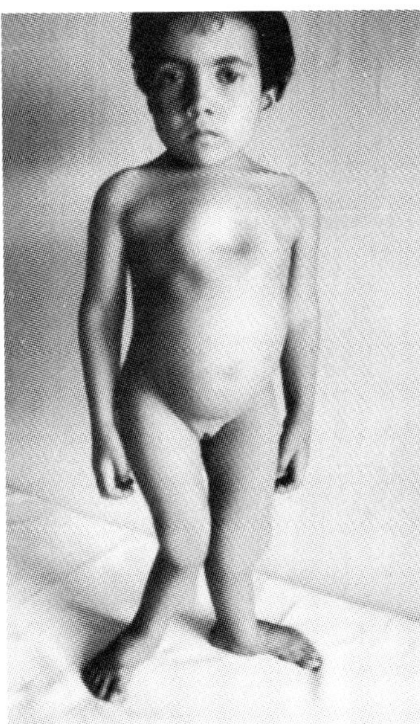

Fig. 13.6E: Bilateral rachitic genu valgum, valgus collapse in ankle region and early toe-in deformities of the feet. Note the associated deformity in the chest wall

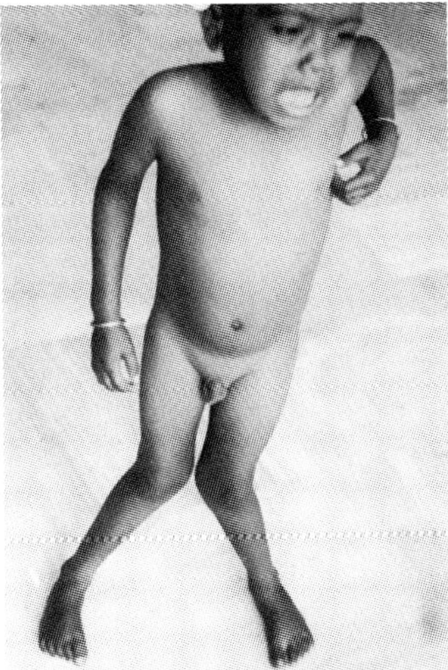

Fig. 13.6F: Bilateral idiopathic genu valgum

How to Assess Valgum or Varum

Patient sits at the edge of the couch with both legs extended. In neutral position of the limb, hold the ankles from behind. Try to approximate both malleoli so that they just touch each other. Normally, they must touch before the inner surfaces of the knees come together, rather, there should be on an average 0.5 cm gap between the medial surfaces of the two knees. If the gap is more, the deformity will be genu varum (bow knee). This is measured and expressed roughly as finger breadth (to be measured in centimeters) between the medial surfaces of the knees. For unilateral varus, the distance between the centre of the medial surface of the affected medial condyle and central plumb line of body is measured.

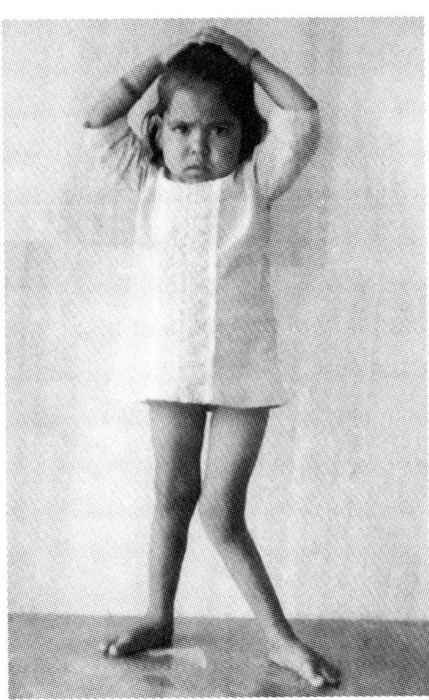

Fig. 13.6G: Genu valgum on left side following chronic osteomyelitis of lower end of femur and damage of outer portion of growth epiphysis. Note also the lengthening of femur

If the medial surfaces of the two knees touch each other before the medial malleoli can come together, the deformity will be called genu valgum (knock knee). Measure the distance between the two malleoli while medial surfaces of knee just touch each other, (do not force or cross the knee). This valgum deformity is expressed by finger breadths as the intermalleolar distance, or is measured in centimeters. In unilateral valgus deformity, the deviation of the medial malleolus from central plumb line will be measured.

Genu valgum and genu varum may be due to pathology in the lower femur and/or upper

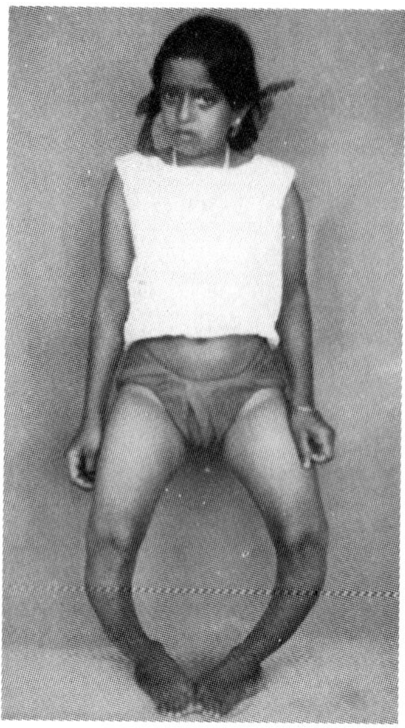

Fig. 13.7A: Bilateral rachitic genu varum (bow knee)

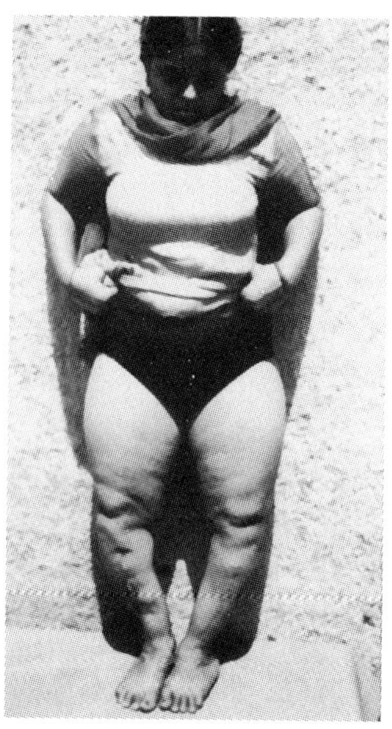

Fig. 13.7B: Same patient 14 years after surgical correction. Note the early recurrence of bowing of knees

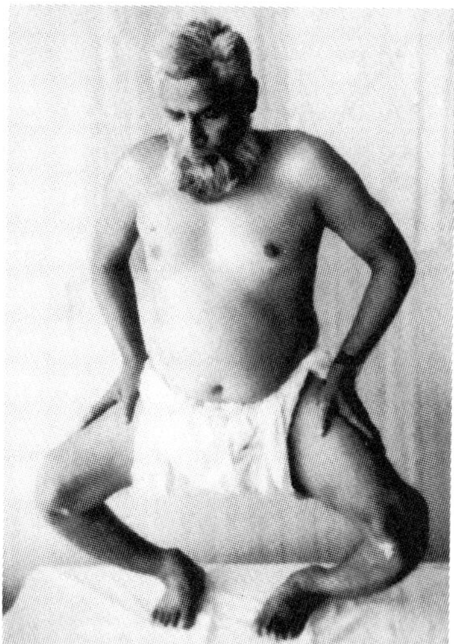

Fig. 13.7C: Photograph of advanced rachitic genu varum (bow knee + bow leg) (patient is standing). Note the secondary adaptive changes at ankles and feet

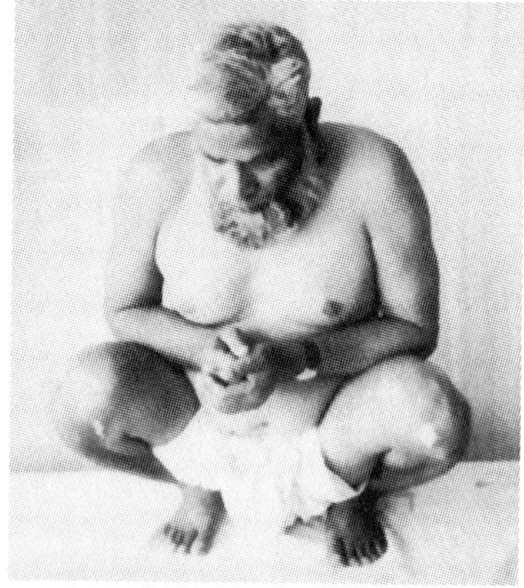

Fig. 13.7D: Same patient in squatting position genu varum partially disappeared, indicating seat of deformity both at upper tibia and lower femur

tibia. The contribution of each of the components can be assessed, by asking the patient to sit in squatting position. If the deformity completely disappears, the total fault lies in the lower femur. If it disappears partially or does not disappear—the fault will be in both components.

Fallacies of Genu Varum

a. Bow leg
b. Anteversion of femoral neck

a. *Bow leg:* Genu varum (bow-knee) can be confused with bow leg since the effect appears to be the same. However, genu varum is a deformity at the knee, while in bow leg, bones are at fault by producing an inwards concavity. Bow

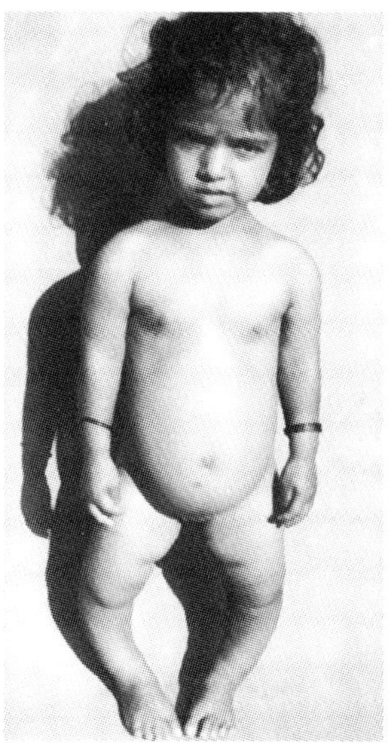
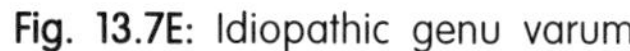

Fig. 13.7E: Idiopathic genu varum

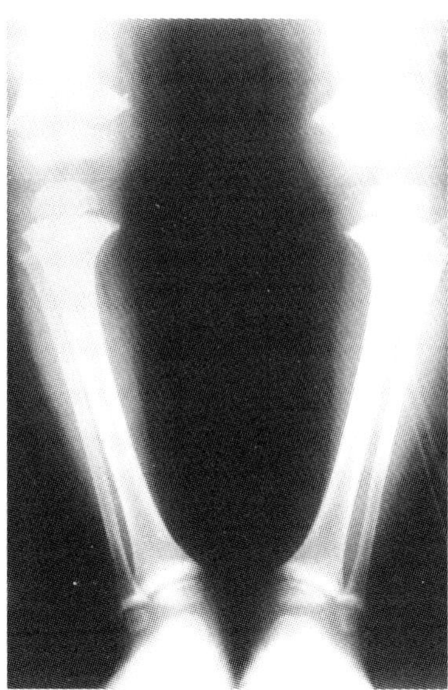

Fig. 13.7F: X-ray picture of idiopathic genu varum

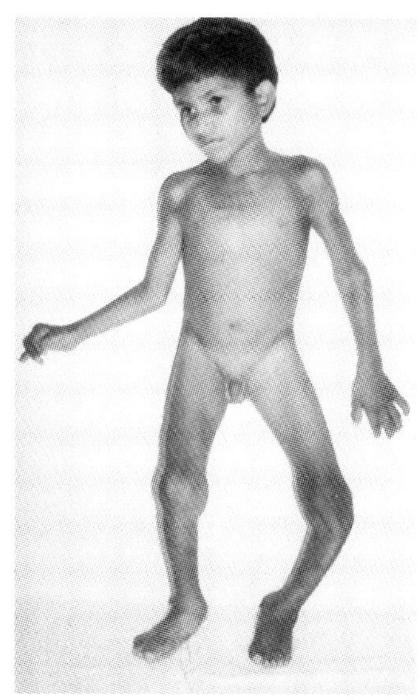

Fig. 13.7G: Marked genu varum on left side following old multifocal (left knee, left shoulder and right knee) septic arthritis

leg can be due to various causes: (i) Normally during infancy, (ii) congenital, (iii) idiopathic, (iv) traumatic—malunited fracture, (v) rachitic—bowing is at about distal third junction (see Fig. 2.5), (vi) syphilitic—sabre tibia, (vii) Paget's disease, (viii) pseudoarthrosis of tibia, (ix) degenerative arthrosis of knee joints—varus collapse, (x) osteogenesis imperfecta, (xi) dyschondroplasia, (xii) Blount's disease—infantile tibia vara (a rare condition mostly seen in black heavy weight children who walk early. Due to irregu larity of growth in the medial tibial epiphysis, there is tibia vara).

Bow leg can be differentiated from genu varum by the following method:

Drop a plumb line from the mid inguinal point. In genu varum, the knee lies outward to this line, whereas in bow leg this line passes through almost the centre of the knee joint.

b. *Anteversion of femoral neck*: The angle between the plane of femoral neck and femoral transcondylar plane is about 40° at birth, and decreases to 10-20° at the maturity. Persistance of increased femoral anteversion leads to internal rotation of the whole leg.

Clinically the range of internal rotation of the extended hips will be greater than the external rotation.

In the opposite deformity, i.e. femoral retroversion there will be preponderance of external rotation over the internal rotation.

Femoral retroversion usually gets corrected automatically by the age of 3 years. However it may persist due to faulty sitting and sleeping postures.

Anteversion of femoral neck can produce the apparent effect of genu varum. While the patient lies supine, the patella is made to face upwards. If in this position genu varum disappears, it indicates anteversion of the femoral neck.

Genu recurvatum deformity: In standing position, a normal knee is straight, i.e. in zero degree vertical pendulum position. In genu recurvatum, it buckles back, i.e. popliteal fossa becomes convex (instead of it being normally concave, because the knee gets recurved in the opposite direction, which is normally not possible), (Figs 13.8A to D). For all practical purposes, it can be measured from zero degree of extension. However, allowance must be given for the normally possible hyperextension of the knee in certain individuals (in which case the other knee will also be the same). It can be measured in the weight bearing position of the limb from the lateral side. The long axis of thigh (tip of trochanter to centre of the lateral surface of lateral femoral condyle) and the long axis of the leg [tip of head of fibula to lateral mid point of ankle, i.e. tip of lateral malleolus (for all practical

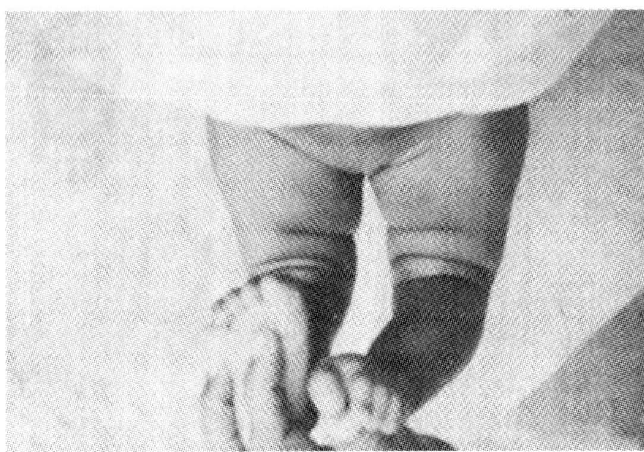

Fig. 13.8A: Bilateral genu recurvatum due to congenital quadriceps contracture

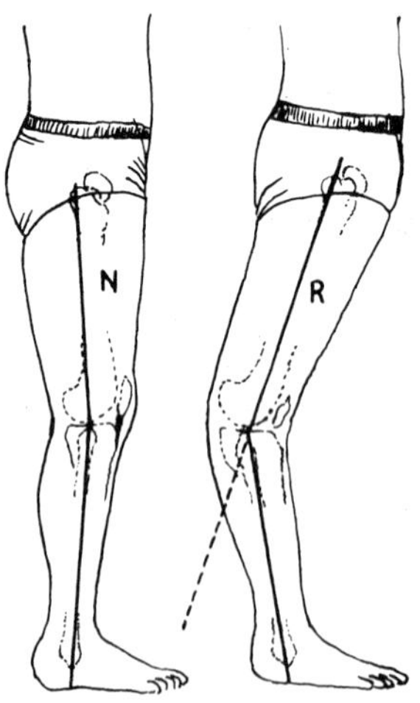

Fig. 13.8B: The axis of leg and thigh are cutting much posteriorly rather than having an anterior inclination in a normal limb. N = normal, R = genu recurvatum

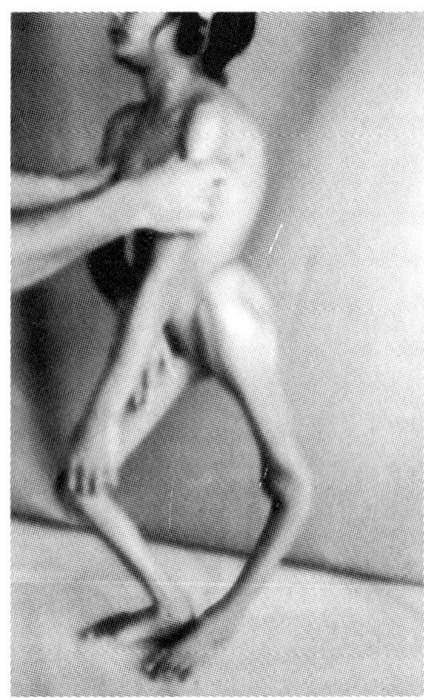

Fig. 13.8C: Unilateral (left) genu recurvatum following polio paralysis

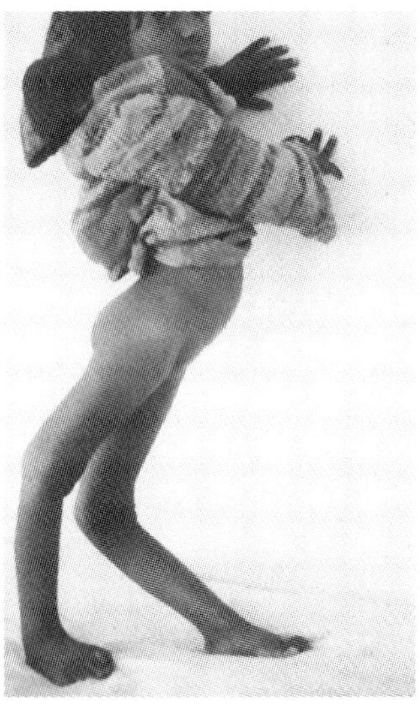

Fig. 13.8D: Bilateral genu recurvatum following polio-paralysis. In such cases hyperextension of hips and calcaneous at ankle-heel level develops

purposes) should be in same line. In genu recurvatum, the long axis of the leg will drift anteriorly and will make an angle with the thigh axis at the knee level (Fig. 13.8B). The supero-inferior angles (which will be equal), will be angle of genu recurvatum.

Inspection

Inspect both knees simultaneously from the front, the sides and from behind (Fig. 13.9).

From the front (Fig. 13.9i): Mark the normal contour, i.e. quadriceps prominence/bulge; position, shape and size of patella; patellar ligament; supra- and infra-patellar fossae; anterolateral and anteromedial tibial flares; tibial tubercle and shin of tibia. Any skin changes, swelling and sinus, if present, should be examined as in the chapter of Introduction.

From the side (Fig. 13.9ii): Watch for normal contour, i.e. vastus lateralis bulge, tight sloping of ilio-tibial band, bulge of biceps femoris, fibular neck depression and normal bulge of the leg. Any abnormal shift and/or prominence of fibular head must be noted.

From behind (Fig. 13.9iii): Usually, pathology in and around the knee manifests with some degree of flexion of the knee joint. In that case, ask the patient to comfortably extend the knee joint without altering the position of the hip and spine. Mark the residual angle of flexion at the knee joint. It is better to express or measure the amount of flexion from zero position of extension. Note the contour of back of thigh, supra popliteal slope, popliteal fossa flanked on both sides by the prominent hamstrings (biceps femoris on the outer side, accentuated by the iliotibial band; and semimembranosus and semitendinosus on the medial side accentuated by the gracilis and more anteriorly by the sartorius). In the lower part of the floor of the popliteal fossa and upper part of the leg, the gradual bulge produced by the popliteus, gastrocnemius and soleus muscles, in that order, is marked. Look for any varicosity, any pulsation or any other abnormality. Any

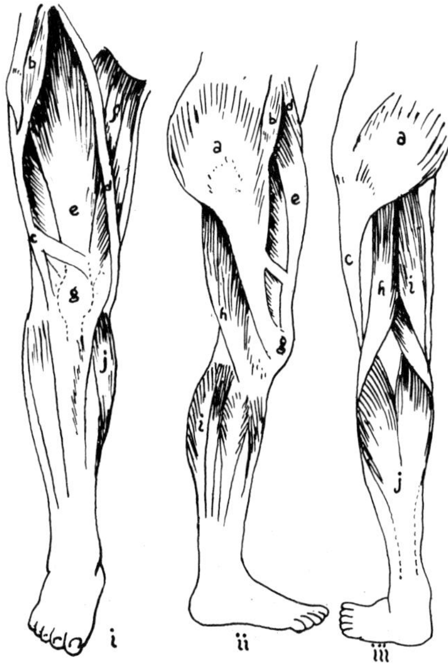

Fig. 13.9: Contour of the limb around, above and below the knee (i) from front, (ii) from side, (iii) from back. a = gluteus maximus, b = tensor fascia femoris, c = iliotibial tract, d = sartorius, e = quadriceps, f = adductors, g = patella, h = biceps femoris, i = medial hamstrings, j = gastroc-soleus

collection in the knee joint or pathology of the posterior part of knee presents with obliteration of the popliteal fossa.

Baker s Cyst

Baker's cyst (a synovial pouch communicating with the knee joint usually through a flap-valve mechanism) appears as the median posterior swelling in the popliteal fossa. Semimembranosus cyst occurs on the more medial side.

Palpation

This should be done from anterior aspect, sides and back (as in inspection).

i. *Superficial palpation:* Note the temperature, skin surface, sensitivity and elasticity of skin, any subcutaneous adhesions, pliability of subcutaneous layer and any superficial tenderness. If there is any swelling or sinus, these should be examined, as in chapter of Introduction.

ii. *Deep palpation*: Mainly concentrate on palpating the (1) Structures surrounding the joint, i.e. soft tissues, (2) Bony components of the joint, (3) Joint line and articular surfaces as far as possible.

Palpation of Soft Tissue

Palpate muscles, tendons, ligaments, capsule, synovial tissue, peripheral nerves and blood vessels in the vicinity.

Muscles and tendons: Note the tone, texture, pliability of quadriceps muscle, quadriceps tendon and ligamentum patellae upto its attachment to tibial tuberosity, and the continuity of quadriceps apparatus. On the two sides, palpate vastus medialis bulge upto adductor tubercle anteromedially, and vastus lateralis merging into quadriceps expansion antero-laterally. Posterolaterally, palpate the iliotibial band, specially from the point of view of its tightness, and behind it, the biceps femoris upto its attachment into the fibular head region. On the posteromedial aspect, the semi-membranosus and semitendinosus should be assessed by asking the patient to flex the knee against resistance.

Palpate the quadriceps expansion on both sides of the patella and ligamentum patellae. Suprapatellar bulge can be due to synovial thickening and/or fluid. Synovial thickening, if present (doughy or earthworms-in-a-bag feel) may be palpated in the infrapatellar and suprapatellar fossae. Palpate on both sides to ascertain the continuity, thickening and any tenderness of the collateral ligaments. Palpate for some irregular or regular bony mass at the upper attachment of medial collateral ligament (Pellegrini Stieda disease). Posteriorly, it is difficult to feel any synovial thickening because it lies quite deep. In the popliteal fossa, especially palpate the popliteal artery pulsation, any glandular enlargement or any cyst (Morrant Baker's cyst). Lateral popliteal nerve should be palpated by rolling it against the neck of the fibula and note for any tenderness, thickening or beading.

Palpation of the joint line: The knee joint line (both on the lateral and medial side) should be palpated for its sharpness, any tenderness, presence of any cyst (usually attached to the meniscus) or synovial thickening. Sometimes the torn part of the meniscus may be felt as a firm, tender, irregular mass. Upper tibiofibular joint should also be palpated for any capsular and/or synovial thickening and tenderness (at times tuberculosis or any of the synovial neoplasms have been seen to specifically arise in this area). The capsule of the knee joint is mostly blended with the quadriceps expansion, collateral and other enforcing ligaments, hence palpation of the above mentioned structures will amount to palpation of the capsule in that zone.

Palpation of the articular surfaces: Most of the articular surfaces are not palpable. However, the margins can be well palpated and thus can provide an idea about any existing pathology.

Bony Palpation

It should be done on both the non-articular, as well as the articular parts of the participating bones. Note for normal congruity, presence of any abnormal knob like or irregular swellings and any tenderness, starting from the patella, medial femoral condyle, medial tibial condyle, lateral femoral condyle, lateral tibial condyle, fibular head and neck and tibial tuberosity.

Patella: Extend the supported knee and ask the patient to relax the quadriceps. Now, holding the patella from the side, push it to the other side. Maintaining this position, the opposite index finger can palpate the articular surface to a variable extent. Reverse the direction of push and repeat the palpation on the other side of the articular surface (Fig. 13.10).

Femoral condyles: Anteroinfero-lateral and antero-infero-medial portion of the articular surfaces of the femur can be palpated while gradually flexing the knee to the fullest possible extent (Fig. 13.11).

Tibial condyle: Articular surfaces of the tibial condyles can usually be palpated anterolaterally

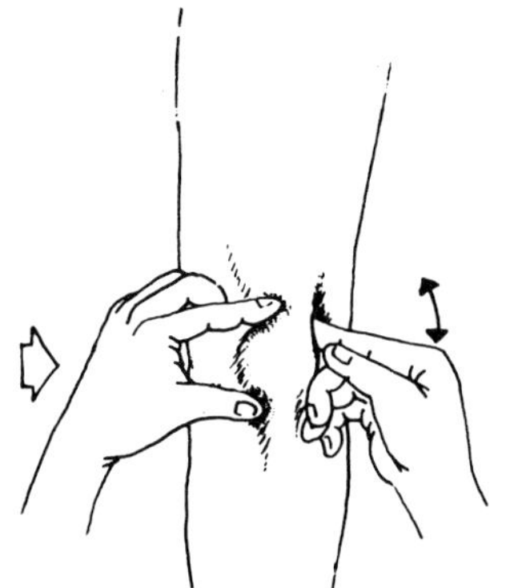

Fig. 13.10: Palpation of under surface of patella (articular surface)

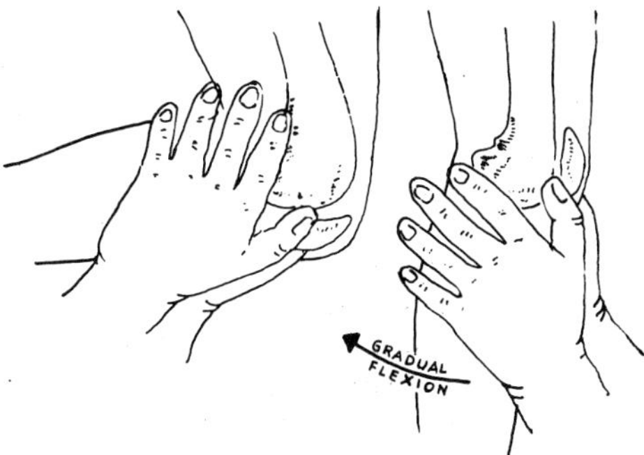

Fig. 13.11: Palpation of accessible articular surface of femoral condyles

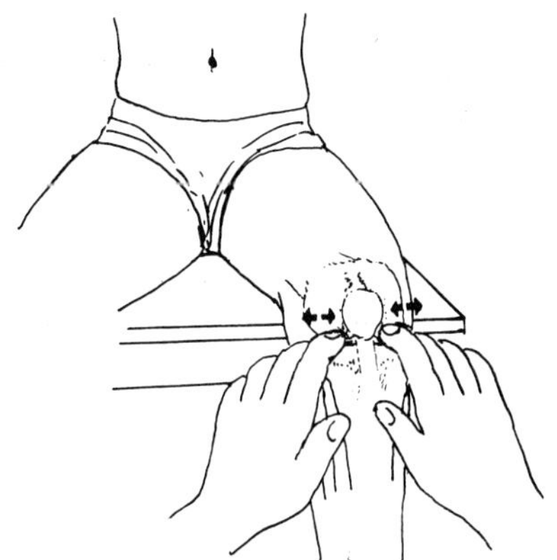

Fig. 13.12: Palpation of accessible articular surface of tibial condyles

and anteromedially in 90° flexed position of the knee. Insinuate the index fingers on both sides of the ligamentum patellae. With side to side rolling movements, any irregularity and tenderness of the articular surfaces can be palpated to some extent (Fig. 13.12).

Ascertaining the Presence of Fluid in the Joint

Anatomically, the knee being a composite joint has many crevices and folds, which can conceal varying amounts of fluid before it is manifested. Presence of little amount of fluid manifests as obliteration of the infrapatellar fossae. Usually, fluid in the knee accumulates in the suprapatellar pouch which is lax and accommodative. Thus, if the amount of fluid is more, the suprapatellar swelling becomes tense and presents the look of a shiny, ballooned-up knee. At this stage, or even earlier, synovial swelling must be differentiated from swelling due to fluid in the joint.

Features of Synovial Swelling

- The feel of synovial swelling is usually doughy or earthworms-filled-in bag.
- Usually, it is warm.
- There can be pseudofluctuation, i.e. fluctuation in only one axis.
- The edge of the synovial swelling can be palpated and rolled under the fingers.
- The swelling cannot be squeezed out to another compartment of the knee joint.
- Transillumination will be negative in synovial thickening.

Tests for Fluid in Joint

a. *If quantity is small*: The infrapatellar fossae appear comparatively full. Now compress the infrapatellar fossae. The fluid will be initially displaced, but slowly refills the area after the release of pressure.
b. *If only localized in the suprapatellar pouch* (Fig. 13.13a): Extend the knee as far as practicable. Fix the patella up and posteriorly towards femur by pressing the little and ring fingers over it. Now hold the lower part of the swelling with the thumb

and index finger of the same hand. Pressing with the thumb and index finger of opposite hand over superior part of swelling, elicit cross-fluctuation.

c. *If fluid is moderate*: Elicit cross-fluctuation across under surface of patella (Fig. 13.13b), i.e. put the thumb and index finger of one hand on both sides of the ligamentum patellae at infrapatellar fossae. Pushing the fluid by the thumb and index finger of the opposite hand placed over the suprapatellar pouch region, elicit cross-fluctuation.

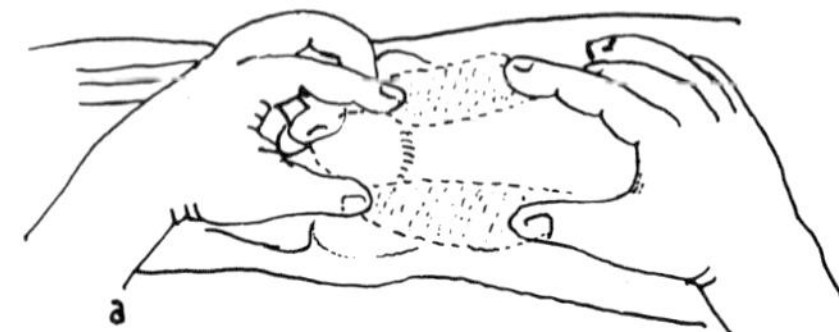

Fig. 13.13A: Testing of fluctuation in suprapatellar pouch (when fluid is less)

d. *Patellar tap*: It cannot be elicited if there is little fluid. It further cannot be elicited if there is massive amount of fluid. It can only be elicited when there is enough of fluid, without it being in much tension. In such a condition the patella floats anteriorly.

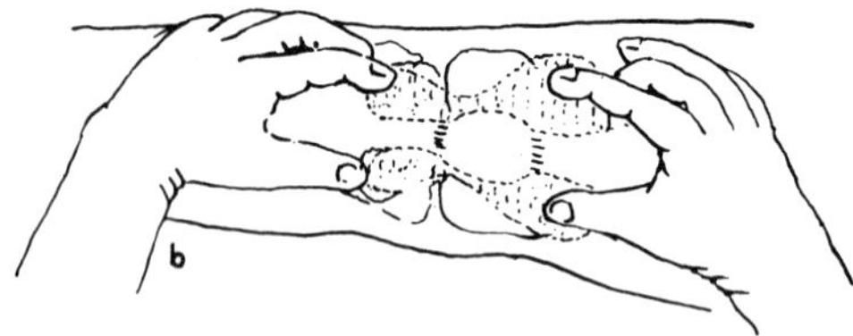

Fig. 13.13B: Testing of cross-fluctuation from suprapatellar pouch to infrapatellar fossae

Method (Fig. 13.13C): Knee should be extended. Now squeeze the suprapatellar pouch region towards the knee by the widely separated first web of the hand. Put the conjoint tips of the thumb and index finger of the opposite hand over the anterior surface of the patella. Give a gentle jerk posteriorly. The articular surface of the patella, displacing the fluid underneath, taps over the anterior articular surface of the femur and immediately comes back (rebounds) to its position thus producing the characteristic 'tap'.

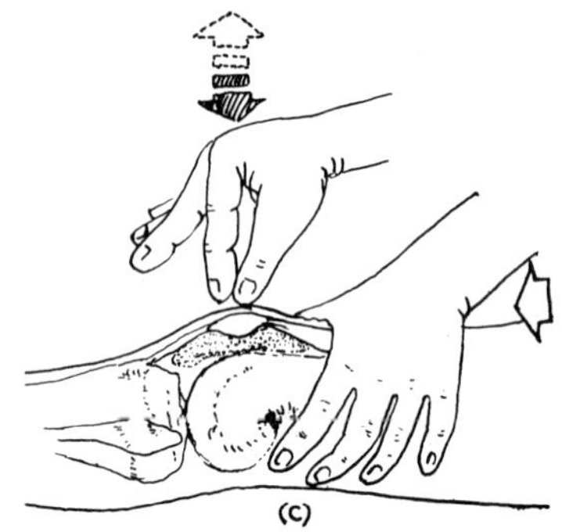

Fig. 13.13C: Demonstration of patellar tap

Transillumination

Depending upon the clarity of fluid, transillumination can be positive to a varying extent (Figs 13.14A and B).

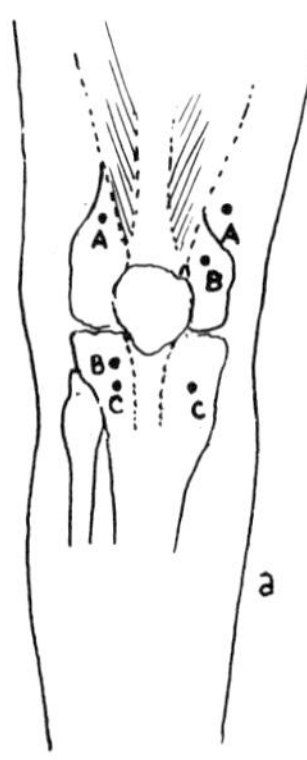

Fig. 13.14A. Sites of transillumination. A to A = across suprapatellar pouch, C to C = across infrapatellar fossae, B to B = suprapatellar infrapatellar fossae

Method: It can be done across the two sides of the suprapatellar pouch. If the fluid is much more, it can be demonstrated across the under surface of the patella, from the suprapatellar pouch to the infrapatellar fossae. Thirdly, it can

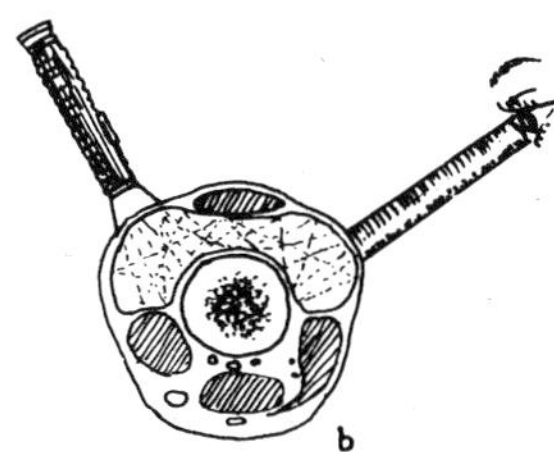

Fig. 13.14B: Transillumination test: method of transillumination

also be demonstrated across the two sides of the infrapatellar fossae. It is better to demonstrate this in a dark room. However, it can be done in an ordinary examination room too. Take a black foldable sheet or X-ray plate, and fold it in a tube form. Put its one end firmly adapted over the skin surface, illuminate from the contralateral side and visualise the glow through the upper end of the dark folded tube. This transillumination test is of much value in differentiating synovial swelling (negative) from fluid in joint (positive) and also in clinically ascertaining nature of the fluid—in serous collection the glow will be bright, whereas in haemorrhagic collection there will be no glow.

Cystic Swellings Around Knee

Smaller localized collections can be confused with different cystic swelling,. (the bursitis is most frequent).

Cystic swellings around the knee are:

Anteriorly:

a. Suprapatellar bursa—Superior extension of synovium beneath the quadriceps tendon.
b. Prepatellar bursa (Housemaid's knee)—lies subcutaneously in front of lower part of patella.
c. Infrapatellar bursa (Clergyman's knee)—lies in between the ligamentum patellae and anterior surface of tibia.

Laterally

a. Biceps bursa—lies between biceps tendon and fibular collateral ligament.
b. Posterolaterally lie two bursae: (i) between popliteus tendon and lateral condyle of femur, (ii) between popliteus tendon and fibular collateral ligament.

Medially

a. Bursa anserinus between the tendons of sartorius, gracilis, semitendinosus and upper medial part of tibia and the medial collateral ligament.
b. Cyst of medial meniscus.
c. Besides these, there can be several unimportant bursae, which are not of much clinical importance.

Posteriorly

a. Morrant Baker's cyst (In the year 1877 Baker described it in association with tuberculosis)—A midline synovial herniation, which usually presents as an oval, fluctuant swelling in the intermuscular to subcutaneous planes.
b. Semimembranosus bursa (commonest)—lies posteromedially between the medial head of gastrocnemius and the musculotendinous mass of the semimembranosus.
c. Popliteal aneurysm can also be confused as a cystic swelling.

MOVEMENTS (Table 13.2)

Before ascertaining the movement, the power of thc following muscles should be tested individually and graded according to MRC scale: quadriceps, biceps femoris, semitendinosus, semimembranosus, iliotibial tract, gastrocnemius, gracilis and sartorius.

Normal Range

From zero position of full extension of the knee, flexion is possible till the upper part of back of the leg touches the lower part of the back of thigh, (varies according to musculature and fat, average 120°-130° however the normal range of movement can be accepted from 10° of

Table 13.2: Knee movements

Movement	*Range of movement*	*Axis of movement*	*Prime movers*	*Nerve supply*	*Accessory muscles*	*Limiting factors*
1. Flexion	0° to 120°-130° (may be 10° hyper-extension to 140° of flexion)	The axis, around which the movement occurs, is not fixed, but shifts upward and forward during extension of the leg on the thigh, and backward and downward during flexion	i. Biceps femoris ii. Semitendinosus iii. Semimembranosus	L4, 5, S1, 2, 3 -do- -do-	Popliteus Sartorius gracilis Gastrocnemius	i. Tension of extensors of knee ii. Contact of upper calf with posterior part of lower thigh
2. Extension	From full flexion to 0°, i.e. 120°-130° to 0°	The flexion and extension are not as those of a true hinge joint	Quadriceps femoris	L2, 3, 4	Some assistance from tensor fascia latae	i. Tension of oblique popliteal, cruciate and collateral ligaments of knee. ii. Tension of flexors of knee
3. Medial rotation of flexed leg	Few degrees		i. Popliteus ii. Semimembranosus iii. Semitendinosus	L4, 5, S1, 2, 3 L4, 5, S1, 2, 3	Sartorius Gracilis	i. Position of knee and type of rotation reverses in flexion and extension depending upon whether the foot is on the ground or off the ground
4. Lateral rotation of the flexed leg	Few degrees					ii. Tightness of the opposite group of muscles
5. Accessory movement	i. A wider range of rotations and anteroposterior gliding in semi-flexed position—by passive movement ii. Limited abduction and adduction in slightly flexed knee iii. Distraction of tibia on femur on strong traction iv. Locking of knee in full extension by popliteus					

hyperextension to 140° of flexion). With the knee in about 90° flexion, some amount of adduction and abduction as well as lateral and medial rotation (medial more than lateral) elements can also be demonstrated passively in a normal limb. Even in normal flexion 8 to 12° of rotational movements can occur throughout the entire arc. However, they are not important.

Start from zero position of knee, i.e. fully extended knee. If the patient cannot extend and you also cannot make him extend to zero position, this indicates a *"fixed flexion deformity"*. If the patient cannot extend beyond a certain range but you can help him to achieve zero degree position, this indicates *"quadriceps lag"*. Fixed flexion deformity is to be measured from zero degree position to the position of the leg from where it cannot be extended. Beyond the position of fixed flexion deformity, ask the patient to flex the knee as far as practicable by himself. This will be "active free flexion". Beyond this, assist further possible flexion by holding the lower part of the patient's leg. The range of motion gained by this method will be that of "passive free flexion". If the leg still has not flexed upto full range, the deficit will be the "limitation of terminal flexion".

If the joint is not ankylosed, description of the movement should be recorded under following headings:

a. Quadriceps lag (or extension lag) if any.
b. Fixed flexion deformity.
c. Free active flexion.
d. Free passive flexion.
e. Range of utility or activity (free active flexion).
f. Range of possibility (= free active flexion + free passive flexion). This should be modified accordingly if there is fixed flexion deformity.
g. Limitation of terminal flexion—i.e. from end of free passive flexion to full flexion (as in normal knee).
h. Critical arc—The range of 0°-90° at the knee is the most useful range. If the patient has got this range of useful motion, one should be very cautious in performing any surgery, at least for improving on the range. 0°-30° motion at the knee is critical arc required for walking.
i. Abnormal movements: (in lateral and antero-posterior plane) it can be elicited in the presence of: (i) repeated collection of fluid in the joint; (ii) lax ligaments (congenital or acquired); (iii) neuropathic changes (Figs 13.14C and D).
j. Abnormal sounds during movement—While the knee is being moved, actively or passively, place your hand over the knee and try to feel and hear any abnormal sound.
   - Fine crepitations in a young girl suggests chondromalacia patellae; Coarse crepitations occur in degenerative arthrosis and neuropathic joint; while a click denotes meniscal tear or cyst.
   - A thud especially on anterolateral aspect indicates discoid lateral meniscus.
   - If with flexion-extension of the knee, a snap is felt while the patella slips out laterally and then relocates back, it denotes habitual dislocation.

MEASUREMENTS

a. Linear measurement
b. Circumferential measurement

a. Linear Measurement

To ascertain the limb length disparity, linear measurement should be done in the same way as in hip examination, i.e. apparent length measurement and true length measurements (total and segmental lengths).

b. Circumferential Measurement

It is done—(i) to ascertain any shrinkage or swelling at knee level, (ii) to ascertain wasting and swelling of thigh and leg at their mid levels.

Measurement of genu valgum and genu varum: As described earlier in this chapter (page 291).

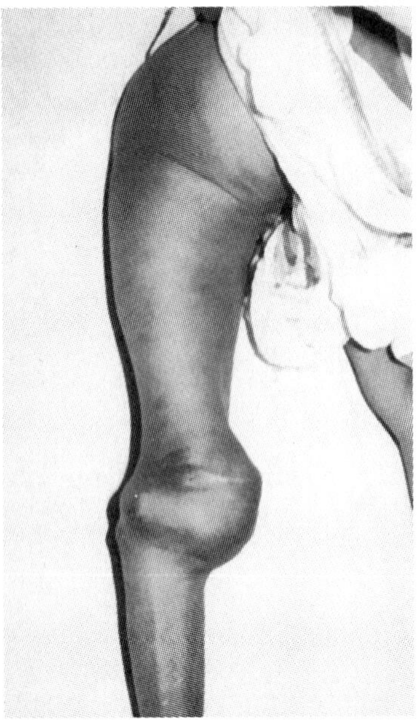

Fig. 13.14C: Charcot's arthropathy of knee and hip

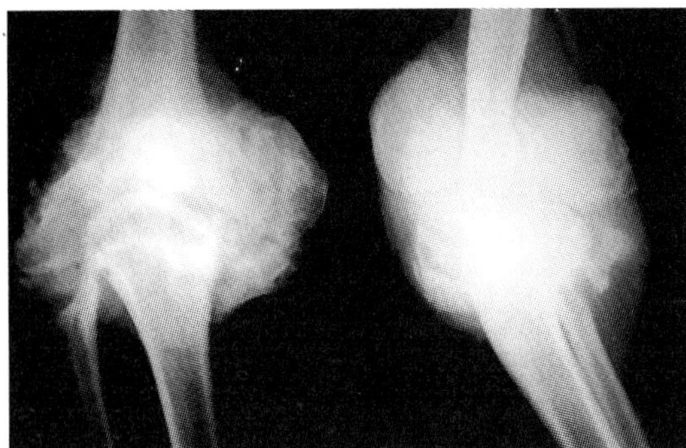

Fig. 13.14D: X-ray picture of Charcot's arthropathy of knee

ASSESSMENT OF INTEGRITY OF THE QUADRICEPS APPARATUS

The quadriceps apparatus is most important for controlling the knee. It consists of—(i) quadriceps muscles, (ii) quadriceps tendon, (iii) patella, (iv) medial and lateral quadriceps expansions (retinaculum), (v) patellofemoral and patello-tibial ligaments, (vi) ligamentum patellae, and (vii) tibial tuberosity. Biomechanically the resulting forces traversing the quadriceps tendon, patella and ligamentum patellae usually exceed five times of body weight.

Any of these parts are likely to be affected due to direct or indirect violence (Fig. 13.15). Quadriceps muscle tear and avulsion of the patella are well known injuries in athletes. In fracture patella, perhaps the consideration of tear of the quadriceps apparatus as a whole, is much more important than the fracture of patella itself, specially from the treatment and functional recovery point of view.

The quadriceps apparatus can be disrupted due to violence, at any place, in any age. However, commonly the quadriceps muscles get torn in young atheletes; patella fracture mostly occurs in the age group of 35 to 60 years; ligamentum patellae gets torn in the age group of 25 to 40 years; and avulsion of tibial tuberosity occurs in late teens and early twenties.

The external violence (like a heavy blow) over the quadriceps muscles causes 'dead leg' or 'Charley horse' syndrome due to local bleeding. Patient has local pain, swelling, tenderness, and difficulty in walking.

1. *Incomplete Quadriceps Tear*

There will be history of sudden pain and swelling anywhere in the mass of quadriceps muscle, specially in the middle third. A gap can be felt in between this mass and the remaining part of the quadriceps. In the extended position of

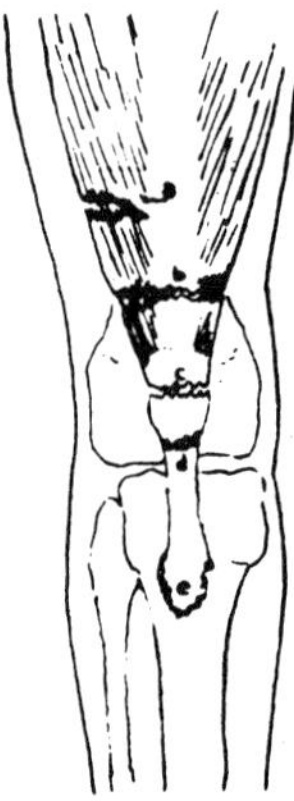

Fig.13.15: Quadriceps apparatus injuries. a = incomplete quadriceps tear, b = complete quadriceps tear, c = fracture patella, d = avulsion of ligamentum patellae, e = avulsion of tibial tuberosity.

the knee, when the patient is asked to contract and relax the quadriceps, this swelling will move proximally and distally with contraction and relaxation of the muscle.

The power of the quadriceps muscles as a group should be tested according to MRC scale. The action of the rectus femoris can be eliminated by fully flexing the hip. Ask the patient to extend the knee. He can do it with the help of the vasti, except for terminal 15°-20° which can be only achieved when the hip is extended to some extent (with the help of rectus femoris). If he cannot do so, it indicates tear of the rectus femoris component.

2. *Complete Quadriceps Tear*

Here a gap can be felt above the upper pole of the patella. In extended position of the knee, ask the patient to contract the quadriceps. This gap will be more prominent.

3. *Fracture Patella* (Fig. 13.16)

In complete fracture of patella with tear of the expansion, a gap is always felt in between the two fragments of the patella. Similar gaps are felt at upper and lower pole region in upper and lower pole avulsions respectively. Simultaneously, pass the fingers on both the sides of the patella in front of the knee joint. You will be able to feel breach in the continuity of the quadriceps expansion, if there is a tear in it. Then ask the patient to contract the quadriceps. If the contraction is communicated to the tibial tuberosity, along with feeling of a gap either in patella or expansion, the tear is an incomplete one. If the contraction is not communicated beyond the gap, it is a complete tear. Incomplete tear may not need surgery.

4. *Ligamentum Patellae*

Being a short and stout tendon, it hardly even tears in the middle. However, if at all it tears

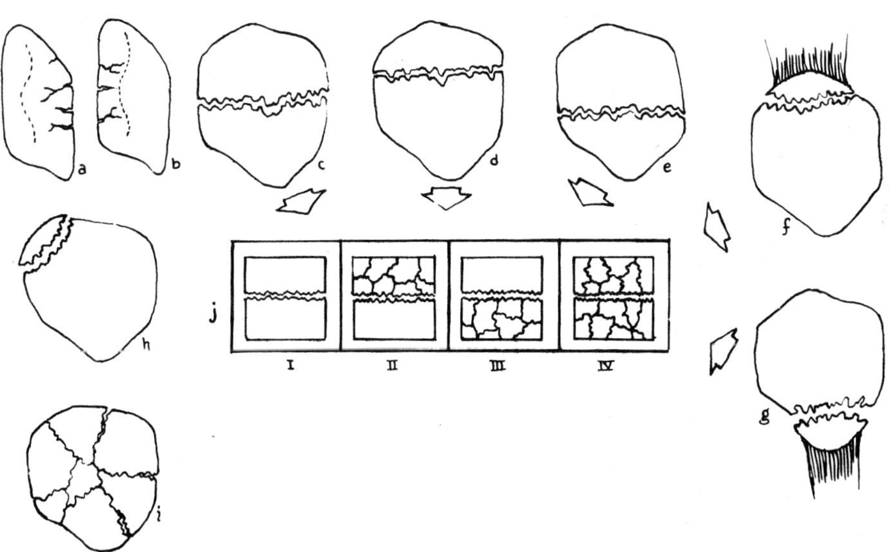

Fig. 13.16: Types of fracture patella. a = Incomplete fracture anterior cortex, b = Incomplete fracture posterior surface, c = Transverse fracture through middle, d = Transverse fracture through upper 1/3rd, e = Transverse fracture through lower 1/3rd, f = Upper pole avulsion, g = Lower pole avulsion, h = Marginal avulsion, i = Stellate fracture, j = Subtypes of c, d, e, f, and g. (i) Both fragments not comminuted, (ii) Upper comminuted lower not comminuted, (iii) Lower comminuted upper not comminuted, (iv) Both comminuted

by direct sharp violence, a clear gap can be felt beneath the lower pole of the patella. Further, quadriceps contraction is not communicated to the tibial tuberosity.

5. *Avulsion of Tibial Tuberosity*

It is mostly incomplete, in which case, there will be local tenderness, broadening and prominence of the tibial tuberosity. Same findings, if found without any history of injury in adolescents, suggest the diagnosis of Osgood-Schlatter's disease (due to traction or stress injuries osteochondritis of tibial tuberosity develops.

INTERNAL DERANGEMENTS OF KNEE JOINT (IDK) (Table 13.3)

The term "internal derangement" originally coined by William Hey (1784) is loosely used to describe the abnormalities in the knee functions due to any cause, but mostly traumatic. Anatomically, no joint contains as many intra-articular structures as the knee does. They are mostly the vestigial parts, but they subserve important functions in maintaining the integrity of the knee. They are strong, but perhaps not to the extent so as to sustain violent rotational and sweep stresses at the knee. Except for the anterior and posterior tendon, and muscles groups, the knee is mainly controlled by these static structures. Hence, in any injury to the knee is mainly controlled by these static structures. Hence, in any injury to the knee joint it is imperative to assess the integrity of these internal structures.

Truly speaking, real IDK (internal derangements of knee) should include—

A. Articular Proper

1. Cruciate avulsion/tear.
2. Semilunar cartilage (menisci—Greek word meaning thereby crescents) tear.
3. Collateral ligament tear.

Rarely in severe knee injury, the three conditions (medial meniscal tear, rupture of anterior cruciate ligament and rupture of medial

Table 13.3: Internal derangement of knee joint

Bony lesion	*Soft tissue lesion*
— Sliced fracture of articular cartilage	Semilunar cartilage lesions
	— tear
— Epiphyseal fracture	— discoid
— Condylar fracture	— cyst
— tibial	Cruciates tear or avulsion
— femoral	— Anterior cruciate.
— Tibial spine fracture or avulsion	— Posterior cruciate.
— Bony loose bodies	Synovial folds entrapment
— Chondromalacia patellae	Synovial calcinosis
— Osteochondritis dessicans (Fig. 13.17) (transchondral fracture or separation of a loose piece of articular cartilage).	—Nipping of infrapatellar pad of fat—Hoffa's disease
— Chondrocalcinosis	
— Pellegrini Steida's disease (few weeks after injury, new bone forms at the avulsed femoral attachment of medial collateral ligament)	Loose bodies— — fibrous loose bodies — Cartilaginous loose bodies — Synovial chondrocalcinosis
— Osgood Schlatter's disease (due to traction or stress injuries osteochondritis of tibial tubercle develops).	
— Sinding-Larsen-Johansson's disease (Reverse Osgood Schlatter's disease—Traction osteochondritis of lower pole of patella)	
— Recurrent subluxation/dislocation of patella	
— Fabella(?)	

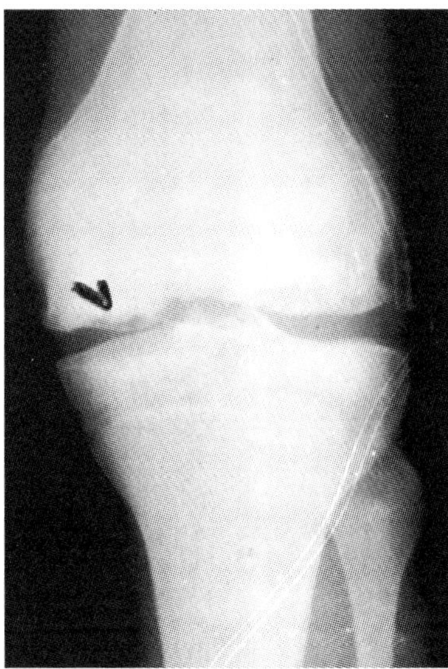

Fig. 13.17A: Osteochondritis dissecans in AP view note the crater-like appearance on the lower end of medial condyle of femur

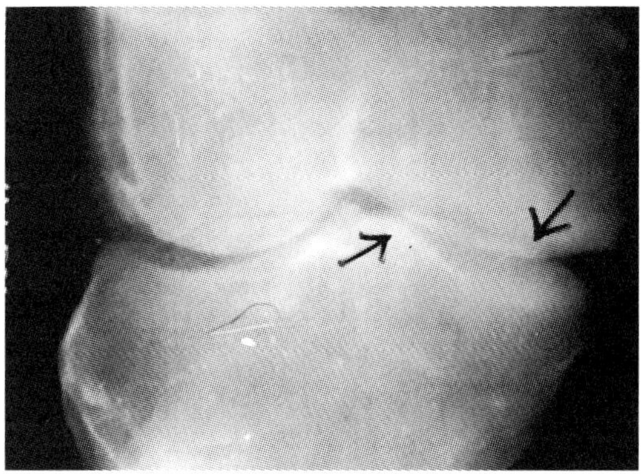

Fig. 13.17B: Osteochondritis dissecans. Note the separated mass

collateral ligament) may co-exist, which is called the "terrible triad of O'Donoghue."

However, symptoms produced by several other conditions, as listed below, mimic the presentation of IDK. Hence in the broader sense, the following may be included in IDK.

B. Walls of the Joint

— Lesions of the capsule with its reinforcing ligaments.

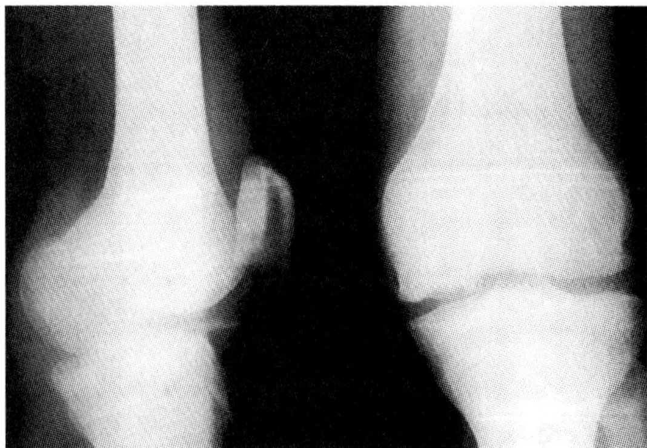

Fig. 13.17C: Osteochondritis dissecans. Note (in the lateral view) the anterior ejection of separated dissecans portion

— avulsion or rupture of:
- collateral ligament
- oblique ligament
- quadriceps expansion
- arcuate ligaments.

— quadriceps apparatus lesions:
- quadriceps tendon rupture
- fracture of patella
- avulsion or rupture of ligamentum patellae
- avulsion/fracture of tibial tuberosity.

The functions of the intra-articular structures are interdependent. Therefore, it is very much likely that two or three conditions of internal derangements of knee may co-exist. Atheletes, specially the footballers have been subjected to internal derangements of the knee most commonly, but these may occur in any type of violence where the knee is subjected to rotational or sweep stresses.

Clinically, most of them present with more or less similar manifestations, i.e.—(i) history of injury (usually twist/rotational strains), (ii) immediate pain, (iii) swelling, (iv) slight flexion of knee, (v) inability or disability in weight bearing, (vi) history of locking, (vii) history of feeling of instability or "giving way", (viii) in many cases, associated features of degenerative changes predominate, (ix) later on, various, deformities may develop.

In the acute stage, patient is usually in agony. Thus, it would perhaps not be proper to subject that knee to various clinical tests only to satisfy the academic needs. However, wherever practicable (acute patients may be put under general anaesthesia for performing the tests), the individual tests must be done for assessing integrity of the various structures.

ASSESSMENT OF THE INTEGRITY OF CONTROLLING GROUPS OF LIGAMENTS

Stress Tests

These are of special importance to assess the integrity of the joint, i.e. for collaterals, the cruciates and semilunar cartilages by side to side, anteroposterior and rotational stress tests respectively. None of the stress tests can be performed without patient's cooperation in acutely injured knee mainly due to two fallacies—acute pain and haemarthrosis. However in such circumstances, these tests can be better performed under general anaesthesia. In internal derangements of the knee, one must endeavour to search for additional injuries, since combined injuries are seen frequently.

Test for Posterior Cruciate Integrity

It has been found practical to start as follows—keeping the palm on the outer side of the fully extended knee, apply an abduction/valgus stress. If the gap on the inner side of the joint is more as compared to normal, it indicates posterior cruciate tear, with or without posterior capsular tear. At this stage, it is not possible to say clearly whether the medial collateral ligament is torn or not.

Posterior cruciate tear can be further confirmed by performing the drawer test (Fig. 13.18). Keep the hip flexed 45°, and the knee flexed 90°, while the patient firmly fixes his buttock on the couch in a lying down position. Sitting on the patient's planted foot, hold the upper end of the leg firmly with both hands and glide it both backwards (posterior drawer) and forwards (anterior drawer) over femoral condyles. It will glide more posteriorly as compared to normal. If the drawer sign is inconclusive, and the medial side of the joint opens up more with valgus stress applied on the extended knee, it strongly suggests posterior cruciate tear. If the medial side of the joint opens up markedly (across both medial and lateral compartments of the knee) in both extension and flexion, it indicates tear of both cruciates (after Muller, W 1983).

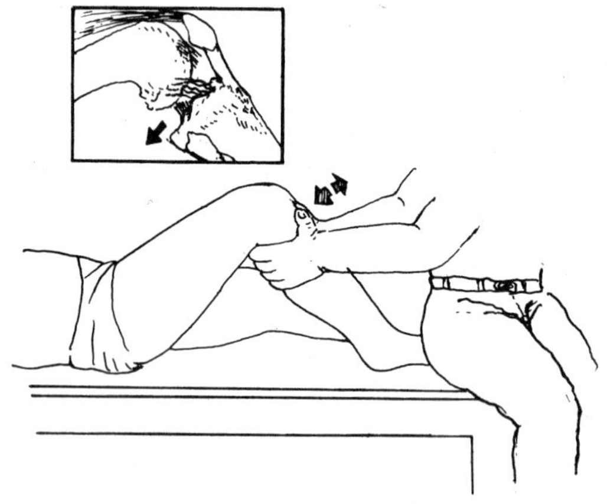

Fig. 13.18: Drawer test

Test for Integrity of the Collateral Ligaments

Flex the knee to about 30° (to make the collaterals maximally tense) and apply valgus stress. If the inner side of the joint opens more as compared to the normal side, it indicates medial collateral ligament tear, which can be felt as well. Reverse the hands and stress for testing the lateral collateral ligament integrity, which is comparatively less frequently torn as compared to the medial collateral ligament (Figs 13.19A and B). However, comparatively more opening of the joint on varus stress, applied both in flexion and extension, indicates disruption of lateral stabilising structures as well as insufficiency of posterior cruciate ligament (Hughston 1969).

Tests for Anterior Cruciate Integrity (Fig. 13.20)

Lachman test is perhaps the most sensitive test to elicit anterior cruciate disruption. Flex the

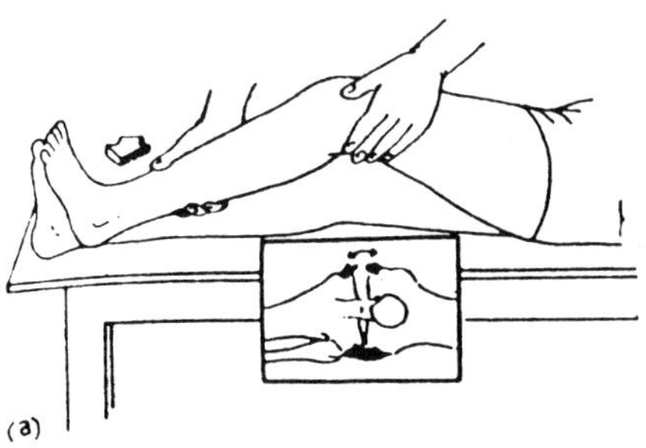

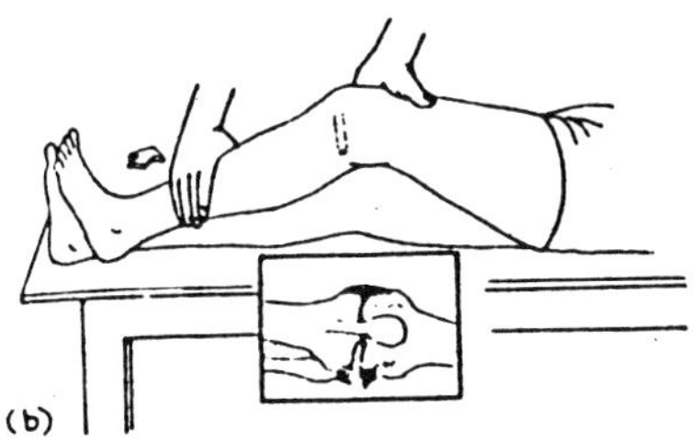

Figs 13.19A and B: Stress test for collateral ligaments A = for medial collateral, B = for lateral collateral

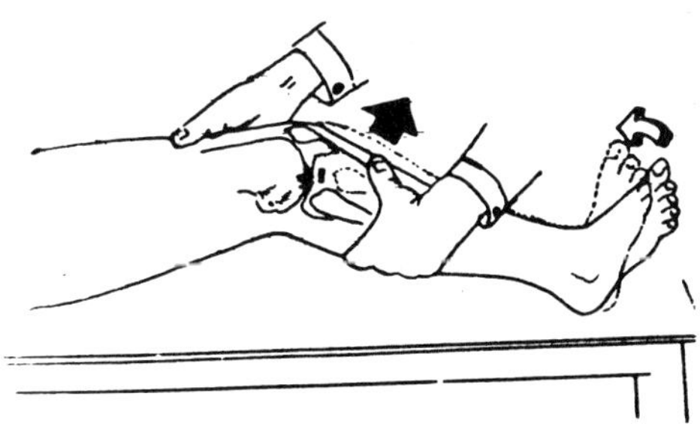

Fig. 13.20: Testing for anterior cruciate integrity

knee by 10°, keeping the lower thigh fixed with the opposite hand. Hold the upper end of the leg and try to glide the tibia over the femur anteriorly. The tibia will sublux anteriorly with a tendency to rotate internally (Lachman's sign). Increasing the flexion to 30°, the tibia will be autolocated back (jerk test), indicating integrity of the medial collateral ligament. Thus, it signifies isolated anterior cruciate avulsion, laxity or tear. If tibia can be subluxed anteriorly without any tendency of rotation, when the knee is flexed more than 30° (upto 90°), it indicates inadequacy of the anterior cruciate, along with the tear of the medial collateral ligament.

Anterior drawer sign, cannot be a conclusive test for isolated anterior cruciate tear. In 90° bent position of knee, anterior gliding of upper end of tibia by 5 mm can be possible in a normal knee. If it is 6 to 8 mm greater than the opposite knee, then it indicates anterior cruciate tear, along with medial collateral ligament tear or laxity.

Sometimes there may be discrepancy between the Lachman test and anterior drawer test. This has been explained by the differential injury of the anteromedial and posterolateral bundles of the anterior cruciate ligament.

A negative Lachman test indicates an intact posterolateral bundle, whereas a positive anterior drawer test indicates the disrupted anteromedial bundle.

Rotational Stress Tests (test for menisci)

They are mainly directed towards diagnosing tear of the menisci. Though no clinical sign is of diagnostic accuracy, rotational stresses in which the menisci are subjected to stretching and/or squeezing, can lead us to suspect meniscus tear, if positive.

Mc Murray's test—Method (Fig. 13.21)

The patient lies supine with his hip flexed 90° and knee fully flexed. Hold the knee with the hand from the dorsal aspect so that your thumb is on the lateral, while the other fingers are on the medial aspect. With the other hand, hold the heel and ankle. Fixing the knee by one hand, and while gradually pulling, externally rotating and abducting the leg as far as practicable, extend the knee. The patient feels sharp pain on the medial side of the joint line and the examiner feels a click on about the same site while the pulling position is maintained. In flexing and

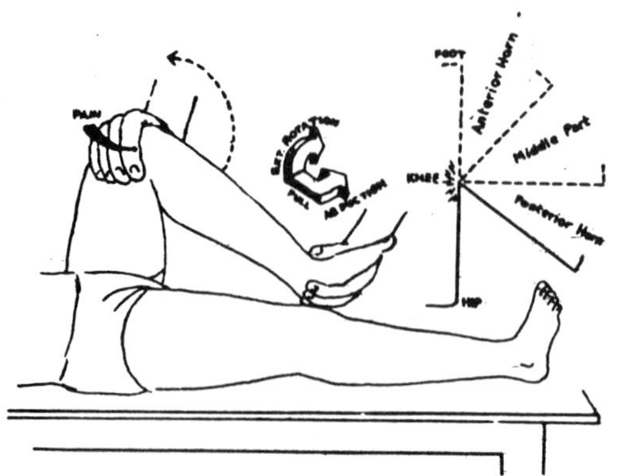

Fig. 13.21: Rotational stress test—McMurray's test

extending the knee in quick successions, every time the knee is extended, the patient will feel pain. This will be a positive stress test for medial meniscus tear. In this manoeuvre, eliciting the painful click in the initial range of extension indicates posterior horn tear, while in the middle range it indicates injury of the middle part. For anterior horn injury, one has to give more stress on eliciting tenderness at the medial side of ligamentum patellae and then to go for eliciting the painful click. In testing for lateral meniscus tear, other manoeuvres remaining the same, the hand holding the heel and ankle, will pull, internally rotate and abduct the leg as far as practicable. However, this test is not always positive.

Apley's Test (distraction test and grinding test)

In the light of monumental works on the knee joint, this test has very limited value, specially in acute cases. However, in late cases, quick assessment can be done before proceeding further for confirmation.

Method (Figs 13.22a and b)

Initially, patient lies prone, firmly planting his thigh on the couch. Bend the knee 90°, press the patient's thigh with your bent knee and with both hands hold the ankle and foot region firmly. Now distract the leg upwards and rotate it internally and externally. If there is collateral ligament injury, the patient will complain of pain at the particular site. Then compress the leg downwards and repeat the rotatory motions. In case of semilunar cartilage tear, the patient complains of pain over the corresponding site.

Squat Test (after Sisk, 1980)

For quick assessment of meniscal tear, ask the patient to fully squat, with the leg and foot alternately fully internally and externally rotated. If there is pain in the joint line on the lateral

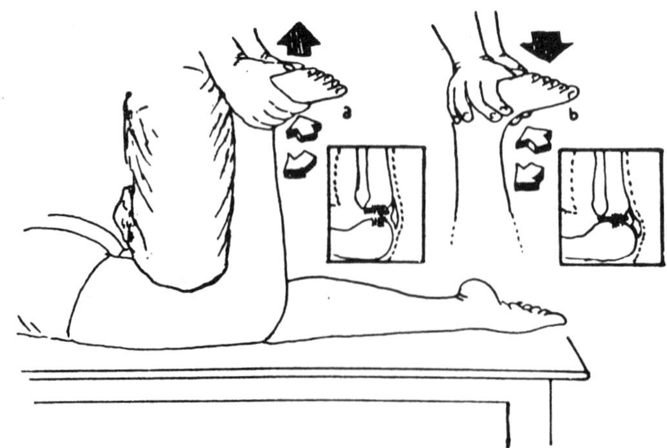

Fig. 13.22: Apley's test. a = distraction test, and b = grinding test

side on squatting with internally rotated leg, it suggests lateral meniscus tear; while pain located medially in the joint line on external rotation of leg indicates tear of the medial meniscus.

Wilson's Test

Osteochondritis dissecans can be vaguely represented by local tenderness on the surface of the femoral condyle (especially the medial). However, this can be clinically confirmed by Wilson's test. Here the knee is flexed to 90°, internally rotated, then it is gradually extended. Patient will complain of pain, the moment the raw areas come in contact, which gets immediately relieved if the knee is rotated externally.

'Q' Angle

The predisposition of a patella for subluxation can be roughly assessed by determining the 'Q' angle. Due to the anatomical alignment of femur, its valgus inclination and the origin of the quadriceps muscles, the line of pull of patellar movement is never direct, rather it is guided by the Quadriceps (Q) angle. This angle is formed by intersection of a line joining the tibial tuberosity to the centre of the patella and another line joining the centre of the patella to the anterior superior iliac spine. The normal 'Q' angle is 12° for females and 15° for males. If this angle is more than 15°, it denotes susceptibility of patella for recurrent subluxation.

Friction Test

In extended position of the knee, the patella is pressed and glided up and down over the femoral articular surface. With affection of the central portion of the articular surface of the patella, painful grating can be felt (e.g. in chondromalacia patella; degenerative arthrosis).

Apprehension Test

In recurrent subluxation or dislocation of patella any attempt of subluxing the patella in slightly flexed position of the knee is resisted by the patient.

Loose Bodies in the Knee Joint (Joint mice)

In such cases, there will be history of moving of an object in the joint, occasional sense of "giving way" of the joint, pain and effusion in the joint and loose body may be seen and/or palpated.

Cause

a. *Non-traumatic*

(i) Osteoarthrosis—detached osteophyte, (ii) Osteochondritis dissecans, (iii) Synovial chondromatosis, (iv) Fibrinous organization of haemarthrosis (haemophilia), (v) Rheumatoid arthritis (vi) Tuberculous arthritis.

b. *Traumatic*

(i) Organised haemarthrosis, (ii) Organised, snapped synovial fringes, (iii) Detached flakes of articular cartilage, (iv) Loose fragment from intra-articular fractures (condylar and fracture patella), (v) Loose fragment of torn semilunar cartilage, (vi) Foreign bodies.

Auscultation

As usual, auscultation is of importance in case of vascular osseous swellings and in fulminating malignancy. In the back of the knee, sometimes popliteal artery aneurysm and arterio-venous fistula do occur, where one can hear a systolic bruit. The lower end of femur and upper end of tibia are most common sites for osteosarcomas. In telangiectatic variety of this growth, systolic bruit can be heard. In case of early chondromalacia patellae fine crepitations can be appreciated if the stethoscope bell is kept on the joint while the knee is moved.

Investigations Required for Knee Pathology

1. General—as in the chapter on Introduction.
2. Local—
   i. Plain X-ray—(a) Anteroposterior, (b) Lateral, (c) Oblique, (d) Sky line (tangential), (e) Stress radiography.
   ii. Tomography
   iii. Aspiration and aspiration biopsy
   iv. Arthrography
   v. Arthroscopy

vi. Cine radiography
vii. Arthrotomy
viii. Radio-scintography
ix. Arteriography

How to Take X-ray Projections

Weight bearing position: Patient stands with equal weight distribution on both legs keeping knees in symmetrical position.

Lateral view: In full weight bearing position and relaxed (lying down) position.

Anteroposterior view: In full weight bearing position and in relaxed position (in lying down position).

Oblique view: Specially to visualise femoral condyles.

Sky line (tangential) view: Skyline view to see the: (a) patellofemoral articular relation, (b) to assess the development of femoral condyles in relation to patella (of special importance in recurrent dislocation of patella), (c) Osteochondral fractures of patella and femoral condyle.

Technique: With patient sitting at the edge of the table with 45° flexion at knee, the X-ray plate is kept at a distance of 10 cm from the knee level, perpendicular to the shin of tibia. The beam is projected from the superior aspect of the patella, striking the plate at 90° (Fig. 13.23). Or the patient lies supine with the knee flexed over sand bags or pillows and the film supported along the femur. The beam is centred to the patella with the tube tilted 15° to the lower leg.

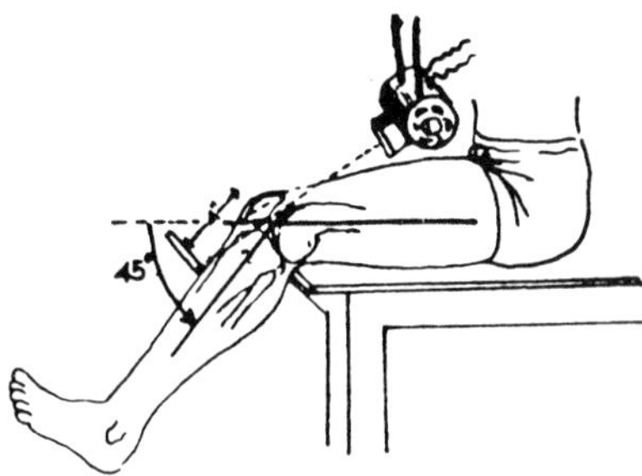

Fig. 13.23: Skyline projection to delineate patellofemoral articulation

Tunnel view: It is taken mainly to display osteochondritis dissecans, the intercondylar notch, and the loose bodies. The patient kneels on the affected side with the film placed under the knee. A sand bag supports the ankle. The patient then leans forward so that the femur is approximately 45° to the table. The beam is centred to the knee joint at right angle to the lower leg.

Stress X-ray

If possible it should be done under anaesthesia in acute cases. However, in chronic cases it can be done as such.

Method: *For antero-posterior stress,* patient sits on the edge of X-ray table at one end with knee flexed in 30° position with plate kept on the outer side of the joint, the examiner pulls the upper end of tibia forwards, and pushes it backward alternately as much as possible.

For side to side stress, patient stands with full weight bearing on the affected limb. With the knee in maximum possible valgus and varus strain, alternately, anteroposterior X-ray projection is shot to delineate any ligamentous inadequacy on medial or lateral aspect of the knee.

In anaesthetised or lying down position, strap both approximated thighs together at the lower end. The plate is kept behind the knees. The examiner then forcibly abducts the legs at the knee while X-ray is shot from anterior aspect. This will demonstrate any medial ligamentous inadequacy.

Cine-Radiography

This is usually of value in assessing the gait of the patient with knee pathology, as well as the integrity of the stabilising ligaments. Here, the movie camera is fixed with sliding X-ray tubes along the wall of the X-ray room, from where pictures are taken while the patient walks in a definite pattern.

Tomography

With the help of the pre-adjusted scale attached in the X-ray machine, the X-ray is taken at a measured depth penetration.

Arthroscopy

Arthroscopy, first performed by K Takagi in the year 1918, has now become an essential investigation, especially with the development of sports medicine. It is mostly used in the knee joint. However, it cannot be a substitute for thorough clinical examination.

It is being used to directly visualise the menisci, articular surfaces of patella and femur, joint capsule, cruciate ligaments, loose bodies, and synovium. Therapeutically it is utilised to remove or suture torn meniscus, to rapair/replace anterior cruciate ligament, to fix detached osteochondral surface, in plica syndrome, to take out biopsy material and joint lavage. The findings can also be simultaneously photographed and video-recorded. However, it has its limitations in having 'blind spots' in its visual field (i.e. posteromedial and posterolateral part of knee and inferior surface of meniscus).

Contraindications to its use: (i) stiff knee, (ii) infected knee, (iii) recent haemarthrosis.

Arthrography

This is a contrast study of the joint space. It can be done either by using a radio-opaque dye directly injected into the joint or injecting air or both (double contrast arthrography). It is valuable in assessing menisci tear, cruciate tear, and presence of any space-occupying lesion. Its special advantage lies in delineating the blind spot areas of arthroscopy. Contraindications—(i) pyoarthrosis, (ii) haemophilia, (iii) dye allergy.

Vibration arthrography is a recent advancement in this technique.

Radio-Scintography

Radio-scanning is not of much value as a diagnostic aid in knee pathology. However, it can be of academic usefulness for various neoplasm and for investigating blood supply of a bone (affected by any pathology).

Genucom

By this instrument, precise non-invasive computer based 3D measurement of total knee stability (for ligaments, patella and knee prosthesis) can be done and analysed.

Arteriography

It is more or less of only academic value, except in vascular lesion related to the posterior part of knee joint. Research workers do utilise this investigation to study rheumatoid pathology and various neoplastic conditions and severe injuries around the knee joint which threaten the vascularity.

Key Diagnostic Points of Common Knee Pathology

Non-Traumatic

1. *Congenital conditions* (Figs 13.24A to E)
   - Usually associated with other congenital defects.
   - Bilateral symmetrical defects.
   - History since birth.
   - At knee, absence of femoral or tibial condyles; congenital quadriceps contracture; genu recurvatum; high placed, low placed, bipartite or absence of patella are the usually known congenital defects.

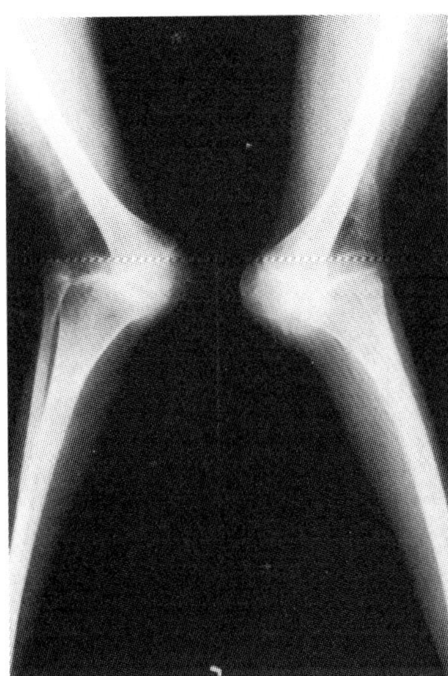

Fig. 13.24A: Bilateral congenital posterolateral dislocation of knee

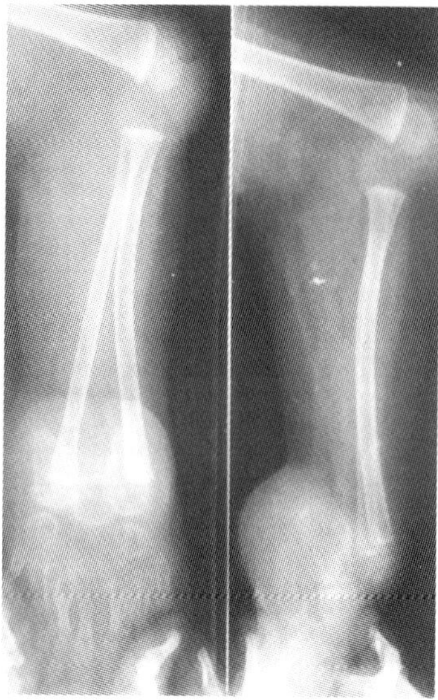

Fig. 13.24B: Congenital unilateral posterior dislocation of knee associated with disorganised ankle and foot

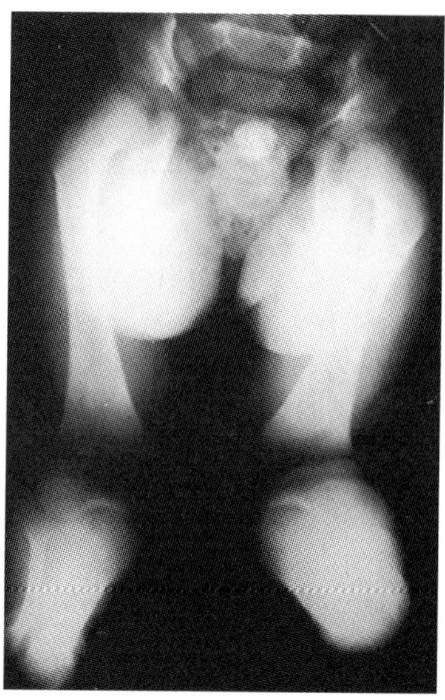

Fig. 13.24C: Bilateral congenital absence of lower end of femora and bilateral congenital below knee amputee

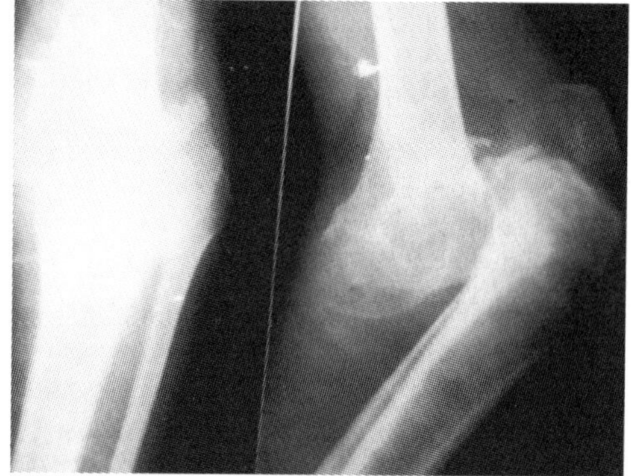

Fig. 13.24D: Traumatic neglected anterior dislocation of knee

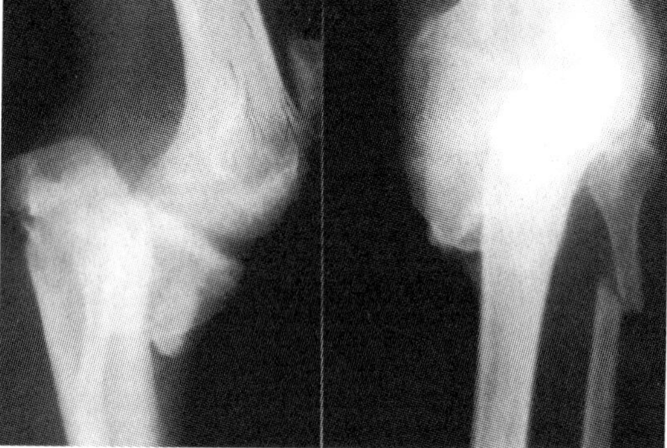

Fig. 13.24E: Traumatic neglected posterior fracture dislocation of knee

2. *Metabolic Diseases and Deficiency States*

Rickets (it occurs due to deficiency of vitamin D or to a defect in its metabolism)

Usually comparatively listless child, with flabby look, irregular bowels, delayed walking, retardation of growth, deformities.

Usual findings: Poor tone of muscles, delayed closure of fontanelles and cranial sutures, craniotabes, bossing of forehead, thickened and everted look of lips, decaying of teeth, broadening of lower radial epiphysis, pigeon chest, Harrison's sulcus, rachitic rosary, pot belly, widening of perineum, anterolateral bowing of lower third of femora, bow knee (Figs 13.5c, 13.7A to C), bow leg (lower third), genu valgum, widening of growing ends of long bones, wind sweep (tackle) deformity (Fig. 13.25).

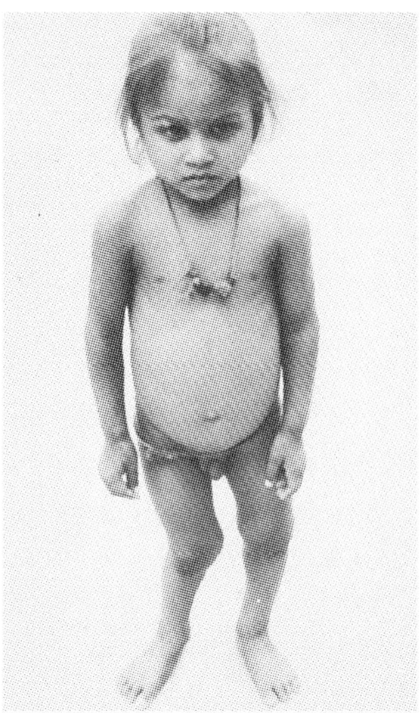

Fig. 13.25A: Rachitic wind sweep deformity

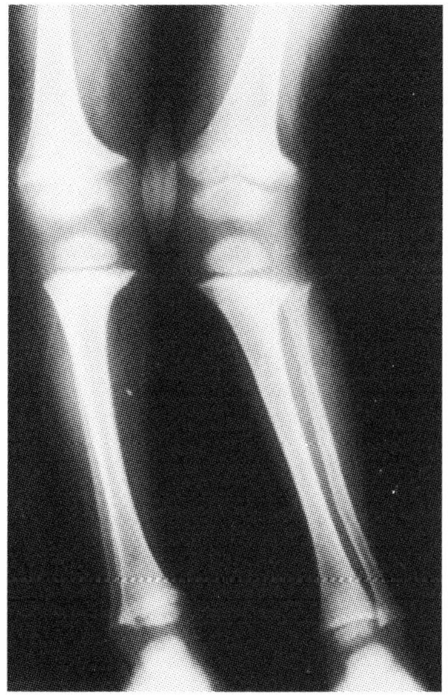

Fig. 13.25B: X-ray of rachitic wind sweep deformity of both legs

X-ray

I. *Florid (acute) stage*: Poorly defined and smaller epiphysis (irregular calcified areas); epiphyseal end of metaphysis cup shaped, poorly defined and fraying look; generalised broadening of metaphysis with flared cortices (most marked in wrist and knee regions); widened epiphyseometaphyseal junction; generalised rarefied appearance of bones with less sharply defined trabeculations and cortices; bending of long bones.

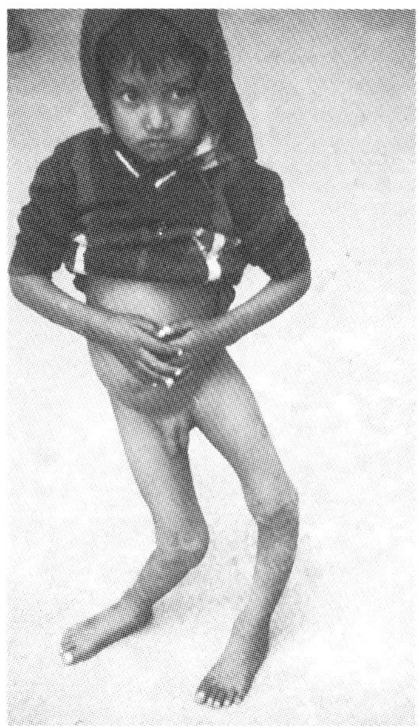

Fig. 13.25C: Bilateral genu recurvatum tendency and wind sweep deformity due to polio paralysis

II. *Healing stage*: Epiphysis gets gradually defined, uniformally calcified, larger epiphyseometaphyseal junction gets narrowed with appearance of denser line; gradual narrowing of metaphysis with flattening of cup and reappearance of transverse trabeculations, gradual restoration of normal bony texture.

III. *Healed stage*: Almost normal epiphysis; denser line at epiphyseometaphyseal junction; legacy of earlier deformities variably persists; normal bony texture.

Scurvy: James Lind discovered its true nature in 1747: It is a deficiency disease due to lack of vitamin C. Acute to subacute presentation, in early childhood (rarely in elderly sailors and soldiers on voyage on sea—'Calamity of soldiers').

— Artificially fed infants and children are more likely to develop scurvy, because vitamin C is destroyed by heat in boiling the milk. Such infants and children may also develop rickets if the milk has not been supplemented with vitamin D.

The combination of rickets and scurvy is known as *"Barton's disease"*.

- Epiphyseal fracture separation at the end of long bone.
- Markedly tender fixed swelling over bone, especially in thigh, due to subperiosteal haematoma (Fig. 13.26).

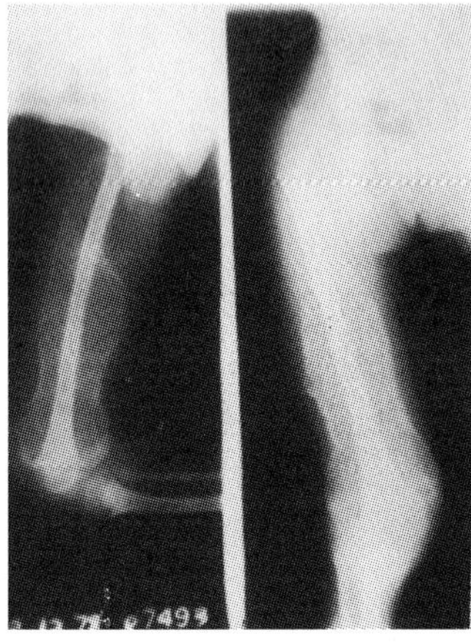

Fig. 13.26: X-ray of scurvy note marked subperiosteal haematoma in femur

- Bluish, spongy bleeding gums, (specially near upper incisors).
- Mild rise of temperature.
- Pseudoparalysis.
- Costochondral separation—presenting as sharp protrusion on anterior ends of the ribs—scorbutic rosary (cf. rachitic rosary—rounded).
- Delayed wound healing.
- X-ray—'pencilling' (thinning) of cortex, marked homogenous rarefaction, subperiosteal or longitudinal bone laying (bone formation). White line of Frankel, scurvy line (irregular radioopaque line caused by calcified cartilage), Wimberger line—the dense line encircling the epiphysis (Ring sign), Pelkan spur—best seen at the ends of rapidly growing long bones, as a small bony spur mostly on the lateral side of metaphysis near its junction with epiphysis.
- The blood ascorbic acid is 0.5 mgm less/dl ml (normal value is 1 mg/dl ml).

3. *Collagen Arthropathy*

Rheumatoid: It is usually a polyarthropathy, in which affection of the smaller joints of the hand and wrist (mainly proximal interphalangeal joints, but doubtful/not the distal interphalangeal joints) is typical.

In Monoarticular Affections

- Knee is commonly affected, with mild inflammatory features.
- Chronic history, wasting of muscles, fluid in the joint, synovial thickening, joint and bony tenderness.
- Gradually, movements get restricted with advancement of disease.
- Deformity—usually triple subluxation of knee.
- Lymph glands usually not enlarged.

4. *Haemophilia*

- May present as acute or chronic haemarthrosis.
- Family history.
- Exclusively in males (X-linked recessive inheritance), except haemophiliac (deficient plasmathromboplastin antecedent-factor XI), which affects both sexes.
- Pseudo tumour (haemophilic cyst) due to intramuscular or parosteal haemorrhage.
- Common joints affected are knee, elbow and ankle.
- History of repeated episodes.
- Patient pale, history of bleeding from other sites too.
- History of prolonged bleeding after any cut.
- Flexion deformity, genu varum, genu valgum.
- In late cases—degenerative changes; ankylosis of joint (usually fibrous).
- Clotting time increased due to lack of antihaemophilic factor (factor VIII)—haemophilia A (30% cases); lack of Christmas factor (Factor IX)—heamophilia B (15% cases).
- X-ray—distended joint, articular surfaces intact but thinned out. In late cases,—genu

valgum and genu varum deformities may be associated due to epiphyseal asymmetry overgrowth, squaring of patella, widening of intercondylar notch of femur. Other non-specific X-ray signs are bone resorption, osteoporosis, cyst formation, etc.

5. *Infective Conditions*
   i. *Acute septic arthritis:*
      — Knee commonest site
      — Usually in children.
      — Acute onset with constitutional features.
      — High fever with rigor.
      — Toxic features.
      — Femoral or tibial metaphyseal affection.
      — Hot inflamed joint.
      — Tenderness specially in joint line.
      — Fluctuant knee swelling (pus).
      — Inguinal lymph glands enlarged and tender.
      — Aspiration of pus clinches the diagnosis.
      — Routine haemogram—polymorphonuclear leucocytosis.
      — ESR raised mild to moderate.
      — Blood culture—positive in limited number of cases.
      — Aspiration culture positive in almost all cases.
      — X-ray—increased joint space, comparatively homogeneous appearance of area around joint with increased soft tissue shadow, generalised rarefaction, localised varying rarefaction due to destruction in the adjacent bones, depending upon osseous pathology.
   ii. *Chronic septic arthritis* (Fig. 13.27)
      — Usually in adults.
      — Presence of active (with purulent discharge) or healed sinuses.
      — Minimal swelling.
      — Usually associated deformities.
      — Varying ankylosis.
      — Adjacent metaphyseal thickening.
      — History of intermittent episodes of flare ups.
      — Inguinal lymph nodes enlarged, firm and may be tender, X-ray joint space distorted and reduced, areas of destruction, bone formation and sequestration. Aspiration may not be of much value. Aspirated material may be sterile. Routine haemogram not of much value.

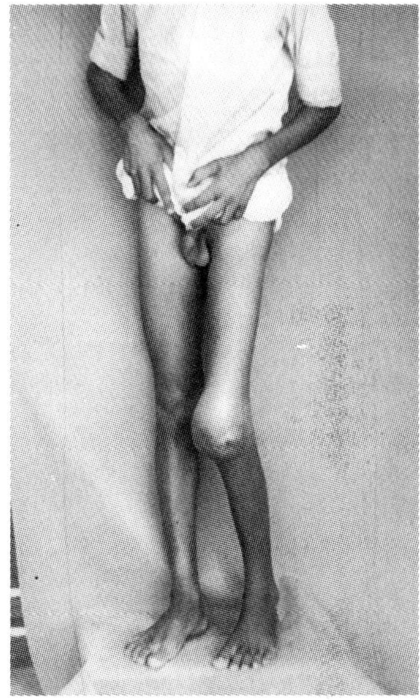

Fig. 13.27: Chronic septic arthritis of knee

   iii. *Tuberculosis knee* (Fig. 13.28)
      In children: Synovial swelling (tumour alba—in white skinned persons), varying flexion deformity, comparatively free movements (as compared to adult affection).
      — Warm, tender, thickened knee.
      — Movements painful, specially at extremes.
      — Wasting of thigh and calf muscles.
      — Triple rather quadruple deformity—in advanced cases.
      — Inguinal lymph glands enlarged, usually matted.
      — Routine haemogram—varying increase in lymphocyte count, raised ESR.

—Mantoux test positive in varying dilutions.
—Aspiration—thin serous/sero-sanguinous—may be positive for AFB.

X-ray—Initially increased joint space due to collection, later decrease in joint space when true arthritis supervenes, generalised rarefaction, localised areas of destruction along with cystic areas, varying ankylosis (usually fibrous ankylosis).

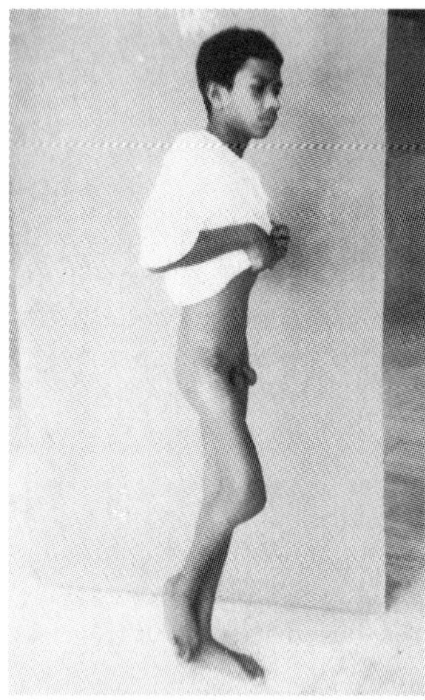

Fig. 13.28: Tuberculosis of knee with sinus

In adults:
—Osseous focus more common (femur, tibia, patella).
—May be synovial swelling.
—Warm, swollen joint.
—Tenderness along the joint line.
—Deformities—usually triple rather quadruple subluxation.
—All movements painful and restricted.
—May be sinuses of tuberculous nature.
—May be shortening of the limb, due to destruction.
—Wasting of thigh and calf muscles.
—Aspiration—thin, serous or serosanguinous—may be AFB positive.
—Synovial biopsy—chronic lymphocytic infiltration; demonstration of typical Langhan's giant cells and epithelioid cells.
—X-ray—reduced joint space, area of subchondral and chondral destruction, generalised rarefaction, varying deformities.

6. *Neoplastic Conditions*

Benign Soft Tissue Growths:
—These are comparatively rare (haemangioma, neurofibroma).
—Small swelling.
—Deep tenderness.
—May be warm if superficial.
—Haemangiomas are usually deep seated (mostly intramuscular).
—X-ray—if growth adjacent to bone—may be localised rarefaction or condensation.
—Lipoma arborescens (tree like) is a very uncommon tumour of synovium, in which there is diffuse replacement of the synovial tissue by mature fat cells, with prominent villous transformation of the synovium. Presenting soft boggy swelling in the suprapatellar pouch needs to be differentiated from pigmented villonodular synovitis, synovial lipoma, synovial chondromatosis, synovial haemangioma, rheumatoid arthritis, xanthoma, amyloid arthropathy.

Malignant Soft Tissue Growths
—Usually young adults in thirties.
—Synovioma—either in relation to synovial reflection, bursae in relation to tendon, or even penetrating adjacent bone.
—Varying size and shape of slowly growing swelling with ill-defined margins.
—Warm, tender.
—X-ray—combination of bone defects and soft tissue swelling like snow storm appearance.
—Usually eccentrically situated according to site.
—Soft to firm in feel.

Benign Bony Growths
Benign bony growth in relation to bone is rare, except for exostosis which may arise from lower

femoral or upper tibial region—as firm to hard, painless knob-like swellings—projecting away from central knee axis. Usually multiple and associated with deformities. May be pressure symptoms, e.g. foot drop due to pressure on lateral popliteal nerve. May turn malignant.

X-ray—exostosis usually projects away from the joint axis, and has a medullary cavity continuous with parent medulla.

Giant Cell Tumour (osteoclastoma)

— Usually in 3rd decade.
— Common sites—condylar regions (upper end of tibia, lower end of femur).
— Eccentric, tender, globular swelling.
— Feeling of yielding on pressure (demonstration of egg-shell crackling should not be attempted as it may produce fracture of the thin expanded cortex, leading to dissemination of the growth into the surroundings).
— Knee movements fairly preserved for a pretty long time.
— Movements only affected due to mechanical obstruction or bursting of tumour into the joint.

X-ray—expansion of the cortex, trabeculations (leading to soap bubble appearance), usually delineation of uppermost end of the expanded segment from the normal medullary cavity (if malignancy supervenes, this delineation is usually not marked), may or may not break into the joint. No area of bone formation.

Osteosarcoma

— The most common sites are the lower end of femur and upper end of tibia.
— Fusiform, painful and comparatively huge swelling.
— In knee region, perhaps osteosarcoma presents the largest swelling.
— All typical features of malignancy.
— Pathological fractures.
— Aspiration—bloody fluid.
— Active movements of knee usually affected due to pain and mechanical reasons, but passive movements are relatively free.

X-ray—soft tissue shadow, areas of bone destruction and bone formation, sun-ray spicules, Codman's triangle formation, cortico-medullary delineation not lost.

7. *Degenerative Arthrosis*

— By far most prevalent form of arthritis. In squatters (as in Asian-Indian culture) about 45% people over 60 years age suffer from osteoarthritis of knee.
— Chronic history—symptoms coming on just after rest, amelioration after mild to moderate activities. May again increase with prolonged activities.
— Coarse crepitations felt over joint with movements.
— Varus/valgus collapse of knee.
— Basically the articular cartilage thins, cracks, and breaks away, often leaving the subchondral bone rough roughened and thickened. The joints are disfigured with various deformities.
— Occasionally, painful or painless soft (or, cystic), mildly warm and tender swelling of the knee—specially localised in supra-patellar area.
— In later stages—limitation of movements; in advanced cases deformities may occur.

X-ray—(i) Condensation of subchondral plates in upper end of tibia depending upon the particular deformity (e.g. under medial plateau in varus collapse), (ii) Subchondral cystic areas, (iii) Osteophytic formation, especially at condylar margins, (iv) Compartmental collapse of joint space, depending on deformity, (v) Loose bodies may be present.

Traumatic Conditions

A. *Extra Articular*

Soft tissue injuries, except disruption of quadriceps apparatus, may manifest as tender swelling of diffused nature. However, one must examine and investigate repeatedly to exclude any intra-articular damage, which if missed, may jeopardise knee functions.

B. *Intra-Articular*

1. *Anterior Cruciate Avulsion*
   - Mild to moderate swelling of knee joint following injury (haemarthrosis).
   - Tenderness mostly localised over the anterior tibial plateau region.
   - Extremes of movement painful.
   - Lag of active terminal extension of knee (by about 15-20°).
   - Posteroanterior stress test positive (Lachman's sign; Drawer test).

X-ray—a triangular flake of bone is seen in between the femoral and tibial condyles in lateral X-ray (Fig. 13.29). In anteroposterior view, fissures in the tibial spine region are noticed. In stress radiography, anteroposterior laxity can be well demonstrated.

— Arthroscopy (diagnostic or even therapeutic).

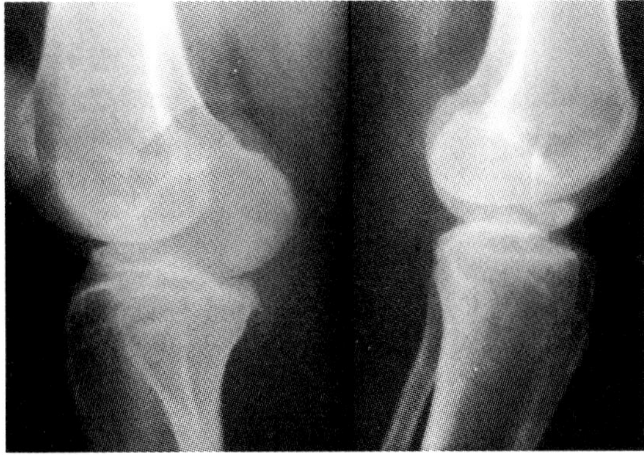

Fig. 13.29: Avulsion of anterior cruciate/fracture of tibial spine open fish mouth appearance

2. *Posterior Cruciate Avulsion* (Fig. 13.30)
   - Features almost comparable to anterior cruciate ligament avulsion except that anteroposterior stress test is positive.
   - In complete disruption, a peculiar 'sagging back' of the tibia is observed as compared to the normal side, while the patient is supine with hip flexed at 45° and knee flexed at 90°.

3. *Medial Meniscus Tear*
   - Usually history of rotational strain in weight bearing and partially flexed knee.
   - Immediate pain.
   - Immediate inability to extend the knee.
   - Mild swelling due to haemarthrosis.
   - Movements of the knee actively possible, but extreme flexed painful.
   - Full range of passive movements possible.
   - Rotational stress tests (including Apley's grinding test) positive.
   - Maximum tenderness at about a point located in the joint line, in the middle of ligamentum patellae and medial side of the knee joint.
   - If there is entrapment of the synovial fringes in between the articular surfaces, tenderness is situated more anteriorly than in meniscal tear.
   - Arthroscopy (diagnostic and even therapeutic).

4. *Lateral Meniscus Tear*
   - Almost identical findings except for reversal of point of tenderness and rotational stress tests.

5. *Fracture Patella* (Fig. 13.16)
   i. Incomplete fracture of patella—In crack fracture of anterior surface, except for tenderness localised in that region and mild to moderate swelling, knee may be nearly normal.
   ii. Complete fracture of patella—In an acute case, besides the findings of an acute traumatic knee (swelling, ecchymosis, bruisings, tenderness and all movements painful) other findings are:
      - Gap at the site of fracture can be palpated.
      - Quadriceps contraction is not communicated through the fracture.
      - Patient can walk (specially in late cases) but with high stepping tendency to clear the ground.

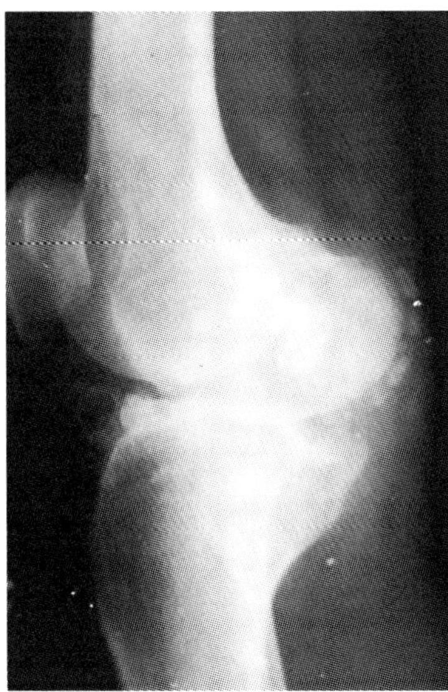

Fig. 13.30: Neglected old case of posterior cruciate avulsion and posterior capsular tear avulsion. Note the calcification along the avulsed capsule

— He may be able to walk on his toes (equinus position) but has difficulty or is unable to walk on his heels.

iii. Comminuted fracture of patella—if without any separation of fragments, the presentation is like that of intra-articular condylar fractures. However, quadriceps expansion and integrity of quadriceps apparatus must be assessed fully in such cases.

X-ray—Confirmatory.

6. *Condylar Fractures (Femoral or tibial)*
   - History of comparatively severe violence.
   - Immediate excruciating pain.
   - Marked swelling due to haemarthrosis.
   - Restriction of movements to a great extent.
   - Depending on the position of the fractured fragments, passive laxity of knee, specially in case of tibial condylar fracture.
   - Maximum tenderness at that particular condylar end.

X-ray is confirmatory.

7. *Recurrent Dislocation of Patella* (Fig. 13.31)
   - Usually in girls of adolescent age.
   - History of recurrent dislocation or subluxation of patella.
   - Many a time, the patient herself reduces the dislocation/subluxation.

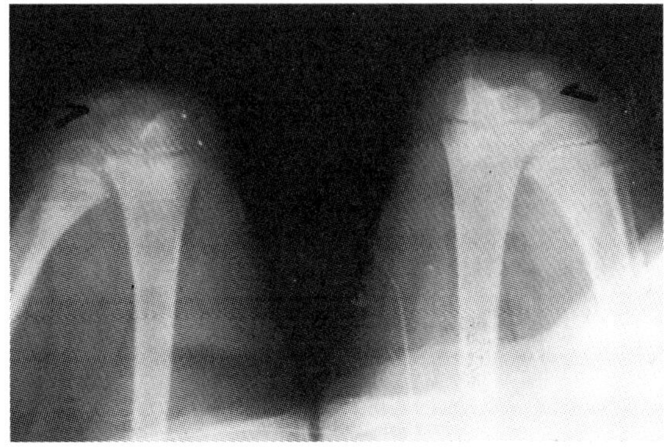

Fig. 13.31: Bilateral recurrent dislocation of patella

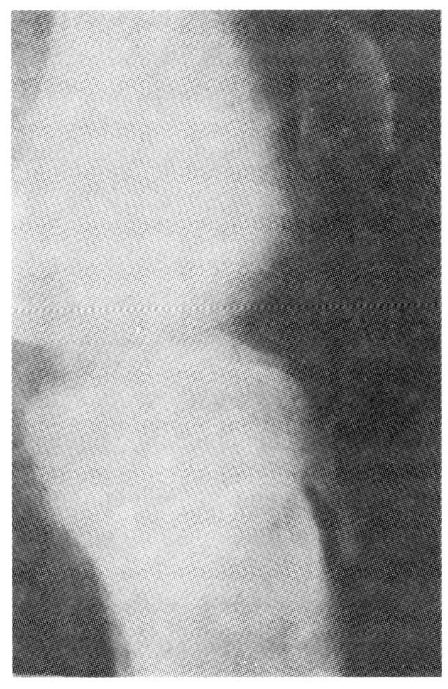

Fig. 13.32: Osgood-Schlatter's disease of tibia

- May be associated with genu valgum.
- Such episodes are followed by mild to moderate pain and swelling which subside in a few days.
- Sky-line view X-ray—may demonstrate the lateral femoral condylar ridge to be flattened as compared to the medial.

8. *Chondromalacia Patellae*
   - Young girl complains of pain deep in the knee, specially behind the patella.
   - Pain more in getting up and down the stairs with occasional effusion.
   - Articular surfaces of patella tender.
   - Anterior surface of medial condyle of femur also tender.
   - X-ray—almost normal.
   - Arthroscopy (diagnostic and therapeutic).

9. *Patellar Malalignment (Chondromalacia Patellae)*

The word 'chondromalacia' (meaning thereby= soft cartilage) has been corelated to define dry patellar pain (mainly the undersurface) or to refer to cartilage changes anywhere in the knee, has become confusing and controversial, and its features have been encompassed within the broder term "Patellar Malalignment" (grelsamer 2000). Such patellar in adults is mostly due to patellar malalignment (translational or rotational deviation of the patella related to any axis). Patellar malalignment is associated with tightness of the following sructures—in order of frequency—the lateral retinaculum, the hamstrings, the ilio-tibial band, the quadriceps, the hip rotators, and the Achilles tendon. In patellar malalignment, the patient usually complains of a sense of giving way and pain when he gets up from seated position, climbs up stairs or uphill or squats, since these activities exacerbate the abnormal pressure distribution above the patella.

Pain in patellar region usually comes after prolonged sitting due to venous congestion and stretching of painful tissue—'prolonged squatting sign' or 'Movie theatre sign' Location of pain should be classically anterior, but it may be medial, lateral or popliteal.

Once diagnosed and confirmed by MRI or scintigraphy (technetium scanning), the management should be principally strecthing of the tight structure and/or braces (to realign the position of patella), and surgery (only for resistant cases).

10. *Osgood-Schlatter's Disease* (Fig. 13.32)
    - Usually adolescents complain of pain in the tibial tuberosity region, specially after strenuous activity.
    - Prominence of tibial tuberosity.
    - Tenderness on tibial tuberosity, especially while pressing from the lateral side.
    - Strong contraction of quadriceps causes pain in tibial tuberosity.
    - X-ray—enlargement with or without fragmentation of tibial tuberosity (Fig. 13.32).

BIBLIOGRAPHY

1. Grelsamer RP: Patellar malalignment. *J Bone Joint Surg* **82A**:1638-1650, 2000.
2. Pandey AK, Pandey S, Pandey P: Results of partial patellectomy. *Archives of Orthopaedic and Trauma Surgery* **110**: 246-249, 1991.
3. Turek, Samuel L: *Orthopaedics, Principles and their Applications* **4**: 1269-1406, 1984.

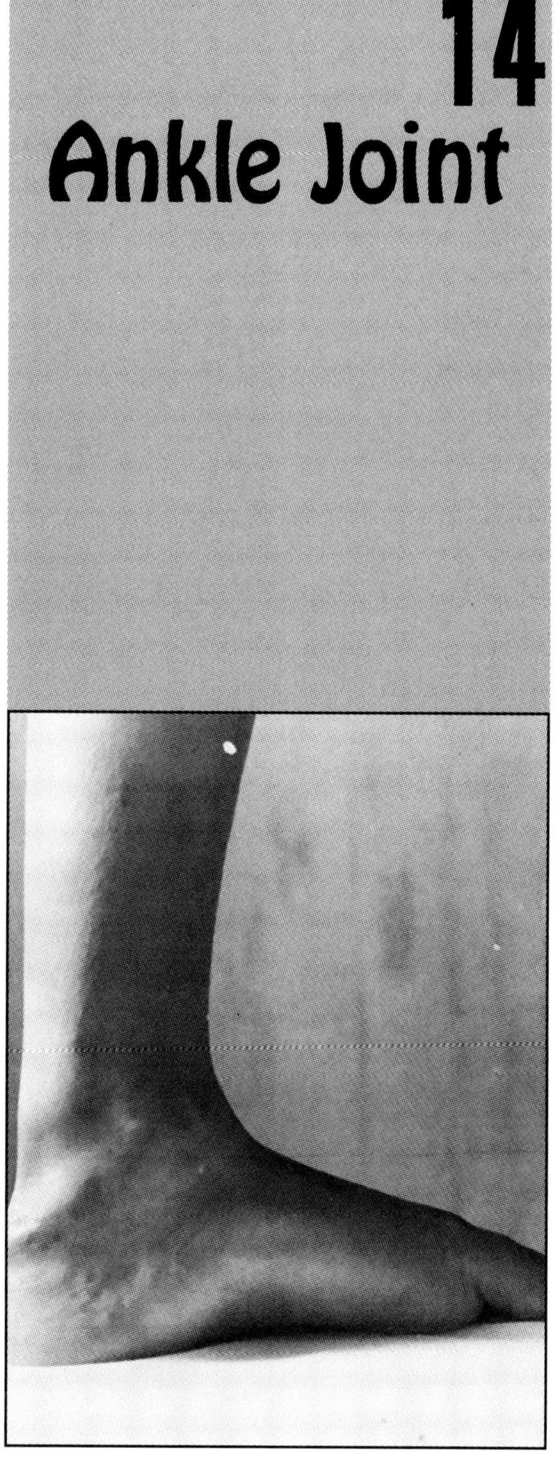

INTRODUCTION

In a biped, each normal ankle assumes the responsibility of transmitting at least 50% of the body weight to the tripod like structure of the foot in such a fashion that the rhythmic gait pattern is not disturbed.

ANATOMICAL CONSIDERATIONS

I. Anatomically the ankle joint (a hinge joint) is the articulation of the dome of the talus into the 'ankle mortice'. The integrity of the ankle mortice is mandatory for normal functioning of the joint.

A. Ankle mortice is made up of (a) bony and (b) soft-tissue components

a. *Bony components are*:

i. Lower articular end of tibia.
ii. Articular surface on medial aspect of lateral malleolus.
iii. Articular surface on lateral aspect of medial malleolus.

b. *Soft tissue components are*:

i. Anterior inferior tibiofibular ligament.
ii. Posterior inferior tibiofibular ligament.
iii. Interosseous tibiofibular ligament.
iv. Inferior deep transverse ligament (i.e. the inferior lower and deep portion of the posterior tibiofibular ligament which is a strong thick yellowish band).

The part of ligaments lying close to the bone have a more or less fibrocartilaginous texture.

II. The ankle joint is peculiar in having no muscular coverage on any of the sides.

III. It has important controlling groups of tendons, almost all around. These are arranged as follows:

a. *Anteriorly*: From medial to lateral the following structures are strapped down by the superior and inferior ('Y' shaped) extensor retinacula just above and at the ankle level.

— Tendon of tibialis anterior.
— Tendon of extensor hallucis longus.
— Anterior tibial artery and vein.
— Anterior tibial nerve.
— Tendon of extensor digitorum longus.
— Tendon of peroneus tertius.

b. *On posteromedial aspect*: Below and behind the medial malleolus the flexor retinaculum straps down the following structures (from medial to lateral side).
— Tendon of tibialis posterior.
— Tendon of flexor digitorum longus.
— Posterior tibial artery and vein.
— Posterior tibial nerve.
— Tendon of flexor hallucis longus.

c. *Posteriorly*, just in the midline, is the stout tendinous mass of triceps surae (tendo-Achilles). In between the posterior capsule of the joint and this tendon lies the slender tendon of plantaris.

d. *On the posterolateral aspect* are the peroneus longus and peroneus brevis tendons in the peroneal sheath and they are strapped down by superior and inferior peroneal retinacula.

IV. The synovial reflection of the ankle joint is not as complicated as that of the knee, but are intercommunicating with those of the other joints of the foot upto the tarsometatarsal joints. The synovial swellings can be palpated on anteromedial, anterolateral, posteromedial and posterolateral aspects of the joint. It is not possible to approach the entire synovial reflections through a single incision.

The tendons around the ankle are surrounded by the synovial sheaths, which are common sites of affection in tuberculosis and rheumatoid arthritis.

V. Integrity of the ankle joint depends mainly on collateral ligaments.

a. The fan shaped deltoid ligament is on the medial side. It is attached superiorly to the tip of the medial malleolus and inferiorly, from in front backwards, to the tuberosity of navicular, spring ligament, neck of talus, the sustentaculum tali and tubercle and body of talus. Thus the components of deltoid ligament are the tibionavicular, anterior tibiotalar, tibiocalcaneal (superficial) and posterior tibiotalar (deep) ligaments. The deltoid ligament assists the spring ligament in holding up the head of the talus, and thus helps to maintain the medial longitudinal arch of the foot.

b. On the lateral side, the lateral ligament consisting of, the three bands of anterior talofibular (thinnest, flattened and most fragile), calcaneofibular (stronger, round and thicker), and posterior talofibular (very strong band), is responsible for maintaining a stout check on the ankle joint. Any disruption in these ligaments lead to sprain of the ankle joint. These ligaments are blended with the capsule of the ankle joint.

Capsule is comparatively loose anteriorly and posteriorly to allow the plantar and dorsi-flexions. However, in extreme range of motion they get stretched and behave like check ligaments.

VI. The ankle forms the fulcrum at which the leg transmits the body weight to the foot. The foot remains in contact with the ground in standing, walking or running. When the foot is caught either on uneven slope or in a pit hole/ditch, even a little imbalance of the body gets accentuated at the distal end of the long lever arm of leg leading to various fractures along with subluxation or dislocation at the ankle level. These have been grouped together as "Pott's fracture".

VII. Within the contour of the ankle mortice, the dome of talus is equally vulnerable in the various injuries of the ankle joint.

Besides the common sequelae of injuries, the talus is also notorious for undergoing avascular necrosis because of its comparatively precarious blood supply.

BLOOD SUPPLY OF TALUS (Fig. 14.1)

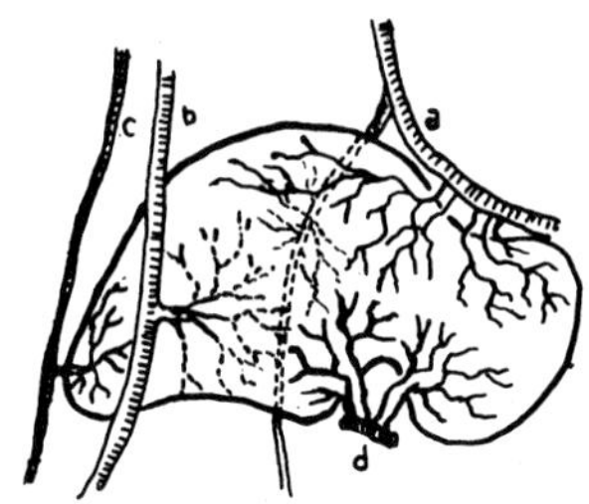

Fig. 14.1: Blood supply of talus; a = anterior tibial artery; b = posterior tibial artery; c = peroneal artery; d = vessels coming through sinus tarsi

The main sources of blood supply to the talus are:

1. Posterior tibial artery
2. Anterior tibial artery
3. Peroneal artery

The braches of these arteries are mainly grouped under two headings:

i. Through anterior capsule of ankle joint, blood vessels enter anterosuperior portion of neck of talus.
ii. The blood vessels coming through the sinus tarsi (tarsal canal) enter from the inferior surface of the neck of talus.

Very few blood vessels enter the postero-inferior portion of the body of talus.

Head of the talus is supplied by vessels entering:	— the superior surface of neck. — the inferolateral surface of neck.
Body of talus is supplied by vessels entering through:	— the superior surface of neck. — the antero-inferior surface of neck. — medial surface of body. — anterolateral surface of body. — posterior tubercle.

In any disruption of the anterior capsule of the ankle joint (e.g. fracture dislocation of ankle joint), the blood supply is likely to suffer, resulting in variable avascular necrosis of talus.

VIII. The main blood vessels going to the foot, i.e. anterior tibial and posterior tibial arteries, are very closely related, anteriorly and posteromedially respectively, to the capsule of the ankle joint. Therefore, major injuries of ankle joint, specially dislocations are likely to press, partially damage or even disrupt the main blood supply, thereby threatening the circulation of the foot.

IX. The skin is very closely disposed over the bony contours almost all around the ankle joint. In dislocation of the ankle joint or similar injuries, the skin gets devitalised due to pressure, and may undergo necrosis.

METHODOLOGY

History

History taking is as in the chapter of Introduction. The main complaints following any trauma or disease in the ankle are pain, swelling, limp, instability and deformity.

General and Systemic Examination

As in the chapter on Introduction.

Any affection of the ankle is likely to affect the gait and posture of the patient. Hence, if it is possible, patient should be asked to walk first, as normally as possible, then on the heels and toes alternately. While standing, if possible, note the posture and mode of weight bearing at the affected ankle and foot. Each step of examination must be compared with that of opposite ankle, however, if both are affected, findings should be noted separately.

Regional Examination

It should be done from tip of the toes to the hip.

It is always paying to examine the leg as a whole along with the ankle, e.g. even ligamentous disruption at the ankle can be associated with fracture of upper end of the fibula—Maisonneuve injury.

Effects of Ankle Pathology on Regional Joints

As already considered while dealing with the knee, various deformities at the knees are likely to affect the ankle, hip and spine and *vice-versa*. Further, ankle has to act as a buffer in any affection of the foot and balance weight transmission at the knee. To avoid pain at the ankle due to any pathology, the patient tries to manoeuvre the intrinsics of the foot, which in turn either produce various clawing effects, or fanning out tendency of the toes. When the muscles controlling the smaller joints of the foot are paralysed, the main brunt falls on the ankle. On the other hand, when ankle movements are affected, the smaller joints of the foot try to accommodate as far as practicable, e.g. if plantar flexion at the ankle is lost, either due to any pathology or following arthrodesis, the mid-tarsal, sub-talar and even tarsometatarsal joints provide for varying amount of workable flexion of the foot.

Except in paralytic conditions (where the overpowering muscles determine the deformities), the ankle has the tendency of postural fixity in the possible position of walking, whereas the smaller joints accommodate to compensate for the loss of ankle movements. Therefore, the overall assessment of the foot and ankle must be done simultaneously.

I. *Varicosities*

Blowing out (dilatation with tortuosity) of the venous channels on the medial side of the ankle should be looked for. The integrity of the deeper valves of the veins in the legs and thighs should be tested for. These varicosities may be responsible for pain around the ankle joint. There may be discolouration of the skin, chronic ulcers and sometimes troublesome bleeding from the ulcers.

II. *Oedema Around the Ankle*

Ankle is the site of oedematous swelling from various causes, ranging from congenital lymphoedema to neoplastic compression. In medical conditions like anaemia, hypoproteinaemia, filariasis, cirrhosis of liver, congestive cardiac failure, nephrotic syndrome, oedema around the ankle may be the first sign. Oedema due to posture, pregnancy and pelvic pathology should also be kept in mind. The nature (pitting or non-pitting) and extent of oedema should be noted.

Examination of Lymph Glands

Palpate the lymph glands in the popliteal fossa and inguinal region and note their character.

LOCAL EXAMINATION

Inspection

Attitude

Typical attitudes (as described in the chapter on Foot) should be looked for.

The attitude of the foot and ankle can also give a clue to the mode of injury and displacement in different types of Pott's fracture.

In most of the pathologies of the ankle, this region is swollen all around. Any swelling of the tendon sheath appears along the long axis of leg and foot beyond the joint level.

Keep both ankles and feet in identical position. Inspect systematically from anterior, lateral, posterior and medial sides.

Anteriorly, Note the Following

i. Relation of the foot to ankle (normal, equinus, calcaneus, valgus and varus).
ii. Interrelation of the malleoli (normally the lateral malleolus lies 1 cm below and behind the medial malleolus) (Fig. 14.2).
iii. Long saphenous vein.
iv. Anterior group of tendons.

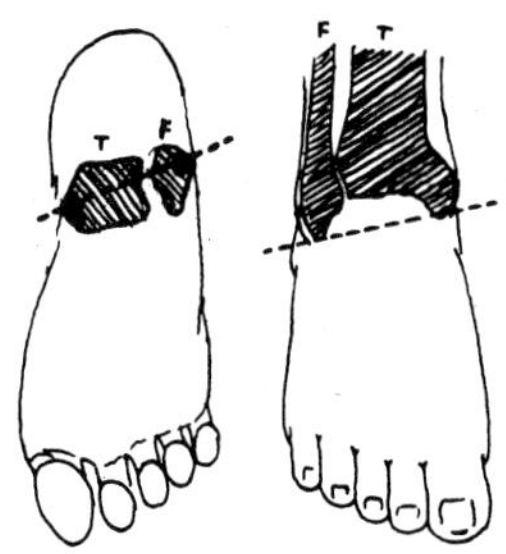

Fig. 14.2: Showing inter-malleolar relation. Note that the tip of lateral malleolus (F-fibula) is distal and posterior to the medial malleolus (T-tibia)

v. Fossae in front of the malleoli (which may be full in swelling of ankle).
vi. Any abnormal finding, like swelling, sinus, etc.

Laterally, Note the Following

The tendons of peroneus longus and brevis lie just behind the lateral malleolus. Note if they are prominent. From here, there is a gradual shallow concavity posteriorly upto the fossa on the outer side of the tendo-Achilles (tendo-calcaneus). Note any abnormal finding.

Posteriorly, Note the Following

i. Prominence of tendo-Achilles, along with the calf bulk.
ii. Any swelling in relation to tendo-Achilles.
iii. Fossae on both sides of tendo-Achilles.
iv. Pattern, position and size of heel, (broadening, or narrowing; tugged up or plantigrade or splashed out; normal, small or large in size).

Medially, Note the Following

The tendon of tibialis posterior lies just adapted to the posteroinferior margin of the medial malleolus—note if it is prominent. From here, upto the fossa on the medial side of tendo-Achilles, a gradual shallow concavity is maintained. Note any abnormality.

Palpation

i. *Superficial (touch)*: In superficial palpation, surface and texture of skin, temperature and any superficial tenderness, anaesthesia, hypoaesthesia or paraesthesia is to be noted.
ii. *Deep palpation (feel)*: It is not easy to palpate the joint margins of the ankle joint all around. Palpate the malleoli and feel for any thickening, tenderness, and irregularity and also note the relation between two malleoli. Palpate and assess individually the tendons around the ankle joint starting from one side. Note their position and continuity and feel for any thickening. Assess their excursion, power of parent muscle and spasm if any. Note any tenderness, synovial swelling and ganglion along their course. On the posterior side, the presence of a soft to firm swelling in relation to the tendo-Achilles is not uncommon. Usually it manifests anterior to the tendo-Achilles as pre-Achilles bursitis or posterior to it as post-Achilles bursitis.

Palpate for anterior tibial arterial pulsation in between the tendons of extensor hallucis longus and extensor digitorum longus, i.e. at about midway between the malleoli (Fig. 14.3A), which may be absent congenitally.

Palpate for posterior tibial arterial pulsation behind the tendon of flexor digitorum longus, i.e. 1 finger breadth behind the medial malleolus. (Fig. 14.3B), which may be congenitally absent or too feeble.

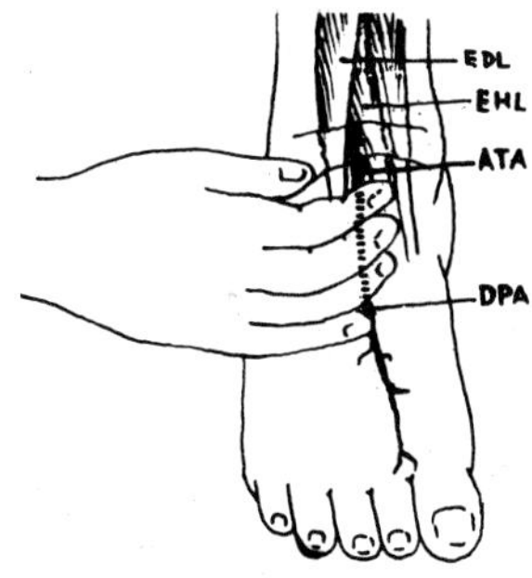

Fig. 14.3A: Palpating the anterior tibial artery (ATA anterior tibial artery, EHL extensor hallucis longus, EDL extensor digitorum longus, DPA dorsalis pedis artery)

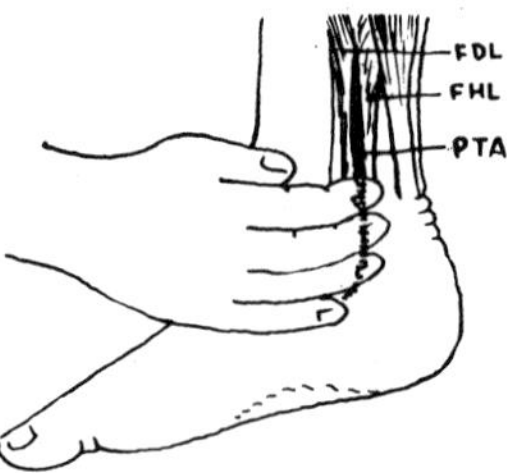

Fig. 14.3B: Palpating the posterior tibial artery (PTA posterior tibial artery, FDL flexor digitorum longus, FHL flexor hallucis longus)

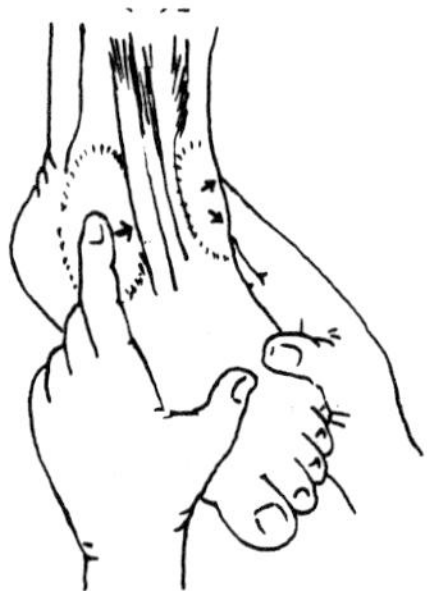

Fig. 14.4A: Cross-fluctuation between anterolateral and anteromedial swelling

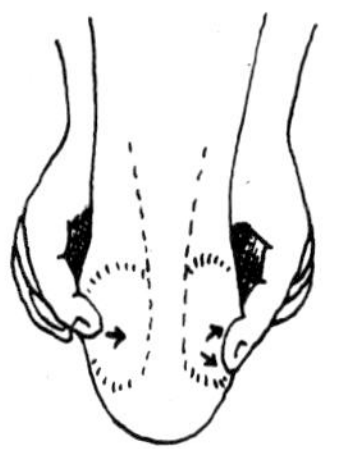

Fig. 14.4B: Cross-fluctuation between posteromedial and posterolateral swellings

Any synovial swelling or fluid in the ankle joint usually manifests as outpouchings around the ankle, mainly on the posterolateral, posteromedial, anterolateral and anteromedial aspects. Synovial swellings are soft and doughy in feel. It is probably impossible to demonstrate the presence of a small amount of fluid in the ankle joint. In presence of moderate to large amount of fluid, cross-fluctuation can be demonstrated.

Method of Demonstration of Cross-Fluctuation in between the Anterolateral and Anteromedial Swellings, (Fig. 14.4A); *and Posterolateral and Posteromedial Swellings* (Fig. 14.4B)

Plantar flex the ankle joint as far as practicable. The dorsal tendons form tight longitudinal straps across the ankle joint. Place both index fingers in front of both malleoli. On pressing from one side, the contralateral finger will feel the impulse in presence of fluid in the ankle joint. Similarly, in between the posterolateral and posteromedial pouchings, fluctuation can be demonstrated if the ankle is kept dorsiflexed (Fig. 14.4B).

Mode of Demonstration of Cross Fluctuation in Between Anterior and Posterior Swellings (Fig. 14.4C)

Ankle should be placed in as much neutral position as possible. The index finger and thumb of one hand are placed anterior to the malleoli. Index finger and thumb of the opposite hand are placed on either side of the tendo-Achilles at slightly lower level. Now, simultaneous pressure by the finger and thumb of one hand propels the fluid to the opposite compartment and therefore an impulse is felt by the fingers of the opposite hand.

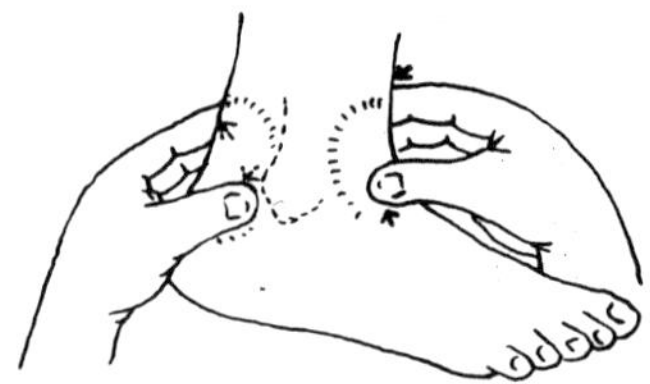

Fig. 14.4C: Cross-fluctuation between anterior and posterior pouchings

Due to circuitous disposition of the ankle, transillumination is usually not positive. However, when the amount of fluid is large, the distended joint is so tense that cross-fluctuation may not be demonstrable effectively. Here, transillumination may be positive. Transillumination may also be positive if done from anterolateral to anteromedial or from posterolateral to posteromedial out pouchings (and *vice-versa*).

MOVEMENTS

Normal movements at the ankle (from 0-position of the ankle, i.e. in right angled position) are:

a. *Dorsiflexion* (15°-30°)

When the joint is dorsiflexed, the widest anterior part of the talus is wedged tightly between the two malleoli providing sound stability to the joint.

Dorsiflexion of foot exerts traction on posterior tibial vein and in case of thrombosis of calf veins, passive dorsiflexion of foot causes pain in the calf—Homan's sign.

b. *Plantar Flexion* (30°-50°)

In fully plantar flexed position of the ankle, the posterior and narrowest part of the dome of talus articulates with the ankle mortice. In this position, some side to side rocking and inversion/eversion of the ankle can be passively demonstrated. Movements should be assessed under different headings, as in the chapter of Introduction. While testing for passive movements at the ankle, stress movements at the ankle should be done to confirm the integrity of the controlling collateral ligaments. Of course, it is better to test dorsiflexion, plantar flexion and stress movements at both ankle joints simultaneously for comparison.

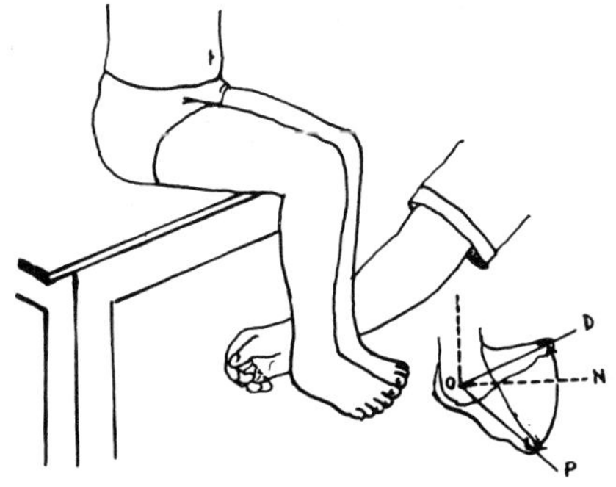

Fig. 14.5: Demonstration of active dorsiflexion and plantar flexion at ankle

Method: Patient sits on the edge of the bed or examination table keeping his knees bent about 90° and both his legs and feet hanging down the edge of the table. Sitting on one side of the patient, support the lower part of the legs from behind. Patient is then asked to alternately dorsiflex and plantar flex both the ankles simultaneously from the zero position (i.e. foot at 90° to the leg axis). Note the excursion of the hind foot in either direction in both feet (Fig. 14.5). Then, holding the mid and fore parts of the foot by another hand, dorsiflex and plantar flex the foot passively, at ankle level, and note the additions possible over the active range.

a. *Assessment for Lateral Collapse of Ankle*

The paralytic foot most commonly goes for valgus in various combinations. Valgus collapse at the ankle becomes quite apparent when the patient bears weight on that foot (Figs 14.6A and B). Cosmetically it is ugly and difficult to correct. It should be assessed separately from valgus at the sub-talar joint.

Method (Fig. 14.6C): Assess the extent of passive valgus at the normal foot under maximum possible stress. In neutral position of the ankle and foot, hold the ankle from dorsum, in between the thumb and index finger. Your first web should firmly grip the dorsum of the talus. Hold the heel, i.e. the body of the calcaneum in between the thumb and index finger of the opposite hand. While the first hand remains firmly static, passively evert and invert the heel as much as possible, using the other hand. This will assess the movements at the subtalar joint. Total valgus of the affected foot, minus the possible valgus at the subtalar joint will be the valgus collapse at the ankle. Similarly, varus collapse of the ankle (rare condition) can also be assessed.

b. *Critical Arc*

15° plantar flexion to 15° dorsiflexion (from 0° position, i.e. neutral right angled position of the foot) is the critical arc for the ankle. This is because an average 15° plantar flexion at the ankle is the minimum required for push off phase of the gait. On the other hand, about 15° of dorsiflexion is the minimum required for

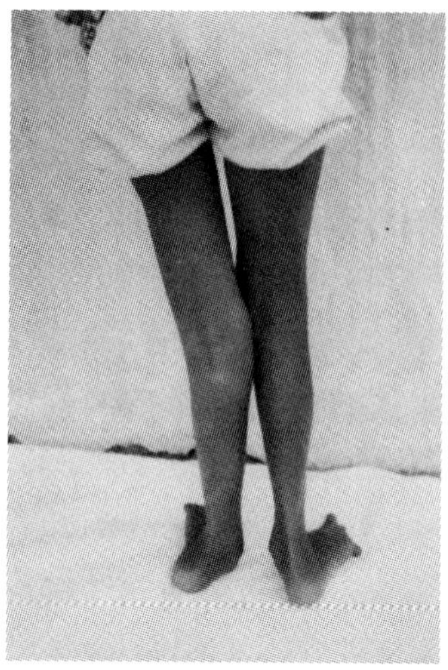

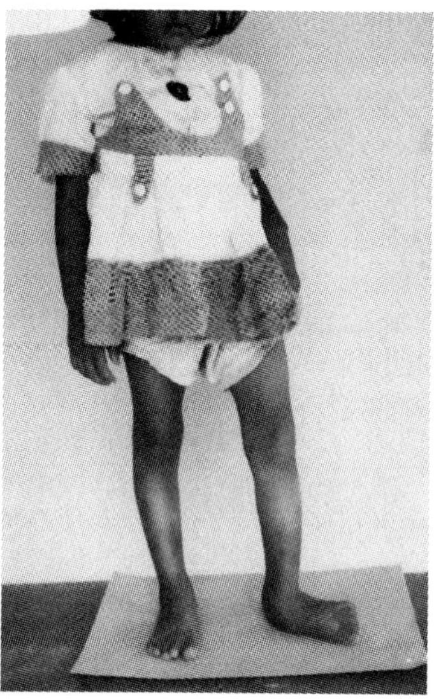

Figs 14.6A and B: Note the early valgus collapse at ankle besides the valgus at subtalar joint

deceleration to heel strike phase of gait and squatting.

c. *Abnormal Movements*

In paralytic and neuropathic ankle and feet and Charcot's arthropathy, abnormal movements are possible. Each type of abnormal movement should be noted separately.

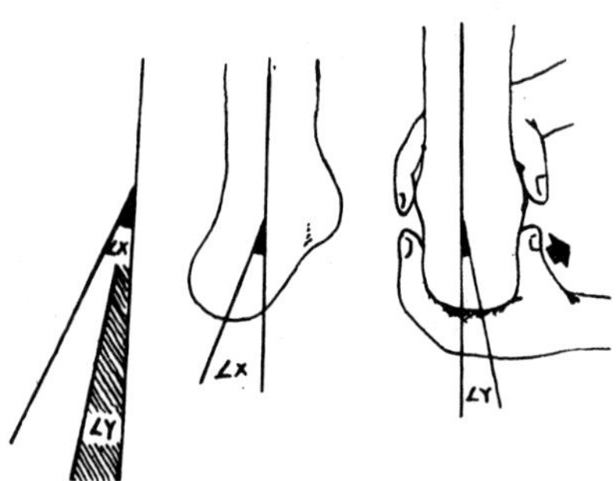

Fig. 14.6C: Method of measuring the valgus collapse at the ankle: angle Y denotes the valgus at subtalar joint, angle X denotes total valgus of foot, so X Y = valgus collapse at ankle

d. *Stress Test (To assess integrity of the controlling group of ligament)*

Method (Figs 14.7A and B): Place the ankle in neutral position. Hold the lower leg firmly from the front, by one hand. Hold the foot at about the level of the head of talus by the opposite hand. For testing the lateral collateral ligaments, (Fig. 14.7A) invert the foot forcibly (within limit of pain tolerance) and note:

i. The yield of the foot.
ii. The gap in front of, beneath and behind the lateral malleolus.
iii. The point of maximum pain.
iv. The range of inversion possible at the ankle.

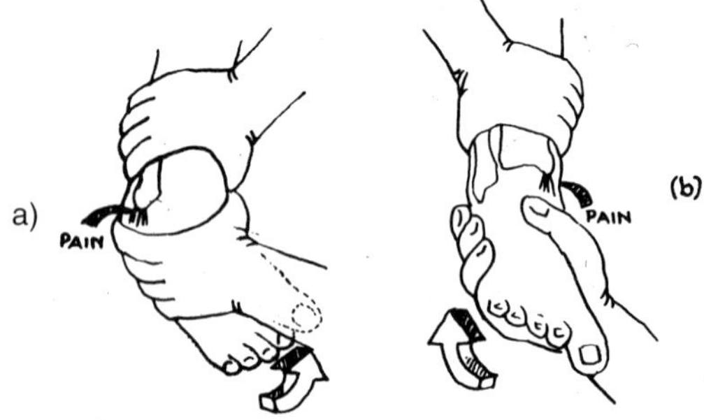

Figs 14.7A and B: Testing the integrity of (a) lateral and (b) medial collateral ligaments of ankle

For testing the integrity of the medial collateral ligament (i.e. deltoid ligament), stress has to be given in the opposite direction. Holding the lower leg in the same position, the foot is everted and the aforesaid points are noted in relation to the medial malleolus (Fig. 14.7B).

Stress tests, for integrity of anterior and posterior ligaments, i.e. capsular reinforcements, are not that important. However, they can be noted as exaggeration of passive dorsiflexion and plantar flexion of the ankle (in laxity or tear of the posterior and anterior capsular reinforcements respectively).

Anteroposterior Stress Test—(Brostrom-1965)—Anterior Drawer Sign

The integrity of the capsule and the anterior talofibular ligament (sometimes calcaneofibular ligament as well) can be tested by pulling the heel anteromedially against resistance applied by the other hand over the anterior aspect of the lower leg. Anterior subluxation of 3 mm of the talus is pathological.

Special Test

Rupture of tendo-Achilles

Tendo-Achilles is the strongest tendon of the body. Achilles the Greek hero was the son of Peleus and Thetis. When he was a child his mother dipped him in the river Styx by holding his heel to make him invincible in battle. But the heel, by which he was held did not get wet, and so it remained unprotected. Achilles died after receiving an injury in the heel at the seige of Troy.

The Achilles tendon usually ruptures 2 to 6 cm proximal to its insertion in os calcis, where the tendon is ischaemic and weaker than normal. It occurs usually in middle aged men as a result of any trivial stumble or a sudden painful snap during walking or negotiating stains.

After rupture dorsiflexion of foot can be done more than normal. Plantar flexion reduces, but never completely even with complete rupture of the tendo-Achilles, since some active plantar flexion is maintained by the combined action of tibialis posterior, long flexors of toes and peroneum longus and brevis.

A. Test for Rupture of Tendo-Achilles (Fig. 14.8A to D)

Ask the patient to stand on tip toe. In case of weak tendo-Achilles, there will be a lag in lifting the heel. In case of partial rupture, the patient will also complain of pain at the site. In complete rupture, the lag will be much more, but standing on tip-toe is never completely absent (since some power of plantar flexion exists due to intact tibialis posterior, long flexors of toes, and peroneus longus and brevis). Along with this, a gap can also be felt at the rupture site in which one can insinuate the examining finger. At both ends of the gap the rounded ends of the ruptured tendon can be felt in late cases. In late neglected cases the ends feel like adder heads.

II. Thompson's Test (1962)

Patient is asked to lie prone with his feet projecting beyond the examining table. On squeezing the calf the foot automatically plantar flexes, if tendo-Achilles is intact or even partially torn. However, in complete rupture flexion is not possible, hence there is no movement of the foot.

III. X-ray

In true lateral view of ankle and foot, taken in possible maximum plantar flexion, the rugosities at the back of ankle will be lacking; and if taken in maximum dorsiflexion, the soft tissue lining at the back of the ankle will be more or less vertical and close to the bone with marked calcaneus effect of the foot (Fig. 14.8B).

IV. Needle Test

Tim O'Brien by performing his "needle test" to dynamically assess the integrity of distal 10 cm of tendo-Achilles has reported very reliable results.

Method: The patient lies prone. Under aseptic conditions a 25 gauge hypodermic needle is pierced through the skin at a point 10 cm above

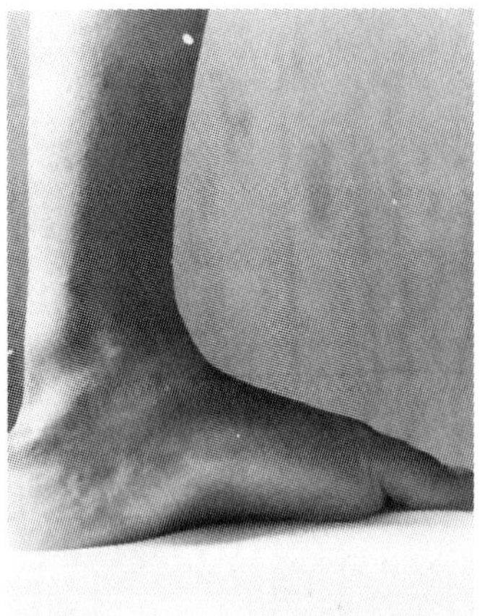

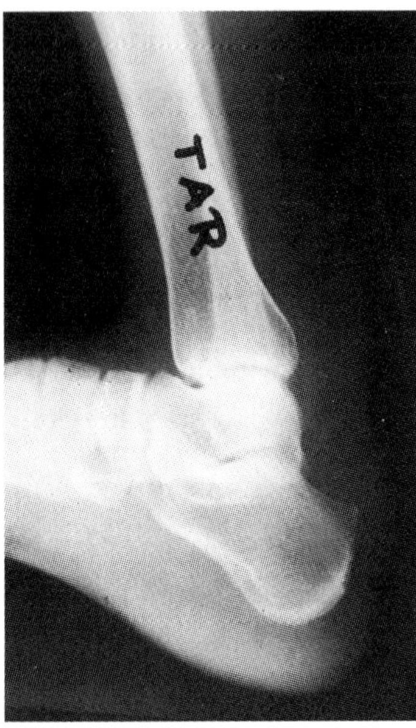

Figs 14.8A and B: Clinical photograph and X-ray showing complete rupture of tendo-Achilles

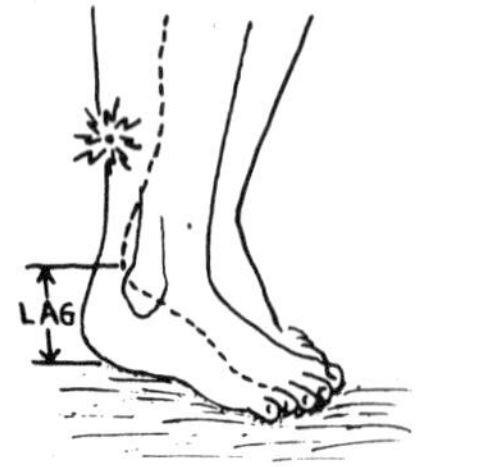

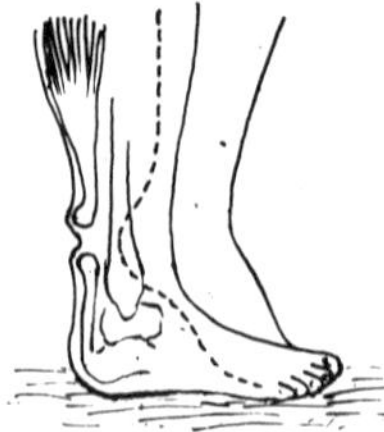

Figs 14.8C and D: (c) Test for partial rupture of tendo-Achilles and (d)Test for complete rupture of tendo-Achilles

the upper end of calcaneum and just medial to the midline of the calf. The foot is then passively plantar flexed and dorsiflexed. With intact tendo-Achilles, the needle will swivel in a direction opposite to the movement of the foot. Absence of this swiveling indicates complete rupture of the tendo-Achilles.

B. *Test for Pre-Achilles and Post-Achilles Pathologies (Mainly Bursitis) and Achilles Tendinitis* (Figs 14.9A and B)

The patient is asked to walk on his toes (with the heel off the ground). He will complain of pain in case of pre-Achilles pathology. The patient is then asked to walk on the heel (with the toes off the ground). There will be pain in post-Achilles pathology.

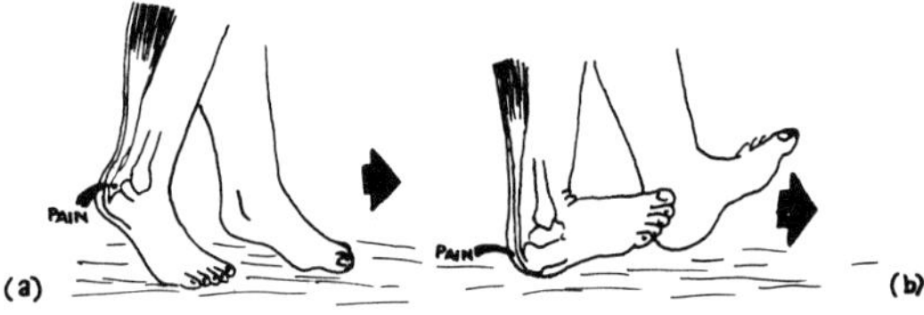

Figs 14.9A and B: Test for pre-Achilles (a) and post-Achilles (b) bursitis

In Achilles tendinitis, pain will be in both mode of walking, but will be more on walking on the toes.

A short tendon or repeated forceful contractions (e.g. in jumping, running, tennis or volleyball playing, etc) may cause Achilles tendinitis.

Clinical features are: pain in and around the tendon, which increases after exercises; gradually morning pain and stiffness in the ankle region and heel develop; forceful plantar flexion against resistance aggrevates the symptoms; tendon is tender on squeezing.

It may be confused with pre and post Achilles bursitis, stress fractures of tibia and fibula, peroneal tendinitis.

Management protocol should avoid corticoid infilteration, since it is liable to produce rupture of the tendo-Achilles.

C. *Test for Tendovaginitis of Tibialis Posterior Tendon* (Fig. 14.10)

Patient sits with his legs hanging from the edge of the table. Ask him to plantar flex his foot to the maximum and then invert it against resistance. Pain will be complained of behind the medial malleolus. At the same site there may be a tender and soft/firm thickening palpable along the tibialis posterior tendon.

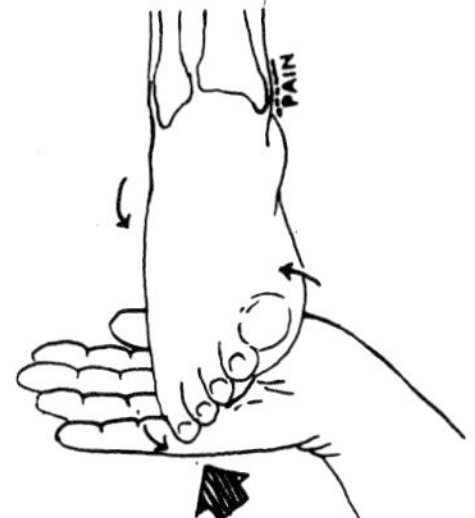

Fig. 14.10: Test for tendovaginitis of tibialis posterior tendon

D. *Test for Peroneal Spasm* (Fig. 14.11)

Patient sits with legs hanging over the edge of the table. Ask him to plantar flex and invert the foot. There will be marked limitations. Forced inversion will lead to pain behind the lateral malleolus.

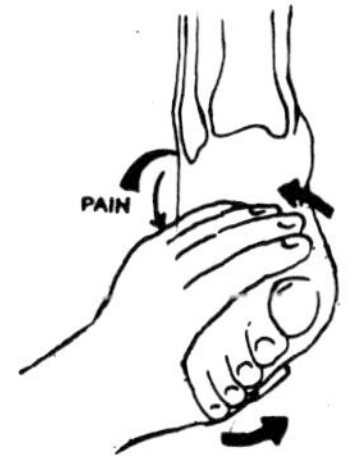

Fig. 14.11: Test for peroneal spasm

Shin splints (Anterior leg pain): This problem is mostly faced by young athletes due to poor conditioning for the event, over-exercises/activities, sudden change in the pattern of sport event. Repetitive traction by anterior and posterior tibialis muscles on the edges of the tibia leads to diffuse linear pain along the anterior or medial edge of the mid shaft or distal one-third of tibia. There is diffuse tenderness along the origin of anterior or posterior tibialis muscles. There may be decrease in the power of dorsiflexors of ankle and foot.

MEASUREMENTS

a. Linear

Affection of the ankle as such is comparatively less responsible for producing limb length disparity. However, severe injuries, advanced tuberculous and pyogenic infections, neoplasms and dyschondroplasia in the ankle region are likely to affect the length of the limb. Chronic pyogenic osteomyelitis of lower end of tibia and fibula has been seen to produce limb length disparity (increase in length more frequently than shortening).

Method: Total and segmental measurements of lower limb should be done as in the examination of hip and knee. The distance between the tip of medial malleolus to the sole (along a line dropped vertically from the medial malleolus) indicates roughly the height of talus, calcaneum and heel pad. Affection of any of these can produce disparity in this measurement.

b. Circumferential Measurement (Fig. 14.12)

It should be done at the level of ankle joint and mid calf. The first indicates any increase or decrease in girth of the ankle, whereas the latter measures any increase or decrease of the muscular bulk.

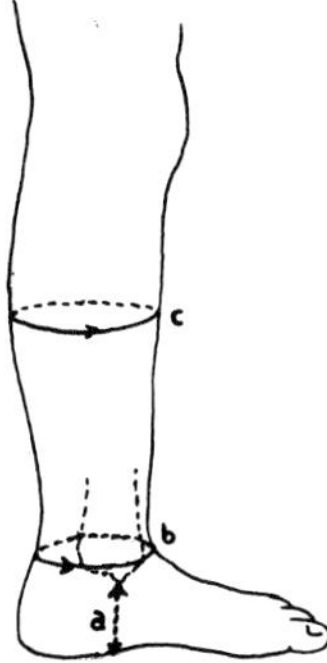

Fig. 14.12: (a) Vertical height of talus + calcaneum + heel pad, (b) Circumferential measurement around ankle, and (c) Circumferential measurement at the mid calf level

C. Oblique Circumferential Measurement (Figs 14.13A to C)

It should be done across the point of the heel and front of the ankle. In calcaneus deformity, this will be increased, whereas in equinus deformity, it will be decreased.

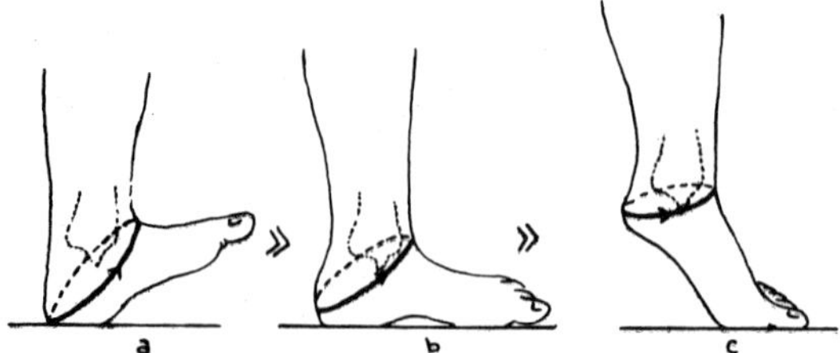

Figs 14.13A to C: Oblique circumferential measurement across the ankle, a = calcaneus, b = normal, c = equinus

Auscultation

It is not important, but suspected swelling around the ankle should be auscultated.

Power

The power of the controlling muscles must be tested and charted separately according to MRC scale. Intrinsics of the foot should also be tested, as they are likely to be variably affected in ankle involvements and *vice-versa.*

INVESTIGATIONS FOR ANKLE PATHOLOGY

A. Routine Investigations

(As in chapter on Introduction)

B. Radiology

Besides routine investigations for various joint affections, stress X-rays of the ankle are important. These are best done under general anaesthesia to avoid pain in various traumatic and pathological conditions. The importance of these X-rays are more in injuries around the ankle region. Of course, anteroposterior and lateral views are mandatory.

Stress Radiology

Patient lies supine with both legs straped together in neutral position. A sand bag is placed beneath the lower leg, both feet are held at the forefoot level. The X-ray plate is placed posteriorly and the beam is focussed at the mid ankle level. Then, while the feet are forcibly inverted, or everted (as per suspicion) to the maximum, the shot is taken (Fig. 14.14). The ankle mortice and talar dome interrelation can be very well assessed in an anteroposterior view.

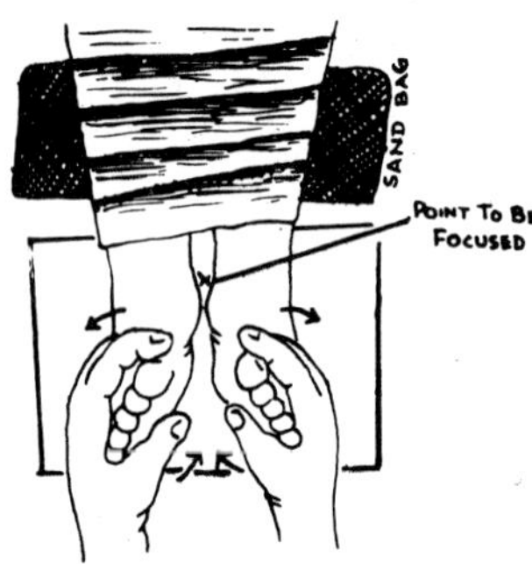

Fig. 14.14: Method of taking stress radiography in fully inverted position (to test the integrity of the lateral collateral ligament, mainly calcaneofibular and posterior talofibular)

Normally, forced inversion can tilt the talus in the mortice by 10°. In a stress radiography taken under general anaesthesia, talar tilt between 10° to 15° is suggestive of rupture of the anterior talofibular ligament alone; between 15° to 30° rupture of anterior talofibular and calcaneofibular ligaments; and more than 30° tilt is suggestive of rupture of all three components of the lateral ligament. To assess the integrity of posterior melleolus, specially in complicated Pott's fracture, an oblique view must be taken, which also clarifies any doubtful fracture of the medial malleolus.

C. Arthroscopy

It is gaining importance in exploring the lesions of the ankle, e.g. loose bodies.

Key Diagnostic Points to Common Affections of the Ankle

1. **Of the Congenital Conditions, Club Foot is the Commonest (Figs 14.15, see also Figs 15.25 to 15.28)**

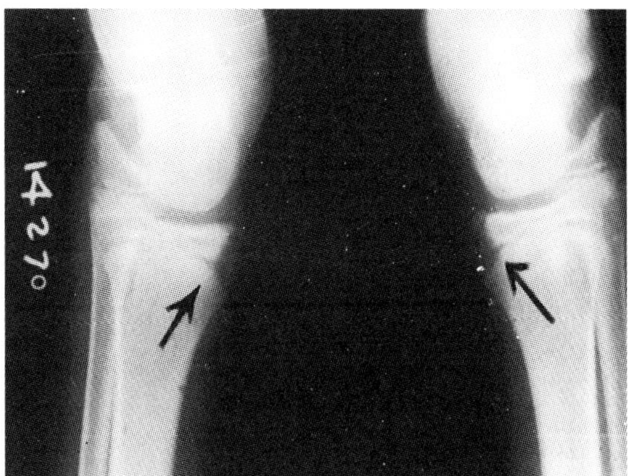

Fig. 14.15: Congenital absence of medial malleolus of both ankles initiating secondary deformity at ankle

2. Tuberculosis of the Ankle (also called as 'Scrophula') (Fig. 14.16)

— Insidious onset.
— Tender, slightly warm.
— Swelling around the ankle (usually doughy feel due to synovial thickening).
— Painful limp.
— Joint line tenderness.

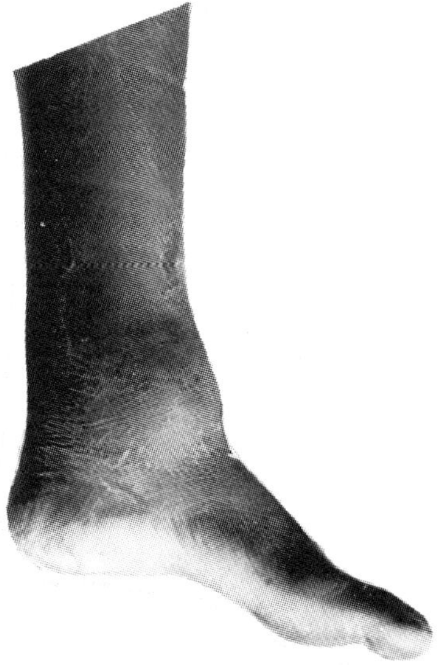

Fig. 14.16: Tuberculosis of ankle. Note the synovial swelling

— All movements restricted.
— Usually equinus/equinovarus deformity.
— Sinuses usually present posteromedially or posterolaterally.
— In comparatively late cases, fibrous ankylosis.
— Wasting of calf muscles.
— Popliteal/inguinal lymph glands may be enlarged and of tuberculous nature.

X-ray

— Comparative increase of soft tissue shadow.
— Generalised rarefaction of adjoining bones.
— Reduced joint space.
— Localised destruction.
— Joint collapse.

3. Pott's Fracture

— History of direct or indirect violence and twisting of ankle.
— Broadening of ankle.
— Disturbed relationship of the malleoli.
— Shape of ankle and foot distorted depending upon the displacements and subluxation.
— Painful limitation of ankle movements.
— Joint line tender at the site of fracture.
— In late cases, degenerative changes supervene comparatively early.

X-ray—Confirmatory (Figs 14.17A and B).

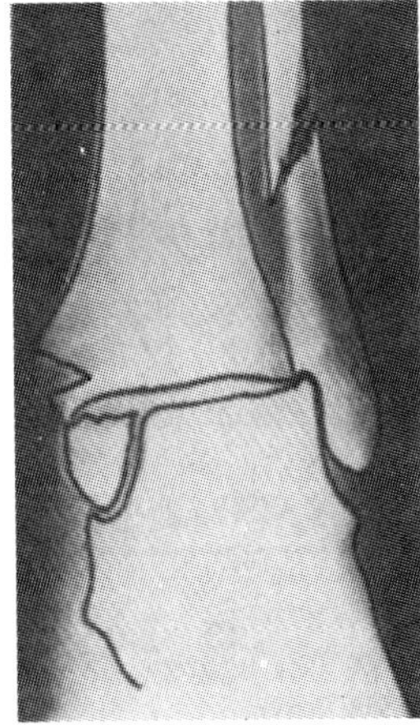

Fig. 14.17A: Pott's fracture—subluxation of ankle

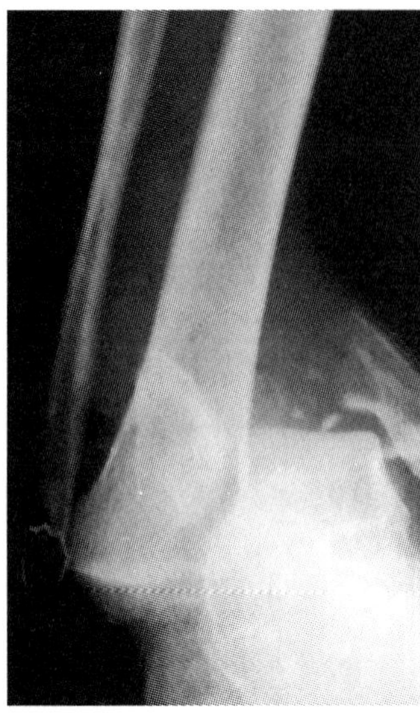

Fig. 14.17B: Fracture dislocation of ankle, such types are usually compound

Cycle Spoke Injury

A common injury in children (5-6 years), who are carried on cycles, either sitting on the front rod or on the back carrier, with their feet hanging or kept on both side of the mudguard. The foot slips and gets caught in between the spokes of the moving wheel. Due to an inversion twist strain, abrasions on proximal dorsolateral aspect of the foot along with swelling of the foot and lower leg develops.

— On X-ray, epiphyseal crush injury and/or metaphyseal fracture (usually of green stick type) of lower end of tibia may be visible.

Sprain of the Ankle

It is the commonest traumatic affection of the ankle. Inversion sprain is much more common than the eversion type, and recurs even on minor strains, if not properly treated.

In Inversion Sprain

— History of inversion twist of the ankle in a plantar flexed foot.

— Swelling on outer aspect of the ankle, especially in front and distal to the lateral malleolus.

— Maximum tenderness at anterior and below the lateral malleolus in the line of the anterior talofibular ligament.

— Attempt at further inverting the foot is resisted due to pain.

— May be accompanying fracture of the base of the 5th metatarsal.

— Stress radiography, putting the feet in maximum possible inversion, must be done to assess the tear of the lateral collateral ligaments of the ankle. In anteroposterior view—there may be avulsion of the tip of the lateral malleolus.

In Eversion Sprain

Maximum tenderness is at the upper attachment of deltoid ligament, i.e. just below and around the tip of the medial malleolus. Swelling is also more in the same region. X-ray may show avulsion of the tip of the medial malleolus.

6. Rheumatoid Arthritis

— Gradual onset, usually in females between 20 to 40 years.

— Usually bilateral affection of the ankle with affections of other joints (especially the smaller joints of the hand) along with typical deformities. In early stage warm and tender synovial swelling around the ankle, more prominent on anterolateral, anteromedial, posteromedial and posterolateral aspects.

— Swelling may appear along the commonly affected tendons (flexor hallucis longus, tibialis posterior, tibialis anterior and the peronei).

— Movements are painfully restricted.

— X-ray

  — Generalised rarefaction and 'pencilling' of the cortex.

  — Joint space maintained till late stage which thence gradually reduces.

  — In late cases degenerative changes supervene.

7. Crystal Arthritis (also see chapter on Joints)

— Males of about 40 or more are mainly affected.

— Ankle is a common site after the big toe.

— Cartilage, tendon, and bursae are main tissues to be affected.

— History of episodes of attack with inflammatory signs usually coming in small hours of the morning.

— In a typical gouty arthritis affecting the first metatarsophalangeal joint, with or without other joint involvement, search for gouty tophi (on and around the greater toe, thumb, lobule of ear, elbow, etc).

— In a typical gout, serum uric acid level is raised.

— In pseudogout—calcium pyrophosphate dihydrate crystals produce chondrocalcinosis usually in the larger joint (symptoms similar to those of gout).

— In pseudogout there may be calcification in the menisci of knee.

— In gout (and crystal arthritis) the inadequately processed waste products collect in the synovial fluid triggering painful inflammation.

— Sodium (Na) biurate accumulate primarily in the big toe.

8. Tailor's Ankle

— Persons regularly sitting in crossed-leg position, develop adventitious bursae over lateral malleolus, e.g. Hindu priests worshipping and tailors working while sitting in cross-legged position on the ground; muslims who offer regular players (Namaz) develop Muslim's callus (Pandey S 1988)—two oval callosities on the upper-outer aspect of proximal foot and lateral malleolus.

9. Poliomyelitis

In poliomyelitis, ankle region can be variously affected. Depending upon the pattern of paralysis, deformities like equinus, calcaneus, varus or valgus individually or in different combinations develop. There may be simultaneous affections/deformities of the foot, knee or hip, or even other parts of the body.

— History of febrile attack in childhood followed by paralysis which usually improves to varying extent.

— Paralysis of lower motor neuron type, which is usually asymmetrical.

— No sensory loss.

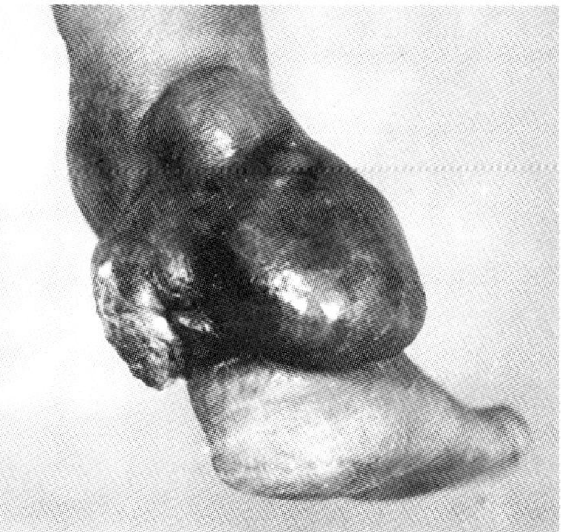

Fig. 14.18A: Ossified villonodular synovitis of ankle, very very rare presentation (Pandey S 1981)

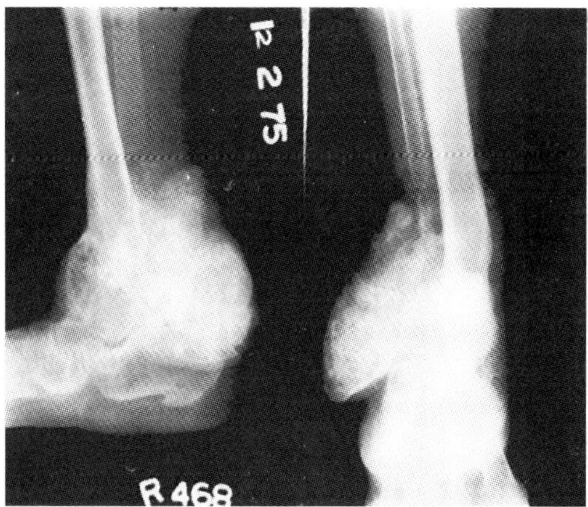

Fig. 14.18B: X-ray of the same patient (Fig. 14.18A)

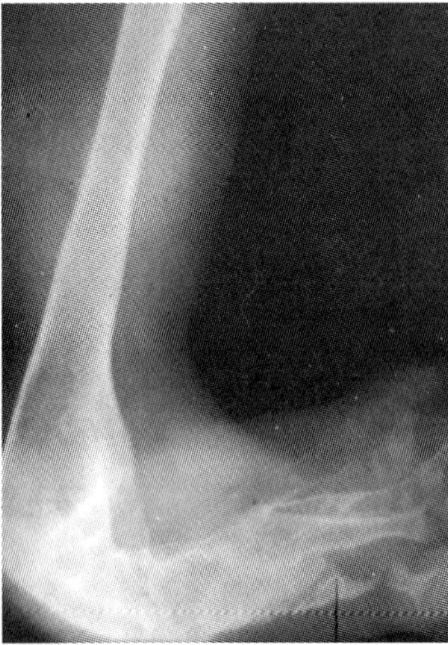

Fig. 14.19A: X-ray of leg, ankle and foot of 10 years aged girl with completely fused ankle and foot joints in grossly deformed position due to severely crushed injury at the age of 2 years

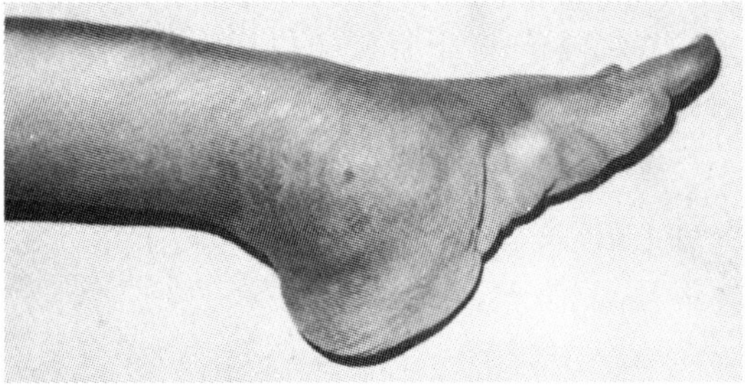

Fig. 14.20: Lymphangioma over ankle, hind foot and lower leg leading to overgrowth of that region

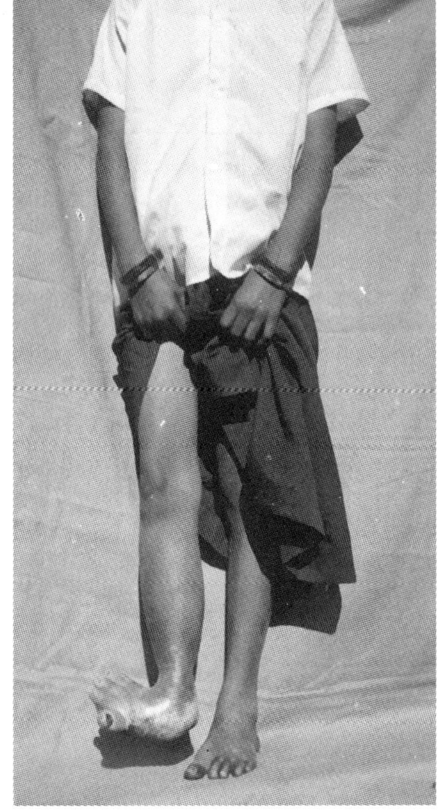

Fig. 14.19B: Same patient six months after possible correction—in first stage nearly plantigrade foot

10. Villonodular Synovitis

- — Chronic synovitis—ankle affection second to knee.
- — Young adults (usually males).
- — Soft nodular swelling (synovial) with effusion.
- — Swelling (rarely ossified), (Figs 14.18A and B).
- — Aspiration of thick orange brown fluid (sterile), containing cholesterol in large amounts—pathognomonic.
- — Arthroscopy reveals the characteristic picture.

BIBLIOGRAPHY

1. Leonard MH: Injuries of the lateral ligaments of the ankle. *J Bone Joint Surg* **31A**: 373, 1949.
2. Lettin AWF: Diagnosis and treatment of sprained ankle. *British Medical Journal* 1, 1956.
3. Mulfinger GL, Trueta J: The blood supply of the talus. *J Bone Joint Surg* **528**: 160, 1970.
4. Potter TA, Kuhns JG: Rheumatoid tenosynovitis. *J Bone Joint Surg* **40A**: 1230, 1958.
5. Pandey S: Pigmented vellonodular synovitis with bone involvement. *Arch Orthop Trauma Surg* **98**: 217, 1981.
6. Pandey S: Muslim's callus. In B Helal, D Wilson (Eds): *The Foot* London: Churchill Livingston, 700-01, 1988.
7. Rose GK: Ankle injuries. In Clark JMP (Ed) Modern Trends in Orthopaedics, **3**: 161. London: Butterworth, 1962.

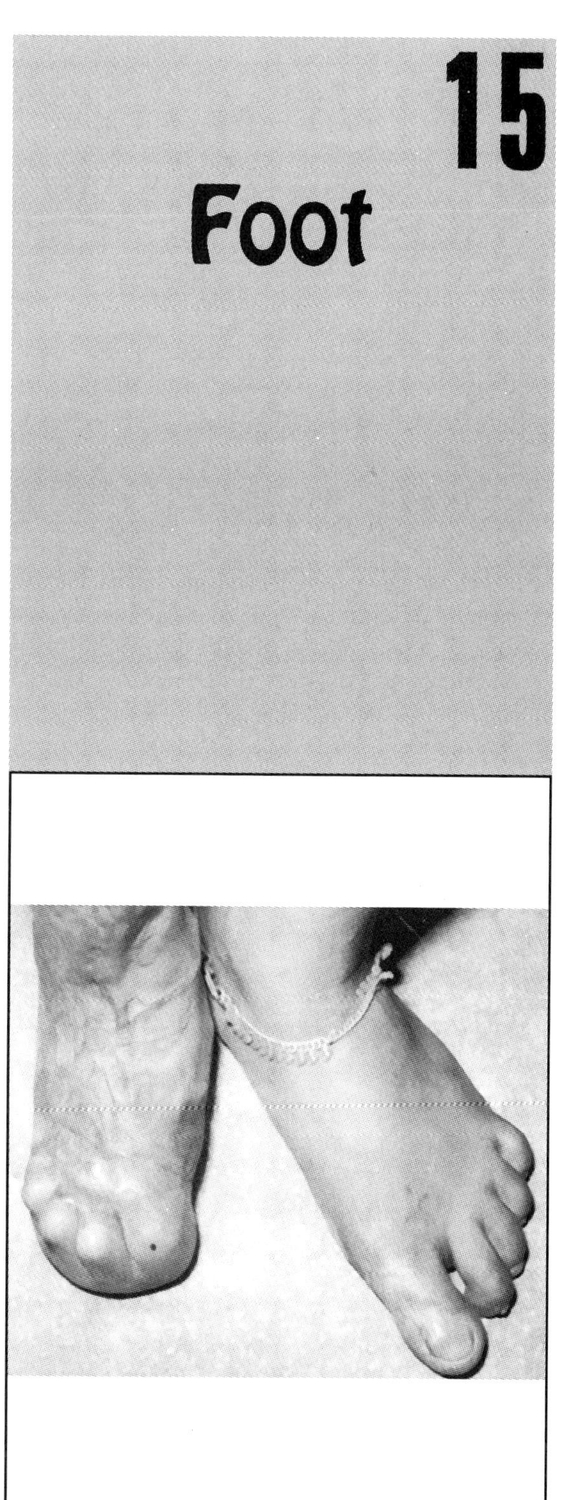

15 Foot

INTRODUCTION

In bipeds the foot takes on the important responsibilities of receiving the weight of the whole body and at the same time stabilizing the individual in changing environmental conditions. A normal foot must—(i) be plantigrade, (ii) have normal anatomical disposition and physiomechanics, (iii) be resilient with proper springiness to provide a rhythmic normal gait. The average person takes 8,000 to 10,000 steps in a day. The average person walks 2,41,350 kms (150,000 miles) on the feet in life time.

There are over 300 identified foot ailments ranging from chronic foot strain/discomfort to those that may put the patient's life, limb or mobility at risk. Serious consequences may arise without careful proper examinations, diagnosis and management of the foot and ankle problems.

Foot disorders tend to be progressive, so catching them early can save a lot of grief.

The ankle along with the foot, functionally forms one unit. Hence, while considering the physiomechanics of a normal foot and pathodynamics of any diseased foot, the ankle must also be taken into account.

Feet are said to be the 'mirror' of an individual's health. Sore foot can impair your concentration, make you irritable, and frequently are responsible for pain in the leg, knee, hip and low back.

ANATOMICAL CONSIDERATIONS

The foot is a complex structure of 28 bones (one-fourth of the bones in body), 33 joints, 57 articulating surfaces, 112 ligaments and 20 muscles.

Neuromuscular control in a rhythmic fashion, is essential to distribute the normal proportion of body weight through different portions of the foot in changing situations of stance and mobility. In the normal weight bearing position, each foot carries 50% of the body weight. In turn, the rough distribution of the weight in each foot is as follows (Fig. 15.1).

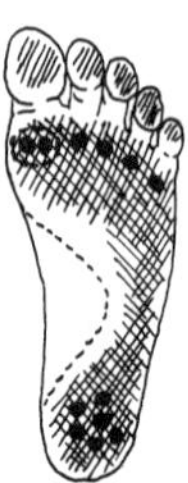

Fig. 15.1: Weight transmission in a plantigrade position. One dot represents one unit

Taking the unit of weight bearing as one, the outer four metatarsal heads carry one unit each, the first metatarsal head carries two units and the calcaneal post carries six units of weight.

Though the concept of "anterior heel" bearing the load upon the five metatarsal heads is a more or less established fact, however, the depiction of weight bearing has remained controversial. Wulf (1988) believes that in bipodal upright position, the load bearing are as follows, i.e. 4 > 3 > 2 whereas in monopodal position, it is 1 > 2 = 3 = 4.

Arches of the Foot

The function, of the longitudinal arch between the heel and the forefoot and the transverse arch between first and fifth metatarsal heads, is to absorb shock, energy and force and to transmit loading.

For suppleness of the plantigrade foot, the arches of the foot must be maintained.

a. *Transverse Arch (Anterior arch)*

The metatarsals and tarsals are arranged with a convex dorsal curve, mainly at the metatarsal heads level, held together by transverse ligament and maintained by transverse and oblique heads of adductor hallucis.

Collapse of this arch may—(i) Press upon the digital nerve (usually the communicating twig between the 3rd and 4th space digital nerves leading to Morton's metatarsalgia, (ii) Produce anterior flat foot.

Recently the existence of 'transverse arch' in a normal foot, has fallen in controversies. It is being observed that there is always a longitudinal arch in a normal foot, whereas there is no distal transverse metatarsal arch during the stance phase, i.e. during weight bearing. Rather a transverse arch indicates a possible pathological deformity like cavus and hallux valgus.

b. *Longitudinal Arches*

Medial longitudinal arch—formed by the calcaneal tuberosity, talus, navicular, three cuneiforms, inner three metatarsals and corresponding phalanges.

Lateral longitudinal arch—formed by the calcaneal tuberosity, cuboid, outer two metatarsals and corresponding phalanges.

Both these arches are maintained by—(i) Fascia—plantar aponeurosis, (ii) Ligaments—spring ligament, long plantar ligament, short plantar ligament, (iii) Tendons—tibialis posterior, peroneus longus, (iv) Muscles—long flexors, intrinsics.

Collapse of these arches result in—flat foot, valgus foot, spread foot. Accentuation of these arches (mainly medial)—results in cavus foot.

For the intricate and finer movements, the foot has multiple smaller joints. These joints have more or less communicating synovial reflections. Hence, any disease starting in one bone or joint is likely to spread and affect the adjoining bones and joints of the foot.

The skin of the sole is tough enough to withstand the pressures and pricks of a rough surface and at the same time is sensitive enough to make the person acquainted with the exact condition of the surface. Hence proper sensation and vascularity of the skin of the sole and subcutaneous pad are of paramount importance for the foot to subserve its proper functions.

Heel pad located beneath the calcaneum is an efficient shock absorber attenuating the peaks of dynamic forces and dampening vibrations. It consists of dense strands of fibrous septa (rich in collagen fibres) which form large sealed compartments packed with fat cells.

Table 15.1: Broad divisions of foot

Part	*Zone*	*Main function*	*Possible deformities*
Hind foot	Behind the mid-plane of sinus tarsi	Stability	Equinus, calcaneus, varus and valgus
Midfoot	From mid-plane of sinus tarsi to tarso-metatarsal joints	Springiness	Cavus, planus, rocker bottom foot
Forefoot	Distal to tarso-metatarsal joint	Piano distribution of weight	Adduction/abduction of metatarsals, claw foot

Control of the foot: Besides the long tendons as considered in the chapter on ankle, smaller muscles of foot are no less important as far as finer functions of the foot are concerned.

Anatomicofunctionally the foot may broadly be divided into *HIND FOOT, MIDFOOT,* and *FOREFOOT* (Table 15.1).

OSSIFICATION OF FOOT BONES (Fig. 15.2)

Tarsal bones usually ossify from one centre, except for the calcaneus, which has an additional epiphysis for its posterior part.

Talus	6 months IUL	Medial cuneiform—2nd year
Navicular	3rd year	Lateral cuneiform—1st year
Cuboid	9 months IUL	Intermediate cuneiform—3rd year
Calcaneum	5 months IUL	

The epiphysis for the posterior part of calcaneum appears at 6-8 years and unites by the 14th-16th years.

Metatarsal bones: Each metatarsal bone ossifies from two centres, one primary for the shaft and one secondary for the base of the first and for the heads of rest of the metatarsal bones.

Phalanges: Each phalanx ossifies from two centres, a primary one for the shaft, and secondary one for the epiphysis of the base.

Congenital Malformations of the Feet

- Congenital talipes equinovarus (club foot);
- Congenital elevation of little toe (the little toe remains hypoplastic and overlies its

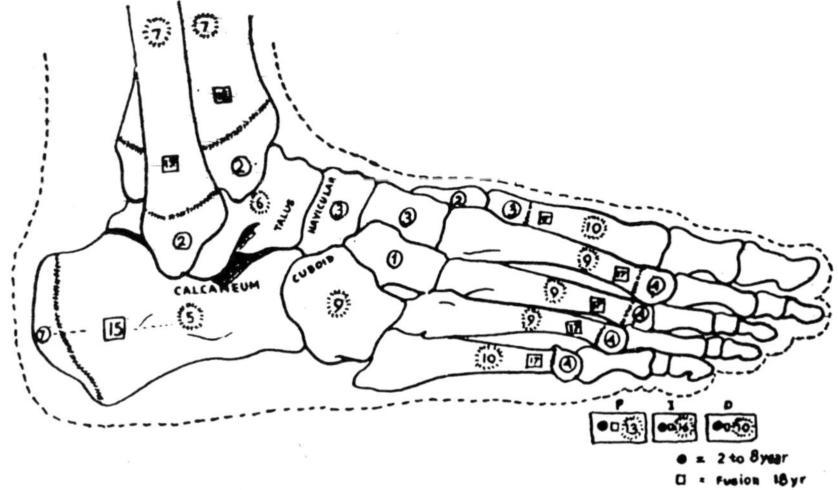

Fig. 15.2: Ossification around the ankle and foot • Dotted circle—primary centre in weeks (IUL) Complete circle—secondary centre in years • Square—fusion in years • P = proximal phalanx, I = intermediate phalanx, D = distal phalanx

neighbour, and causes pain due to rubbing in the shoe);

- Curly toes (3rd and 4th toes are usually affected, and they get flexed at the distal interphalangeal joint);
- Syndactyly usually remain symptom free, unless they are complex syndactyly (when bone is involved with angular deformities causing shoe-fitting problems) (Fig. 15.2A).

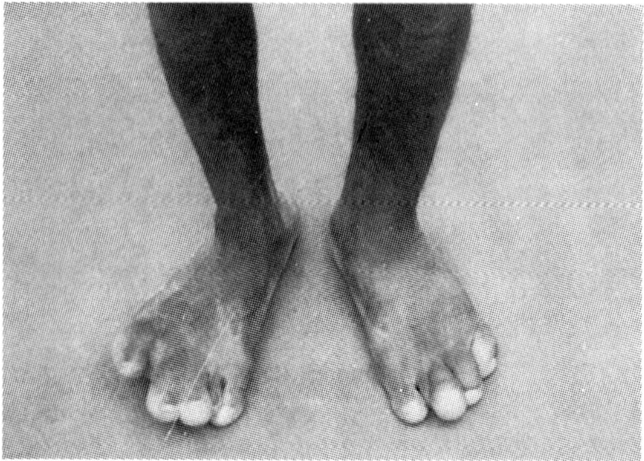

Fig. 15.2A: Syndactyly

- Macrodactyly (may be due to neurofibromatous and congenital vascular anomalies) (Figs 15.39A and B).
- Polydactyly (accessory digits) (Fig. 15.2B). It may be associated with chondroectodermal dysplasia (Ellis-Van Creveled syndrome) in which there are chondrodysplasia, ectodermal dysplasia, polydactyly, congenital heart disease.

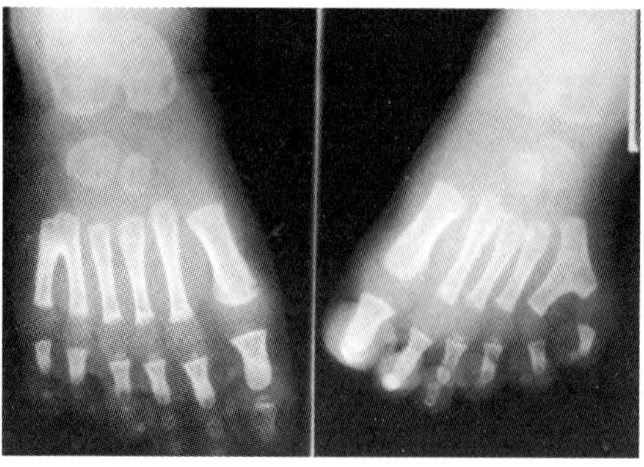

Fig. 15.2B: Polydactyly

- Pobble foot (cf. Apert's syndrome, page 464) (named after Edward Lear's poem about the Pobble, who had no toes). Disarticulation of all the five toes is known as Pobble operation (used to be performed for severe clawing of the toes) (Figs 15.2C1 and 15.2C2).

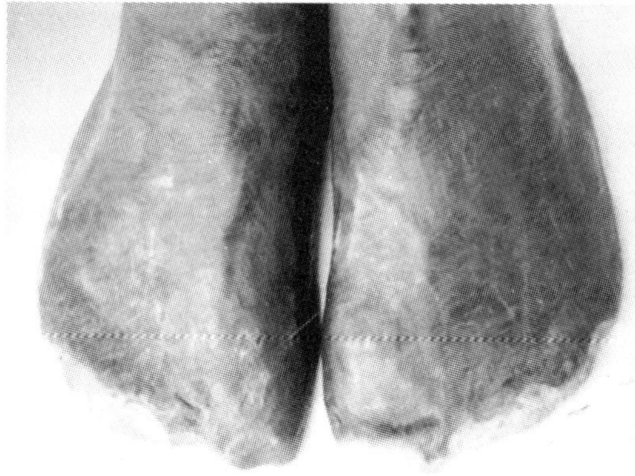

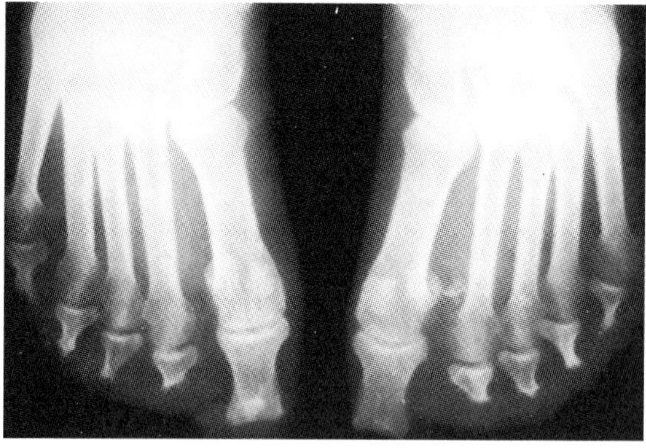

Fig. 15.2C1 and C2: Apert s syndrome (cf. Pobble foot)

- Tarsal coalition (due to failure of differentiation of mesenchymal, there is fusion of tarsal bones.
- Brachymetatarsia (congenital shortening of the metatarsal caused by premature closure of the epiphysis) may be associated with brachymetacarpia. Both may have familial history. Besides the cosmetic complaints, there may be pain around adjacent metatarsal heads while walking. These can be managed by the lengthening of the metatarsals (metacarpals in case of bradymetacarpia).
- Congenital convex pes valgus: Though described first in 1914 by Henkin, it was named

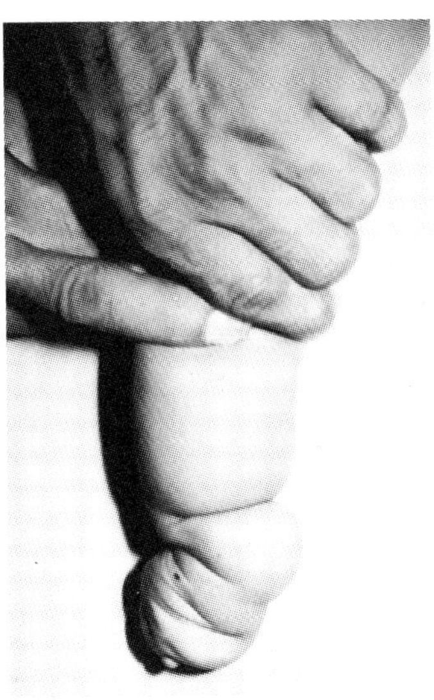

Fig. 15.2D1: Rudimentary foot with deep skin creases in soft tissues

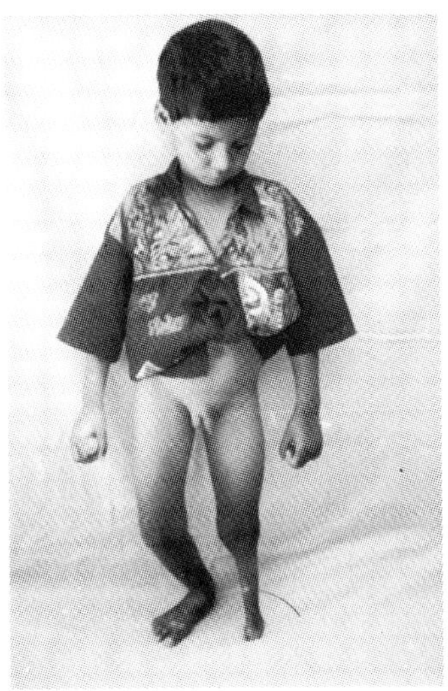

Fig. 15.2D2: Rudimentary foot and ill developed leg

properly by Lamey and Weissman in 1939. The most obvious radiological feature in this deformity is vertical orientation of the talus-congenital vertical talus. Talus is also vertically oriented in other conditions, e.g. congenital pes calcaneovalgus and spastic cerebral palsy. In congenital vertical talus (Fig. 15.4H) there is rocker bottom appearance—due to prominence of the head of talus and equinus of heel.

- Rudimentary foot (Fig. 15.2D1): The leg may also be short with muscular and other soft tissues atrophy (Fig. 15.2D2).

DEFORMITIES OF THE FOOT

Any deviation from the anatomical plantigrade foot (Fig. 15.3a) is a deformed foot. The deformities of the foot can be grouped under the following headings. These may exist individually or in various combinations.

1. Equinus (Fig. 15.3b)

The entire weight is borne by the forefoot, the hind foot remaining off the ground. The latin word equinus means horse, which bears weight on the forefoot only. The equinus deformity may be compensatory to weakness of the quadriceps femoris muscles and/or the gluteus maximus, and/or to shortening of the limb. Hence, the power of the quadriceps femoris and gluteus maximus must be assessed and the limb lengths accurately measured, when examining any case with equinus.

Before the equinus develops, the tendo-Achilles starts becoming tighter. Equinus can be divided into four grades.

Grade I Pre-equinus—Tendo-Achilles tightness. Here patient cannot walk on his heel. He can somehow squat, e.g. by keeping his leg abducted and/or with back markedly bent forward.

Grade II Along with equinus, heel starts becoming smaller and cavus starts developing.

Grade III Heel becomes obviously small and cavus accentuates along with splaying of the forefoot.

Grade IV Clawing of the toes also develops along with the deformities of grade III.

Equinus deformity may be due to contracture of gastrocnemius and/or soleus. If the equinus disappears after flexing the knee by 90° or more, it indicates its cause lying in gastrocnemius; if it persists, the cause is in soleus; and if it gets partially corrected the causes are in both.

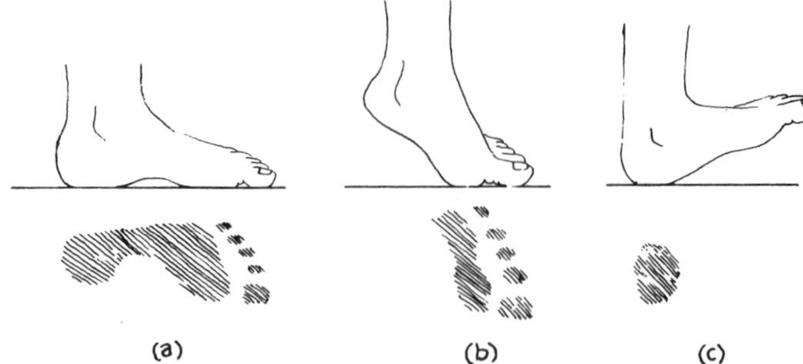

Fig. 15.3: (a) Plantigrade foot with foot print, (b) Equinus foot with foot print, and (c) Calcaneus foot; shaded area below indicates foot print

2. Calcaneus (Fig. 15.3c)

Here the weight is borne mainly by the hind foot. The forefoot may have varying degrees of weight bearing but definitely below normal.

3. Varus (Figs 15.4A and B)

The weight is borne mainly on the outer side of the foot in a gradually increasing amount, from behind forwards. This deformity is mainly at the hind foot.

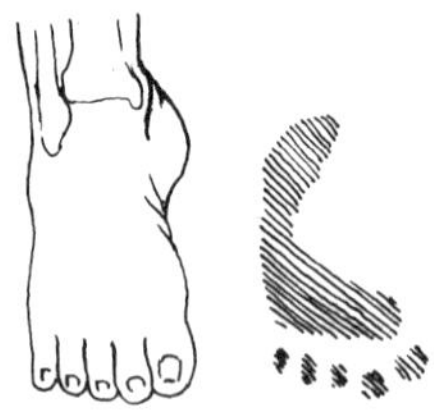

Fig. 15.4A: Varus foot from front with foot print

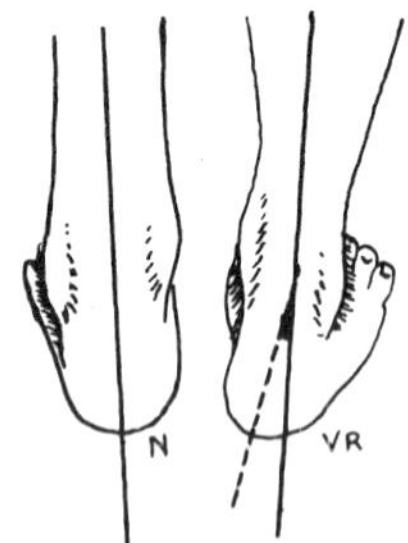

Fig. 15.4B: Varus foot from behind. N = Normal, VR = Varus

4. Valgus (Figs 15.4C to I)

Here weight is mainly borne on the inner side of the foot in gradually increasing amount from before backwards. This deformity is of the hind foot or of both the forefoot and hind foot.

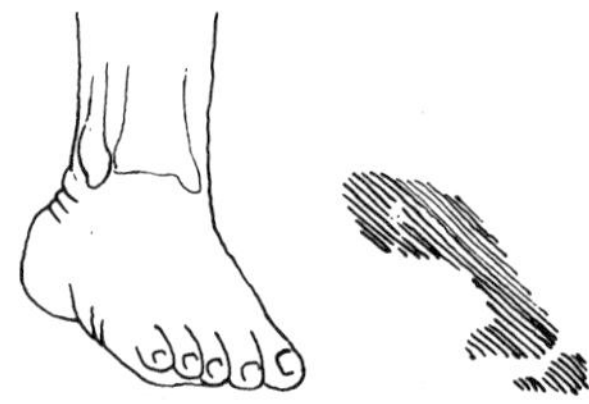

Fig. 15.4C: Valgus foot seen from front with foot print

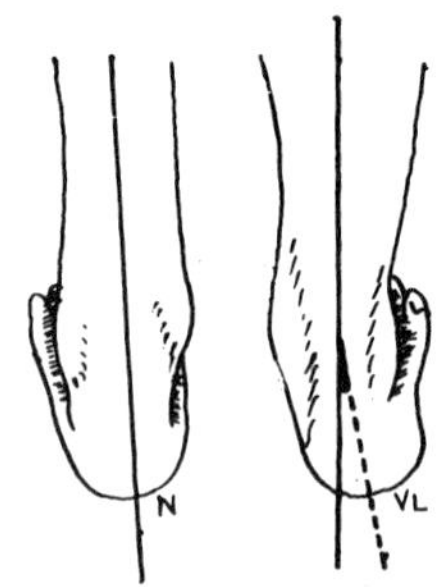

Fig. 15.4D: Valgus foot seen from behind N = Normal, VL = Valgus

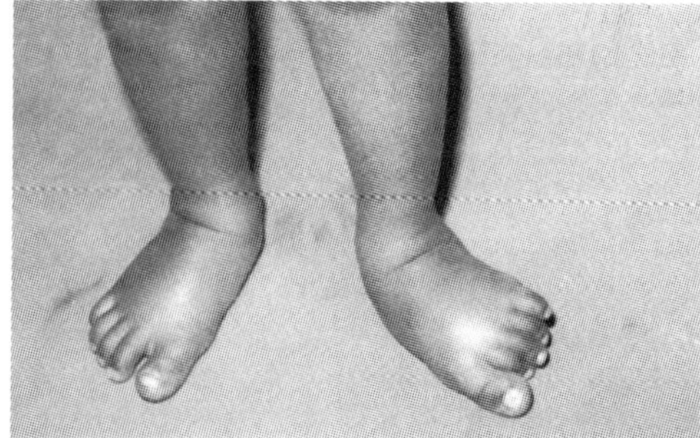

Fig. 15.4E: Left foot pes valgus, right foot pes planus in a child

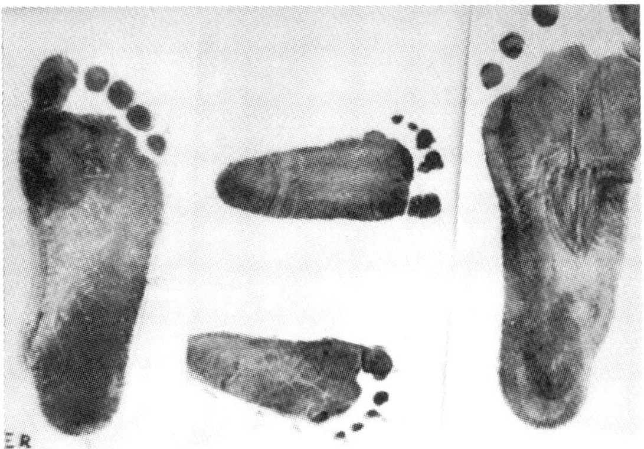

Fig. 15.4F: Foot prints: On the left of mother, on the right of father, in the centre of the son

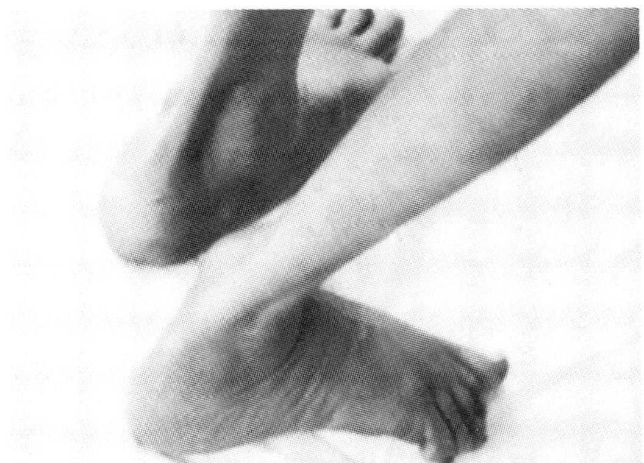

Fig. 15.4G: Pes valgus in adult

5. Inverted Foot (Figs 15.5A to C)

As such, inversion is an act of a particular movement of the foot mainly occurring at subtalar joint, the persistent effect of which manifests in a particular deformity, i.e. 'varus'. However, when the hind and the forefoot both are in varus position, the deformity is termed as 'inverted foot'. The accentuation of this position will gradually turn the sole towards the sky,—'supination of the foot'. In these positions, i.e. in inverted and supinated foot, adduction of the forefoot and the plantar flexion of the ankle will also coexist.

6. Everted Foot (Figs 15.4J and 15.4K)

The eversion is an act of a movement occurring mainly at the subtalar joint, the persistent effect

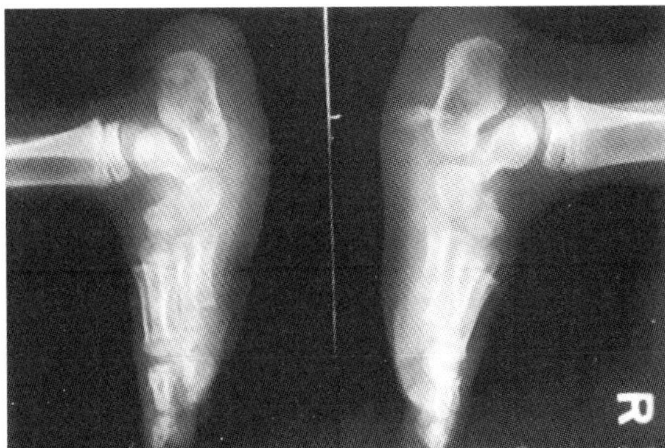

Fig. 15.4H Bilateral congenital vertical talus

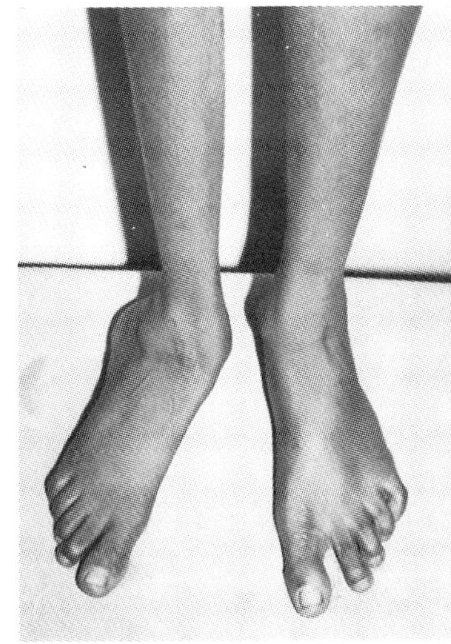

Fig. 15.4I: Valgus collapse at right ankle

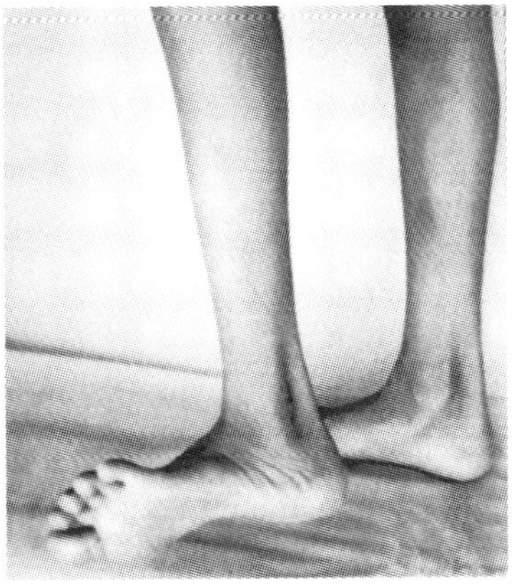

Fig. 15.4J: Everted foot

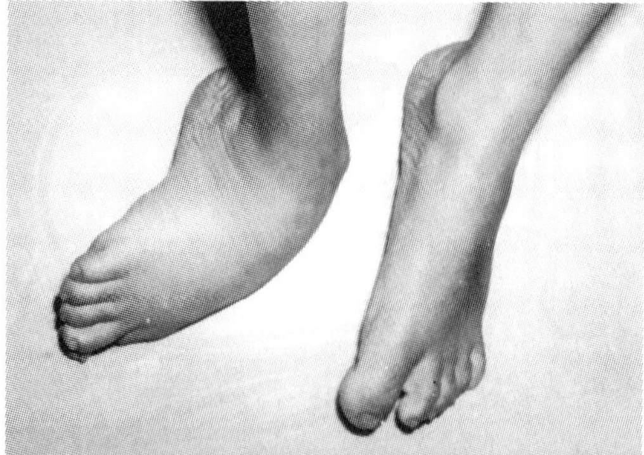

Fig. 15.4K: Markedly pronated foot

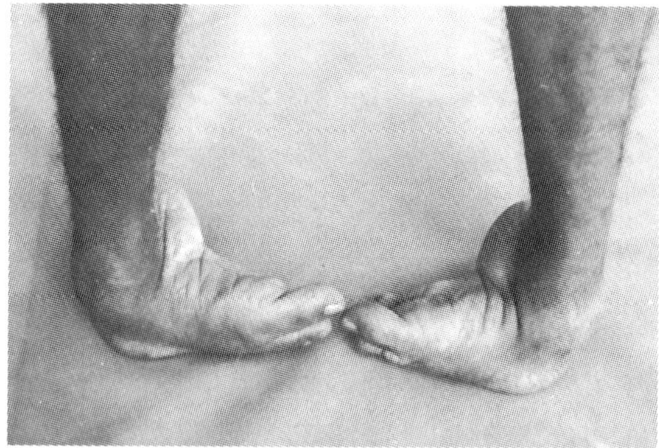

Fig. 15.5B: Neglected very severe club feet (supinated feet)

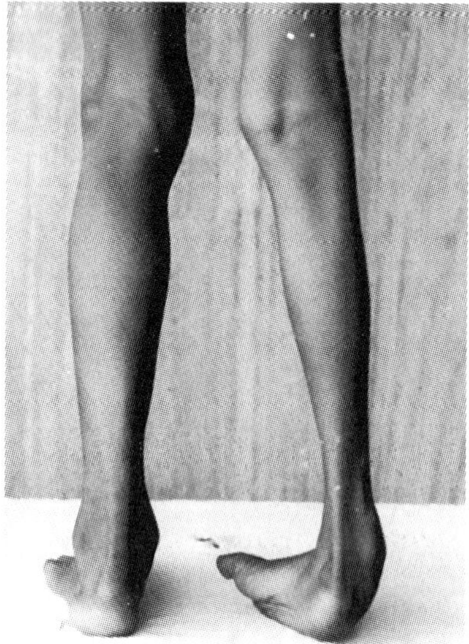

Fig. 15.5A: Moderately inverted foot

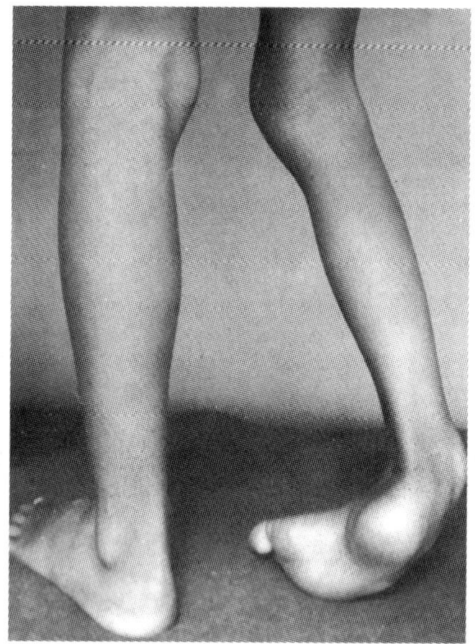

Fig. 15.5C: Severe equino-cavo-varus foot (inverted foot)

of which will result in a deformity, i.e. valgus. However, when the hind foot and forefoot both are in valgus position, the deformity is termed as 'everted foot'. Here the outer part of the sole bears lesser and lesser weight. In the exaggerated situation the outer part of the sole acquires a tendency to face towards the sky. This is called a pronated foot. In these, i.e. everted and pronated foot (Fig. 15.4K), abduction of the forefoot and some amount of dorsiflexion at the ankle will also coexist.

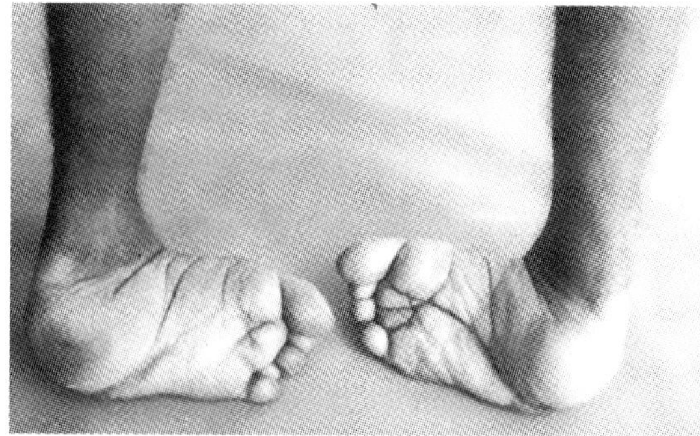

Fig. 15.5C1: Neglected severe club feet (supinated feet)

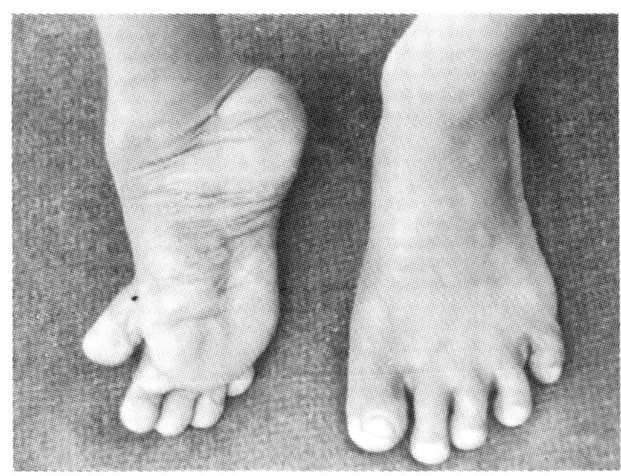

Fig. 15.5C2: Paralytic (polio paralysis) supinated foot (right)

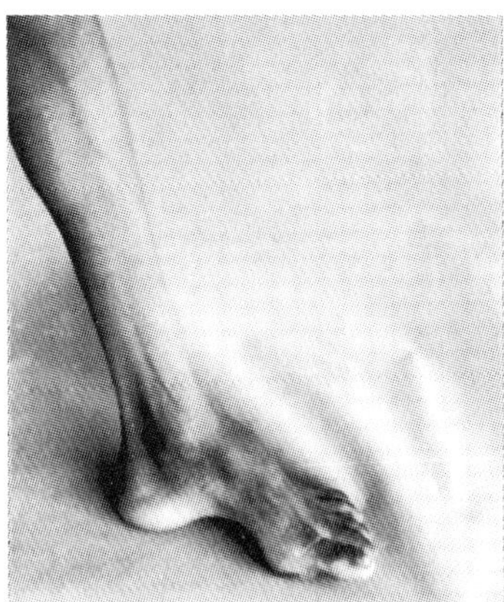

Fig. 15.6B: Clinical photograph of pes cavus with tight tendo-Achilles and smaller heel

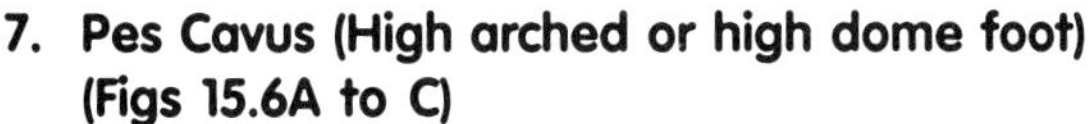

7. Pes Cavus (High arched or high dome foot) (Figs 15.6A to C)

A normal foot has a medial longitudinal arch which is higher than the lateral one. When this normal proportion is accentuated, the medial side of the foot tends to assume the shape of a high arch and looks like a cave. It rarely occurs as a single deformity. It is a common accompaniment of equinovarus, equinus and dorsal subluxation of the metatarsophalangeal joints (claw foot). Pes cavus can be flexible (which can be corrected by pushing the first metatarsal head upwards) or rigid.

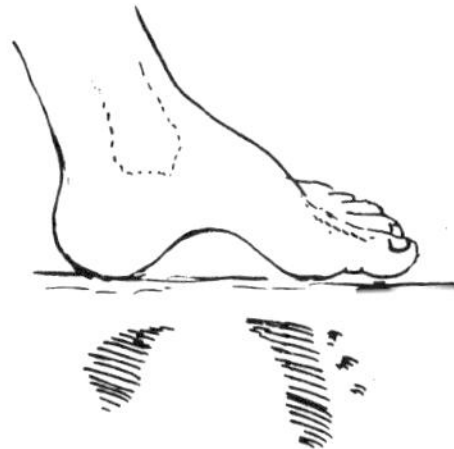

Fig. 15.6A: Pes cavus with its foot print

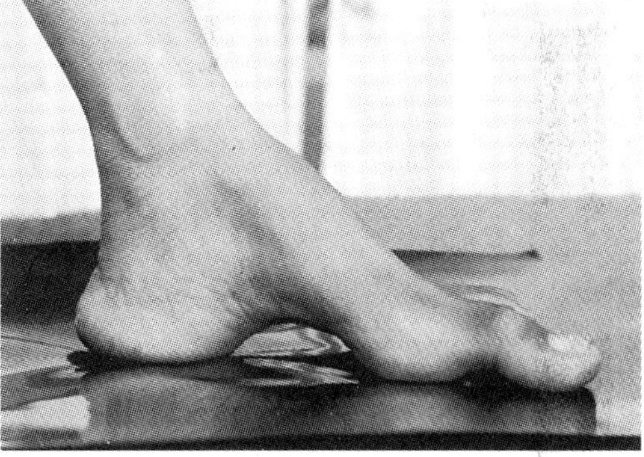

Fig. 15.6C: Calcaneo-cavus foot (note the splashed-out heel)

8. Pes Planus (Flat foot) (Figs 15.4E and F and 15.8)

Collapse of medial longitudinal arch (physiological or pathological) leads to pes planus. The normal concavity due to the medial longitudinal arch is absent and instead the medial side of the foot bulges as a medial convexity, particularly on weight bearing. In physiological or paralytic cases, the flat foot is supple and full passive inversion of the foot is possible. In physiological pes planus, almost normal medial arch appears, when the person attempts to walk on the forefoot or when one attempts to push up the first metatarsal head from the plantar surface or when the foot is not bearing weight. On the other hand, flat foot resulting from the spasm of the peronei is spastic and rigid. It is a protective mechanisms against the painful foot resulting from congenital vertical talus, congenital osseous bars, and irritating bed of peronei. On an attempt to passively invert this type of foot, there will be resistance, and patient will feel pain along the prominently standing peroneus longus and brevis tendons, behind and above the lateral malleolus (Figs 15.9A to C).

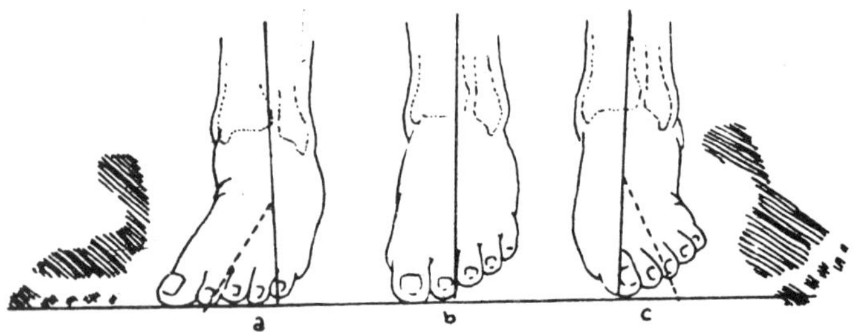

Fig. 15.7: (a) Adduction of forefoot with foot print, (b) normal alignment of forefoot, and (c) abduction of forefoot with foot print

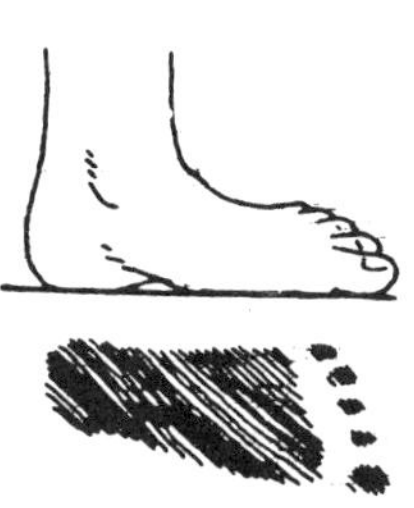

Fig. 15.8: Pes planus (see clinical photograph 15.4E and F—right foot pes planus)

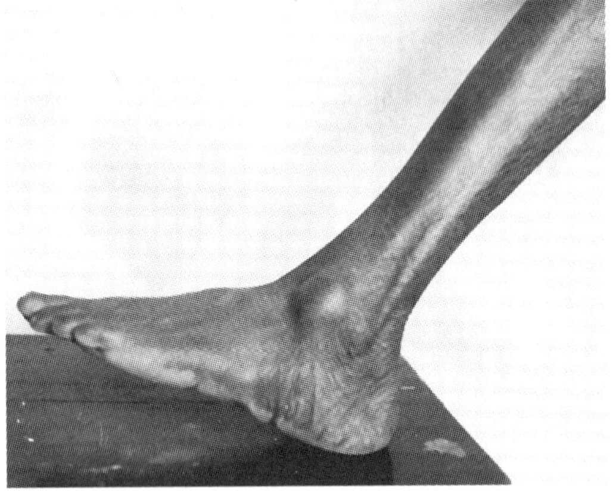

Fig. 15.9A: Spastic flat foot

Exaggeration of the pes planus may result in pes valgus (Figs 15.4E and G)

Test for flexible flat foot: With full weight bearing, if the heel is in valgus position, which changes to varus when child is on tip toe position (bears weight only on fore foot), it indicates flexible flat foot.

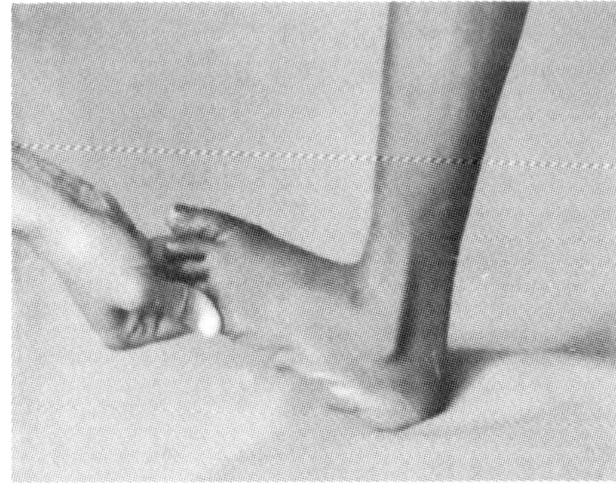

Fig. 15.9B: In spasmodic flat foot, any attempt of passively inverting the foot makes the peroneus longus and brevis tendons more and more prominent

Jack test: Jack's test demonstrates a synchronised activity of the intrinsic and extrinsic musculature and its influence on the physiopathomechanics of the flaccid flat feet. It is performed by passively extending the great toe with the patient standing. If the flat foot is due to collapse of the navicular-cuniform joint, the arch will be restored, the foot tends to be supinated, and there is tendency of external rotation of tibia with inversion of the heel. When these occur, it indicates a flexible flat foot.

9. Congenital Convex Pes Valgus

The most obvious radiological feature in this deformity is vertical orientation of the talus—congenital vertical talus (Fig. 15.4H).

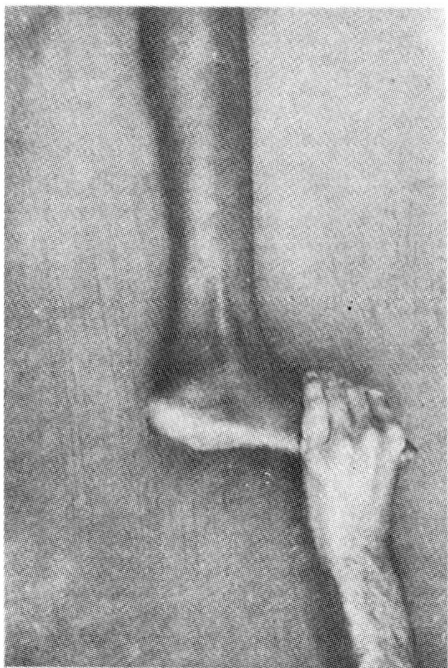

Fig. 15.9C: Note that even with the attempt of forceful inversion, it is not possible to do it and peronei stand prominent

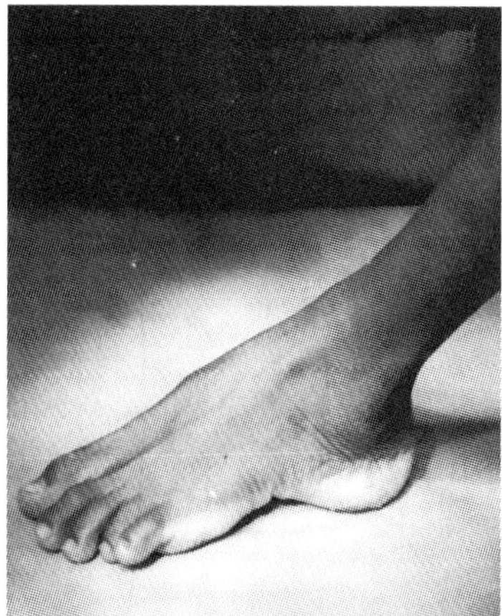

Fig. 15.10A: Pes abductus

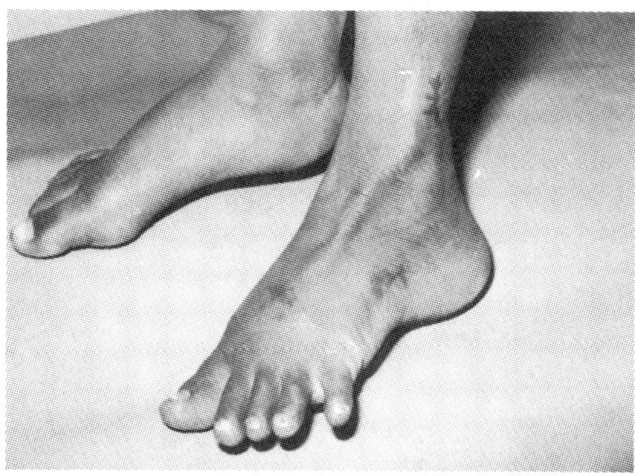

Fig. 15.10B: Pes abductus due to over active transferred peroneus brevis tendon

10. Adduction of the Forefoot (Pes adductus or Sickle foot) (Fig. 15.13H—right foot)

From the transitional zone of mid to forefoot the foot assumes a tendency of deviation towards the inner side. In a normal neutrally aligned lower limb, a line joining the centre point of the patella to the anterior mid-ankle point, if extended distally, passes through the second toe or the second web (Fig. 15.7b). In adduction of the forefoot, this line passes through the toes or webs outer to this.

11. Abduction of Forefoot (Pes Abductus) (Figs 15.10A and B)

From the transitional zone of hind to forefoot the foot deviates to the outer side. Here, the axis (as mentioned in pes abductus) passes inner to the second toe (Fig. 15.7c).

12. Brachymetatarsia (see page 340)

13. Clawing of the Toes (Figs 15.11A and B)

There is hyperextension at the metatarso-phalangeal joint and plantarflexion at the interphalangeal joints. As a result, the pulps of the toes do not touch the ground even in full flexion of the interphalangeal joints. Passively elevating the depressed metatarsal head further exaggerates the plantar flexion of the toe (Fig. 15.11B). Complete paralysis of both plantar nerves causes a 'pied-en-griffe' deformity.

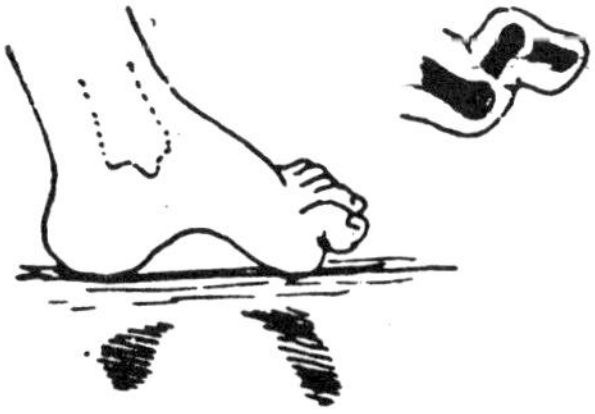

Fig. 15.11A: Clawing of toes

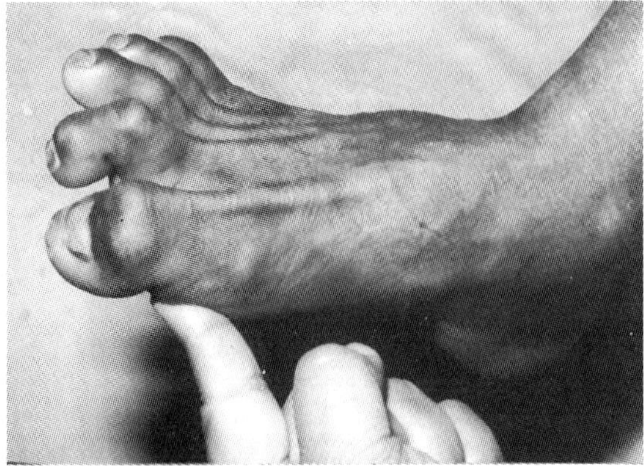

Fig. 15.11B: Clawing of toes

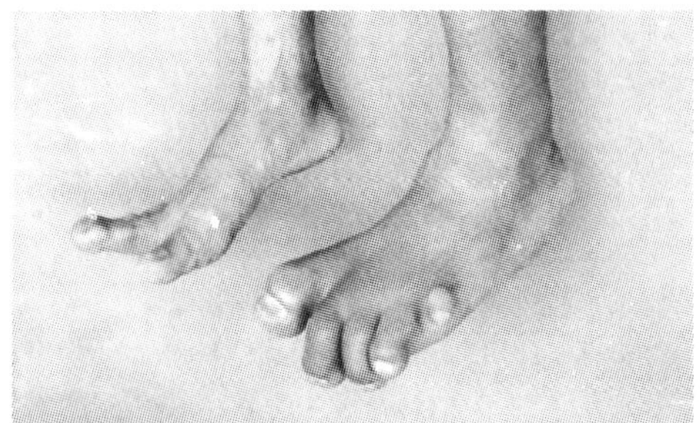

Fig. 15.12B: Clinical photograph: left foot showing hammer toe of big toe, 2nd toe with DIP in extension, 3rd toe with DIP in flexion, 4th toe going for hammer toe, 5th toe subluxated dorso laterally with tendency of hammer toe; right foot-macrodactyly of 2nd toe

14. Hammer Toe Deformity (Figs 15.12A to D)

There is acute plantar flexion contracture at the proximal interphalangeal joint and flexion or extension at the distal interphalangeal joint. (There is no marked change at the metatarso-phalangeal joint; some times metatarsal head may be depressed on the plantar surface). The second toe is usually the one affected.

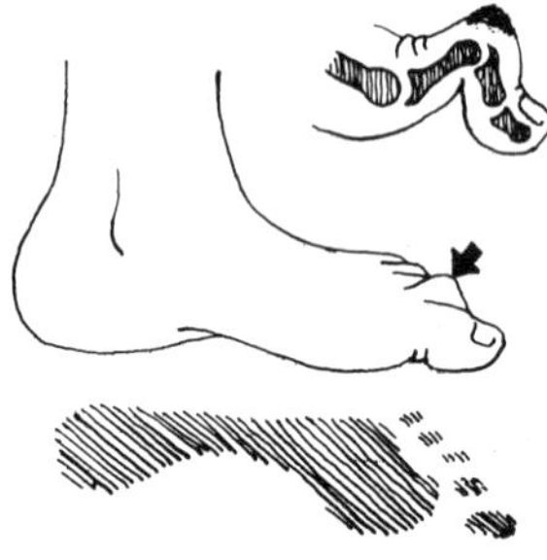

Fig. 15.12A: Hammer toes (line drawing)

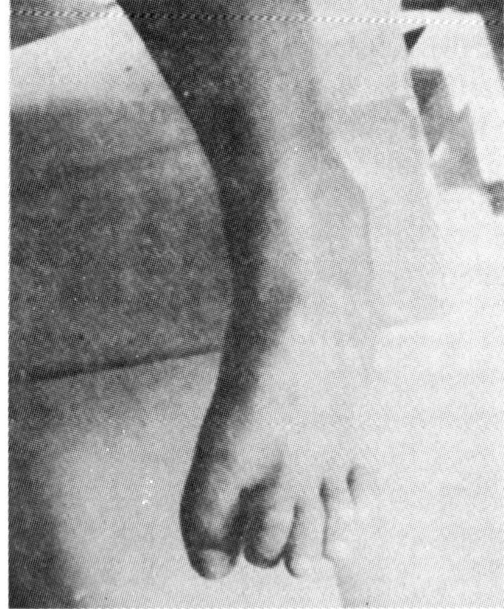

Fig. 15.12C: Hammer toe of first and second toes

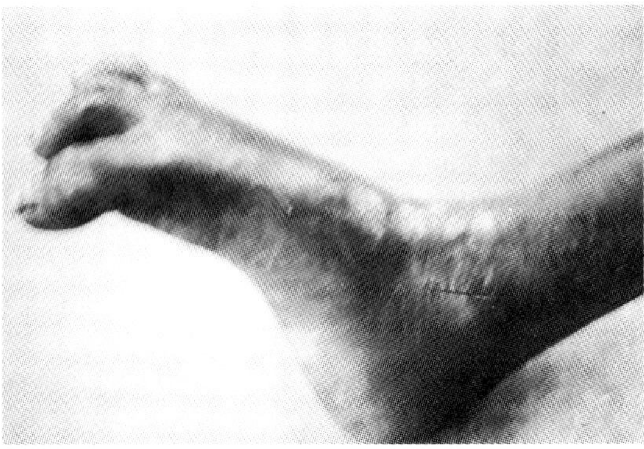

Fig. 15.12D: Hammer toe of all the toes

15. Hallux Valgus (Figs 15.13A and B, E to G)

The long axis of the great toe deviates outwards at the metatarsophalangeal joint. The supero-medial aspect of first metatarsal head, which deviates medially, stands markedly prominent and is usually associated with thickened over-lying soft tissues (bunion, callosity). The great toe in turn may push the other toes (second and even the third) laterally (Fig. 15.13H), and may even override the next toe (Fig. 15.13B). Sometimes second toe may also override the deviated great toe (Figs 15.13A and G).

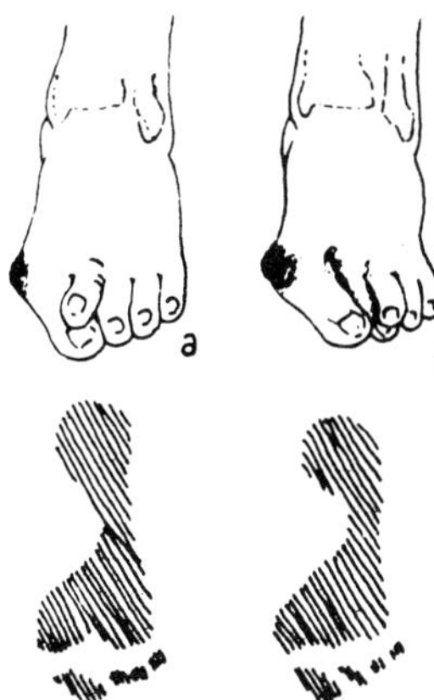

Fig. 15.13A and B: Hallux valgus with foot print

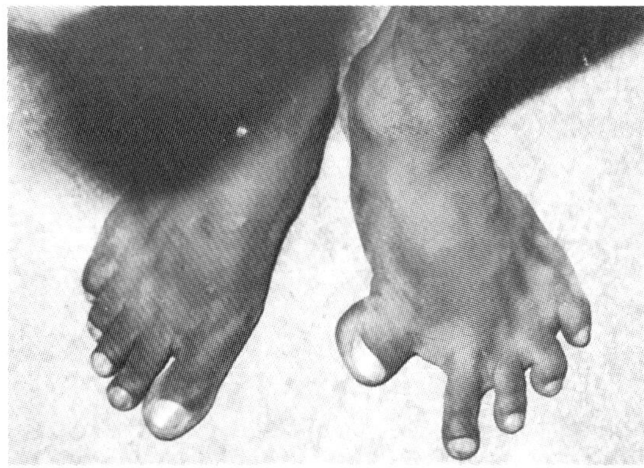

Fig. 15.13D1: Hallux varus deformity. Other toes of the same (left) feet are also deviating inwards

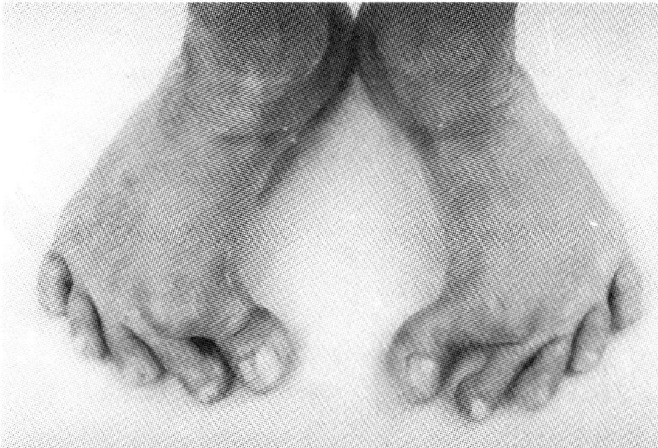

Fig. 15.13D2: Bilateral hallux varus. Note that all the toes in each foot are going for varus deformities

16. Hallux Varus (Figs 15.13C and D2)

The great toe deviates inwards at the metatarso-phalangeal joint. The second toe often follows suit.

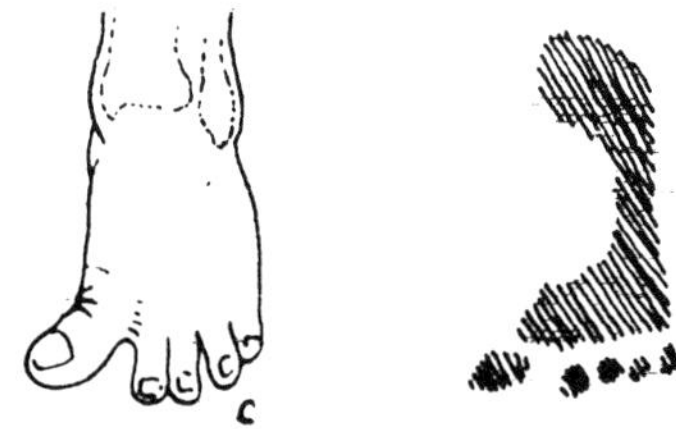

Fig. 15.13C: Hallux varus

16a. Wind Sweep Deformities of the Toes

In rheumatoid arthritis, sometimes there may be wind-sweep deformities of the toes, i.e. valgus deformities of the big toe (followed by others) in one foot and varus in other (Fig. 15.13H)

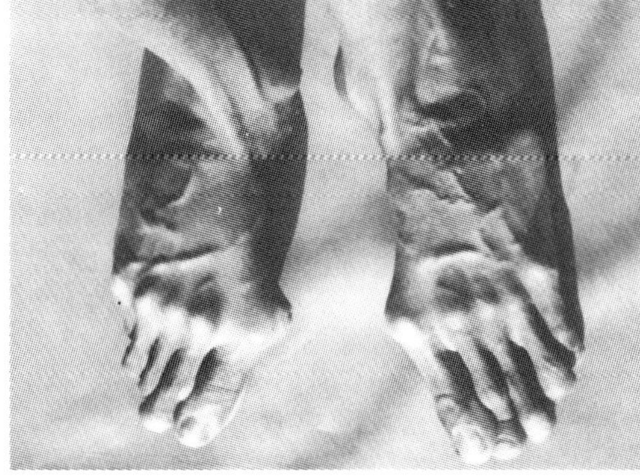

Fig. 15.13E: Clinical photograph of bilateral hallux valgus. Right markedly pronounced with bunion and callosity

17. Hallux Rigidus (Synonyms-hallux fluxus, hallux dolorosus, dorsal bunion, metatarsus primus elevatus)

The word 'hallux-rigidus' was coined by Cotterill, JM in 1888. It is a disorder characterized by a progressive restriction of the first metatarso-phalangeal joint. If during the growing period short shoes are regularly used, the metatarso-phalangeal joint of the big toe becomes stiff

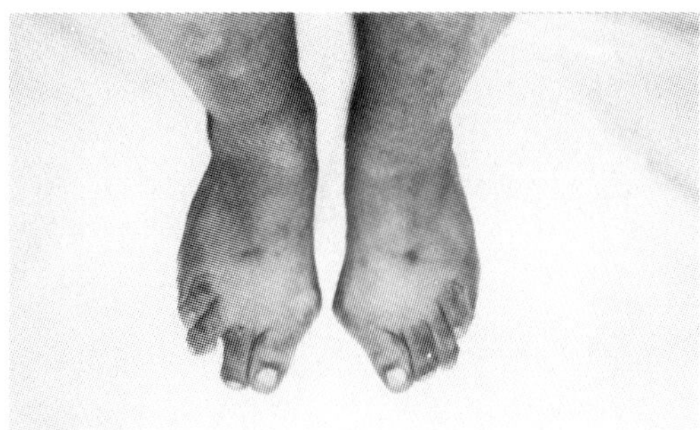

Fig. 15.13F: Hallux valgus in both feet. Note the deviated big toes are overriding their corresponding second toe

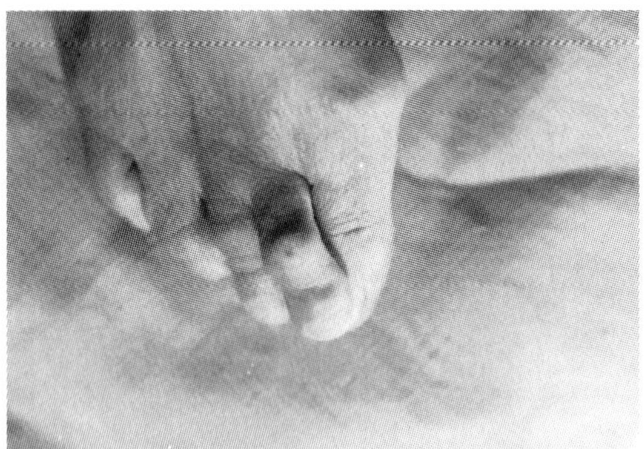

Fig. 15.13G: Hallux valgus. Note the second toe over-riding the deviated first toe

(hallux rigidus) due to osteoarthrosis. This may also result following intra-articular fractures, osteochondritis of the metatarsal head, gout or pseudogout.

18. Hallux Limitus

'Hallux limitus' indicates a decrease or a limitation of the range of motion in the metatarsophalangeal joint of the big toe, while 'Hallux-rigidus' indicates the absence of the movements at that foot. It is often associated with a mechanical block to dorsiflexion caused by periarticular osteophytes with an impingment exostosis of the first metatarsal head against an osteophyte at the base of proximal phalanx.

19. Digitus Quintus Varus

Deviation of long axis of the little toe medially is known as digitus quintus varus (Fig. 15.14A

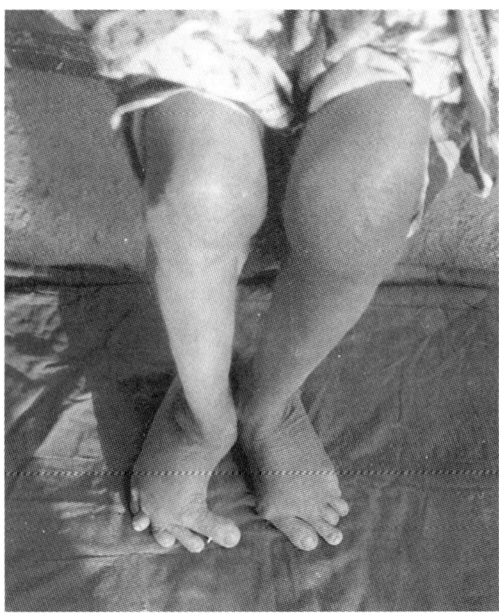

Fig. 15.13H: Wind sweep deformities of the toes. Marked adduction of the forefoot led to sickle deformity of the right foot

A

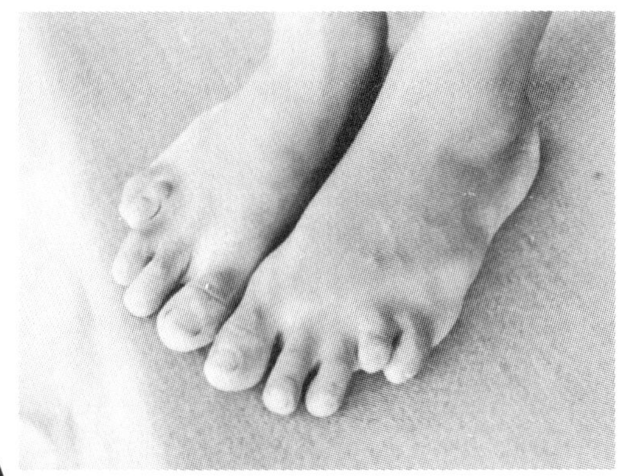

B

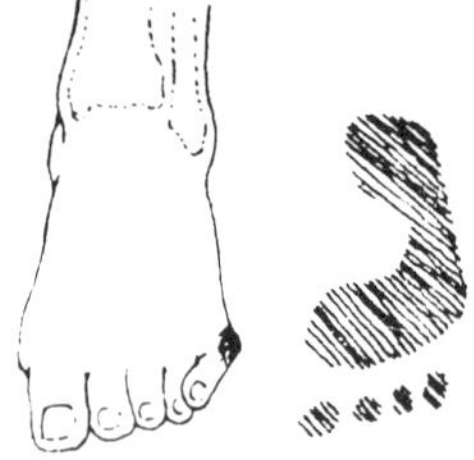

Figs 15.14A and B: Digitus quintus varus super inductus

in right foot). However, when the little toe is so much deviated as to override the fourth toe, this is called 'digitus quintus varus superinductus' (Fig. 15.14B).

20. Pes Transversus or Spread Foot (Fig. 15.15A)

In a normal foot, while weight bearing, the concentration of weight is more on the first and fifth toes (tripod stand concept of foot). Sometimes the third metatarsal head collapses. This can be clinically felt as a bony swelling through the sole in that area. In addition, there is an increase in the breadth of forefoot. The concentration of weight in this area also increases. Such a foot is known as pes transversus or spread foot.

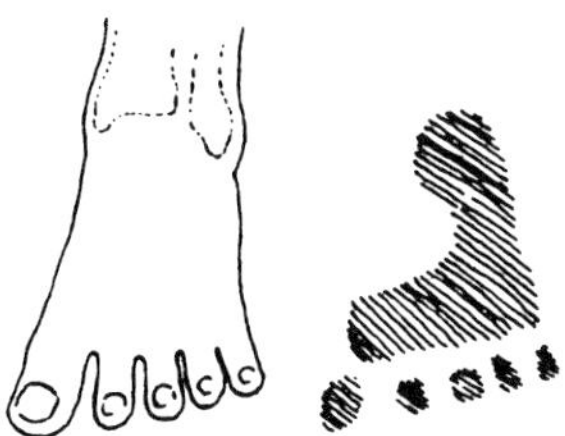

Fig. 15.15A: Spread foot

21. Cockup Deformity of Toes (Fig. 15.15B)

In elderly diabetics and in patients of posterior tibial nerve neuropathy, a deformity, like the clawing of toes, is produced and is known as cockup deformity.

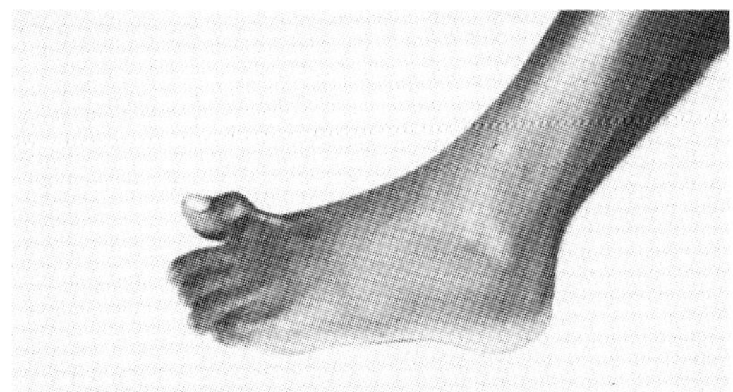

Fig. 15.15B: Cockup deformity of big toe

22. Skew Foot

Here the hind foot is in severe valgus along with adduction of the forefoot. It is cosmetically acceptable.

23. Talus Foot

This is usually a postural moulding defect seen in the neonates. It may be in exaggerated form presenting high arching in midfoot, calcaneus look at hind foot (heel) and hammer-toe position of the big toe. Such cases require corrective splint.

Common Combinations of Deformities

1. Equinus + cavus + varus with or without adduction of the forefoot—Club foot (Figs 15.25 to 15.28).
2. Varus + cavus + adduction of forefoot—Hollow foot (Fig. 15.16A).

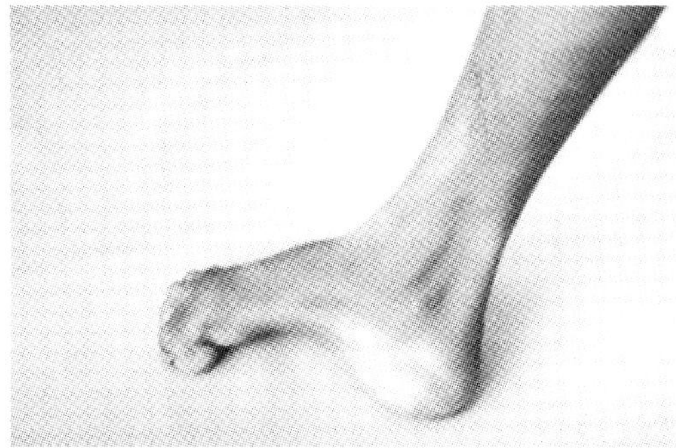

Fig. 15.16A: Hollow foot

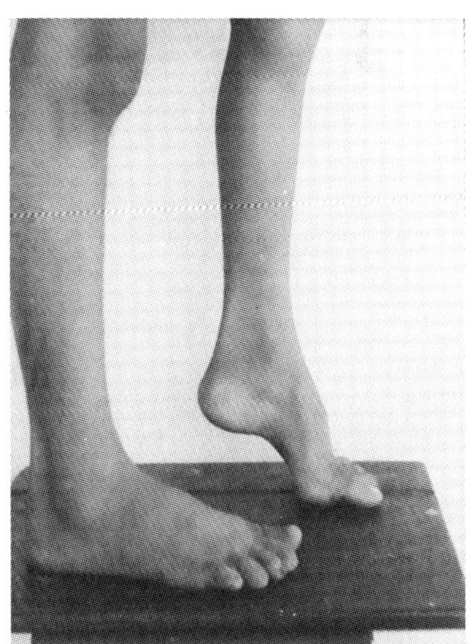

Fig. 15.16B: Equino cavus foot

3. Pes planus + valgus + abduction—Knock flat foot.
4. Cavus + valgus—Knock hollow foot.
5. Cavus + pes transversus—Hollow spread foot.
6. Equinus + cavus—Equino-cavus foot (Fig. 15.16B).
7. Calcaneus + valgus + cavus—Calcaneo-cavo-valgus (Figs 15.17A and B)

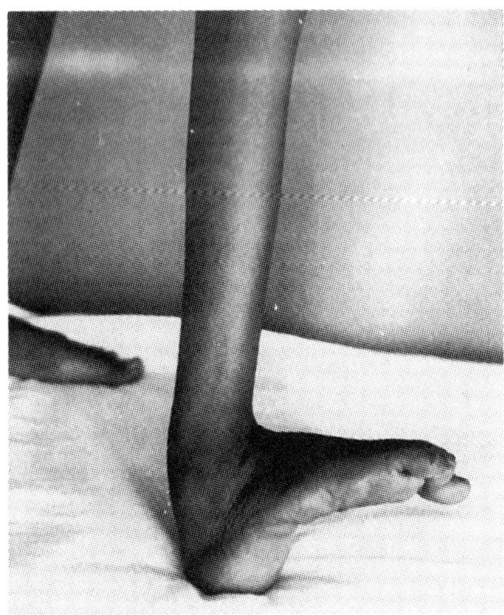

Fig. 15.17A: Calcaneo-valgus foot

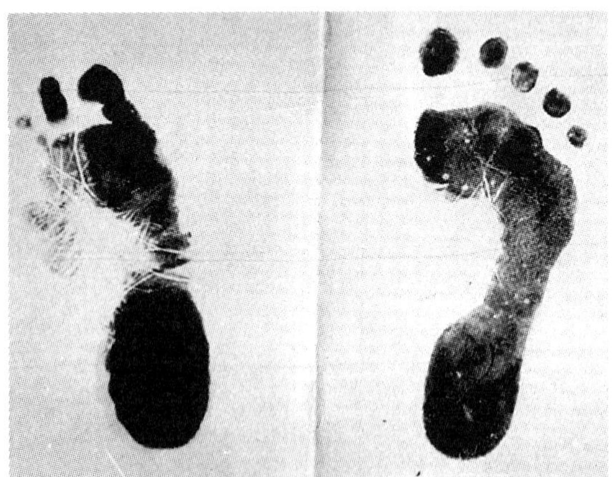

Fig. 15.17B: Foot print of calcaneo-valgus (left) foot

TYPES OF FOREFOOT

The type of forefoot varies according to the relation of the first and second toe. Three common varieties of forefoot have been recognised:

1. Egyptian Type of Forefoot (Fig. 15.18A) (After Debrunner, HU) 1 > 2 > 3 > 4 > 5

The great toe is longer than the 2nd toe, the second toe is longer than the 3rd toe and so on.

2. Intermediate Rectangular Foot/Square Foot (Fig. 15.18B)

The great and second toes are equal.

However, the 2nd toe may be equal or longer than the 3rd toe.

The 3rd toe may be equal or longer than the 4th toe.

The 4th toe may be equal or longer than the 5th toe.

3. Grecian (Greek) Foot (Fig. 15.18C) 1 < 2 > 3 > 4 > 5

The great toe is smaller than the 2nd toe. The 2nd toe is bigger than the 3rd toe. The 3rd toe is bigger than the 4th toe. The 4th toe is bigger than the 5th toe.

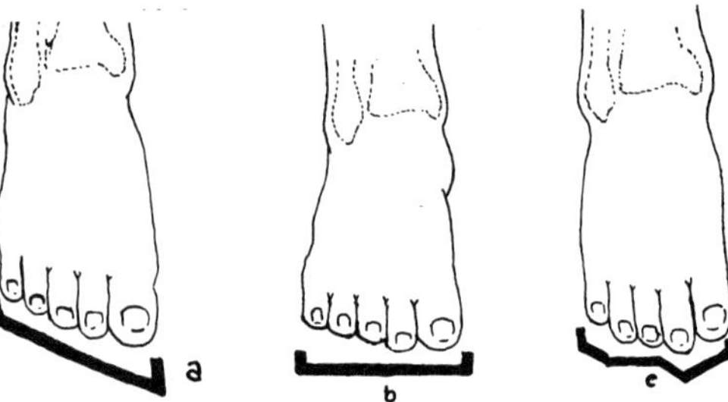

Figs 15.18A to C: (a) Egyptian foot, (b) Rectangular foot, and (c) Grecian foot

There can be abnormal congenital or acquired patterns which must be assessed carefully, e.g. in Marfan's syndrome in which the feet and hands are extremely long and thin with great length of the toes and fingers. The big toe is much longer than the rest the toes and may result in varus or valgus deformities. The marked laxity of the ligaments produce flat foot.

METHODOLOGY

History Taking

(As in the chapter on Introduction)

The main complaints regarding the feet of children are about deformities, while in adults they are mainly regarding pain and swelling. When pain is complained of, enquire about its specific site and relation with standing, walking (distance usually covered before pain starts), and rest. In case of congenital deformities (e.g. club foot), the family history (for such deformities) and obstetrical history (age of mother, drug used during pregnancy, presentation, etc) must be taken in detail.

General and Systemic Examinations

As in chapter on Introduction

If the patient can stand and walk, the gait must be noted. The position of the foot in stance phase should be noted with particular emphasis in the weight bearing pattern of different parts of the sole. While examining the gait, ask the patient to walk on tiptoes (the forefoot), heels, outer border, and inner border of the feet respectively. This gives an overall impression about the function of the foot. If one is able to walk in the above patterns normally, the foot is most probably normal.

Regional Examination

As usual for the lower limb, i.e. from the lumbosacral region to the tips of the toes.

LOCAL EXAMINATION

Prerequisites: (i) Both feet must be examined simultaneously in identical positions as far as possible, (ii) Expose upto the ipsilateral hip or till at least above knee level, (iii) The foot is better examined while the patient is sitting at the edge of the couch, (iv) Examination of the footwear, specially the older used one, must also be done. Also enquire about the type and duration of foot wear used and condition of ground, where maximum walking is done by the patient.

Attitude

The axial relation of the foot with that of the leg should be noted and compared with the opposite side. The attitude of the foot when the patient is in lying down position should also be noted—this has special importance, particularly when examining a paralytic foot. Note the effect of any foot pathology on the ankle, knee and hip.

Inspection

It should be done from the dorsal and plantar as well as the medial and lateral aspects.

Note the anatomical alignment of the foot and toes, interrelation of toe lengths, any overriding of toes, skin condition, oedema, venous prominences, nail beds, the webs and the tips of the toes. Looking from the plantar side, the anatomical disposition, skin condition, presence of any callosities, oedema, corn, shoe bite, trophic ulcer or any other abnormal findings should be noted. Any swelling or sinus in this zone must be examined. The foot may be riddled with multiple sinuses specially in the tropics (e.g. in tuberculosis, mycetoma of foot—Madura foot, Kaposi's sarcoma, tropical ulcer). While looking from behind, note the shape and size of the heel, besides the prominence, alignment and continuity of the tendo-Achilles.

Palpation

Superficial Palpation

Feel the skin surface and temperature. Feel for dorsalis pedis, posterior tibial and anterior tibial arterial pulsation. Note must be made of any superficial tenderness or any anaesthesia/ paraesthesia.

For palpating the dorsalis pedis, gently put two fingers (index and middle finger) over the proximal part of the first inter metatarsal space. For the posterior tibial artery, palpate one finger breadth posteroinferior to the medial malleous. For the anterior tibial artery, palpate at about the centre of a line with a slight upper convexity joining the two malleoli anteriorly or at about half finger breadth lateral to the extensor hallucis longus tendon at the ankle level.

Deep Palpation

Confirm the anatomical alignment of the bony structures. Palpate the tendons individually. If any abnormal finding like swelling or sinus is present, proceed as given in the chapter on Introduction.

Palpate to elicit deep tenderness with certain common conditions in mind.

i. With the index finger, press upwards, backwards and laterally on the medial border of the foot at a point where the medial arch just starts—tenderness indicates calcaneal fascitis.
   Palpate just behind and below the navicular tuberosity—tenderness indicates hyperstretching of the spring ligament (strained foot).
ii. With the index finger tip, press upwards from sole in between 3rd and 4th metatarsal head and also on the adjoining proximal area—tenderness indicates metatarsalgia. Further confirmation can be had by squeezing the forefoot which will trigger the original pain of the patient.
iii. Squeeze in between the thumb and index finger, just in front and above the attachment of the tendo-Achilles at the heel—tenderness indicates pre-Achilles bursitis, while pain on pressing the posterior aspect of tendo-Achilles, indicates post-Achilles bursitis. These can be further confirmed by asking the patient to walk on toes (pain will be complained in case of pre-Achilles bursitis) and heels (pain in case of post-Achilles bursitis). In Achilles tendinitis (e.g. in active ankylosing spondylitis and rheumatoid arthritis), pain in heel region will be there both on heel and toe walking, and tendo-Achilles will be tender on side to side squeezing.

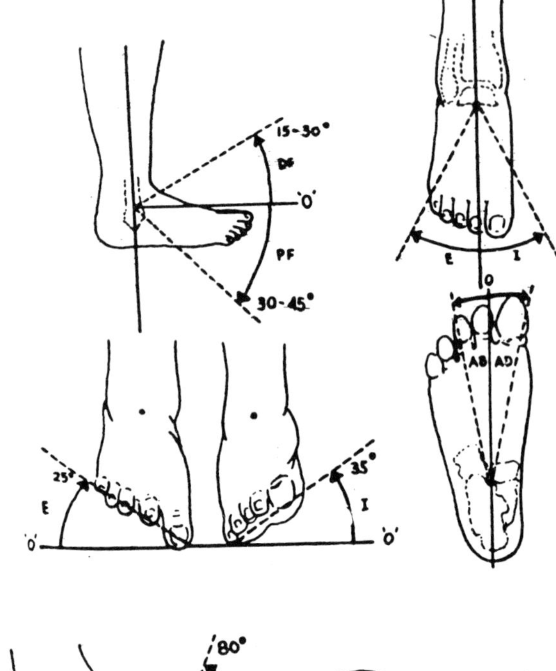

Fig. 15.19: Zero axis and normal range of movements of ankle and foot. Df = dorsiflexion; PF = plantarflexion; E = eversion; I = inversion; AB = abduction; AD = adduction; Ex = extension; F = flexion

MOVEMENTS (Fig. 15.19—zero axis and normal range of movements on ankle and foot)

Though the smaller joints of the foot have been anatomically disposed as to produce certain groups of movements, but in normal physiomechanics of the foot, the movements are more or less inter-related. However, different sets of movements should be tested at different joints. In assessing any movement, the standard pattern (as given in the chapter on Introduction) should be followed but, it may not be easy to evaluate the movements of the smaller joints of the foot under the desired headings.

Method of Eliciting Different Movements and Zero Axis of Ankle and Foot

It is very difficult to test isolated active movements of the foot, hence it is advisable to proceed with accessing the movements passively.

Inversion and Eversion

It can be better tested by making the patient sit on a stool with knee flexed at about 70°. It can be tested also while the patient is lying supine. With one hand, hold the ankle firmly from the dorsum to fix the talus. The other hand holds the body of calcaneum in between the thumb on one side and the index and middle finger on the other. Now try to move the calcaneum on the fixed talus. Turning-in of the heel will demonstrate inversion and turning-out eversion at the fulcrum of the subtalar joint. The axis of movements lies 45° above the horizontal plane and 16° inner to the long axis of the foot and runs upwards, forwards and medially.

Movements at the subtalar joint can also be tested as follows:

Adduction and Abduction of the Forefoot (Fig. 15.20)

Hold the hind foot from the dorsum with one hand, i.e. the first web firmly grips the talus, while the thumb and index finger fix the calcaneum from the two sides. Now with the other hand, hold the forefoot with the thumb on the dorsum and other fingers on the sole. Passively deviating the forefoot inwards demonstrates adduction and outwards abduction. The fulcrum is at the mid tarsal joint, i.e. the talo-navicular on the inner and the calcaneocuboid on the outer side. The axis of these movements runs from behind forwards, more or less, along a line joining the centre of the patella, mid ankle point and second web.

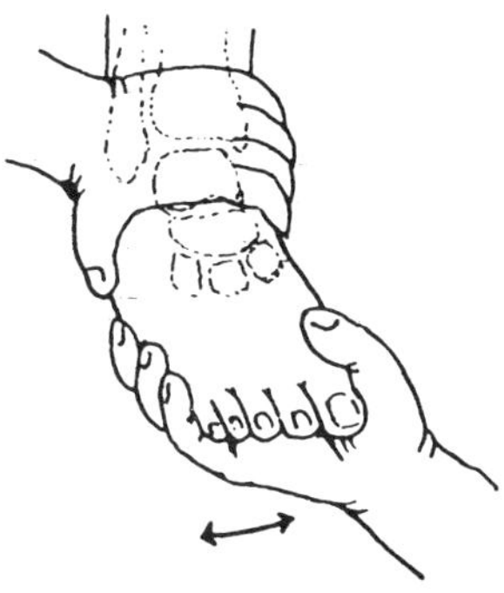

Fig. 15.20: Demonstration of adduction and abduction movements of forefoot

Movements of the toes are not as important as those of the fingers of the hand. However, a gross assessment of active plantarflexion and dorsiflexion of the toes (specially of the big toe) should be done. Beyond the active range, the pliability of the joint should be tested by noting the passive range of movement.

Intrinsic Tests

Hitherto the intrinsics of the foot have been neglected in clinical methodology. As discussed earlier, these small but powerful muscles are essential for the springy and rhythmic pattern of gait. Hence they must be tested as far as practicable. Even if tested as 'group movers' it will be a worthwhile examination.

Closing and fanning out of the webs are produced by the interossei—the dorsal interossei being responsible for fanning out while plantar interossei are for closing the webs, the axis being the second metatarsal.

Method (Fig. 15.21): Hold the forefoot just distal to the midtarsal joint level. The card test as done for the fingers will suffice here too. Put the card in the particular web to be tested. Ask the patient to grip it between the adjacent toes and judge the strength of the grip.

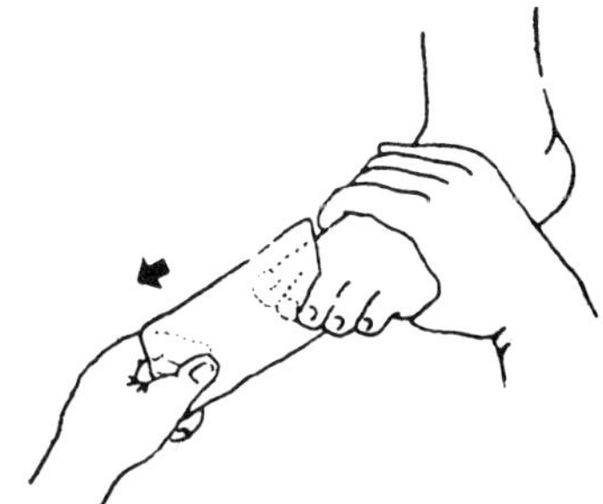

Fig. 15.21: Test for intrinsic muscles—Card test

The lumbricals are difficult to test here individually, since the action of the long and short flexors of the toes are difficult to be neutralized in any particular position. However, a rough estimation can be made of the conjoint of the lumbricals and the interossei.

Ask the patient to plantarflex the toes at the metatarsophalangeal joints, keeping the interphalangeal joints extended as far as possible. The lumbricals, along with the interossei are the prime movers for flexing the toes at metatarsophalangeal joint and extending them at the interphalangeal joints.

Stress Tests

The testing for the exaggerated and passive aforesaid movements will be the stress tests for these joints. These tests are not that important in the foot because the joints are very small and the ligaments of one joint more or less reinforce other joints also. Besides, there are almost two tiers of ligaments holding the main joints.

MEASUREMENTS

These measurements are of paramount importance for chiropodists and orthotists.

i. *Longitudinal measurements give an idea about the length of the foot.*

   a. It should be measured in two axes (Fig. 15.22A) (OX and OY).
   From the most prominent point on the back of the heel (0) to the tip of the greater toe (X) and from the first point to the tip of fifth toe (Y).

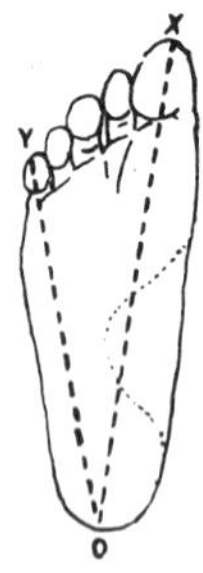

Fig. 15.22A: Longitudinal measurement of foot

   b. The relation of the long lever arm (tip of medial malleolus to tip of the great toe on the inner side, and tip of lateral malleolus to the tip of 5th toe on outer side) and the short lever arm (tip of medial malleolus to the most prominent heel point on medial side, and tip of lateral malleolus to the most prominent heel point on the lateral side) of the foot should be symmetrical on both sides.

ii. *Circumferential measurement* should be done at three levels (Fig. 15.22B).

1. Metatarsal head level (i).
2. Maximum height of the medial arch (ii).
3. Just behind the ankle (iii).

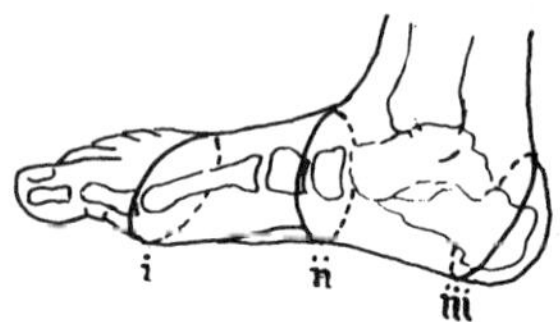

Fig. 15.22B: Circumferential measurement of foot. (i) At metatarsal head, (ii) At maximum height of arch, (iii) Just behind the ankle

The third measurement will be more or less the axial circumferential measurement.

iii. *Vertical measurement* Any variation in the height of calcaneum and the heel-sole-cushion, will disturb the height of the foot, the distance from the tip of the medial or lateral malleolus to the under surface of sole at the corresponding margin.

Measurement of Equinus Deformity

Patient lies on the bed on his lateral side (to eliminate gravity). He is asked to dorsiflex the ankle then further dorsiflex passively as far as possible. Measure the angle between the long axis of the leg (i.e. from mid point of joint line of knee to tip of medial malleolus) and long axis of hind to midfoot (i.e. from tip of medial malleolus to the head of first metatarsal bone). Substract 90° from this angle. The remaining will be the 'angle of fixed equinus deformity'.

Measurement of Calcaneus Deformity

Keeping the feet in zero axis of the legs (mid patella, mid ankle, and second web in one line), dorsiflex them passively as far as possible.

Normally, in an adult, 15° to 30° will be possible. Anything beyond that is due to calcaneus. Measure the total angle of dorsiflexion from 90° position of the ankle. Substract the angle of normal side (if both ankles affected, substract 30°), remainder will be angle of calcaneus deformity, however, for clarity, expression should be of total dorsiflexion from zero position.

Auscultation

If any doubtful swelling exists it should be auscultated.

Examination of the Footwear (Figs 15.22C and D)

The used footwear should be assessed for:

i. Distortion of the shape—indicates underlying rigid deformity of the foot.
ii. Wrinkling of the footwear (specially of the upper-leather or vamp and around the heel). In persistent toe-in there will be exaggerated wrinkling on distal upper medial aspect of the vamp. In persistent heel varus, deep wrinkles may appear on the inner aspect of the heel.

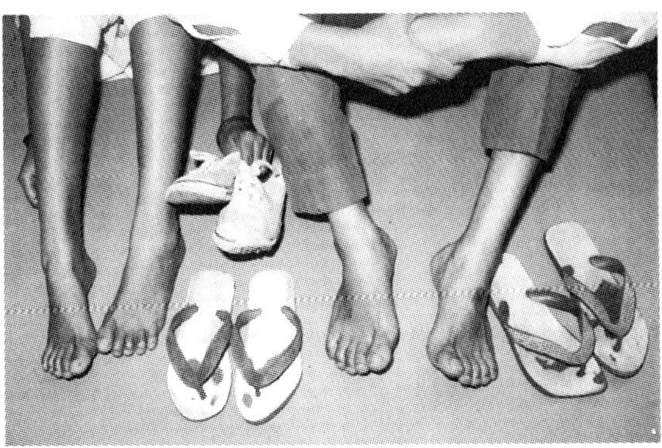

Fig. 15.22C: Examination of footwear

iii. Bulging out and thinning (due to pressure) of the vamp (e.g.—in hallux valgus—bulging on the distal medial side, in valgus foot—bulging on the medial side, in inverted foot—excessive bulging on the lateral side).
iv. Deformation of the sole and the vamp e.g. in neglected or relapsed or resistant club foot.

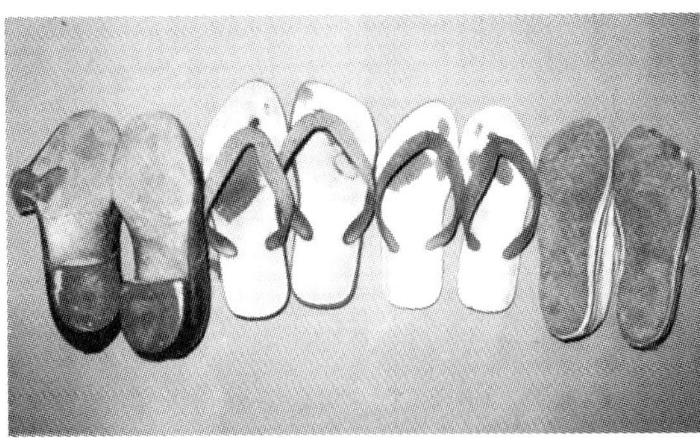

Fig. 15.22D: Examination of footwear

Study of the Sole of Footwear

i. Bulging out of the sole in any particular direction.
ii. Pressure erosion of the sole.
iii. Comparative height of the inner and outer borders (Normally there is tendency of wearing off of the sole on the outer side).
iv. Any pricking point on upper surface of the sole (shoe nail, rough leather margin).
v. Hollowing out or scooping tendency at any particular point of the insole (indicative of localised pressure—of great importance in insensitive foot).
vi. Unused portion on the insole.

INVESTIGATION OF A CASE WITH FOOT PATHOLOGY

1. Routine Investigations

As in the chapter on Introduction.

2. Radiological Investigations

i. *Superoinferior view*: The patient sits with hip and knee flexed 90°. Ask the patient to firmly press his foot on the plate. The whole span of the foot must be focussed on and the beam centred at the mid foot level.
ii. *Lateral view*: While the patient lies halfway on the affected side with that lower

limb rotated outward, the foot is adjusted until the plantar surface is at right angles to the film. The beam is centered to the middle of the foot.

iii. *Oblique view*: This is essential to delineate the inter-tarsal relations properly (Fig. 15.23A).

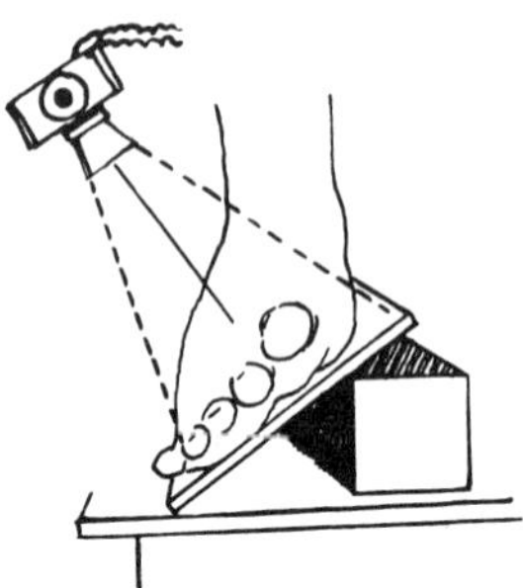

Fig. 15.23A: Positioning for oblique view X-ray of mid and forefoot

Method: The patient sitting with hip and knee flexed at 90°, the inverted foot is placed, on the plate with the forefoot fanned out. The beam should be focussed vertically on the plate.

iv. *Oblique view for the hind foot*: It is also known as axial view for the calcaneum. This view is essential to see the body and posterior part of the calcaneum.

Method: This can be taken with the patient standing or lying down (Fig. 15.23B).

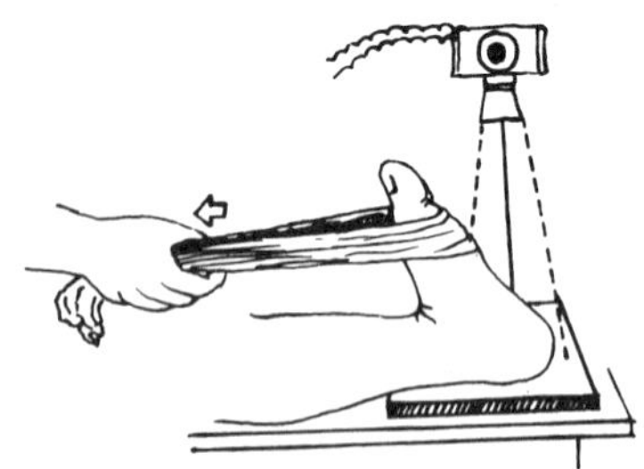

Fig. 15.23B: Positioning for axial view of hind foot (for calcaneum)

While the patient is lying down, the plate is placed beneath the heel. The ankle is passively dorsiflexed as far as possible using a strap. The beam is focussed on the plantar aspect at the midpoint of the junction of the heel with the midfoot.

3. Footprint (Podogram, Ichnogram = imprint of the soles of the feet taken standing)

This is a very useful and cheap method for investigating problems of the foot.

Method: The patient's feet are uniformly painted with duplicating ink and then he is asked to step on a white paper to give his footprint, this may be taken as a static imprint of the foot, when it is desired to assess the weight bearing pattern of one foot.

For studying the gait pattern of the patient, dynamic footprints may be taken, where the patient walks with painted feet on the white papers.

4. Electrical Recording of Footprints

Different electronically controlled devices have been instituted to study the weight bearing pattern of the foot in static or dynamic phase. This has been used especially for studying gait patterns.

5. Image Intensifier Radiography and Cine-Radiography

These devices are useful in studying different gait patterns.

6. Photopodogram

By this method, fine impressions of the skin lines of the sole are obtained on photographic silver bromide paper.

The sole of the foot is coated with concentrated developing solution, and then the foot is carefully put on a silver bromide paper, which is exposed to day-light or lamp light for about 30 seconds. The paper is thereafter removed, fixed and washed.

7. Podoscopy

A sheet of glass is illuminated from beneath. When the foot is placed on it, the sole of the foot can be observed in a mirror placed below. The area of weight bearing, the overall shape of the foot and the condition of arches can be thus studied.

8. Arthroscopy

This has in general not been utilised for joints of the foot. However, in very specialised centres, this is being used for diagnostic as well as therapeutic purposes.

The more developed investigations, like computerized radiopodography, podostatiradiography, pressopodostatiradiography, photoscopic studies, televideopodometry, etc. can be utilised to understand the intricate physiomechanics of a normal foot and the pathodynamics of an abnormal foot.

9. Foetal Surveillance Techniques

These are much helpful for early and accurate diagnosis of malformations (e.g. in spina bifida manifesta and arthrogryposis multiplex congenita.

Key Diagnostic Points of Common Foot Pathology

Assessment of a Case of Club Foot (Tables 15.2 to 15.4)

This has more value in determining the prognosis and the line of management rather than diagnosing the disease, which is quite obvious from the very beginning. Besides general assessment depending upon the clinical grades certain important aspects must be looked into.

NB: Certain MUSTS in an examination of a club foot.

i. Search for evidences of spina bifida (manifesta or occulta) in the lower part of the spine/back (Table 15.3).
ii. Look for other congenital deformities in bone and joints—knees, hips and upper limbs, cleft palate; and in soft tissue—cleft lip, congenital hernia, exomphalus.
iii. Congenital malformation of the vital organs, e.g. heart, liver, lung, etc. should be excluded.
iv. Test for sensation in the foot (specially the sole).

AETIOLOGICALLY CLUB FOOT CAN BE DIVIDED INTO (Table 15.2):

A. *Congenital*

—Idiopathic (commonest).
—Myogenic (imperfect muscle development, e.g. Arthrogryposis multiplex congenita).
—Neurogenic (e.g. spina bifida).
—Osteogenic (e.g. absent tibia).

Club foot can be inherited (Fig. 15.28C); also occurs with few genetically inherited conditions, e.g. diastrophic dwarfism, Freeman-Sheldon syndrome.

B. *Acquired*

—Paralytic (poliomyelitis, myopathy).
—Inflammatory (post-infective contracture of calf muscles).
—Traumatic (injury in leg or ankle or foot, compartment syndrome—VIC)
—Neoplastic (in calf or foot).

In arthrogryposis multiplex congenita (Figs 15.24A and B), club foot exists along with flexion and adduction at hip (may be congenital dislocation of hip), congenital contracture of quadriceps, extension at elbow, adduction and medial rotation at shoulder, etc. in various combinations.

Late cases of club foot can be divided into:

i. Resistant (certain elements of the deformity resist correction).
ii. Relapsed (certain elements of the deformity recur).
iii. Neglected [club foot not taken up for treatment within 9 months (Figs 15.28D and E).

The idiopathic congenital club foot can be differentiated from acquired specially the poliotics on the points mentioned in the Table 15.2

Callosities

Callosities are circumscribed plaques of hyperkeratosis induced by intermittent trauma. They

Table 15.2: Clinical differences between congenital and acquired equinovarus (club foot) deformities

Congenital	*Acquired*
1. History since birth	1. Deformity appears after birth
2. Usually bilateral (about 60%) These types more common in boys	2. Usually unilateral Not such preference (sexwise)
3. Set pattern of deformity i.e. equinovarus with adduction of forefoot and cavus	3. Usually only equinovarus
4. Congenital groove mostly present	4. Not present.
5. Heel looks smaller and tugged up	5. Heel maintains its shape and size except in severe and neglected cases
6. Look of calf—in severe and very severe type—looks more or less cylindrical	6. Configuration of calf usually maintained
7. Feel of calf usually tough	7. Calf is usually supple
8. In severe and very severe type, subcutaneous tissue has tight and adherent feel on posteroinfero-medial aspect and atrophied on dorsolateral aspect	8. Except in neglected cases, sub-cutaneous tissue feels softer more or less on all aspects
9. May be associated with other congenital deformities	9. Associated paralytic deformity in same leg and/or other leg and/or other part of body
10. Neurological examination—normal	10. Motor and/or sensory deficit

Table 15.3: Clinical differences between idiopathic club foot and club foot associated with spina bifida

Idiopathic club foot	*Club foot with spina bifida*
1. Present since birth	1. Appears later, usually after 2 years of age
2. Cause not known	2. Neurogenic, due to paresis/paralysis of the roots controlling the muscles on the dorsolateral aspect of the leg and foot
3. Sensation intact	3. Affected
4. Trophic ulcers–not present	4. Present
5. Associated congenital deformity may be present in other joints	5. Usually other joints remain free
6. Management to be started at the earliest	6. Wait and watch for the progress of the deformities
7. Deformities are fixed from beginning	7. Deformities are usually not fixed till late

can be usually of four types according to the causative factors (Table 15.5).

Corns

Corns are localised callosities over bony prominences of foot and occasionally of the fingers. They occur due to friction and pressure. Corn consists of a central hyperkeratotic spike projecting downwards towards the dermis and forming a hard 'core' on the surface, surrounded by an area of semi-opaque thickening of horny layer. The pressure of the core on the nerve causes exquisite pain which is worse in high humidity. In diabetese or after faulty paring it may get infected.

Soft corns are more persistant hyperkeratotic lesion between 4th and 5th digital interspace mostly as kissing lesions. There may be underlying bony spur. Removal of cause, ring pad, shoe-padding, metatarsal bar may be useful. Salicylic acid application and cautious paring may help. Any underlying bony spur should be removed.

Injection of silicon fluid underneath the corn (silicon prosthesis) can cure many corns.

Table 15.4: Clinical grades of club foot

Clinical findings	*Grades of club foot*			
	Mild (Fig 15.25)	*Moderate (Fig. 15.26)*	*Severe (Fig. 15.27)*	*Very severe (Fig. 15.28)*
Skin Condition	Normal	Almost normal	Stretched on superolateral aspect, crowded skin creases on posteromedial aspect. Congenital grooves on the inferomedial aspect of the foot and rarely in the lower leg. Thin callosities on the dorso-lateral aspect	Atrophied skin, congenital groove always present in inferomedial aspect of foot and lower leg, thick callosities
Attitude of the foot	Mild equinovarus	Equinus element more dominating than the varus. Associated adduction of the fore-foot	Varus, adduction of forefoot, equinus and cavus in that order	Inverted foot, equinus element comparatively less, foot turns almost inwards at right angles to the leg alongwith marked cavus
Stretchability of the deformity	Fully correctable on passive stretching	75-50% correctable on passive stretching	Correctable by 50-25% on passive stretching	Less than 25% correctable, on passive stretching
Effect of stretching on vascularity	No effect	Blanching of the toes after 75-50% correction.	Blanching of the toes after 50-25% correction	Blanching of toes after less than 25% correction
Heel	Almost normal	Comparatively smaller	Small, moderate heel varus	Small, severe heel varus
Calf	Normal	Almost normal	Tendency to become tapering and cylindrical	Almost cylindrical (peg like)
Feel of calf muscles	Normal	Almost normal	Firm	Markedly firm, and presents the feel of fixity
Treatment	Manipulative massage and maintenance with orthotics	Manipulative massage, serial strapping, serial plaster cast, maintenance orthotics. For resistant cases—posteroinferomedial soft tissue release	Trial of serial plaster casting. Several of these type require soft tissue release, External fixator	Soft tissue release, maintenance with orthotics, regular stretching and physiotherapy—even then recurrence is common External fixator Combined soft tissue release and bony operation

NB—For neglected, resistant and relapsed club foot presenting beyond 3 years of age, bony operations are usually needed for satisfactory correction.

Table 15.5: Types of callosities

Type of callosity	*Site*	*Cause*	*Presentation*	*Management*
Orthopaedic callosities	Sole, beneath metatarsal heads	Structural-abnormality of foot; unsuitable footwear; abnormal gait; trophic disorders	Abnormal look, tenderness, fissuring	Treat underlying cause; calus softened by salicylic acid and gently pared away; regular supervision of susceptible region, chiropodist care
Callosities due to repeated pressure, appliances, and wears	Sites of straps of calipers; front of lower thigh in hand to knee gait.	Repeated pressure in calipers; Ill-fitting trusses		
Occupational callosities	Sites affected are according to occupation, e.g. muslim callus on forehead and upper outer aspect of foot (Figs 15.24C and D).	Repeated pressure at particular site (e.g. in muslim prayer positions)		
Callosities due to habits and tick	Gnaw-warts on fingers, back of hands	Regular biting habit of certain child or mentally ill person		

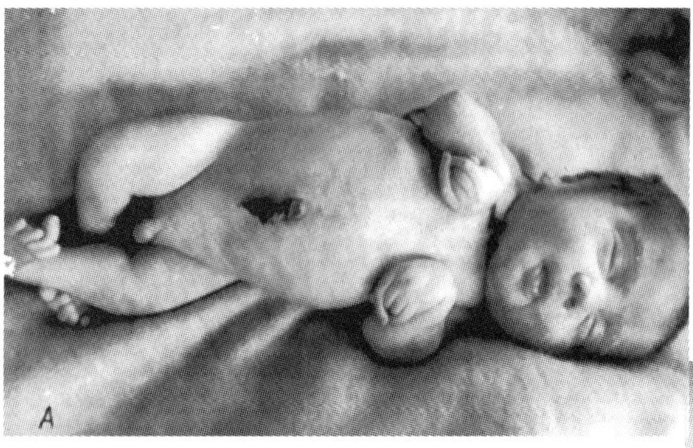

Fig. 15.24A and B: Arthrogryposis multiplex congenita

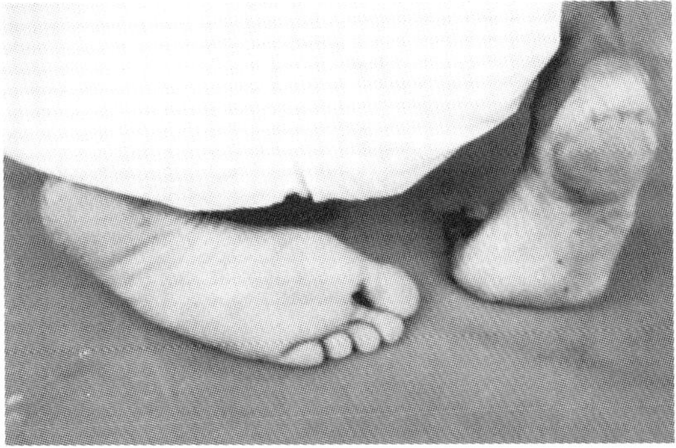

Fig. 15.24C: Prayer-position of feet by Muslims which add to the formation of Muslim's callus

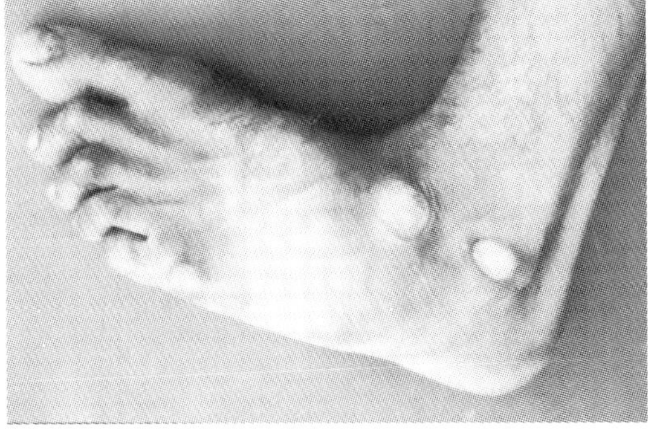

Fig. 15.24D: Muslim's callus

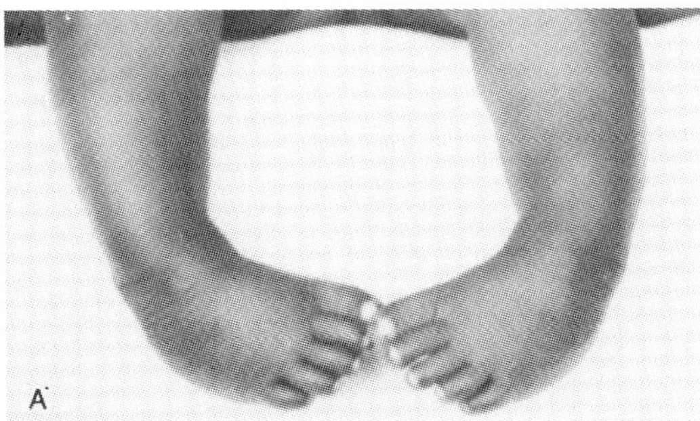
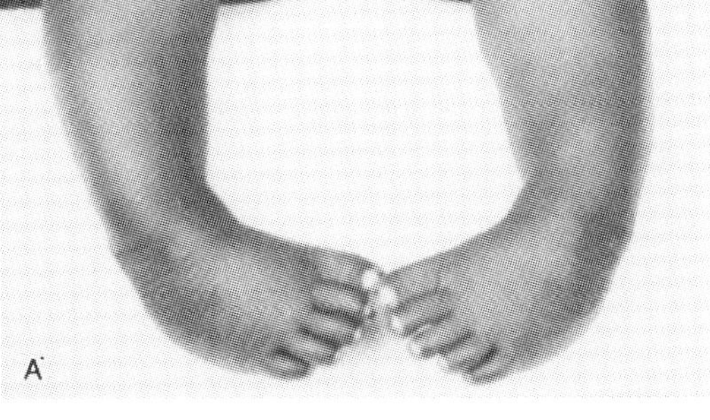

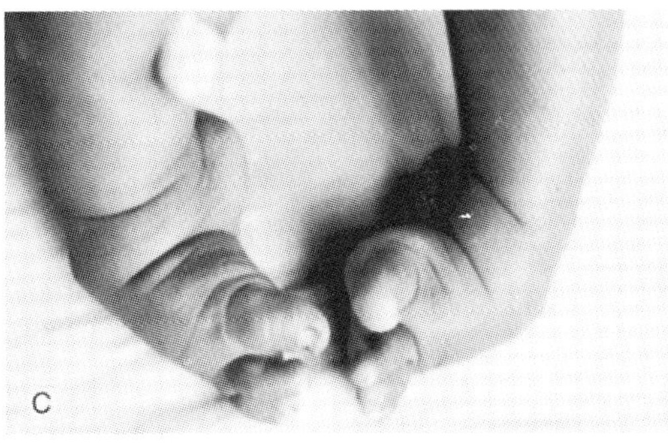

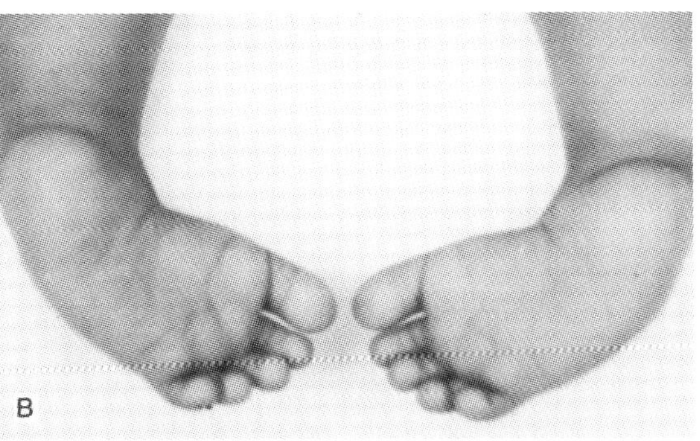

Figs 15.25A and B: Mild club foot

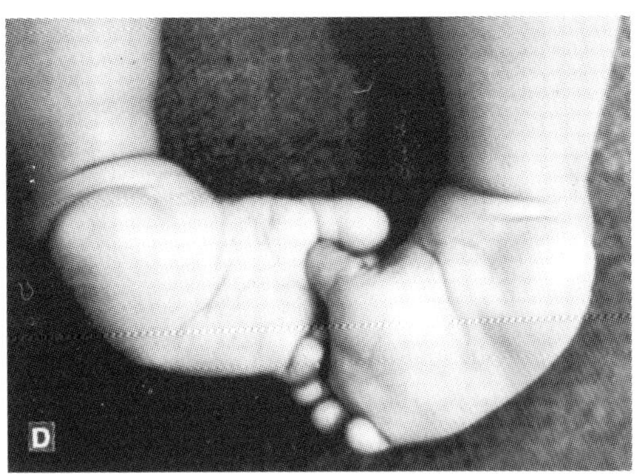

Figs 15.26A and B: Moderate club foot

Causes of Pain in the Heel: (As shown in Fig. 15.29)

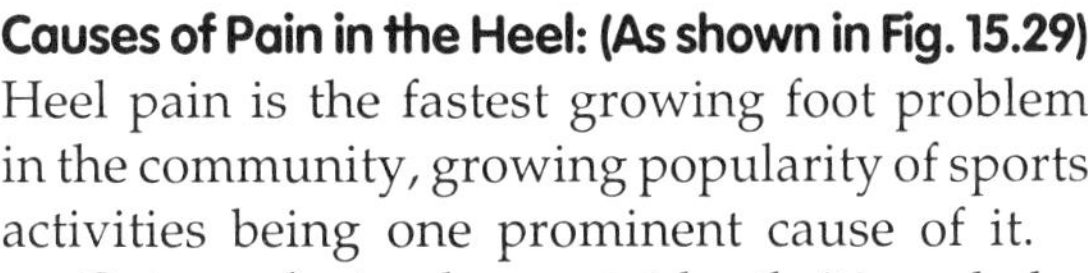

Heel pain is the fastest growing foot problem in the community, growing popularity of sports activities being one prominent cause of it.

Osteomalacia, rheumatoid arthritis, ankylosing spondylitis, prolonged standing, diabetes, faulty footwear, protozoal and helminthic infections of gut can also produce pain in the heel.

Causes of Pain in Midfoot

Besides the pain due to injuries, infections, and neoplasm, conditions like pes planus, accessory navicular, osteochondritis of navicular (Kohler's disease), congenital coalition of the tarsals leading to spastic flat foot, may cause pain in the midfoot.

Table 15.6: Differentiation between wart and callosity of foot

	Wart	*Callosity*
Cause	Infection with human DNA papilloma virus	Thickening of the skin at the points of excessive pressure
Common sites	More in the forepart of the sole	Beneath the heads of the metatarsals. Also on the dorsum of the foot, e.g. in club foot, hammer toe, etc.
Basic pathology	Lesions are intra-epidermal, Dry, friable papillomatous projections	Hyperkeratinisation
Tenderness	Marked	May be tender
Surface	Mosaic like	Thickened, smooth surface
Relation to surrounding skin	Can be clearly demarcated from the surrounding skin	Blends with the surrounding skin

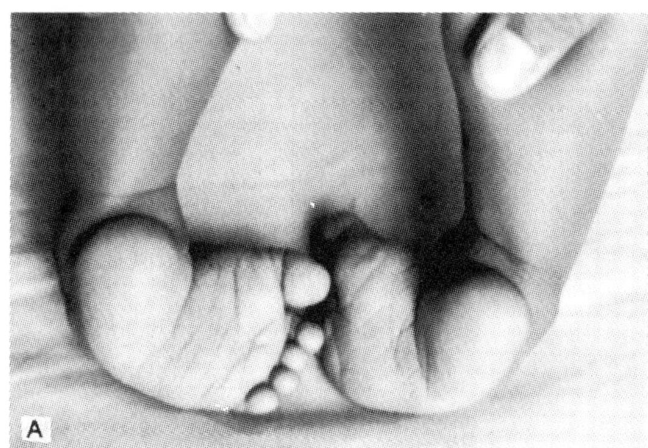
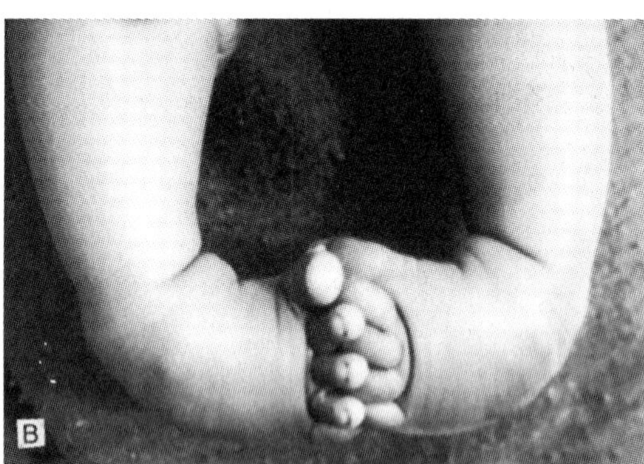

Figs 15.27A and B: Severe club foot

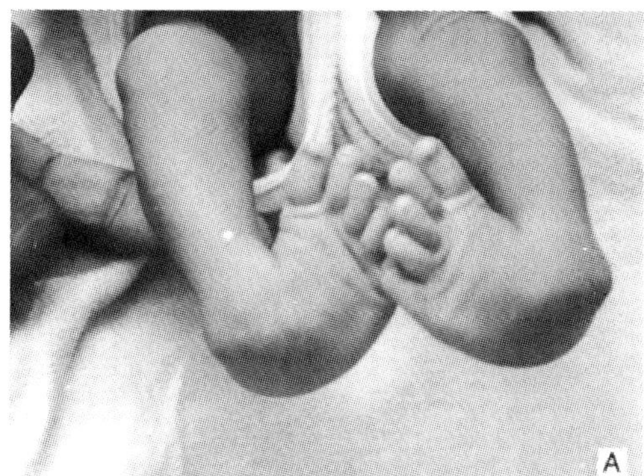
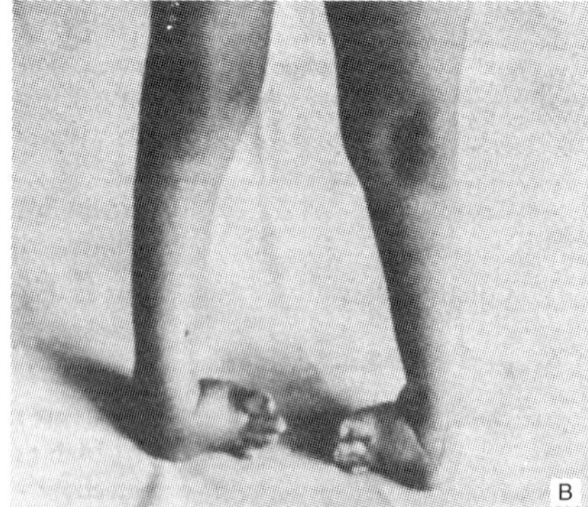

Figs 15.28A and B: Very severe club foot

Causes of Pain in the Forefoot

i. *Metatarsalgia*

a. March fracture—stress fracture usually occurs in the neck of second metatarsal; history of unusual amount of walking; tender swelling on the dorsum of the foot, at the site of fracture.

b. Morton's metatarsalgia—Middle aged women; severe pain in the forefoot radiating to the adjacent sides of 3rd and 4th

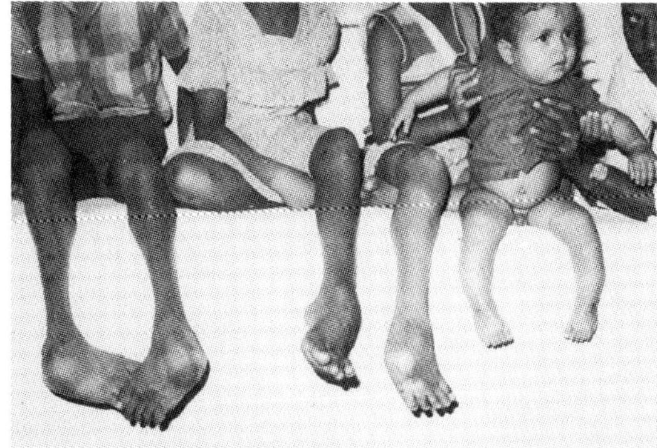

Fig. 15.28C: Club foot in a family. Father and three children (out of four) have club foot

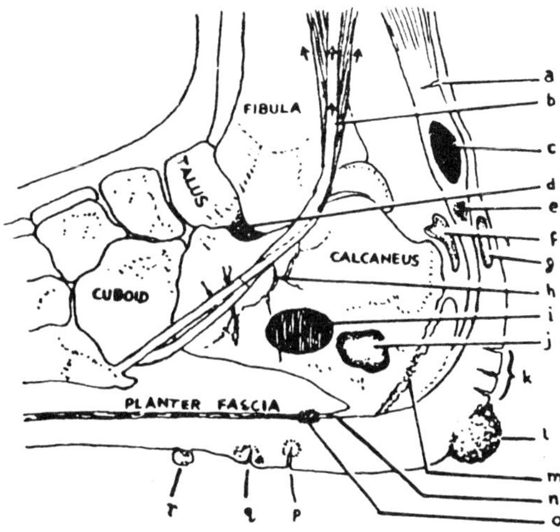

Fig. 15.29A: Painful heel: a = partial rupture of tendo-Achilles, b = peroneal spasm, c = xanthoma, d = sub-talar arthritis, e = Achilles tendinitis, f = pre-Achilles bursitis, g = post-Achilles bursitis, h = fracture calcaneum, i = neoplasm of calcaneum, j = cyst/tuberculosis of calcaneum, k = fissures, l = melanoma, m = traction or stress injuries induced osteochondritis of posterior calcaneal apophysis—apophysitis—(Sever's disease—Fig. 15.29B) calcaneal apophysitis, n = calcaneal spur, o = plantar fascitis, p = thorn prick, q = corn, r = wart

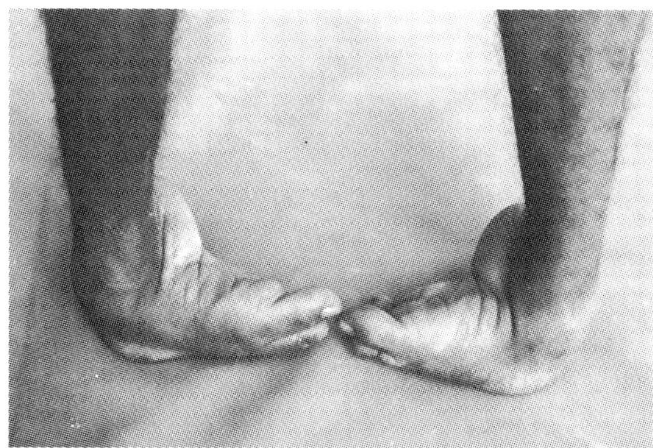

Fig. 15.28D

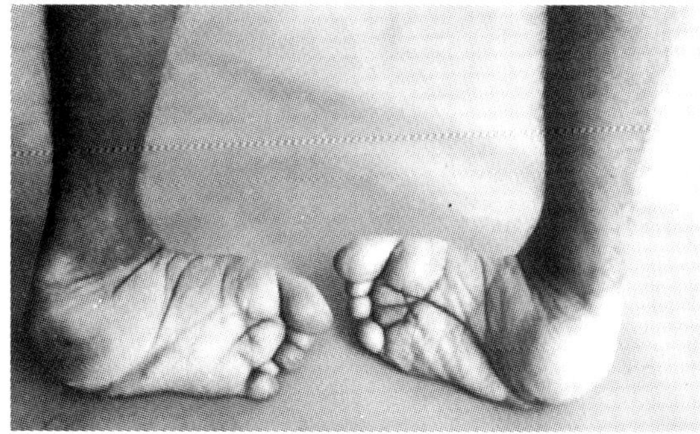

Figs 15.28D and E: Neglected very severe club foot

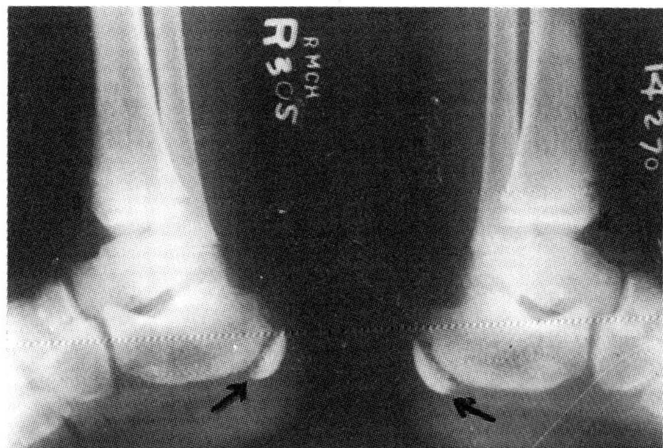

Fig. 15.29B: Calcaneal apophysitis (Sever's disease)

toes or 2nd and 3rd toes; tenderness on pressing the sole between the 3rd and 4th metatarsal heads; squeezing of the forefoot triggers the pain.

c. Dropped transverse arch (anterior flat foot)—is a common cause of pain in the forefoot. Here there is broadening of the forefoot, callosities beneath the metatarsal heads and weakness in raising the metatarsal heads.

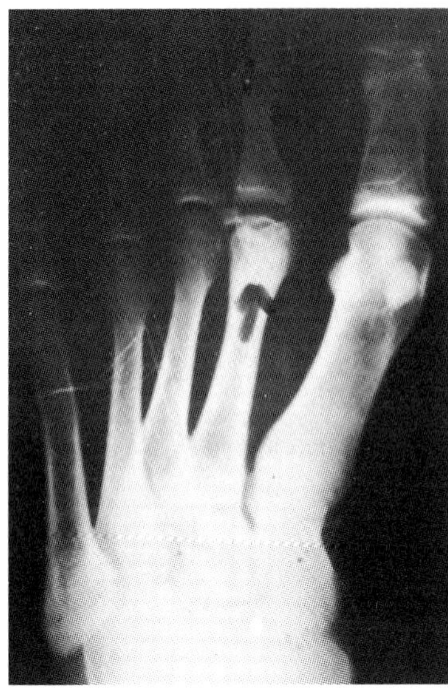

Fig. 15.29C: Freiberg's disease

ii. *Freiberg's Disease*

Osteochondritis of the distal epiphyses (metatarsal head) (usually of the second metatarsal), in adolescent or adult males (Fig. 15.29C)

iii. *Fractures of Metatarsals*

iv. *Gouty Arthritis*

Middle aged men, complain of acute onset of pain with or without burning sensation usually in the region of 1st metatarsophalangeal joint (in pseudogout, the ankle is more affected).

- —Symptoms usually precipitate in the small hours of the morning.
- —Local inflammatory features.
- —Other joints, like ankle, knee, small joints of hands and feet may be affected.
- —Serum uric acid level raised.
- —In chronic cases gouty tophi occur on big toe (Figs 15.30A to C) pinna of ear, fingers, elbow, etc.
- —Joint aspirate from joint, tophi, ligaments, etc—may show presence of sodium biurate salt (cf. in pseudogout—calcium pyrophosphate crystals).

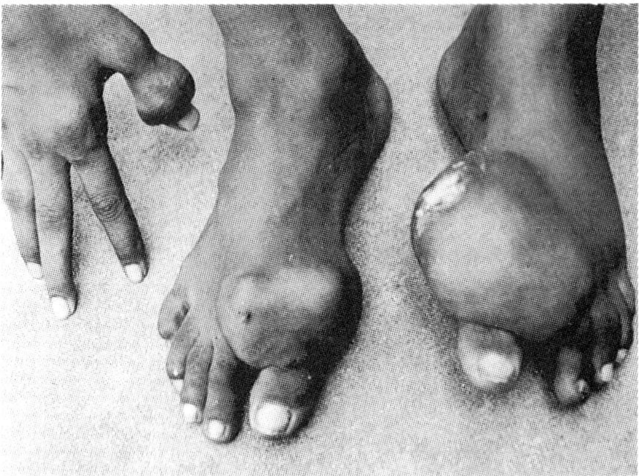

Fig. 15.30A: Typical gouty tophi on both 1st metatarsophalangeal joint of both feet and also on the right thumb and base of index finger

Causes of Ulcers in the Soles

- i. Trophic ulcer—Hansen's disease (Figs 15.31A to E), sciatic or medial popliteal nerve palsy, spina bifida (Figs 15.32A to E), paraplegia (traumatic).
- ii. Diabetic ulcers—Twenty per cent or even more hospitalised diabetic patients are admitted for the foot problems, mainly the ulcers.
- iii. Ulcers of vascular origin—Buerger's disease
- iv. Arteriosclerotic ulcers.
- v. Neurosyphilitic ulcer.
- vi. Infective—Actinomycotic (Madura foot) (Figs 15.33A to C), pyogenic.
- vii. Post-traumatic.
- viii. Post-burn.
- ix. Neoplastic, e.g. melanomatous (Fig. 15.35A).

v. *Tuberculosis of Foot* (Figs 15.34A to C)

- —Mostly affects tarsals (talus and calcaneum) and intertarsal zones.
- —Chronic gradually increasing pain and mild to moderate swelling (may even fluctuate) on the dorsal aspect of foot.
- —Tuberculous sinuses (usually more than one with indrawn, puckered margin, discoloured surrounding, serosanguinous or thin straw coloured discharge).
- —Tenderness at affected bones and joints.

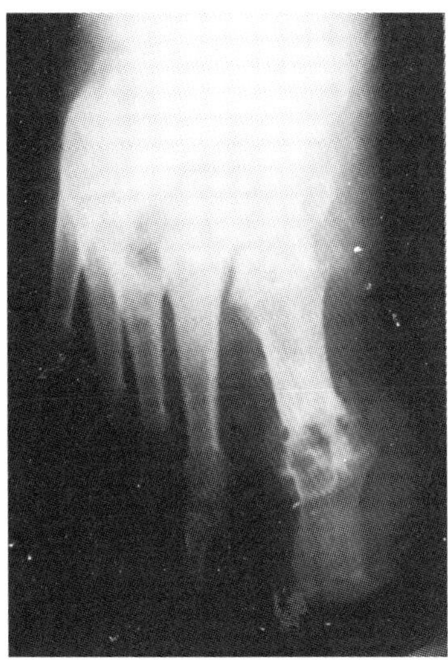

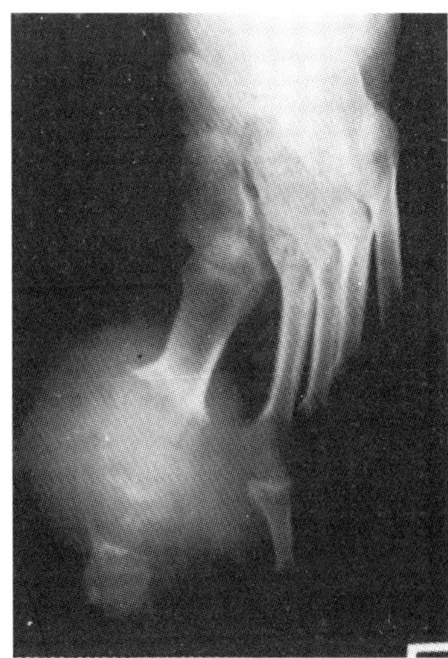

Fig. 15.30B and C: X-ray photograph of same patient (Fig.15.30A). Note the destruction in the first metatarsophalangeal zones due to deposit of urate crystals

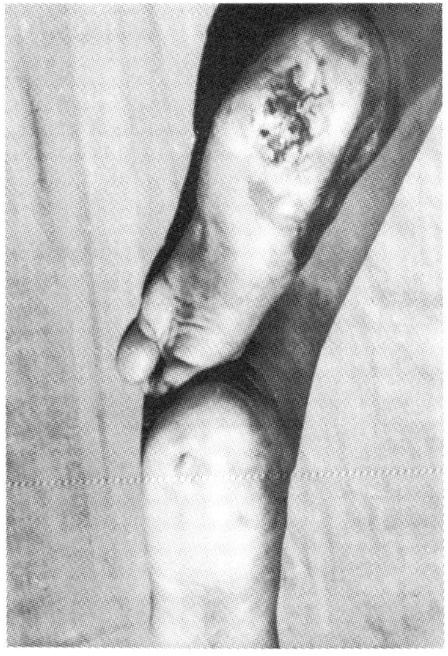

Fig. 15.31A: Trophic ulcers (Hansen's disease)—on left heel healed; on right still very active

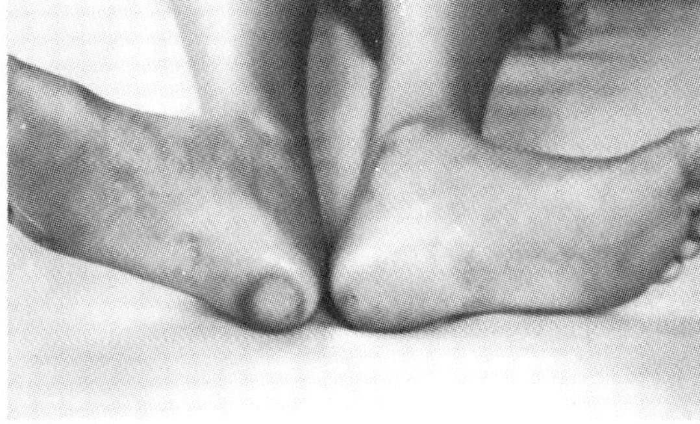

Fig. 15.31B: Pre-ulcerative appearance of trophic ulceration in the both of heels due to Hansen's disease

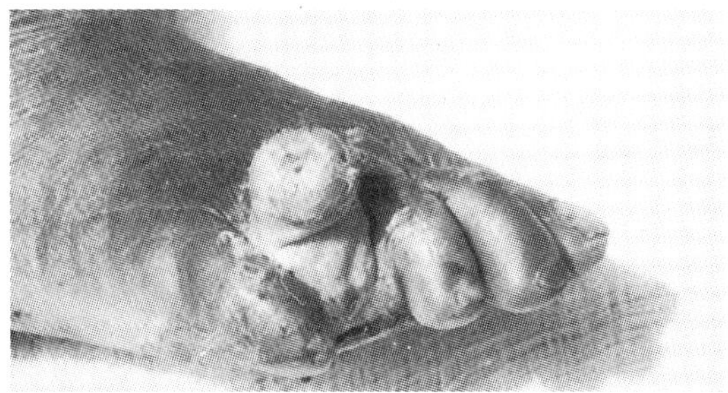

Fig. 15.31C: Destroyed and dislocated stump of 4th toe and trophic ulcer at the distal outer end of foot due to Hansen's disease

— Regional lymph glands may be enlarged and matted.

CERTAIN RARE BUT INTERESTING CONDITIONS

a. Ainhum (Fig. 15.37)
b. Xanthomatosis (Fig. 15.38)

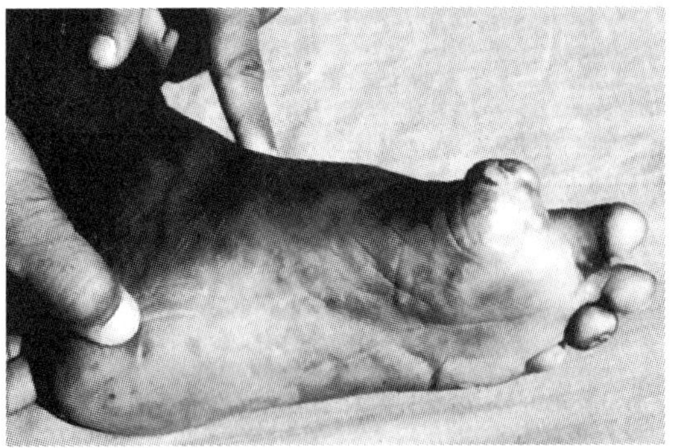

Fig. 15.31D: Trophic ulcer in heel and destroyed and fallen off big toe due to Hansen's disease

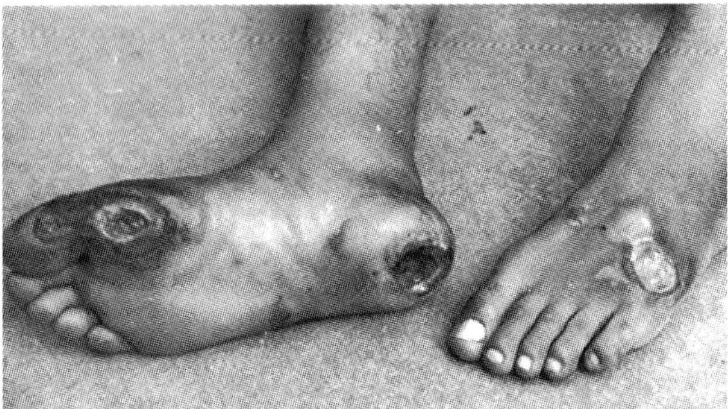

Fig. 15.32A: Trophic ulceration on both desensitised feet due to spina bifida

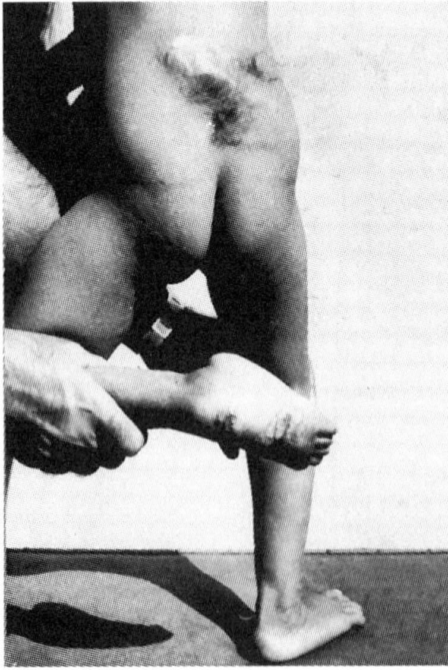

15.32B: Neglected equino-varus deformity with trophic ulcer on the dorsum of foot due to spina bifida

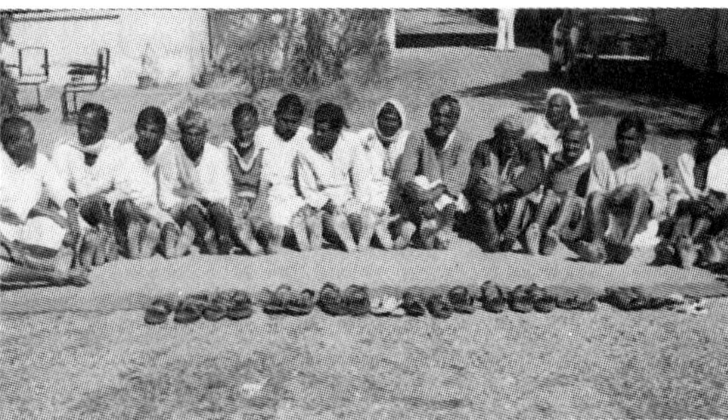

Fig. 15.31E: Group of the patients of Hansen's disease with trophic ulcerations in the feet

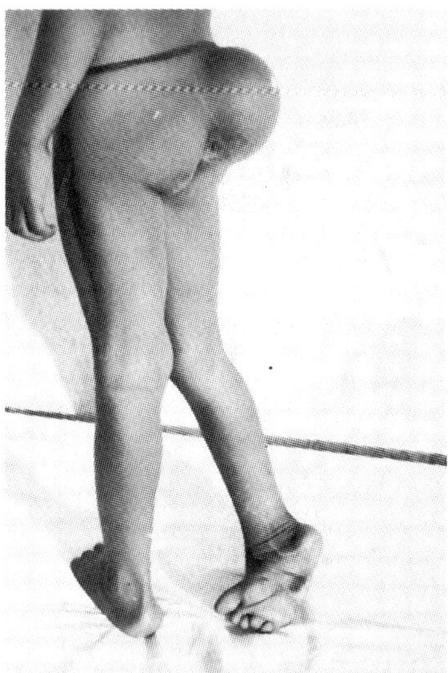

Fig. 15.32C: Neglected equino-cavo varus deformity of right foot with ulceration on the dorsum of foot associated with spina bifida manifesta

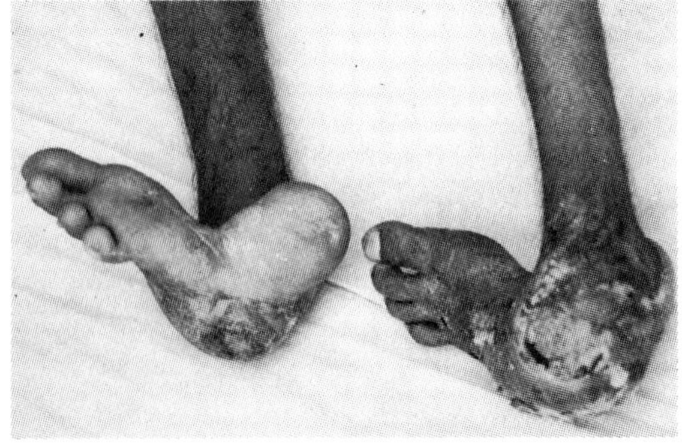

Fig. 15.32D: Neglected severe equino-cavo varus deformities with extensive ulcerations associated with spina bifida

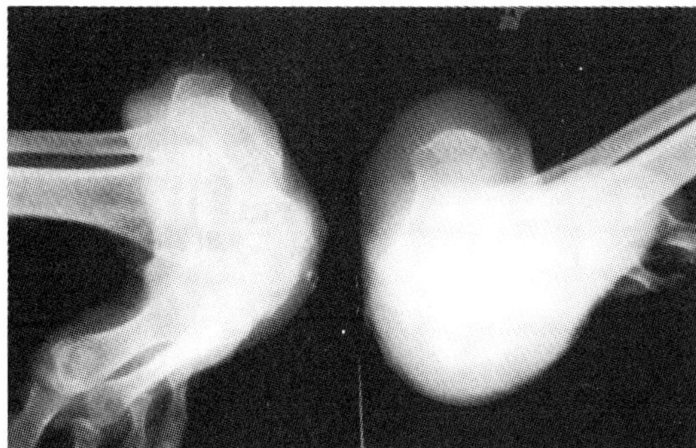

Fig. 15.32E: X-ray of the same patient (Fig. 15.32D)

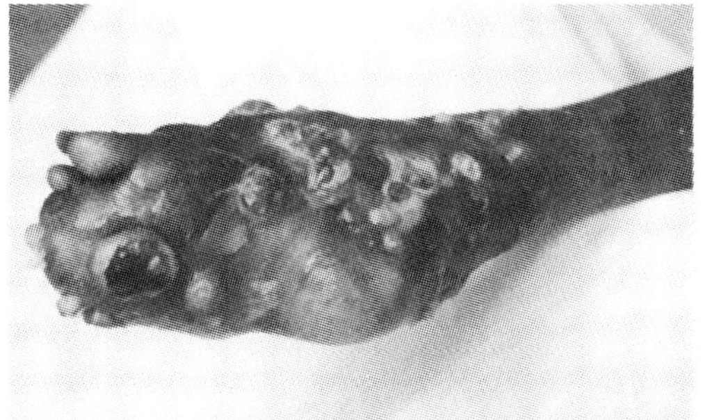

Fig. 15.33A: Advanced Madura foot

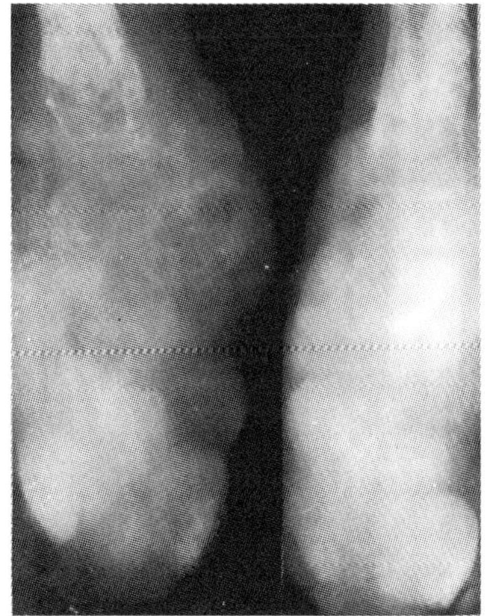

Fig. 15.33B: X-ray of the same patient (Fig. 15.33A)

c. Hyperplasia of foot (Figs 15.39A and B)
d. Ewing's sarcoma of talus (Fig. 15.35B)
e. Haemangiosarcoma of foot (Figs 15.36A and B)

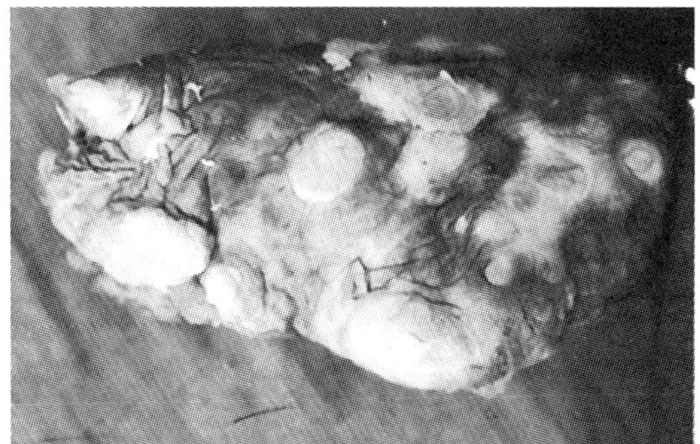

Fig. 15.33C: Amputated foot ridden with extensive Madura foot ulcers

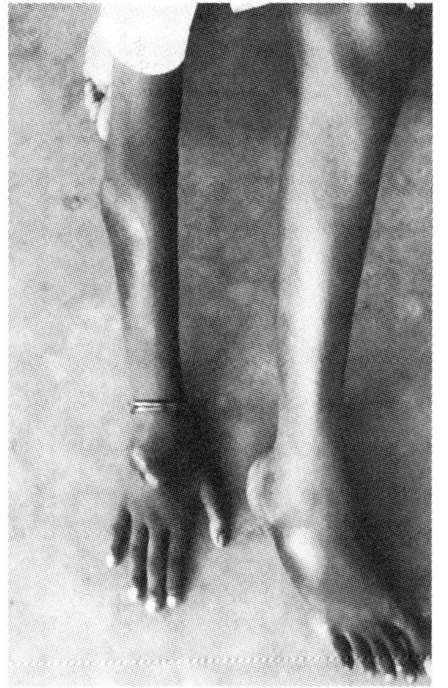

Fig. 15.34A: A lady aged 27 with multi-focal tuberculosis (right elbow, hand, right upper tibiofibular joint and right foot

Disorders of Toe Nail

Nails are exo skeleton. Their disorders include congenital affections to neoplasm.

Common affections are: traumatic, usually blunt crush;

Acute infections are usually sub or para-ungal.

Chronic infections are usually fungal in origin.

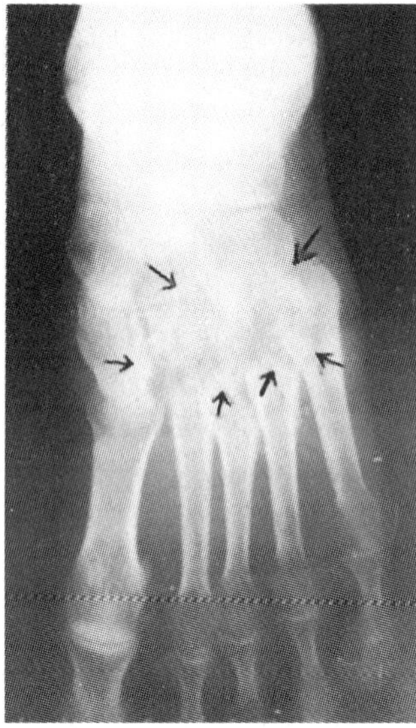

Fig. 15.34B: X-ray photograph of her foot lesion (Fig. 15.34A) (photo taken on reverse film)

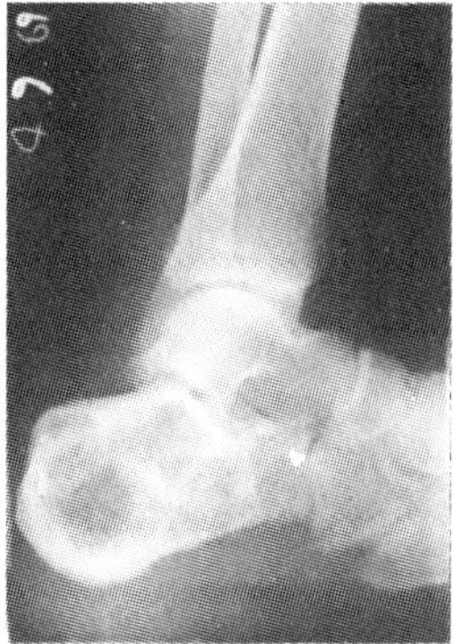

Fig. 15.34C: Giant cell tumour of calcaneum

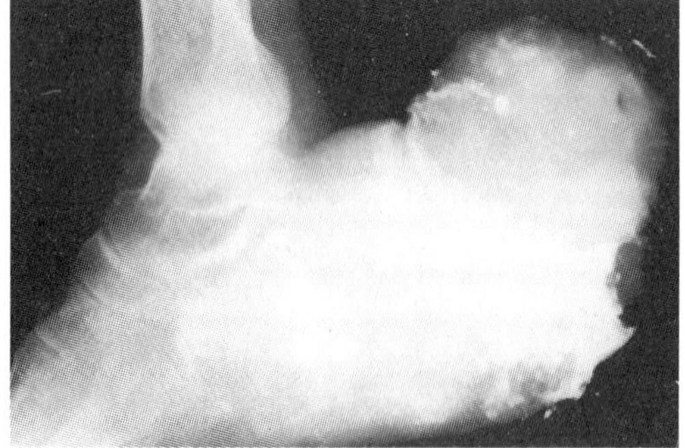

Fig. 15.35A: X-ray of advanced malignant melanoma of calcaneum

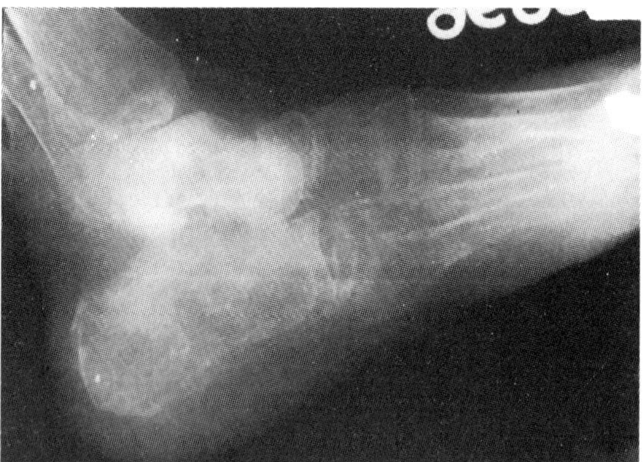

Fig. 15.35B: Ewing's sarcoma of talus which may be misdiagnosed as avascular necrosis

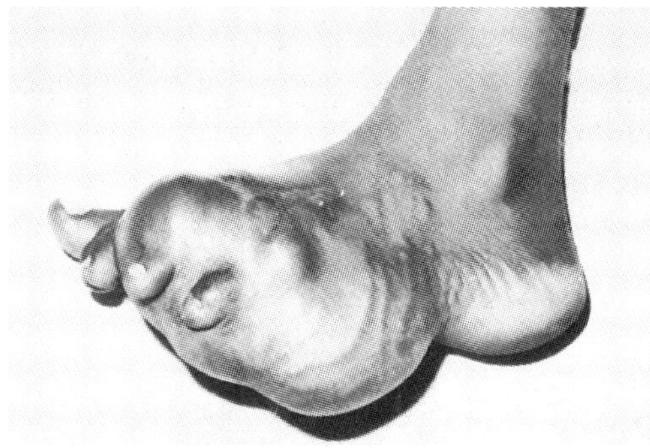

Fig. 15.36A: Haemangiosarcoma of foot

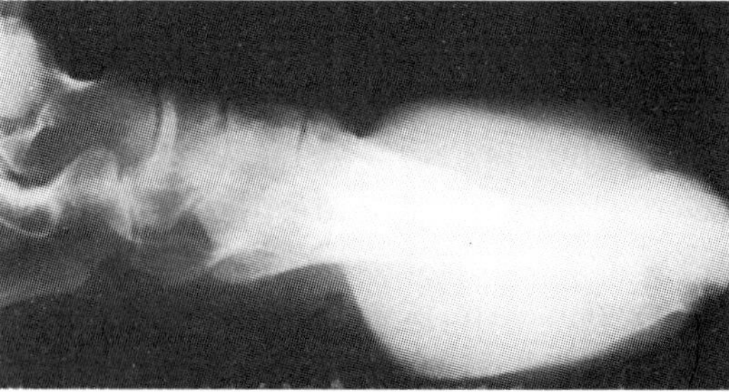

Fig. 15.36B: X-ray of the same foot (Fig. 15.36A)

Acute infections are extremely painful and usually require surgery. Chronic infections are extremely difficult to eradicate.

Ingrowing of toe nail (embedded toe nail) of the big toe (Fig. 15.40) may be familial. It can result from using tight shoes with crowded toe-box.

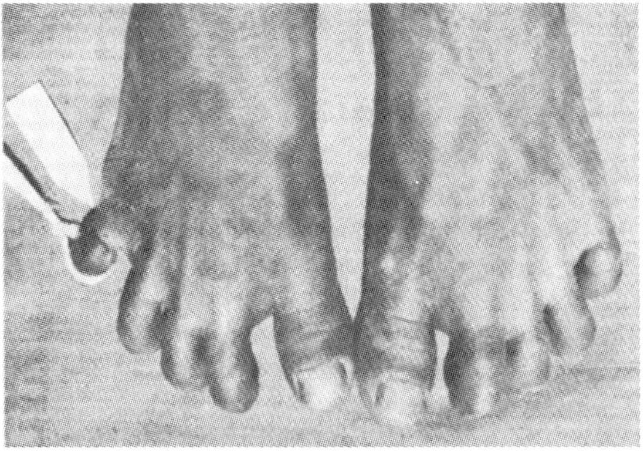

Fig. 15.37: Ainhum. Note the constriction around the base of little toe beyond which the toe is going for gangrene

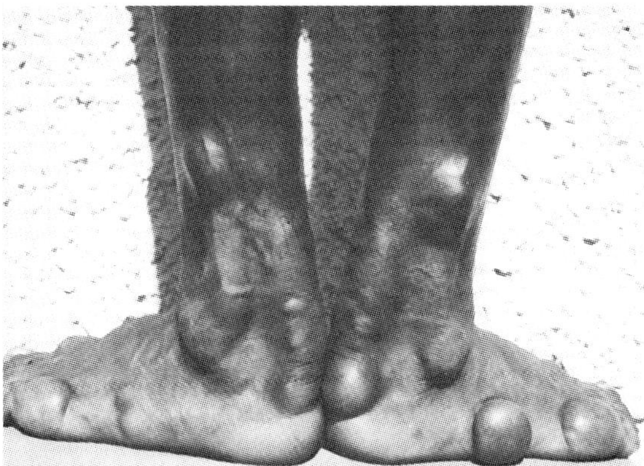

Fig. 15.38: Multiple xanthomatous swellings over both feet and around ankles

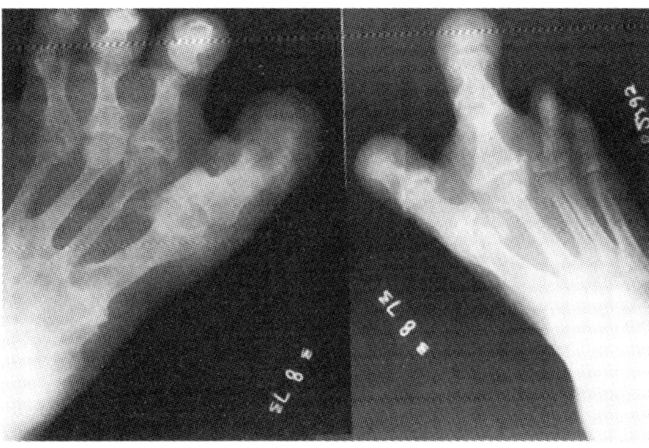

Fig. 15.39A: X-ray of hyperplasia of both feet. Note the giant development of short long bones

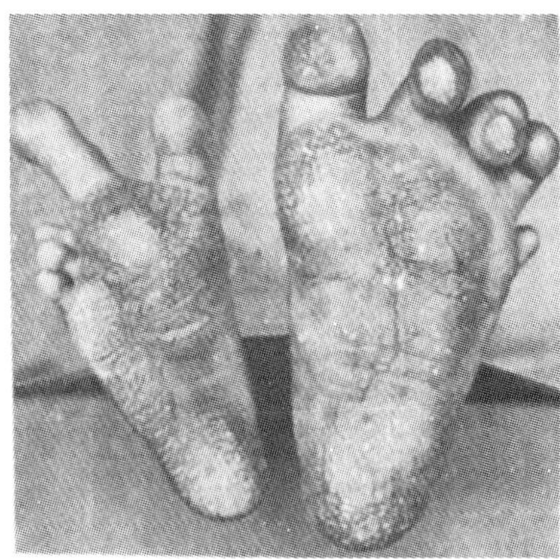

Fig. 15.39B: Hyperplasia of foot. Note the sole aspect of hyperplastic foot with hyperkeratosis

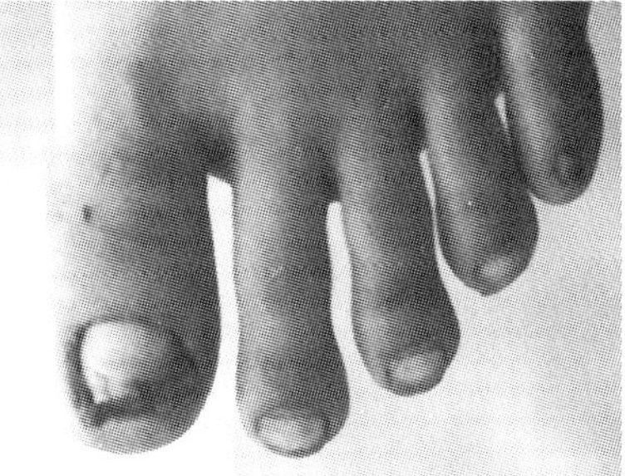

Fig. 15.40: Ingrowing nail of big toe

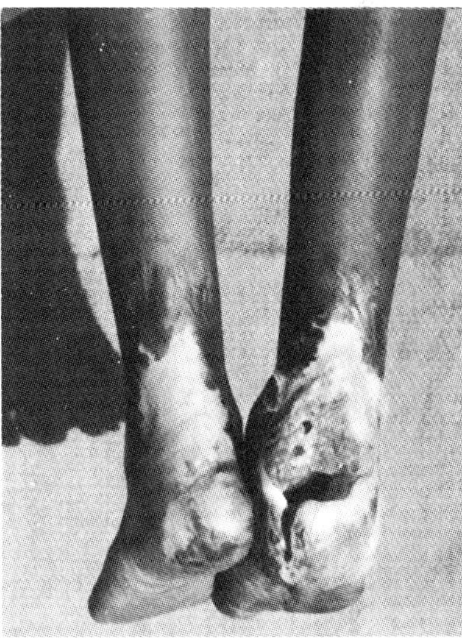

Fig. 15.41A: Cold fire burn effects on the back of heels (used for heating the feet in winters)

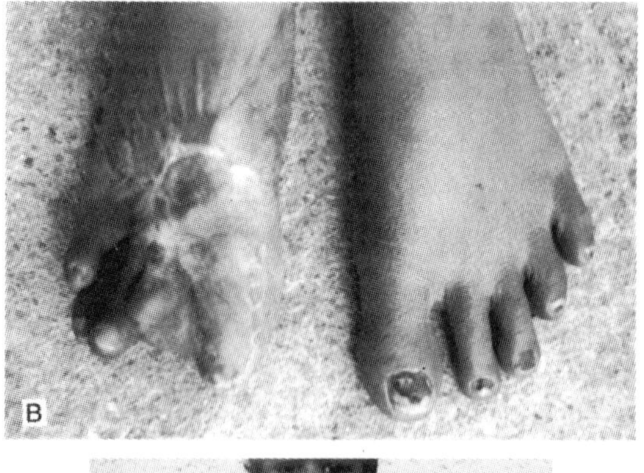

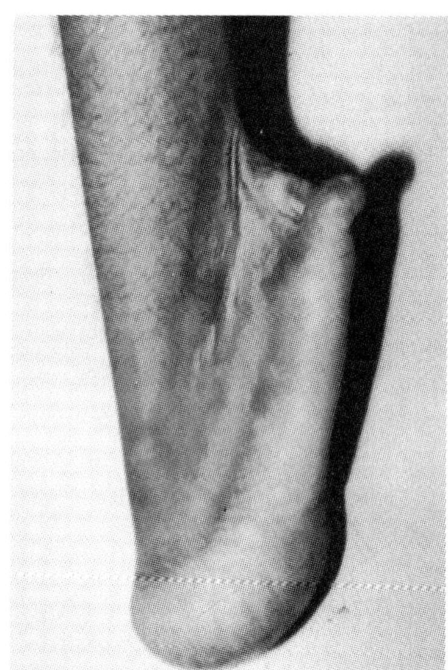

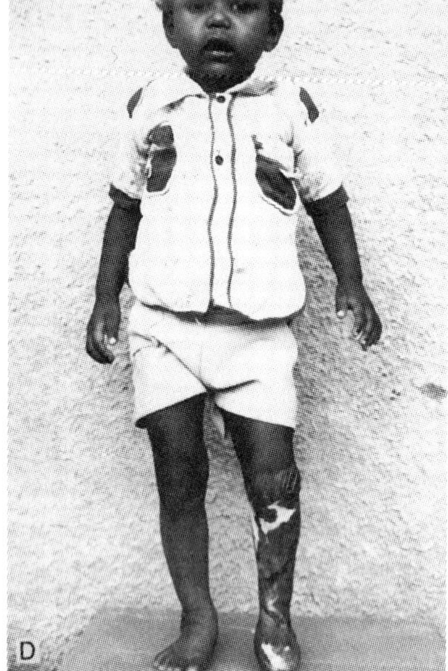

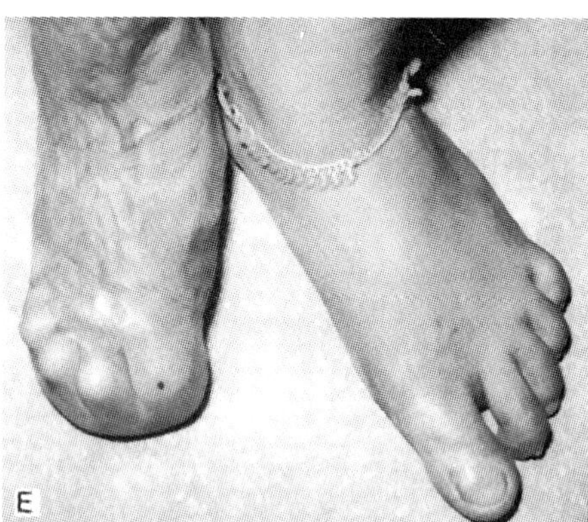

Figs 15.41B to E: Postburn contractures

Lateral nail-fold is commonly affected. Patients with fleshy nail folds and thin nail plates are more vulnerable. Patient presents with burried tender side margins of the nail with frequent/ recurrent features of inflammation/infection with or without discharge of thick beads of pus.

Paronychia is the infection (which is subcuticular and under eponychium) around (and may be under) the nail. The affected digit is usually acutely inflamed at the distal end, painful and markedly tender.

Onychogryphosis is the thickened and crooked (may be curly) overgrowth of toe nail.

The big toe of an elderly bed-ridden people is more vulnerable.

Accessory Ossicles

The accessory ossicles of the foot are developmental in origin and are inconstant, independent well defined bones with regular margins in an otherwise normally developed foot. They may be symptomatic in themselves or may misinterpretated as a fracture (which may create medicolegal problems).

The accessory ossicles can be visualised on:

a. Medial aspect: (i) OS trigonum, (ii) OS subtentaculi, (iii) accessory navicular, (iv) OS supranaviculare, (v) Os inter cuneiform; (vi) OS intermetatarseum.
b. Lateral aspect: (vii) OS calcaneus secundarius, (viii) OS peroneum, (ix) OS vesalianum, (x) OS infranaviculare, (xi) OS accessorium supracalcaneum, (xii) OS subcalcis.
c. Superior aspect: Nos (i), (iii), (iv), (v), (vi), (vii), (viii), (ix) are seen.
d. In anteroposterior view of ankle: (xiii) OS subfibulare, (xiv) OS subtibiale, and (xv) Inter calary bone.

BOUND FOOT DEFORMITY

In China between the age of 3 to 7 the feet are bound in stout iron boots to make it short and to give them the shape which is thought to be erotic. The deformities complex consist of cavus foot + flexion contractures of the toes. Hibb's angle on average remains about 75° and Meary angle 128°. The cause of the deformities can easily be levelled as iatrogenic. This system continued till 20th century.

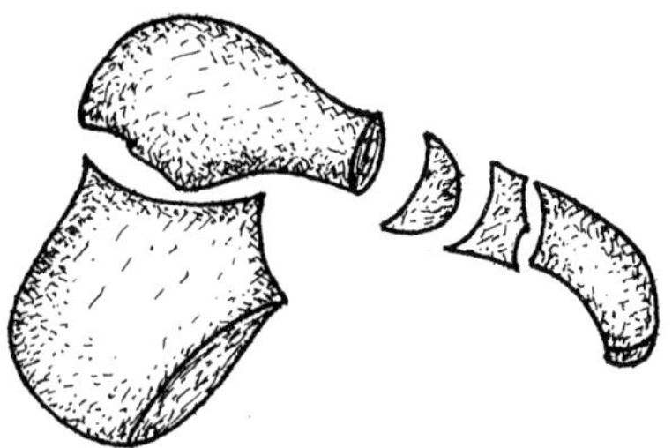

Fig. 15.42: Bound foot deformity

BIBLIOGRAPHY

1. Balkin SW. *Arch Derm* **111**: 1143, 1975.
2. Jack EA: Naviculocuneiform fusion in the treatment of flat foot. *J Bone Joint Surg* **35-B**: 75-81, 1955.
3. Luger EJ, Nissan M, Karpf A *et al*. Pattern of weight distribution under the metatarsal heads. *J Bone Joint Surg* **81-B**: 199-202, 1999.
4. Pandey AK, Pandey S: Calcaneal osteotomy and tendon sling for the management of calcaneus deformity. *J Bone Joint Surg* **71-A**: 1192-98, 1989.
5. Pandey S: Ewing's sarcoma of talus. *Jr of Bone Joint Surg* 1971-A......
6. Pandey S. 'Infections and Infestations'. In Helal B, Rowley DI, Gracchiolo III A *et al* (Eds). *The Surgery of Disorders of the Foot and Ankle* 630-51, 1996.
7. Pandey S. Tropical Diseases. In Helal B, Wilson D (Eds) *'The Foot'* London: Churchill Livingston 642-702, 1988.
8. Pandey S, Jha SS, Pandey AK: 'T' osteotomy of the calcaneum. *International Orthopaedics* (SICOT) **4**: 219-24, 1980.
9. Rook, DS Wilkinson, FJG Ebling: Oxford, London: Blackwell Scientific Publication 485-87, 1979.
10. Wilkinson DS: Cutaneous reaction to mechanical and thermal injury. In Arthur (Ed): *Textbook of Dermatology* (3ed).

16 Peripheral Nerve Injuries

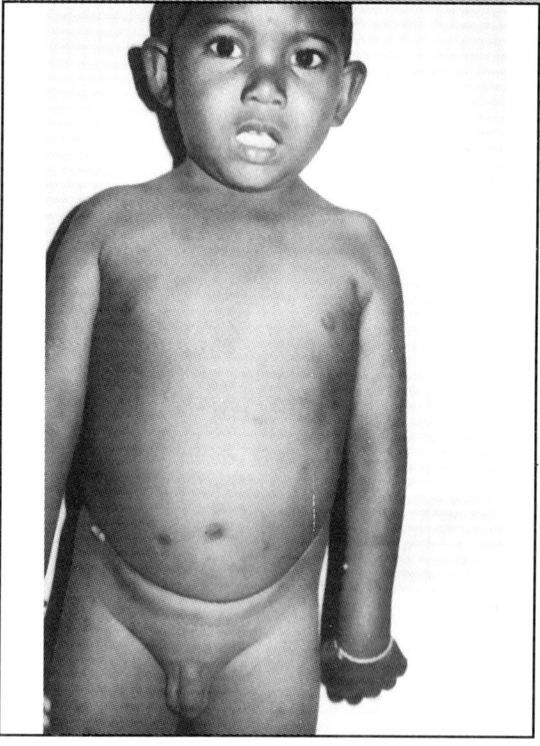

INTRODUCTION

The peripheral nerves are formed from the spinal nerves which emerge in 31 pairs, representing each segment of the spinal cord. These spinal nerve roots either branch directly or through a network (plexus) as the peripheral nerves.

Peripheral nerve affections usually leave legacies, sometimes quite disabling to the patient and even affecting his ADL (activities of daily living). Though peripheral nerves are mixed nerves, but the main disabling factor is the residual motor weakness. However, complete sensory loss is none the less disabling.

ANATOMICAL CONSIDERATIONS

The main nerves in the upper limb are ulnar, median and radial. In the lower limbs the sciatic and its two main branches, lateral and medial popliteal nerves, are the main motor nerves.

All these nerves have more or less the same anatomical structure. The main structural and functional unit of a peripheral nerve is the axis cylinder. This is surrounded by myelin sheath, which in turn is surrounded by a fine neurolemma sheath (Schwann's cell sheath). This forms a nerve fibre. Multiple nerve fibres are loosely connected together by a fine network of collagen—endoneurium, which contains fine vascular and lymphatic capillaries. These together form a nerve bundle or funiculi which is surrounded by an epithelial layer—the perineurium. Multiple bundles are bound together by a fibrous sheath—the epineurium in which run the main blood vessels and lymphatics of the nerve.

Except for the ulnar nerve behind the medial epicondyle and lateral popliteal nerve winding around the neck of the fibula, the rest of the peripheral nerves are well protected.

In their course, most of the peripheral nerves have to pass through some myofascial or fibro-osseous tunnels where they are likely to be entrapped in certain pathologies of the surrounding tissues—*entrapment neuropathy*, e.g. (Fig. 16.1) (Table 16.1).

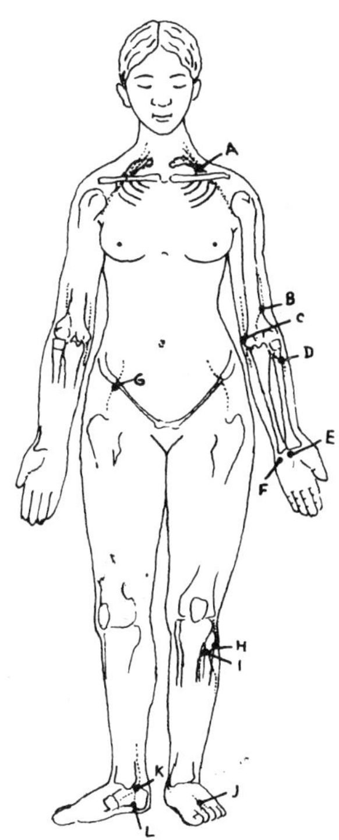

Fig. 16.1: Sites of common entrapment neuropathy. A = thoracic inlet, B = radial nerve, C = ulnar nerve, D = posterior interosseous nerve (supinator tunnel), E = carpal tunnel, F = Guyon s canal, G = lateral cutaneous nerve of the thigh (meralgia paraesthetica), H = common peroneal nerve (lateral popliteal nerve), I = deep peroneal nerve (anterior tibial nerve), J = Morton s metatarsalgia, K = posterior tibial nerve (tarsal tunnel syndrome), L = medial calcaneal branch of posterior tibial nerve

The peripheral nerves are commonly affected due to injuries. The nerve injuries have been classified by Seddon (1943). Later on Sunderland (1951) suggested another classification, which is more practical and helpful in determining the prognosis (see Table 16.2).

History taking: General and systemic examinations to be done as in chapter on Introduction.

ASSESSMENT/INVESTIGATIONS OF PERIPHERAL NERVE INJURY

Clinical

Inspection: Note any typical attitude and any abnormal finding in the area supplied by the concerned nerve.

Palpation: Besides palpating on usual lines, feel for the texture and pliability of subcutaneous tissues and muscles supplied by the concerned nerve.

Palpation of the Nerve

i. If there is tenderness on pressure along the course of the nerve, it indicates irritational stage of the nerve, which is present in an incomplete lesion, or inflammation of the nerve.
ii. In the course of a nerve, where complete division of nerve is expected, feeling of a neuroma (a firm, tender, nodular mass at the distal end of the proximal segment) and a glioma (a firm, almost non-tender, fibrous mass at the proximal end of the distal segment) almost confirms the diagnosis.
iii. Tinel's sign (Jules Tinel, 1917)

The importance of Tinel's sign is in determining:

a. Whether a nerve is interrupted.
b. Whether a nerve is in process of regeneration.
c. Rate of regeneration.
d. Whether a nerve suture has succeeded or failed. However, even in incomplete regeneration this sign may be positive.

Method: Press the nerve gently or percuss about 2.5 cm below the site of lesion or nerve suture. If young axis cylinders are present, the patient will feel a sensation of "pins and needles" *(formication)* for a few seconds, along the course of the nerve. According to the progress of regeneration of the axis cylinder, the site of formication also advances. Tap along the course of the nerve, starting from the periphery. The moment the level of regeneration is reached, pain and/or tingling will be felt along the course of the nerve.

Assessment of the Muscle Power According to MRC Scale

(See chapter on Introduction)

In peripheral nerve injury all motor functions distal to the level of injury get abolished. The

Table 16.1: Common entrapment neuropathies

Nerve	*Site*
• Ulnar nerve	—In between the medial epicondyle and the Osborne's ligament—a tight fibrous band forming an arch joining the origin of the two heads of the flexor carpi ulnaris—*Elbow tunnel syndrome or Cubital tunnel syndrome.* In this tight myofascial-osseous tunnel, the ulnar nerve becomes vulnerable to injury —At the hook of the hamate (Guyoń's canal—pisiform hamate tunnel). F Guyon (1861) described a fibro-osseous tunnel in the proximal medial aspect of palm. It is bounded by the piseform medially and proximally, and the hook of the hamate laterally, and posteriorly by the transverse ligment. JR Hunt was the first to describe ulnar nerve entrapment at this site
• Median nerve	—Median nerve entrapment/compression can occur at three places: 1. Pronator teres syndrome is most proximal 2. Anterior interosseous syndrome in proximal forearm 3. Carpal tunnel syndrome at the most distal end of forearm and in front of wrist (in the carpal tunnel)
• Radial nerve	—At about the junction of the lower fourth and upper three-fourth of the arm where it enters from posterior to anterior compartment
• Posterior interosseous nerve	—Where it passes through the supinator muscle from anterior to posterior compartment in the upper forearm
• Thoracic inlet syndrome (Scalene syndrome; cervical rib syndrome)	—A vice like action compresses the brachial plexus and subclavian artery
• Sciatic nerve—compression sciatic neuropathy; Piriformis syndrome (See page 177 in the chapter on Spine)	
• Lateral popliteal nerve	—Lateral popliteal compartment (at the neck of fibula)
• Peroneal nerve entrapment or fibular tunnel syndrome	—The nerve is compressed under the fibrous arch in the region of the bifurcation of the nerve into its deep and superficial branches
• Medial calcaneal branch of posterior tibial nerve	—At anteroinferomedial aspect of the calcaneum
• Posterior tibial nerve (Tarsal tunnel syndrome)	—Posterior tibial nerve gets compressed in the fibro-osseous tunnel formed between the medial malleolus and flexor retinaculum
• Lateral cutaneous nerve of thigh (Meralgia paresthetica)	—Beneath the outer end of the inguinal ligament
• Morton's metatarsalgia	—Due to regular, intermittent pressure on 3rd or 4th digital branch of the medial plantar nerve, a granuloma develops at the level of the metatarsal neck, causing plantar hyperaesthesia of 3rd and 4the toes, mainly in females
• Suprascapular nerve entrapment described by Koppel and Thompson (1963)	—Can occur in throwing athlete who complains of pain in shoulder region, confusing with tendinitis, rotator cuff tear, cervical disc disease

Table 16.2: Gross differentiation of three types of nerve injuries (After Seddon 1943)

1	*Neuropraxia* 2	*Axonotmesis* 3	*Neurotmesis* 4
Definition	— Shock of the peripheral nerve suspending the physiological conduction (Nerve concussion or transient nerve lesion)	— Damage/section of axons, sheath remaining intact	— Complete damage/section of the nerve, i.e. axon and its sheath
Pathology	— Local demyelination of the nerve fibres. No Wallerian degeneration Axis cylinders are intact	— Axons distal to site of damage degenerate — Wallerian degeneration occurs	— Axons distal to damage degenerate Wallerian degeneration occurs — Neuroma at distal end of the proximal segment, palpable after 8 weeks — Glioma at the proximal end of distal segment, palpable after 8 weeks
Aetiology	— Pressure over the nerve, mild stretch	— Prolonged, marked pressure — Moderate to severe stretch — Entrapment in surrounding fibrosis — Friction neuritis — Injection neuritis	— Cut injuries — Avulsion injuries
Depth of paralysis	— Mild, mainly motor palsy, may be varying temporary sensory loss	— Moderate to severe (mostly severe) — Motor, sensory, vasomotor, pilomotor and sudomotor	— Always severe — Motor, sensory, vasomotor, pilomotor, and sudomotor
Electrical excitability	— Normal (both galvanic and faradic)	— Altered (only responding to long duration stimuli) — Reaction of degeneration	— Altered (only responding to long duration stimuli) — Reaction of degeneration
Nerve conduction	— Possible	— Ceases	— Ceases
Recovery	— Complete	— Evident in 6-8 weeks may be complete	— Never complete (complete recovery only possible after proper surgical anastomosis)
Usual time taken for recovery	— Days to weeks	— Months to year (at the rate of 1 mm a day)	— After surgical repair—months to year (the rate more sluggish than axonotmesis) (In closed injuries, difficult to differentiate from axonotmesis in first three months)
Treatment	— Wait and watch. — Splintage of paralysed parts. in functional position	— Splintage — Wait and watch — If no recovery in three months, • Exploration • Neurolysis • Resection and anastomosis • Nerve grafting	— Exploration; Neurolysis — Primary suturing — Secondary suturing followed by splintage — Nerve grafting — Reconstructive procedures — Tendon transposition — Bone shortening — Joint stabilisation

NB—Sunderland (1951) has classified the nerve injuries into five degrees depending upon the depth of the damage: damage of myelin sheath; damage of myelin sheath and axon; further damage of endoneurium; further damage of perineurium; and complete division of nerve trunk.

Sunderland	**Seddon**
First degree: No anatomical disruption. Only physiological	Neuropraxia
Second degree: Only axon disrupted, sheath intact	Axonotmesis
Third degree: Axon + Schwann's cell sheath + endoneurium disruption. Intact perineurium May be neuroma in continuity. Prolonged uncertain recovery	Axonotmesis (+)
Fourth degree: Axon + Schwann's cell sheath + endoneurium + part of perineurium: Part of epineurium, though intact in continuity, but almost no recovery	Neurotmesis
Fifth degree: Complete section	Neurotmesis

muscles supplied by that nerve distal to the injured level, are paralysed, become atonic and get wasted. Spontaneous fibrillations may become evident by 2 to 4 weeks. With proper regeneration of the nerve, variable muscle-power recovers. The extent of recovery can be assessed clinically by grip meter, pinch meter, evaluation of endurance, speed of movement and individual muscle power and function.

Elicitation of Reflexes

(See chapter on 'Spine')

Mapping out the Deficits in Sensations

(See chapter on 'Spine')

Vasomotor Assessment

Sweat test: Using iodine/starch, this can be done to map out the anaesthetic areas as dry and devoid of sweating.

Guttman's test: Quinizerine powder turns purple when it comes in contact with sweat.

Skin and Nails

Note the condition of the skin supplied by the affected nerve. Especially look for the: (i) texture, any discolouration, (ii) presence/absence of normal skin folds, and rugosities, (iii) atrophic changes, (iv) trophic ulcerations, (v) condition of nail bed, and (vi) condition of finger/toe tips.

Investigations

1. *Electrodiagnosis*

These provide more or less quantitative assessment of the nerve deficit. The important ones are:

a. Motor nerve conduction test,
b. Strength duration curves,
c. Electromyography.

However, 'Nerve stimulation' and 'Nerve action potential recording' have also been suggested (Seddon, 1972).

a. *Motor nerve conduction test*: Basis of the test—Ability of the nerve to transmit an electrical impulse.

Method: Firstly calculate the approximate threshold of the current strength required to cause a muscular contraction, by stimulating the nerve on the sound side. The stimulating electrode is then applied on the affected nerve, distal to the possible site of lesion. If a current strength twice as great as the calculated threshold fails to produce a muscular contraction, nerve conduction is absent. Slow rate of conduction suggests damage to the nerve. The site of an incomplete lesion can also be located by this test. So long the stimulating electrode lies distal to the lesion, the conductivity is good, but this nerve conductivity is markedly reduced or even absent when the stimulating electrode is placed proximal to the lesion.

b. *Strength duration curve:* Basis—Depending upon the excitability of the nerve and muscle, a graph is prepared by plotting the minimal voltage required for the muscle to contract, against duration of the stimulus in milliseconds. The status of a muscle as regards innervation, denervation or reinnervation can be indicated by these curves.

If the voltage is kept constant, a normal muscle will respond to an electrical stimulus given for a duration of 300 milliseconds to less than a millisecond, even down to 0.1 milliseconds. The strength-duration curve obtained for such a muscle has been named as 'nerve-curve', since the stimulation becomes effective through the motor nerve of that muscle.

In a completely denervated muscle, a low voltage stimulus can only be effective if the electrical stimulus is given much longer, e.g. 100 milliseconds or more. The curve for such a muscle is called 'muscle-curve', since muscular contraction has been obtained from direct stimulation of the muscle fibres. The partly innervated muscle is characterised by superimposition of the two basic curves (nerve and muscle curves) producing an upward kink in the plotted graph.

c. *Nerve conduction monitor* is a noninvasive diagnostic aid, which can effectively perform

Table 16.3: Features of different nerve affections of upper limb

Nerve 1	*Muscles supplied* 2	*Sensory area* 3	*Vasomotor effect* 4	*Mode of injury* 5	*Presentation* 6	*Tests* 7	*Prognosis* 8	*Treatment* 9
Brachial plexus (upper type—Erb-Duchenne $C_{5,6}$) (Figs 16.2A and B)	Deltoid, teres minor, supraspinatus, infraspinatus, clavicular head of pectoralis major, biceps, brachioradialis, supinator, brachialis	May be some sensory loss on outer aspect of arm and forearm	Nil	—Obstetrical palsy —Traction injury —Vehicular accidents —Fall on shoulder point —Fire arm injury —Stab injury	Typical policeman tip position, i.e. arm internally rotated, adducted, elbow extended, forearm pronated, wrist in mild flexion and flexion of the fingers	—	Varying; may recover to workable extent	Wait and watch, splintage, (palm to sun splint) exploration, neurolysis, primary suturing of the nerve, nerve graft, nerve transfer
Brachial plexus (lower type-Klumpke's paralysis C_8, T_1)	Intrinsic muscles of the hand, flexion and extension of fingers are controlled by lower trunk	Ulnar side of forearm and hand and a narrow strip over arm	Horner's syndrome	-do-	Claw hand, i.e. metacarpophalangeal joints hyperextended and interphalangeal joints flexed. If occulopupillary paralysis occurs due to affection of 1st thoracic nerve before its communication with white ramus—Horner's syndrome (apparent endophthalmos, ptosis, contraction of pupil with absence of dilatation on shading the eye or on instillation of coccaine, loss of ciliospinal reflex and often absence of sweating on corresponding half of face and neck	—	Usually bad	-do-
Brachial plexus (whole arm or mixed type $C_{5,6,7,8}$, T_1) (Figs 16.3A and B)	Complete paralysis of all muscles of arm, forearm and hand	Part of arm, whole of forearm and hand	May be present. Occulo-pupillary paralysis may occur	-do- —Pancoast tumour —Hypercallus in fracture clavicle —Aneurysm of subclavian artery	Presentation varies according to roots involved.	—	Constantly bad	-do-
Nerve to serratus anterior $C_{5,6}$ (Figs 16.4A and B)	Serratus anterior	—	—	Root avulsion, root pressure, iatrogenic	Winging of scapula	Ask the patient to press with hands against the wall. The medial border of scapula on affected side stands prominent (wings out)	—	Wait and watch, tendon transfer (teres major, pectoralis major) —Osteopexy (Fix medial border of scapula to vertebra)

Contd.

NB. Neglected brachial plexus birth palsy usually develop internal rotation contractures leading to glenoid deformities (flat glenoids, biconcave glenoids, pseudoglenoids) with or without posterior subluxation or dislocation of the glenohumeral joint, which are severely advanced by the age of two years. It should be investigated early by imaging. MRI can be done from the early age; and CT after five years of age. Arthrography helps to visualise the skeletally immature glenohumeral joint.

Currently available choices of management are: microsurgical nerve reconstruction in infants; secondary reconstruction with tendon transfers or osteotomy (e.g. humeral derotation osteotomy)

Table 16.3: Contd.

Nerve 1	*Muscles supplied* 2	*Sensory area* 3	*Vasomotor effect* 4	*Mode of injury* 5	*Presentation* 6	*Tests* 7	*Prognosis* 8	*Treatment* 9
Circumflex humeral or axillary $C_{5, 6}$	Deltoid, teres minor	A small area on the lateral side of upper arm overlying the insertion of the deltoid *(regimental badge area)*	—Dislocation of Shoulder, fracture of neck of humerus, fracture-dislocation of shoulder. —Infective neuritis —Operations on shoulder and upper arm. —Injection palsy	Inability in actively abducting the shoulder. (Sometimes with the help of supraspinatus and rotation of scapula, full abduction can be possible)	The patient is asked to abduct the shoulder, while the examiner observes and palpates the deltoid for any contraction	—	—	Wait and watch. —Splint (shoulder abduction splint) —Neurolysis —Nerve repair —Tendon transfer (Trapezius) —Arthrodesis of shoulder
Median nerve $C_{6, 7, 8,} T_1$	In forearm-pronator teres, palmaris longus, flexor digitorum superficialis, flexor carpi radialis, flexor digitorum profundus (lateral half), flexor pollicis longus, pronator quadratus. In hand—-Abductor pollicis brevis, opponens pollicis, flexor pollicis brevis (partly), Ist and IInd lumbricals	In both high and low lesions—Palmar side—radial 3 fingers, corresponding part of palm. Dorsal side—terminal phalanges of thumb and 2 fingers. Autonomous supplies zone: dorsal and palmar surfaces of the distal phalanges of index and middle fingers	Causalgia (irritative syndrome of varying degree) is a common development Trophic disturbances specially in terminal phalanx of index finger	*Injury:* Supracondylar fracture, penetrating and glass cut injuries. *Entrapment Neuropathy:* Carpal tunnel syndrome; VIC Disease: Leprosy	—Ape thumb —While the patient raises his arm with palm facing forwards, he is asked to make a fist, the index finger stands outstretched while the other fingers go for serial flexion (Benediction attitude) —Trophic changes, ulceration on tip of index finger —Wasting of thenar muscles. —*In lesion above the wrist:* Loss of pronation of forearm, flexion of wrist, flexion of index and middle fingers, flexion and opposition of thumb —*Lesion near wrist:* Loss of opposition of thumb	1. Ask the patient to clasp both hands—the index finger of the affected hand remains extended due to loss of power in flexor digitorum profundus and superficialis of the index finger, which flex the interphalangeal joints (Fig. 16.5A) other fingers can be flexed by the intact medial half of flexor digitorum profundus (supplied by the ulnar nerve). The above two tests indicate lesion near about the cubital foosa 2. Ask the patient to make a tight fist—index finger remains extended (Fig.16.5B) 3. Ask the patient to oppose the thumb to the ring finger. This opposition and flexion of terminal phalanx is lost 4. While the dorsum of the patient's hand rests on the table, put the ulnar border of your fisted hand with extended index finger over the proximal part of his palm. Ask the patient to touch your index finger by the radial border of his thumb—	Bad	—Wait and watch —Neurolysis —Nerve pedicle graft —Nerve cable graft —Reconstruction procedures specially for opponens of the thumb

Contd.

Table 16.3: Contd.

Nerve 1	Muscles supplied 2	Sensory area 3	Vasomotor effect 4	Mode of injury 5	Presentation 6	Tests 7	Prognosis 8	Treatment 9
						this will not be possible due to paralysis of abductor pollicis brevis (most important) (Fig. 16.6). Another test is 'Pen test', in which while the patient rests his hand on the table with palm facing the ceiling, a pen is held over his thumb and he is asked to touch the pen with the tip of his thumb. It will not be possible due to weakness of abductor pollicis brevis. Besides special tests, individual muscle should be tested, e.g. (i) Flexor pollicis longus—while the PIP is kept steady, the patient is asked to flex the terminal phalanx against resistance. (ii) Flexor carpi radialis—Ask the patient to flex the wrist, it deviates to ulnar side due to unopposed action of flexor carpi ulnaris (due to weakness of flexor carpi radialis). Further flexor carpi radialis tendon does not stand prominent nor it can be felt taught on attempting to flex the wrist against resistance.		

Contd.

Table 16.3: Contd.

Nerve 1	*Muscles supplied* 2	*Sensory area* 3	*Vasomotor effect* 4	*Mode of injury* 5	*Presentation* 6	*Tests* 7	*Prognosis* 8	*Treatment* 9
						Kiloh-Nevin sign: To test terminal function of the digits against resistance, ask the patient to form an "O" with the tips of the thumb and index finger. In anterior interosseous nerve deficit (syndrome), fine pinch posture is abnormal. The index finger becomes extended at the distal interphalangeal joint, as it makes contact with the pulp of the thumb, which also gets hyper-extended at the interphalangeal joint, due to weakness of flexor digitorum profundus and flexor pollicis longus muscle respectively (supplied by anterior intero-sseous nerve).		

Contd.

Table 16.3: Contd.

Nerve 1	Muscles supplied 2	Sensory area 3	Vasomotor effect 4	Mode of injury 5	Presentation 6	Tests 7	Prognosis 8	Treatment 9
Ulnar nerve C_8T_1	In forearm—ulnar half of flexor digitorum profundus, flexor carpi ulnaris. In hand—palmaris brevis, flexor digiti minimi, abductor digiti minimi, opponens digiti minimi all interossei, IInd, IIIrd and IVth lumbricals, adductor pollicis, flexor pollicis brevis (part)	Ulnar 1 finger—palmar and dorsal aspects, corresponding part of palm and dorsum of hand. Autonoms supply: dorsal and palmar aspect of middle and distal phalanges of little finger	Insignificant Trophic changes over the desensitized part of tip of little finger.	Injury: At the elbow— Medial epicondylar fractures, Supracondylar fractures, fracture-dislocation —Stretch tardy ulnar palsy following ununited lateral condylar fracture. At the wrist: —Glass cut. —Penetrating injury, Entrapment: behind the medial epicondyle or immediately distal to it between two heads of flexor carpi ulnaris. Entrapment in muscles of hypothenar eminence. Disease: Hansen's neuropathy	—Ulnar claw hand (see Fig. 7.9A) —Flattening of the palm. Shrunken intermetacarpal spaces and back of first web. N.B. i. In lesions at elbow, flexor carpi ulnaris is also involved resulting in loss of flexion and ulnar deviation at wrist, while in wrist lesions it is spared. ii. In high ulnar palsy, action of ulnar half of flexor digitorum profundus is lost. So the terminal interphalangeal joints are not flexed (ulnar paradox). Ulnar nerve compression at elbow (e.g. cubital tunnel syndrome; tardy ulnar nerve palsy): one of the earliest diagnostic sign is interosseous atrophy, disturbed sensation in the 4th and 5th fingers, inability to seperate the fingers. Even gentle pressure on the cubital tunnel reproduces the pain. Nerve conduction studies show slowing of the ulnar nerve conduction velocity as it crosses the elbow. *Ulnar nerve compression at the wrist:* Usually both superficial and deep branches are affected simultaneously. Compression of superficial branch causes	1. Froment's sign (Fig. 16.7). Ask the patient to hold a newspaper between his thumb and other fingers, while you pull it firmly away. Normally the distal phalanx of the thumb is extended when holding the newspaper firmly. On the affected side, the distal phalanx of the patient's thumb become markedly flexed and the newspaper is held by the very tip of the thumb, due to, paralysis of adductor pollicis and intrinsics. 2. Card test—Put the card in between the fingers and ask the patient to hold it firmly between the fingers. In ulnar nerve affection, the hold will be very loose or not possible (Fig. 16.8) In ulnar nerve damage certain individual muscle can be tested: e.g. (i) Flexor carpi ulnaris: Ask the patient to keep the dorsum of the hand flat on the table and to palmar flex the wrist, in flexor carpi ulnaris weakness, the hand deviates radial wards. Abductor digiti minimi: With the hand position as in 'flexor carpi ulnaris test', ask the patient to abduct the little finger; it will not be possible in abductor digiti-minimi paralysis.	Variable, usually bad.	—Treat primary cause if any —Decompression —Anterior transposition —Medial epicondylectomy —Reconstructive surgery for ulnar claw-hand

Contd.

Table 16.3: Contd.

Nerve 1	*Muscles supplied* 2	*Sensory area* 3	*Vasomotor effect* 4	*Mode of injury* 5	*Presentation* 6	*Tests* 7	*Prognosis* 8	*Treatment* 9
					sensory disturbances, e.g. burning sensations in 4th and 5th digits. Compression of deep branch causes motor loss, e.g. weakness in abduction of little finger and thumb and decreased pinch (Fig. 16.11). Pressure over the Guyon's canal (pisiform-hamate tunnel) causes distal pain if the sensory branches are affected. *Ulnar Dominence and Median Dominence* At times the ulnar and median nerve supplies intermingle, hence even if there is complete damage of one nerve its effect is not complete due to its intermingled supply. To confirm it, inject xylocaine in the median nerve (in case of ulnar nerve damage and *vice versa*). If the paralytic effect becomes complete, then the confused picture was due abberant supply.	Further while palmar flexing the wrist apply resistence over the distal part of palm and fingers, the tendon of flexor carpi ulnaris does not stand prominent, as it does normally.		
Radial nerve $C_{5,6,7,8}$ T_1	In arm—Triceps, anconeus, brachioradials, extensor carpi radialis longus, extensor carpi radialis brevis, brachialis (lateral half). In forearm—Supinator, extensor pollicis longus, extensor pollicis brevis, extensor indicis, extensor digitorum, extensor digiti	Back of the thumb and 2½ of radial fingers (except terminal phalanges) and corresponding area on the dorsum of the hand. Autonomous supply: stamp shaped area on dorsum of 1st web.	Insignificant	*Injury: In axilla and arm:* —Axillary crutch palsy; pressure in spiral groove—against any hard object, e.g. saturday night palsy, operation table palsy, fracture of shaft of humerus; Penetrating injury; Elbow region-	Wrist drop (Figs 16.9A and B) In radial nerve, compression at the elbow region, if the superficial radial nerve is involved, there will be pain and sensory disturbances in the area of distribution. If deep branch is involved, there may be pain in the lateral epicondylar region. The nerve trunk is tender	1. Support the head of the metacarpals and ask the patient to extent the fingers at metacarpo-phalangeal joints—not possible. (Fig. 16.10A) 2. Hold the thumb at its root—ask the patient to extend terminal phalanx of thumb-not possible (Fig. 16.10B) 3. In above elbow	Comparatively good.	—Treat the primary cause. —Wait and watch —Splintage for wrist drop by cock-up splint —Neurolysis —Primary suture. —Secondary suture —Resection anastomosis. —Reconstruc-

Contd.

Table 16.3: Contd.

Nerve 1	*Muscles supplied* 2	*Sensory area* 3	*Vasomotor effect* 4	*Mode of injury* 5	*Presentation* 6	*Tests* 7	*Prognosis* 8	*Treatment* 9
	minimi, extensor carpi ulnaris, abductor pollicis longus. In posterior interosseous nerve (deep branch of radial nerve) affection the muscles supplied by radial nerve in arm are spared. Hence there will be only partial wrist drop.			—Supra condylar fracture, fracture head and neck of radius, iatrogenic (excision of head of radius), VIC *Entrapment* —at the junction of lower 1/4 of arm —Where posterior interosseous nerve passes through supinator *Disease* Chronic lead poisoning, leprosy may cause partial wrist drop. Wartenberg's disease (cheiragia paraesthetica) is an entrapment syndrome at the point where the sensory branch of the radial nerve emerges from beneath the edge of the brachioradialis tendon (about 7 cm proximal to the radial styloid process). This entrapment occurs due to previous oft repeated trauma or from repeated pronation and supination of the forearm	near the proximal portion of the extensor muscle origin. Extension of the fingers increases the pain. Since the extensor carpi radialis brevis tendon inserts at the base of third metacarpal and it helps in stabilising the wrist during the extension of the middle finger, elevation of this finger against resistence with elbow extended causes the typical pain	injury (radial nerve injury), total wrist drop. In below elbow injuries (posterior interosseous nerve injury)—Partial wrist drop, i.e. partial dorsiflexion and radial deviation possible due to spared extensor carpi radialis longus 4. Flex the elbow at 90° with forearm in midprone position Ask the patient to flex elbow further. Brachio radialis will not stand prominent, as in normal cases. 5. Ask the patient to take the flexed elbow over the head and then extend the elbow. —not possible with paralysed triceps		tive procedure for wrist drop. —Jone's triple tendon transfer —Stabilization of wrist
Sciatic nerve L4, 5 and S1, 2, 3	Hamstrings and all muscles of leg and foot	Outer 3/4-4/5 of leg anteriorly and posteriorly, and whole of the foot	—Trophic ulcers specially beneath balls of 1st and 4th metatarsals and calcaneum	*Injury* —Fracture dislocation of hip —Fracture acetabulum —Posterior dislocation of hip —Iatrogenic-	—Foot drop to flail foot —Clawing of toes. —Trophic ulcers. —Features of lower lumbar (L_5 or S_1) compressive	• Ask the patient to dorsiflex the ankle and toes—not possible. In flail foot no active movement possible • In straight leg raising there will	Variable	—Treat the primary cause —Wait and watch —Neurolysis —Stabilization operations of the foot

Contd.

Martin-Gruber anastomosis is an anomaly. In few patients there may be crosslinks among the three peripheral nerve of the upper limb. In this anomaly the motor nerve fibres, normally entirely carried in the ulnar nerve, enter the ulnar nerve from the median nerve via the branches in the forearm. In this condition the dysfunction or disruption of the ulnar nerve above the level of anastomosis may not result in motor loss of muscles in the hand typically supplied by the ulnar nerve

Table 16.3: Contd.

Nerve 1	*Muscles supplied* 2	*Sensory area* 3	*Vasomotor effect* 4	*Mode of injury* 5	*Presentation* 6	*Tests* 7	*Prognosis* 8	*Treatment* 9
			—Causalgia	(posterior approach of the hip). —Penetrating—gun shot injury of thigh. —Injection paralysis	radiculopathy in which usually multiple segments are involved (cf. in disc herniation usually one segment is involved.	be limitation (mainly in traumatic and compression neuropathy) • Differentiation from lumbar radiculopathy (e.g. disc prolapse): straight leg raising is done just short of discomfort. In this position pain caused by sciatic neuropathy is increased by internal rotation of hip, and relieved by its external rotation (this is not in lumbar radiculopathy)		—Protective orthotics
Lateral popliteal nerve L 4, 5, S, 1, 2	Tibialis anterior, extensor hallucis longus, extensor digitorum longus, peroneus tertius, peroneus longus, peroneus brevis	Outer 3/4 of dorsum of leg and middle half of dorsum of foot	Insignificant.	*Injury* —Fracture head and neck of fibula, fracture tibial condyles Penetrating or cut injuries. Iatrogenic. Pressure by neoplasm of underlying bone, e.g. giant cell tumour, exostosis. Entrapment at the neck of fibula. In anterior tibial compartment syndrome. *Disease:* Hansen's neuropathy.	—Foot drop In traumatic condition of nerve, the patient may complain of pain in the lateral aspect of the leg and foot.	Ask the patient to dorsiflex the ankle and toes—not possible. Ask the patient to stand on heel—not possible. Ask the patient to evert the foot—not possible Pressure over the nerve may cause local and referred (along the sensory distribution) pain	Variable	—Treat the primary cause —Wait and watch —Decompression —Neurolysis. —Orthotics with dorsiflexion assist. Tendon transfer (tibialis posterior) —Stabilization of foot; (Lambrindudi's triple arthrodesis)
Medial popliteal nerve L4, 5 S 1, 2, 3	Gastrocnemius, soleus, tibialis posterior, flexor digitorum longus, flexor hallucis longus, intrinsics of the foot	Sole of the foot.	—Causalgia —Trophic ulceration	*Injury:* Penetrating injuries, open fractures *Entrapment:* Posterior compartment syndrome.	—Clawing of toes —Calcaneus and/or valgus foot	Ask the patient to stand on the toes—not possible. Ask the patient to plantar flex the ankle and toes—not possible.	Not good.	—Treat the primary cause —Decompression —Orthotics—for calcaneus deformity —Tendon transfer —Correction of clawing —Stabilisation of ankle and foot

Contd.

Table 16.3: Contd.

Nerve 1	*Muscles supplied* 2	*Sensory area* 3	*Vasomotor effect* 4	*Mode of injury* 5	*Presentation* 6	*Tests* 7	*Prognosis* 8	*Treatment* 9
Posterior tibial nerve compression (Tarsal tunnel) syndrome			Compression due to tenosynovitis venous engorgement; Hansen's neuritis; sustained valgus deformity of foot		Burning pain in sole; retrograde pain along medial popliteal nerve even up to the buttock; clawing of toes (decreased flexion at MPJs and extension of IPJs)	Palpation of nerve on posterior to medial malleolus causes pain in sensory distribution of the nerve.		Treat the cause; Release of flexor retinaculum to decompress the nerve; Explore the area of abductor hallucis
Lateral cutaneous nerve of the thigh	—	Lateral part of front of thigh	—	Entrapment (meralgia paraesthetica)	Pain along distribution.	Hypoaesthesia	Variable	—Local xylocaine and hydrocortisone injection —Decompression —Section of nerve
Femoral nerve L 2, 3, 4	Quadriceps, pectineus, sartorius	Front of middle and lower thigh	Insignificant	—Intrapelvic neoplasm —Stab or gun shot injury in upper thigh.	Disturbed gait.	i. While lying down ask the patient to extend the knee from flexed position—not possible ii. Loss of knee jerk.	Poor.	—Treat the primary cause —Wait and watch —Quadriceps reinforcement (Hamstring to quadriceps transfer)
Obturator nerve	Adductors of thigh	Sensory fibres to hip joint; small area on the lower medial aspect or thigh		Pelvic injury, entrapment: compression or irritation of obturator nerve initially leads to obturator neuritis, causing pain on the medial aspect of thigh; atrophy or spasm or weakness of adductor muscles. Abscence of adductor reflex		While lying down supine, ask the patient to abduct the thigh and then adduct it—it will be deficient	Poor	Wait and Watch exploration, decompression if required.

Vulnerable Anatomical Sites in the Upper Limb

Brachial Plexus Roots coming out of intervertebral foramina may be avulsed. Upper roots at the Erb's point: lower roots in supra-clavicular lesions, posterior triangle of neck.

Axillary Nerve: Underneath the deltoid, around the surgical neck of the humerus.

Median Nerve: 1. Infront of the lower end of the humerus, e.g. supracondylar fracture; after exit between two heads of pronator teres, e.g. Volkmann's ischaemic contracture.
2. In the carpal tunnel.

Ulnar Nerve: Behind the medial epicondyle and beneath the Osborne's ligament (epicondylar tunnel); above the wrist joint where it lies superficial to the flexor retinaculum; in proximal hypothenar region where it lies lateral to the pisiform bone—Guyon's tunnel.

Radial Nerve: In the base of the axilla, e.g. crutch palsy; spiral groove, e.g. fracture shaft of humerus; while piercing lateral intermuscular septum; in front of elbow capsule.

Posterior Interosseous Nerve: While passing through the supinator around the neck of the radius.

Vulnerable Anatomical Sites in Lower Limbs

Sciatic Nerve: Behind the hip capsule, e.g. fracture and/or dislocation of hip.

Lateral Popliteal Nerve: Around the neck of the fibula.

Lateral Cutaneous Nerve of Thigh: Behind the outer end of the inguinal ligament, near anterior superior iliac spine.

Femoral Nerve: During its intrapelvic course at the base of Scarpa's traingle

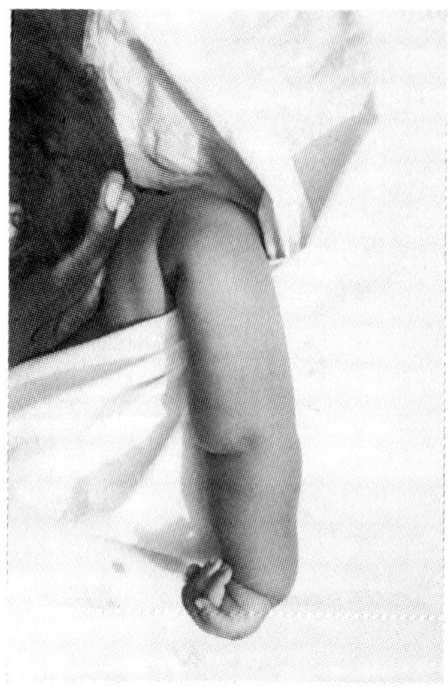

Fig. 16.2A: Erb's palsy at birth

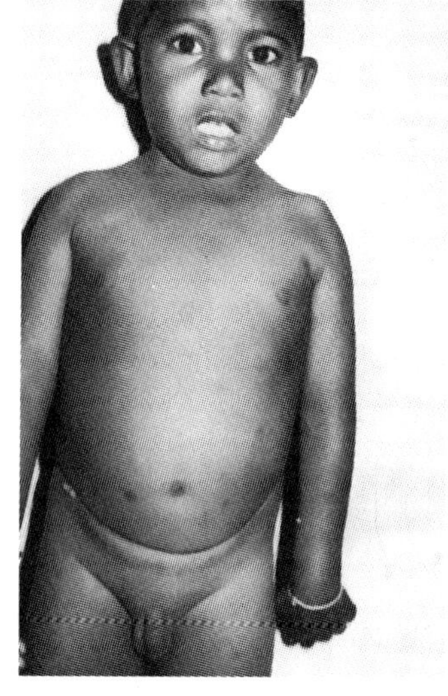

Fig . 16.2B: Patient of neglected Erb's palsy showing typical deformity. Note the wasting of the shoulder muscles

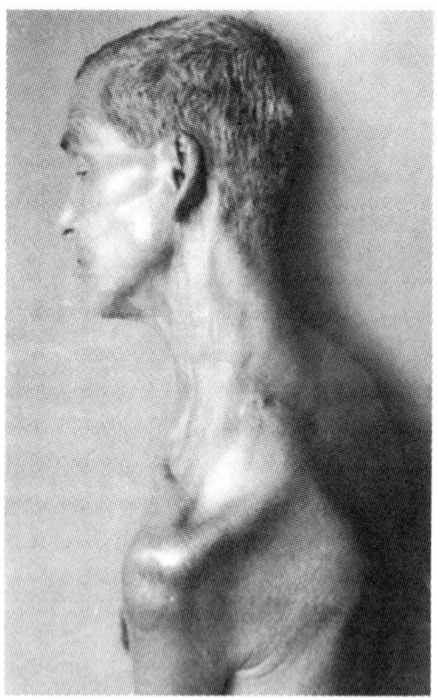

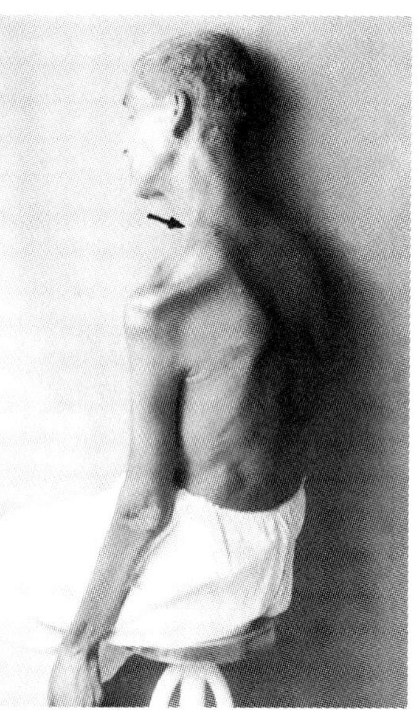

Figs 16.3A and B: Complete brachial palsy—following a stab injury in the supra-clavicular region (arrow showing the site of stab)

motor and sensory latency testing in the upper and lower extremity. It can be of much use for testing the peripheral neuropathies such as carpal tunnel syndrome. Immediate printed test results are obtained which can be correlated to standard electrodiagnostic testing.

d. *Electromyography*: Basis—The electrical changes going on in a muscle are suitably amplified and assessed in the form of sound patterns or recorded in the form of tracings. While a normal muscle is electrically silent at rest, partially/completely denervated muscle

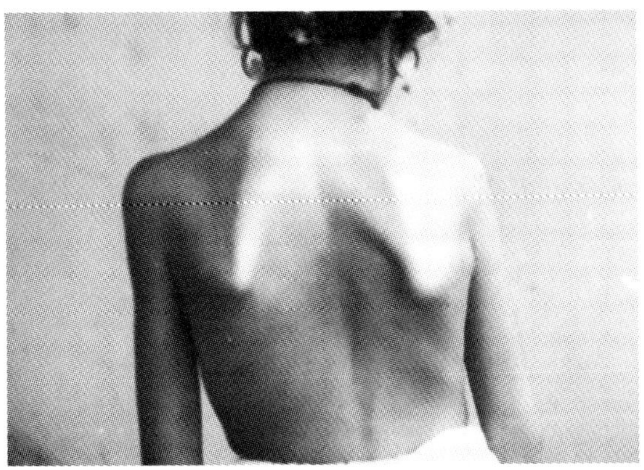

Fig. 16.4A: Typical bilateral winging of the scapula due to paralysis of serratus anterior (a patient of myopathy)

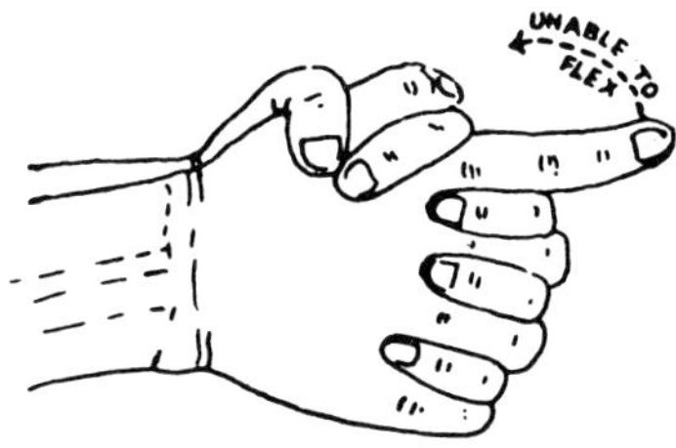

Fig. 16.5A: Method of demonstration of Oschener's clasp test

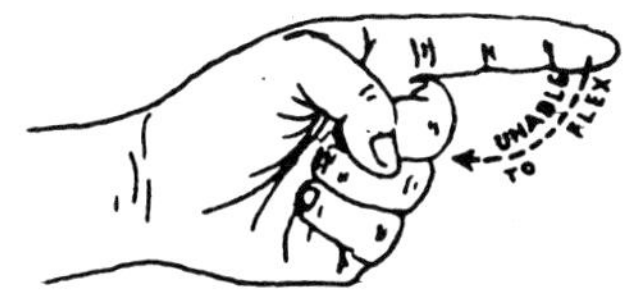

Fig. 16.5B: Test for median nerve injury

shows spontaneous fibrillatory contraction of individual fibres (fibrillation potential). Comparing with the standard wave forms and sound patterns in various disorders, the electromyographic record is studied. This investigation can accurately determine the site of the lesion, i.e. anterior horn cells, peripheral nerves or muscles.

2. *Biopsy*

Biopsy of the affected muscle may help in differentiating whether the effect is of denervation or of ischaemia. The ischaemic muscle shows sudden infarction with early fibrosis,

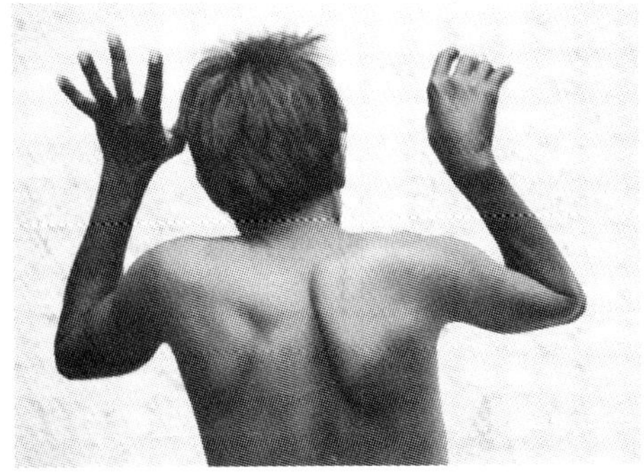

Fig. 16.4B: Winging right scapula due to traumatic serratus anterior paralysis

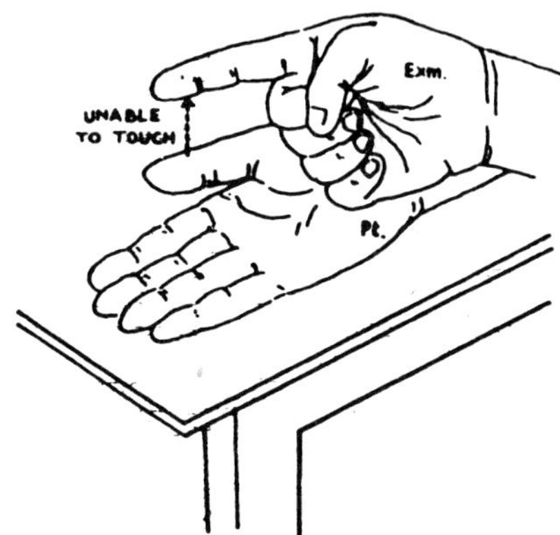

Fig. 16.6: Testing for abductor pollicis brevis muscle in median nerve injury

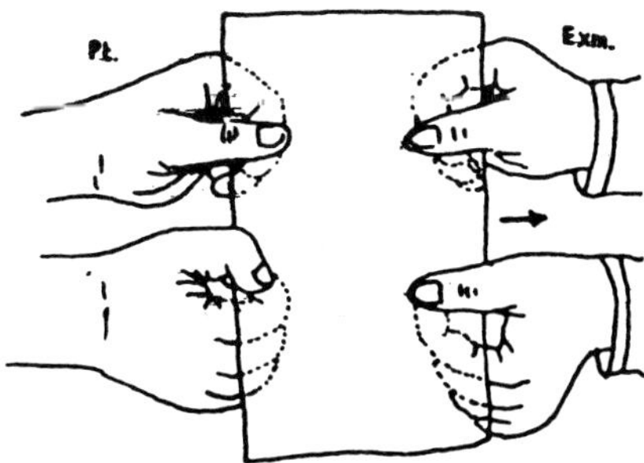

Fig. 16.7: Method of demonstration of Froment's sign for ulnar nerve injury. Note the patient's right thumb acutely flexed to grip the newspaper

whereas, in denervation, gradual diffuse atrophy is followed by late fibrosis.

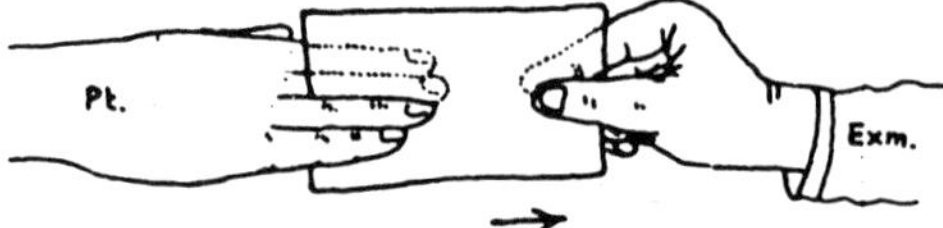

Fig. 16.8: Card test to assess the power of interossei for ulnar nerve injury

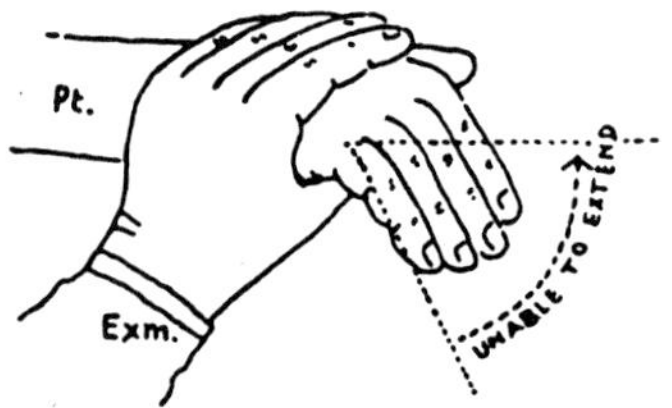

Fig. 16.10A: Testing for the extensors of the fingers of metacarpophalangeal joint (In median nerve injury, patient is unable to extend the fingers of metacarpophalangeal joints)

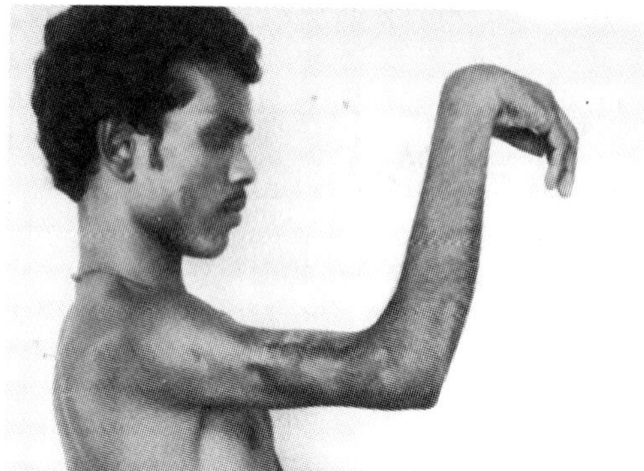

Fig. 16.9A: Typical complete wrist drop following open fracture of humerus

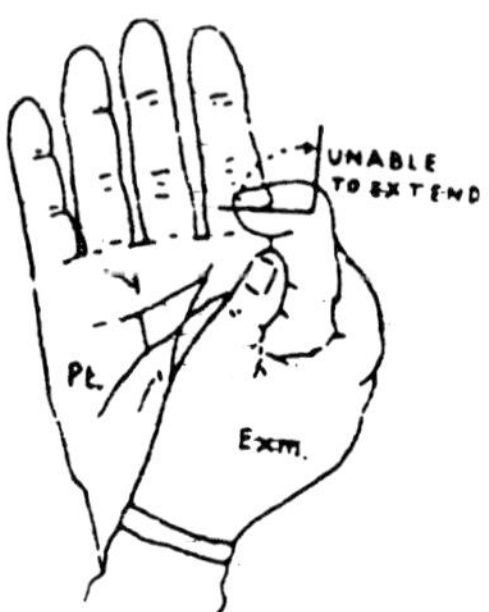

Fig. 16.10B: Testing the power of the extensor pollicis longus—lost in median nerve injury

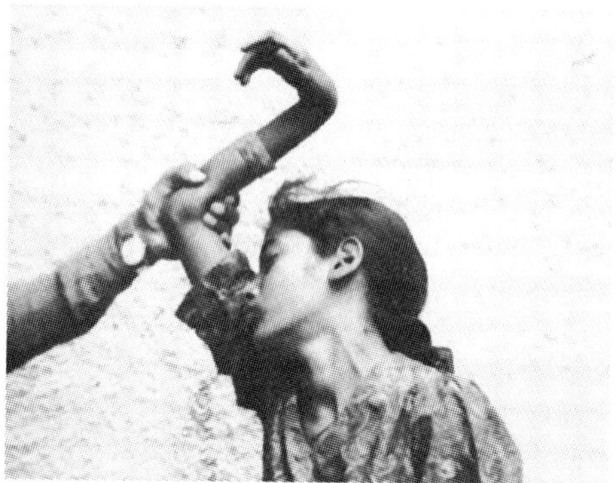

Fig. 16.9B: Wrist drop due to Hansen's disease

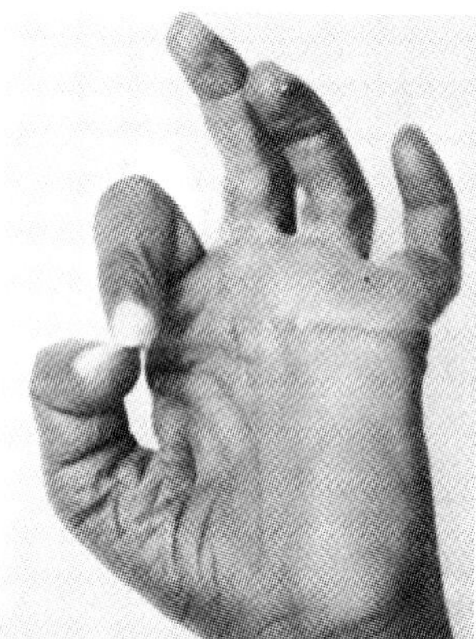

Fig. 16.11: Decreased pinch in ulnar nerve damage

BIBLIOGRAPHY

1. Eversmann WW Jr: Entrapment and compression neuropathies. In Greep DP (Ed). *Operative Hand Surg* (3rd ed) New York: Churchill Livingstone 1341-85, 1993.
2. Gelberman RH, Eaton R, Urbanik JR: Peripheral nerve compression. *J Bone Joint Surg* **75A**: 1854-78, 1993.
3. Koppel HP, Thompson WAL: Peripheral entrapment neuropathies. Baltimore: Williams and Wilkins 131-42, 1963.
4. Pearl ML, Edgerton BW: Glenoid deformity secondary to brachial plexus birth palsy. *J Bone Joint Surg* **80A**: 659-67, 1998.

17 Bone Tumours

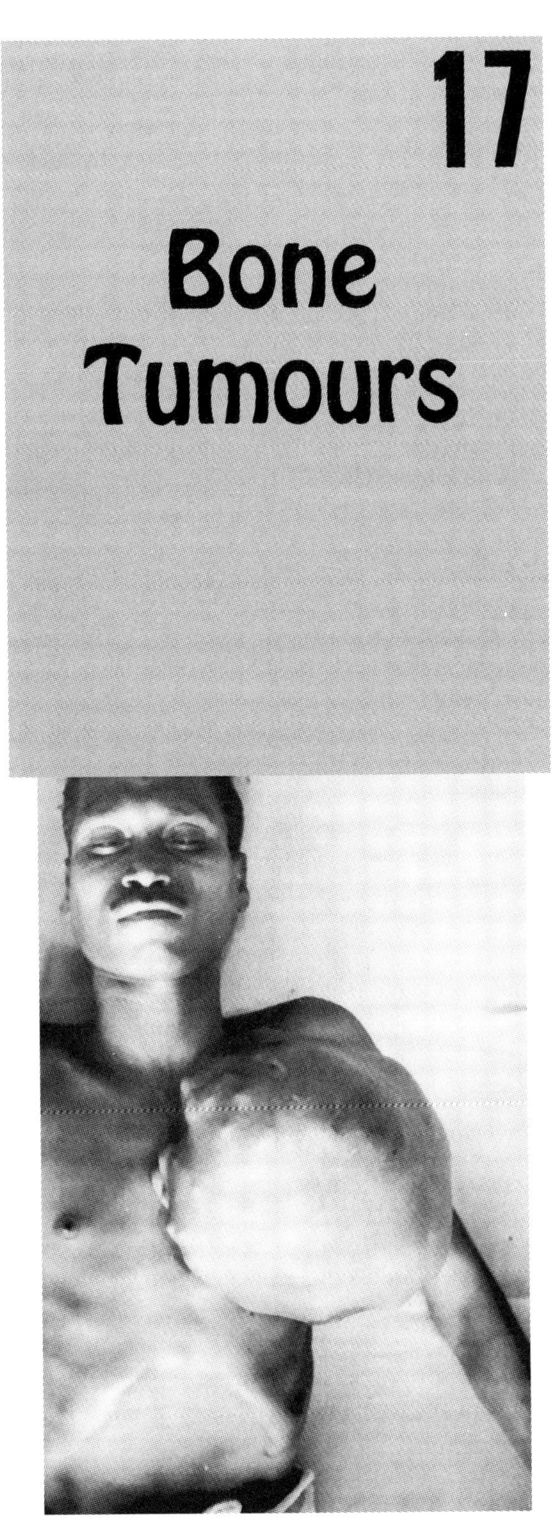

INTRODUCTION

Literally, any tumour means swelling, and its examination implies all norms of examining a swelling but while examining a tumour, a few points deserve special considerations.

Tumours are usually of unknown cause, non-inflammatory and develop independent of and unrestrained by normal laws of growth and morphogenesis.

Except for vague cases of growths which are confined to the marrow, most of the tumours manifest obviously and there is hardly any doubt in making up our mind that one is proceeding to examine a tumour. The problem which remains is that of assessing the type, nature and extent of the growth.

PRIMARY AND SECONDARY BONE TUMOUR

A primary tumour always originates due to hyperactivity of the pleuripotent neoplastic cells (not as a result of secondary implantation). It is almost always solitary, except in extremely rare conditions like multiple exostosis, multiple myelomatosis, skip lesion in osteosarcoma.

A secondary tumour is a malignant neoplasm, occurring as a result of implantation of neoplastic cells, in bone or soft tissue, coming from a primary malignant growth (of soft tissue or bone), and may occur at one or several sites. The primary may be manifest or occult.

The usual primary sites are prostate, breast, bronchus, thyroid, kidney, stomach, adrenals and skin. Usual manifestations are complications of neoplasm, for instance pathological fracture and paraplegia, besides pain, swelling, anaemia and cachexia.

Benign tumours are comparatively less harmful, except for the cosmetic deformity and the mechanical pressure effects. However, features suggestive of a transition to a malignant stage must be thoroughly enquired and looked into. These features are:

1. Sudden rapid growth.
2. Appearance of pain in a swelling, which was painless earlier.

3. Evidence of increased vascularity (venous prominence).
4. Warm overlying skin surface.
5. Clinically invasive nature, e.g. lack of clear demarcation, comparatively warm.
6. Regional lymph gland enlargement of neoplastic nature (i.e. hard but not tender).
7. Above all, affection of the general health of the patient (cachexia, anaemia).

Right from the beginning, it is essential to boost up the morale of the patients suffering from malignancy. While examining a tumour, one must be very gentle. This is essential not only on compassionate grounds, but also due to the fact that while roughly examining a malignant neoplasm, one can produce disastrous consequences like pathological (micro or macro) fractures, and local and/or distant dissemination of the growth. Features of malignancy are usually so obvious that they do not require much handling. Passing the hand gently over and around the growth can acceptably delineate the extent, dimension and relations of the growth. Through advances in diagnostic imaging, histological evaluation, staging procedures, operative strategies, adjuvant (postoperative) and neoadjuvant (chemotherapy also in pre-operative setting) chemotherapies, there appears to have a great future in managing the various skeletal neoplastic growths. Therefore, it is imperative that a very careful and gentle assessment of the neoplasm be done, especially with regard to its relations with surrounding soft tissues and adjoining joints.

While examining a benign neoplasm, all possible mechanical pressure effects must be searched for. Even with the slightest doubt of malignancy, the possible sites of metastasis must be sought for. Unfortunately, the pulmonary bed, working as a filter for circulating neoplastic cells, is a common site for implantation of metastatic tissues. Hence, thorough examination of the pulmonary system is essential. Then, various possible osseous foci (e.g. vertebral column, skull, ribs, pelvis, femora and so on) should be looked for.

In certain neoplasms like multiple myelomatosis, there may not be any obvious swelling any where. The only manifestations may be general systemic features, vague generalised pain, progressive anaemia or other complications like renal failures and paraplegia.

Carcinoma and Sarcoma

- —Carcinomas are malignant tumours arising from epithelial or endothelial tissues.
- —Sarcomas are tumours arising from mesoblastic tissues. Sarcomas of bone and soft tissue are uncommon malignant lesions, characterised by a diversity (varigated) in presentation and biological behaviour.

Post-irradiation Neoplasms

Irradiation therapy was a very popular treatment till the sixth to early seventh decade of this century, but it is getting unpopular because of the advent of more promising chemotherapeutic agents and irradiation hazards. In certain situations like benign giant cell tumour and ankylosing spondylitis, therapeutic irradiation has been blamed for malignant transformations.

CLASSIFICATION OF BONE TUMOURS

A lot of controversy exists regarding the classification and nomenclature of bone tumours, probably because of disagreement between the clinicians, radiologists and pathologists. The controversy regarding the cell origin of different tumours, varying behaviour of certain tumours and confusing histopathological changes in different fields of same tumour also complicate the issue. However, in the year 1972 a World Health Organization sponsored meeting of radiologists, pathologists and clinicians agreed to classify bone tumours on the basis of histological typing. At the same time, certain facts presented in the classification of 'bone registry' cannot be denied.

Staging is the process of classifying a tumour, especially a malignant tumour with respect to its degree of differentian as well as its local and distant extent, in order to estimate the prognosis and to compare between groups of patients.

Staging is done on the basis of clinical findings, imaging and histopathological studies, basically to guide, the operative procedure, goal of treatment (curative or palliative), the extent of excision, the perceived efficacy of adjuvant therapy, prognostise the ultimate outcome.

The first staging system was developed by League of Nation based on TNM system (T = extent of primary tumour; N = presence or absence of nodal metastasis; M = distant metastasis). At present the most commonly used system of staging of the malignant soft-tissue tumours is that of American Joint Committee on Cancer. However the Musculoskeletal Tumour Society adopted a staging system, as described by Enneking *et al* (1980, 1983) for both benign and malignant bone tumours. This system has been more or less agreed upon by AJCC with minor adaptations for malignant bone tumours.

History Taking

In history taking, the following points should be noted in detail:

1. Onset of symptoms in chronological order.
2. Duration of each symptom.

   The usual symptoms of bone tumours are:

   I. *Symptoms due to Primary Growth*
      a. *Local symptoms*: Swelling, pain, affections of joint movement to varying extent, wasting of adjoining muscles, ulcers.
      b. *Constitutional symptoms*: Occasionally constitutional symptoms like fever, weakness, loss of weight, anorexia, progressive anaemia.
      c. *Pressure symptoms:* Like weakness in the distal parts and other symptoms due to pressure on the vital part and neurovascular structures.

   II. *Symptoms due to Metastatic Lesions*
      a. Common complaints due to secondaries in lungs are—cough, haemoptysis, and pain chest.
      b. Secondaries from primaries of the secreting glands (e.g. thyroid, adrenals, salivary, pituitary) may induce the manifestations of hyperfunctional effects of primary glandular secretions.
      c. Sometimes, the patients primarily present with severe complications, e.g. paraplegia due to secondary deposits without any obvious complaints regarding the primary tumours.
3. Rate of growth.
4. Fluctuations in symptoms with or without any treatment, e.g. lessening or exaggerations of swelling and/or pain.
5. Treatment given and its results—Usually the modes of treatment tried are:
   - Indigenous medicines, local applications, radiotherapy (doses, period and sittings of applications), chemotherapy (drugs used, doses and duration) and surgical treatment (for biopsy or ablation).

   The details of the treatment should be noted as far as possible.
6. Family history may not be of that significance in the examination but with the proven role of genetic transmission in certain cases of neoplasms (familial or diaphyseal aclasis, neuroblastoma, etc.), the detailed family history should be taken (Figs 17.1A to D).
7. Occupation of the patient, especially with reference to radiation exposure, regular use of certain chemicals, inhalation of certain obnoxious vapours, exposure to any irritant—physical, chemical or others, should be noted. Certain relations of these irritating substances with neoplastic growths have been proved, e.g. radium, responsible for osteogenic sarcoma, coaltar as a carcinogen, etc.

EXAMINATION

General Examination

The early stages may not be of much significance,

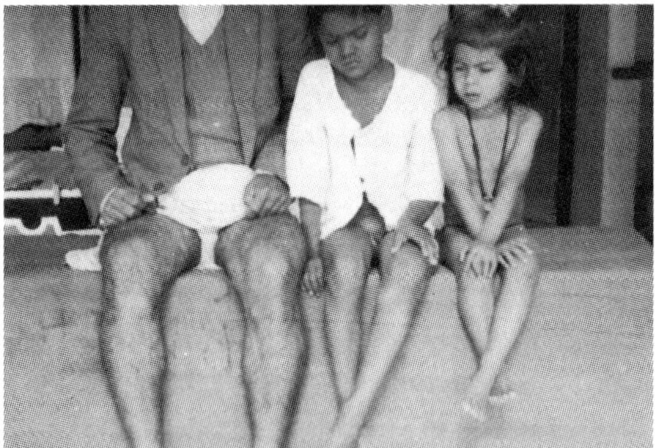

Fig. 17.1A: Familial exostosis (multiple osteochondroma). Father having exostosis in both upper tibiae and other places; first son having exostosis in left upper tibia, left lower femur and ribs; second son having exostosis in left upper humerus, left middle finger, right upper tibia and ribs

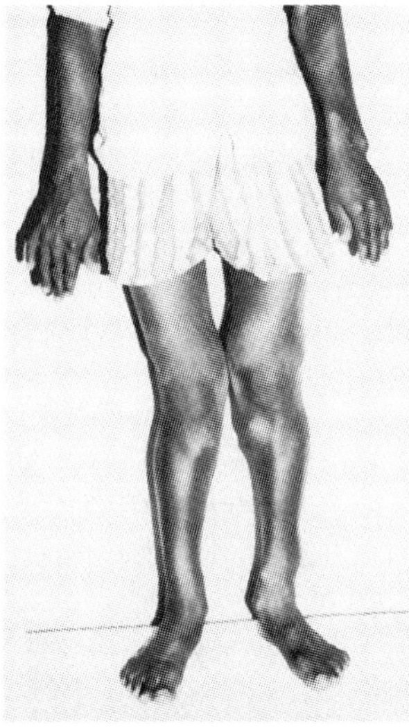

Fig. 17.1B: Multiple exostosis

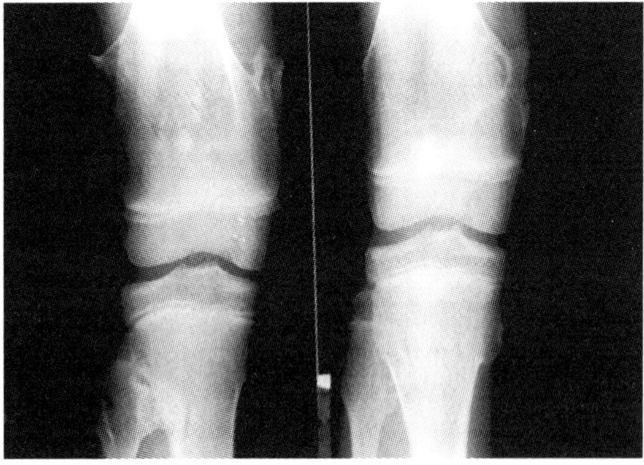

Fig. 17.1C: Diaphyseal aclasia

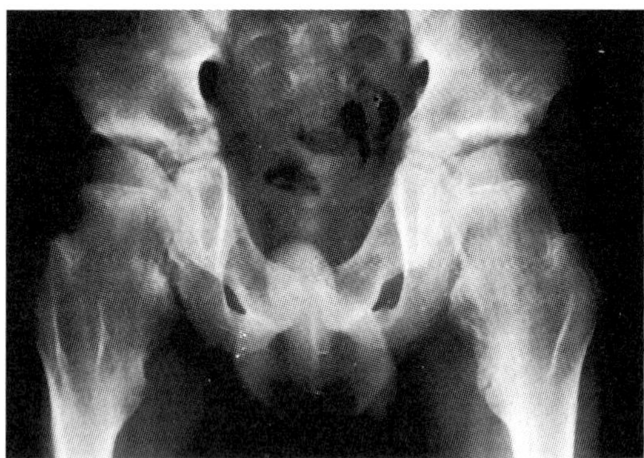

Fig. 17.1D: Diaphyseal aclasia

but in long standing cases of malignant tumours, general effects of cachexia and anaemia may be obvious. The effects of tumour on general behaviour, attitude, gait, posture and functional abilities of the patient should be noted clearly. Any obvious deformity (e.g. in multiple exostosis, chondroma, etc.), should be noted. As a general rule, the hand should be passed from the skull down to the face, chest, pelvis, spine and limbs, in any case of suspected neoplasm. Sometimes various swellings in the skull or pelvis may be masked by hairs and undergarments.

Systemic Examination

As a routine, respiratory system, cardiovascular system, abdominal examination and urogenital system should be examined. Whenever indicated examination of the central nervous system and endocrinal assessment should be done.

Local Examination

Swelling must be categorically and systemically examined.

Inspection

Look for site, size, shape, extent, direction of

growth, engorgement of veins, skin condition, any pulsation, stretching of overlying soft tissue, any scar or ulcer, any movement of the swelling with movement of the limb or part, encroachment of the swelling over adjoining joints and muscle wasting in relation to the swelling.

Palpation

Superficial palpation (touch): Temperature, pliability of skin and superficial tissue, hyperaesthesia, or analgesia or anaesthesia, superficial tenderness, surface of the swelling, and confirmation of the findings of inspection.

Deep palpation (feel): Assess surface of the swelling, extent, margin, deep tenderness, consistency of different areas, fixity of the tumour to superficial tissue, deeper tissues and the underlying bone. The adjoining joint should also be palpated specially because the joints may be affected directly or mechanically. The movements of the adjoining joints must be noted clearly. While palpating, if one gets obvious crepitus or yielding it should be noted. But one should not attempt to demonstrate any crepitus (e.g. egg shell crackling in giant cell tumour). Crackling is due to fracture of thinned out bony shell. In an attempt to demonstrate this crackling repeatedly, the chances of producing further pathological fractures of the thinned out cortical shell increases. This is very likely to disseminate the neoplastic tissues into the surrounding soft tissues and/or distantly.

Examination of the regional lymph glands is mandatory. Almost all malignant neoplasms have glandular disseminations. The nature of the glandular enlargement should be noted categorically.

Examination for any skip lesions: Usually, it is a radiopathological diagnosis. However, in rare instances there may be other palpable swellings in the same bone. The intervening bone may appear clinically normal. This 'skip-lesion' (as in osteosarcoma), is probably due to medullary spread and implantation of neoplastic tissue at that site. However, multifocal neoplasms have also been reported.

Auscultation

This ritual should not be forgotten while examining the neoplasm. In highly vascular tumours (e.g. telangiectatic osteosarcoma, or even any secondaries with high vascularity), systolic bruit may be heard.

Examination of the possible sites for secondaries, specially the lungs, liver, spine, skull, pelvis, ribs, orbital region and other long bones is mandatory.

Search for complications: Possible complication must be kept in mind and search must be made for pressure effects, pathological fractures, paraplegia, hormonal manifestations, etc.

Investigations

1. Routine haemogram.
2. Routine urine examination.
3. Plain X-ray in different views.
   Points to look for in the X-rays:
   i. Disproportionate increase in soft tissue shadow.
   ii. Breach in the continuity of the cortex or any other obvious pathological fracture.
   iii. Amount of destruction.
   iv. Evidence of new bone formation and its appearance.
   v. Any reactionary bone formation (e.g. subperiosteal longitudinal bone laying).
   vi. Corticomedullary delineation (sharp or lost).
   vii. Any evidence of expansion of the cortex.
   viii. Obvious infiltration into joints.
   ix. Skip lesions.
4. Tomography.
5. Contrast radiography.
6. Angiography.
7. Scintography—Radioactive isotope studies.
   Radioactive isotopes are being utilised for localising the neoplastic tissue. Technetium-99m, Strontium 85, Fluorine 18, Strontium 87m, Phosphorus 32, Calcium 45,

Iodine 131 and gold have been used for various neoplastic conditions. The results of these investigations are of much help in ruling out any secondaries, (which may not be obvious otherwise).

8. Computerised axial tomography.
9. Nuclear magnetic resonance (NMR/MRI).
10. Cytological examination—Confirmation can only be by histopathological examination. The material for this examination can be obtained by—
    a. Fine Needle Aspiration Cytology (FNAC).
    b. Needle biopsy.
    c. CT guided needle biopsy.
    d. Open biopsy.
    a. *Fine needle aspiration cytology*: It is an almost painless outdoor or ward procedure with a very high rate of accuracy (97-98%) with the added advantage of obtaining a result within a few hours. In this a fine needle (18, 20, 22) is passed into the suspected tissue and negative pressure is created and maintained in the syringe. The needle is then passed in three to five different directions through the same entry. After completing the aspiration, the pressure in the syringe is equalised, and the needle withdrawn. Contents of the needle are then expressed on a glass slide, smeared and fixed immediately with cytofix. It is then stained for study for Papanicolaou or Haematoxyline.
    b. *Needle biopsy:* With a wide bore needle, aspiration is done from the contents of the neoplasm. Aspiration should be done from various sites of the neoplasm. In a thick smear, the nature of the cells can be studied. This may be almost of confirmatory value (e.g. sternal puncture in multiple myeloma). Unfortunately, in other neoplasms the aspirate study may not be of confirmatory value on several occasions.
    c. *Open biopsy*: Open biopsy, of course, can be authentic but a word of caution is due before embarking on it. As far as the medicolegal aspect is concerned open biopsy can confirm the diagnosis and one must not embark on ablation surgery without confirmation of the diagnosis. But when one thinks of primary resection of neoplasm followed by a possible reconstruction, open biopsy may come in the way. Not only it does damage to the area of operative exposure, but also carries the grave risk of dissemination of neoplastic tissues to the surrounding area. This dissemination may nullify the basic benefit of primary resection, and recurrence of the growth becomes almost a rule rather than an exception. However, the evolution of multiagent chemotherapy provides a comparatively safer umbrella for this procedure. Still, this issue is not that easy and it should be left entirely on the discretion of the surgeon whether or not he should decide to go in for an open biopsy before embarking on primary resection and reconstruction procedures. A thorough gentle clinical examination, supplemented by various investigations can often give very helpful clues in circumventing this tricky problem.

       Peroperative frozen section study is worthwhile. Depending upon the report about the nature of the growth, the surgeon may proceed for definitive surgery.
11. Tetracycline staining studies.
12. Various biochemical tests:
    a. Serum acid phosphatase.
    b. Serum alkaline phosphatase.
13. Renal function tests.
14. Paper chromatography.
15. Electrophoresis of serum for various protein components.
16. Proton emission tomography (PET).
17. Tumour embolisation.

Table 17.1: Classification of primary bone tumours
(Based on WHO classification (1972) (Ackermann, Sison and Schajowicz)

Cell of origin	*Benign*	*Intermediate or indeterminate*	*Malignant*	*Tumour like lesions*
Osteoblasts	— Osteoma — Osteoblastoma — Osteoid osteoma		— Osteosarcoma — Juxta-cortical osteosarcoma (Parosteal osteosarcoma)	— Solitary bone cyst (Unicameral bone cyst) — Aneurysmal bone cyst — Juxta articular bone cyst (Intraosseous ganglion)
Chondroblasts	— Chondroma — Chondroblastoma — Osteochondroma (The most common benign tumour) — Chondromyxoid fibroma.		— Chondrosarcoma — Juxta-cortical chondrosarcoma	— Non-ossifying fibroma (Metaphyseal fibroma). — Fibrous dysplasia. — Eosinophilic granuloma — Brown's tumour of hyperparathyroidism
Osteoclasts	— Osteoclastoma (Giant cell tumour) (Locally malignant)		— Malignant osteoclastoma (Giant cell tumour)	
Medullary tumours			— Ewing's sarcoma — Reticulum cell sarcoma — Multiple myeloma.	— Hodgkin's disease — Lymphosarcoma
Vascular tumours	— Haemangioma	— Haemangiopericytoma — Haemangioendothelioma	— Angiosarcoma of hand can develop with regular contact with polyvinyl chloride (pipes and cement)	
Fibrous tissue 'Adipose tissue 'Nerve tissue	— Desmoplastic fibroma — Lipoma — Neurofibroma — Neurolemmoma		— Fibrosarcoma — Liposarcoma — Neurofibrosarcoma	

Contd.

Table 17.1: Contd.

Cell of origin	*Benign*	*Intermediate or indeterminate*	*Malignant*	*Tumour like lesions*
*Lymphatics	— Lymphangioma		— Lymphomas	
*'Inclusion tissue		— Adamantinoma (of tibia, etc.)	— Chordoma (from notochordal remnants in the sacral region and sella turcica of the skull)	
Synovium	Synovioma	Synovioma	— Synovial sarcoma	

'These (*) marked growths have not been included in classification but it appears logical to include them.

Secondary bone tumours—Primary from breast, prostate, bronchus, thyroid, kidney, stomach, adrenals, and skin.

NB. To facilitate the selection of surgical procedure and comparing the results of different modes of managing malignant musculoskeletal lesions, Enneking *et al* (1980) suggested staging of these lesions basing upon physical, radiological, radioisotopic and histophathological examinations. The system suggested by them is as follows:

IA	—	Low-grade intracompartmental (lesion confined to a single anatomical compartment)	A local procedure with dissection carried out through normal tissue
IB	—	Low-grade extracompartmental (lesion extends beyond a single compartment)	Amputation at proper level.
IIA	—	High-grade intracompartmental	Radical excision with removal of all normal tissues of the involved compartments.
IIB	—	High-grade extracompartmental	
III	—	Lesions (low or high grades intra or extracompartmental) with regional or distant metastasis	

WHO classification system, as modified by Enzinger and Weiss, recognises 82 distinct benign and malignant soft tissue lesions and tumours of 10 major histogenic types, which can arise in the distant part of leg (besides other regions)

Table 17.2: Table showing diagnostic features of important bone tumours (*Benign*)

		Osteoma	*Osteochondroma*	*Osteoid osteoma*	*Osteoblastoma*
	1	*2*	*3*	*4*	*5*
1.	Synonyms	A true osteoma is ivory exostosis	Familial exostoses. Multiple exostoses, Diaphyseal aclasis, Biotrophic osteoma (osteoid) Metaphyseal aclasia, Exostosis (single or multiple).	Jaffe's tumour, Aspirin tumour	Giant osteoid osteoma; osteogenic fibroma of bone
2.	Cell of origin	Osteoblast	Chondroblast, arise from growth cartilage cells	Views of origin: —Jaffe (1935)—a slow growing neoplasm. —Infective origin of self limiting nature (because of sclerosed bony shell, characteristic location, in some cases organisms cultured). —A vascular lesion —Embryonic rest —Hamartoma	Osteoblast
3.	Age, sex	Starts in childhood, manifests in adults	Occurs during adolescence, never after epiphyseal fusion Equal in both sexes	Usually males (10-30 years)	Any age group usually less than 30 years, male more than females (2:1)
4.	Bones affected	Membranous bones—cranial bones, orbit, nasal bones, external auditory meatus, mandible	Bones of cartilage origin. Most Common at the extremities of long bones—lower end of femur, upper end of tibia, upper end of femur. Frequently from epiphysis of flat bones—scapula, innominate. Arise from growth cartilage cells	Any bone (except skull) predominantly in bones of lower extremities (5%), e.g. tibia, femur, vertebrae.	Rare tumour. In vertebrae, limb bones, e.g. femur
5.	Clinical presentation	Hard, immovable, small, sessile, single, slowly growing, smooth surface, may be nodular, growing within may cause pressure on the brain	Usually pedunculated with bulbar extremity projecting towards diaphysis away from epiphyseal plate and is capped by a detached fragment of epiphyseal cartilage Comparative broadening of metaphysis due to base of growth. With cessation of growth the cartilaginous cap shrinks even up to degenerative disappearance	Usually pain (dull ache) at night, relieved by salicylates, may be a tender swelling if superficially located in tibia. May be limp (in lower limb affection). If near joint—effusion, stiffness, contracture	Pain and tenderness. Vertebral involvement may cause weakness and paraesthesia of lower limb
6.	Pathology	Tumour usually composed of bony tissue as dense and hard as ivory	Grows till fusion of adjacent epiphysis, summit often covered by adventitious bursa. When fully developed, the marrow of the shaft is continuous with that of exostosis. May be familial. Symptoms—cosmetic, pressure	Lesions very vascular with numerous nerve fibres. Histology—an inner region of vascular granulation tissue containing osteo-	Cuts with gritty sensation, vascular. Histology—fairly regular orientation of new bone formation with trabeculation. Osteogenic cells

Contd.

Table 17.2: Contd.

		Osteoma	*Osteochondroma*	*Osteoid osteoma*	*Osteoblastoma*
	1	*2*	*3*	*4*	*5*
			effect, local pressure upon nerves (lateral popliteal), vessels, e.g. in popliteal fossa. May turn malignant (chondrosarcoma, osteosarcoma). When fully developed, growth consists of shell of compact bone enclosing cancellous tissue with a cap of cartilage. Cut section—central core of cancellous tissue continuous with medullary canal of parent bone, containing a central blood vessel with branching up to tip of the growth.	blasts, outside which calcification and osteoid formation surrounded by trabecular formation of bone	having look of malignancy. Predominantly osteoid and primitive bone trabeculae, giant cells; distinct and uniform stromal cell, which rarely show mitotic figures (cf. GCT).
7.	Investigation X-ray	Sessile rounded densely opaque shadow	Pedunculated or sessile out-pouching of the trabeculated corticocancellous bone from the metaphysis. Size of growth comparatively smaller than felt clinically (due to cartilaginous cap).	Central radiolucent nidus surrounded by a zone of sclerosed bone, further surrounded by normal adjoining bone	Circumscribed expanding osteolytic lesion with some radio-paque mottling.
8.	Complications	Mainly cosmetic problems Very rarely early intra-cranial pressure symptoms	General—cosmetic, stunted growth; Local—turn malignant (osteochondrosarcoma or chondrosarcoma. —Pressure/stretch neurovascular complication (lateral popliteal nerve). —Fracture	—Radicular irritation —Psychic depression. Entrapment neuropathy (e.g. posterior interosseus neuropathy following osteoid osteoma of upper end of ulna	May turn to malignant growth
9.	Differential diagnosis	Foreign body (bullet, etc)		—Brodie's abscess. —Sclerosing non-suppurative osteomyelitis of Garre. —Non-ossifying fibroma. —Syphylitic osteitis. —Osteogenic sarcoma. —Ch. osteomyelitis with annular sequestrum (e.g. pintract infection)	Osteoid osteoma Osteogenic sarcoma Giant cell tumour
10.	Treatment	For pressure symptoms or cosmetic reasons. Excision with normal bone margin.	Excision with wide base for cosmetic improvement, any pressure symptoms, and the slightest doubt of malignancy (sudden increase in growth rate, warm, pain).	Complete resection—cures, symptomatic—salicylate for pain. —Partial removal. Percutaneous ablation with radiofrequency is preferred treatment for extraspinal osteoid osteoma (Percutaneous computed tomography guided ablation with a radiofrequency electrode introduced through the cannula of the biopsy needle, and the electrode connected to a radiofrequency generator)	Resection cures. Curettage with bone grafting. Radiotherapy for inaccessible lesions, e.g. vertebrae

Table 17.3: Diagnostic features of important bone tumours (*Malignant*)

	1	*Primary osteosarcoma* 2	*Ewing's sarcoma* 3	*Multiple myeloma* 4	*Giant cell tumour* 5	*Secondary growth* 6
1.	Synonyms	Osteogenic sarcoma	Ewing (1928) described; Endothelial myeloma, perithelioma, undifferentiated round cell sarcoma	Plasma cell myeloma; myelomatosis; Multiple myelomatosis; Monoclonal gammopathy; Plasmocytoma (solitary)	Osteoclastoma	Metastatic growth
2.	Age	Predilection for 2nd decade though may occur at any age	5-15 years	Above 40 years	After fusion of growth plate. 3rd-4th decade	Usually elderly age group
3.	Sex	Most common in males than females	More common in males	More common in males	Almost equal	Sex—depending upon the nature of primary
4.	Cell of origin	Osteoblast	—Reticulum cells of marrow —Endothelial elements in marrow (Ewing) —Secondary from adrenal neuroblastoma (Willis) —A variant of reticulum cell sarcoma —On the whole it is the most common malignant bone tumour with multicentric origin	—Neoplastic proliferation of cells which normally produce gamma globulins. —Plasma cell	Osteoclast	Cells of parent tumour
5.	Most common sites in bone	Metaphysis	—Diaphysis Most common malignant tumour of flat bone	Grow over whole extent of mature bone. Of the primary malignant bone tumours, multiple myeloma is the commonest	Epiphyseometaphyseal, area	Usually bone containing the red marrow are the sites of secondaries. In long bones, upper metaphyseal ends and proximal part of diaphysis are more affected than distal bones
6.	Bones affected	Lower femur, upper tibia, upper humerus, radius, ulna. Scapula, small bones (very rare).	Long bones—tibia, femur pelvis, fibula, humerus, clavicle, also short bones, e.g. calcaneum, talus	Usually flat bone containing red marrow—sternum, ribs, vertebrae, skull, pelvis. Long bones, extremely rare distal to knee and elbow.	50% about the knee (upper end of tibia, lower end of femur), lower end of radius, upper end of fibula, lower end of tibia, vertebrae	a. Bones affected—vertebra, pelvis, cervicotrochanter region of femur, ribs, skull, humerus, (almost negligible in below knee and below elbow bones) b. Soft tissues of affected lung, liver, lymph gland, spleen, skin, etc.
7.	Clinical presentation —general and —local	Pain, followed by swelling Rapidly growing, later on cachexia, anaemia and symptoms due to mechanical pressure	Features mimic sub-acute osteomyelitis—pain, fever, mild swelling, pathological fracture	Generalised slowly increasing pain, weakness, progressive anaemia, pathological fracture, paraplegia, renal dysfunction	Swelling, followed by mild pain, tumour tissue prevented from entering the joint space by even thinned out articular cartilage, but may affect joint movements mechanically. May be pathological fracture	Usually manifests as complications like pathological fracture, paraplegia, pressure symptoms besides pain, pallor and cachexia

Contd.

Table 17.3: Contd.

	1	*Primary osteosarcoma* 2	*Ewing's sarcoma* 3	*Multiple myeloma* 4	*Giant cell tumour* 5	*Secondary growth* 6
8.	Salient features	Warm, fusiform swelling with variegated feel, highly vascular, near by joint free except in affections due to mechanical reasons, pathological fractures, features of metastasis. Swelling tender (more at margin)	Fusiform, warm, firm, mildy tender, diaphyseal swelling	Rarely presents as mild swelling, e.g. in clavicle, upper end of the femur and rib. Generalised tenderness specially of the flat bones, e.g. rib, sternum, pelvis, scapula, etc.	Eccentric swelling, hard to firm in feel, slightly warm, near by joint may be affected, egg-shell crackling	Usually comparatively less warm than primary tumour. Diffuse swelling, no respect for joint
9.	Vascularity	Mostly high, even may be pulsating malignant bone aneurysm.	Moderate to severe	Mild to moderate	Low grade, except when it turns frankly malignant, when it increases proportionately	Vascularity depending upon nature of primary growth but comparatively less
10.	Regional lymph nodes	Occasionally enlarged	Moderately to severely enlarged	May or may not be enlarged.	May be enlarged but in very few cases (about 7%)	Regional gland usually involved
11.	Possible sites of metastasis	Lung (diffuse bronchitis, cough, fever, haemoptysis)	Lungs, skull, other bones.	Dissemination to different bones is controversial. Perhaps never settles in lung. May block the renal tubules by protein casts.	All growths expand locally. Frankly malignant ones may metastasise to lung	Itself a metastatic tumour
12.	Investigations general	Nothing significant ESR raised	Leucocytosis even with moderate polymorphonuclear count, confusing picture with subacute osteomyelitis	Normocytic and normochromic anaemia, Microcytic and hypochromic anaemia when there is bleeding, haemoglobin level is lowered, ESR is raised. Routine examination of urine —30% cases may show Bence Jones protein; albuminuria and casts because of renal involvement.	Nothing significant	Macrocytic hypochromic anaemia, ESR raised
13.	X-ray	Increased soft tissue shadow, sun-ray spicules, Codman's reactive triangle, corticomedullary delineation maintained, evidence of bone destruction and bone formation, respect to joint—no penetration into joint.	Expansion of diaphyseal medulla (destructive enlargement) by cystic destruction, onion-peel appearance, mainly due to reactionary sub-periosteal bone formation	Round punched out clear cut areas in a number of bones	Cortical expansion, growth traversed with multiple septae giving soap-bubble appearance; may be breach in the thinned out cortex; about 25% may break into joint. Usually expanded growth margin is sharply demarcated from normal marrow but with malignant transformation this sharpness is not obvious and thin septae area also less visible giving a homogenous ground glass appearance	Irregular, distorted lytic lesions except secondaries from prostate or scirrhous carcinoma of breast, stomach, etc.

Contd.

Table 17.3: Contd.

	1	*Primary osteosarcoma* 2	*Ewing's sarcoma* 3	*Multiple myeloma* 4	*Giant cell tumour* 5	*Secondary growth* 6
14.	Naked eye appearance	Greyish white tumour which does not transgress the cartilage of epiphysis. In mature bones it extends up to the end, but does not penetrate the articular cartilage; variegated appearance, soft, fleshy, vascular with areas of haemorrhage and necrosis	Greyish white, firm from outside	Soft gray tumour of marrow, multiple circumscribed areas of destruction of marrow, pure rarefying lesion, no new bone formation, later marrow cavity filled with tumour tissue	Tumour is encapsulated, firm to hard in feel except when soft tissue is invaded, where it may even be soft	Irregular variably nodular surface with firm to soft or cystic feel
15.	Cut section	Cuts with gritty or variegated feel, greyish white variegated look or cut section presents fleshy to sinusoidal appearance	Cuts with soft feel—resembling cutting of brain tissue, or very soft cake areas of necrosis and haemorrhage with cyst formation; necrotic lamellae (cf. osteomyelitis.)	Presents localised or multiple honey-combed appearance. In one variety known as chloroma, cut surface turns green (due to a pigment), which gradually fades off	Cuts with gritty sensation. Multiloculated maroon coloured cut surface	Cuts with gritty sensation, cut surfaces present look mimicing the primary growth
16.	Histological examination a. Dominant cells (mostly seen in peripheral zone)	Most frequently seen cells are small spindle shaped with hyperchromatic nuclei. Pleomorphism—cells may be polyhexoid, round, cuboidal or columnar, variously arranged in—band, pallisade, columns; multinucleated giant cells, even osteoclast type of cells	Markedly cellular, almost no intercellular substance, Cells—round or polyhedral, uniform cytoplasm, indistinct in appearance (cellular monotony), arranged in cords or sheets, may be arranged around central blood vessels/spaces giving angioendotheliomatous appearance—pseudorosette (cf. in true rosette, cells arranged around central core of neurofibrils), nuclei—prominent and round	Cellular tumour. Plasma cells with abundant cytoplasm, and eccentrically placed nucleus, i.e. typical cart-wheel nucleus, with abnormal features (no perinuclear halo, and polychrome methylene blue stain negative)	Histological grading (I, II, and III) of not much value unless, biopsy material obtained from different sites. Dominant cells—oval shaped stromal cells containing small, elongated darky stained nucleus, stroma cells may manifest features of malignancy. *Osteoclastomatous giant cells* with multiple centrally placed nuclei, may be even 100 in number. (cf. In tuberculosis—in *Langhan's giant cell,* nuclei are peripheraly arranged, about 20 in numbers; in *foreign body giant cell*—usually less than 15 centrally placed variously sized nuclei)	Similar to parent growth
	b. Matrix	In osteosclerotic type—extensive irregular new osteoid and bone with few stromal cell. In osteolytic type—blood containing spaces without endothelial lining lying in anaplastic stromal and necrotic cystic areas. Usually scanty may be myxomatous, cartilaginous, osteoid, fibromatous.	Almost no matrix	Almost no matrix	Scanty, fibrous tissue	

Contd.

Table 17.3: Contd.

	1	*Primary osteosarcoma* 2	*Ewing's sarcoma* 3	*Multiple myeloma* 4	*Giant cell tumour* 5	*Secondary growth* 6
	c. Vascular pattern	Blood vessels are numerous and thin walled, may be lined with cells.		—	Mild or moderate	—
17.	Special features if any		Rosette arrangement pseudo-rosette are common, osteoclasts never found.	—	—	—
18.	Mode of metastasis	Direct to surrounding soft tissues. Along medullary canal Lymphatics Blood vessels—emboli Skip metastasis—direct along the medullary canal	Direct along medullary canal, Via lymphatics—lymph nodes; Via blood vessels—to other bones (skull, vertebrae, ribs), lung	Through blood vessels principally to other bones; to internal organs like liver, spleen, almost never to lungs	Direct to surrounding tissue, also through blood vessels, lymphatics	—
19.	Radio-sensitivity	Radio resistant in average doses, may respond to higher doses.	Highly radiosensitive, but reappears soon after	With irradiation tumour responds markedly but reappears.	Moderately sensitive	As primary tumour
20.	Complication	Huge growth, pathological fracture, metastasis, malignant cachexia.	Distant metastasis, cachexia, pathological fracture	Anaemia, bacterial infection, paraplegia, pathological fracture, renal damage, amyloidosis in 10% cases	Joint affection, frank malignant transformation, (about 10%), pathological fracture	Pathological fracture, pressure symptoms
21.	Chemotherapeutic sensitivity	Definite role Multiagent chemotherapy—methotrexate in high doses, doxorubicin and cisplatin. More recent protocols include iphosphamide with or without etoposide.	Successful regimen have used combinations of vincristine, actinomycin D, doxorubicin and cyclophosphamide	Chemotherapy by melphalan (alone or with prednisolone) and cyclophosphamide has increased survival rate	Nothing specific	As primary growth
22.	Special investigation	As in chapter of Introduction Alkaline phosphatase—raised	As in chapter on Introduction To distinguish from reticulum cell sarcoma—PAS positive diastase soluble glycogen granules in cytoplasm of cells of Ewing's sarcoma	Serum calcium raised, hyperproteinaemia (serum protein rising to 10 gm/liter, or higher). Distorted serum electrophoretic pattern with marked inversion of albumin/globulin ratio. Demonstration of monoclonal paraproteinaemia. Low normal alkaline phosphatase in spite of bony destruction. In 5% of cases—Bence Jones protein in urine (this is also seen in leukaemia, skeletal carcinomatosis, nephritis). Red cells-rouleaux formation in blood and in marrow ESR high	Acid phosphatase raised	Estimation of acid phosphatase or alkaline phosphatase. Increased acid phosphatase usually seen in secondaries from prostate.

Contd.

Table 17.3: Contd.

	1	Primary osteosarcoma 2	Ewing's sarcoma 3	Multiple myeloma 4	Giant cell tumour 5	Secondary growth 6
23.	Survival rate (more than 5 years)	Patients with localised osteosarcoma with adequate chemotherapy—50 to 76%. Patients with metastatic lesions—excision of primary tumour + wedge ressection of lung lesions + chemotherapy—20 to 40%.	Multimodal therapy (Intensive combination of chemotherapy + radiotherapy) of non-pelvic Ewing's sarcoma —50 to 70%	Variable (2-10 years). Bad prognostic features: Raised serum protein more than 10 gm/liter; Bence Jones proteinuria; Involvement of vertebrae, kidney; severe anaemia; severe reversal of AG ratio	Of all the malignancies of the bone, this has the best prognosis	Depending upon nature of primary growth but usually less than 10%
24.	Differential diagnosis	Among the primary and secondary malignant bone tumours. Subacute and chronic osteomyelitis; synovioma	Neuroblastoma (vanillyl mandelic acid in urine) VMA. Reticulum cell sarcoma (silver stain positive reticular fibres)	Unexplained anaemias; Polycystic disease of bone in elderly; senile osteoporosis; secondary carcinoma	Earlier cystic lesions of bones; lesions containing tumour giant cell	
25.	Surgery	—Disarticulation —Amputation (being favoured based upon concept of tumour immunity) —Resection with reconstruction/endoprosthesis —Resection of metastatic lesion (lobectomy in lung) —Limb preservation surgery (rotationplasty)	Radiotherapy followed by resection and reconstruction in very early case (still prognosis poor)	Only for complications, e.g. for pathological fractures; paraplegia	—Thorough curettage with or without filling with acrylic cement or bone grafting. Recurrence is about 35% within 2 yrs. Excision of growth with or without reconstruction or fusion of the neighbouring joint; or endoprosthetic replacement. —Amputation. —Cryosurgery (curettage + liquid nitrogen cryotherapy)	Total excision with or without reconstruction and replacement can prolong comparatively comfortable life under cover of radiotherapy, hormonal therapy and chemotherapy
26.	Radiotherapy	—Only for inaccessible or inoperable lesion. To be given in higher doses	Tumour almost dissolves with radiotherapy but recurrence is the rule	Mainly palliative	Only for inaccessible region and unoperable lesions, e.g. vertebrae.	Depending upon nature of primary tumour.
27.	Possible ideal treatment.	Neoadjuvant (pre-operative induction of chemotherapy) multiagent chemotherapy with limb preservation surgery	Trials of multimodal therapy consisting of intensive combination chemotherapy and radiotherapy	Chemotherapy, palliative irradiation	Excision and reconstruction	Treatment of the primary growth, radiotherapy for secondaries, and suitable chemotherapy
28.	Any genetic relation	Price (1958) noted significant similarity between osteochondroma and osteogenic sarcoma regarding male predominance, peak incidence between 15-20 years, and anatomical distribution. This is of interest because of hereditary background shown by osteochondroma.	Nothing particular	Nothing particular	Nothing particular	In recent years there has been significant improvement in the prognosis of patients with bone metastasis, mainly due to advances in chemotherapy and hormonal treatment. Postoperative radiotherapy should be considered in all cases once initial wound healing occurs after reconstructive surgery

Contd.

Table 17.3: Contd.

	1	*Primary osteosarcoma* *2*	*Ewing's sarcoma* *3*	*Multiple myeloma* *4*	*Giant cell tumour* *5*	*Secondary growth* *6*
29.	Subclassification	Aetiological: 1. Primary osteosarcoma 2. Secondary osteosarcoma on: • Paget's disease • Osteochondroma • Chronic osteomyelitis • Post-irradiation osteosarcoma in ankylosing spondylitis				
30.	Immunotherapy	Immunological approach for managing lethal metastasis is still in experimental stage. Osteosarcoma has been shown to possess specific tumour associated antigens.				

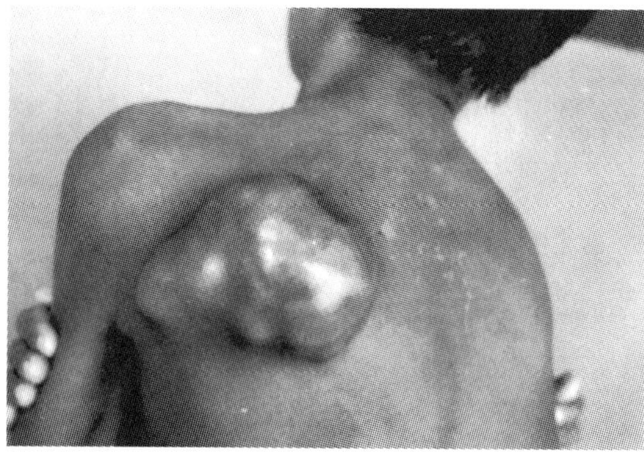

Fig. 17.2A: Osteochondroma of scapula producing mechanical disability in lying down

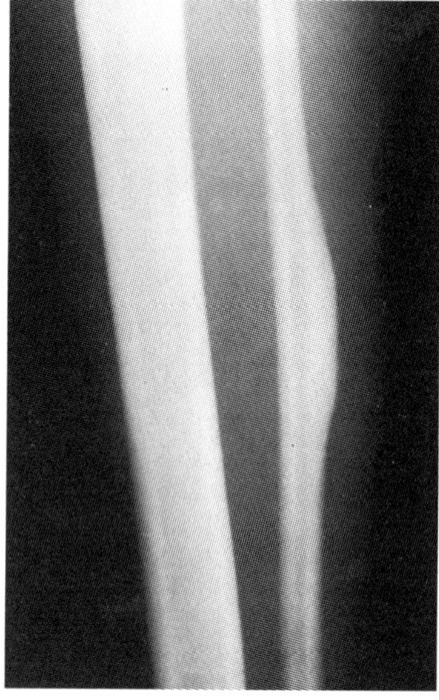

Fig. 17.2B: Osteoid osteoma from fibula

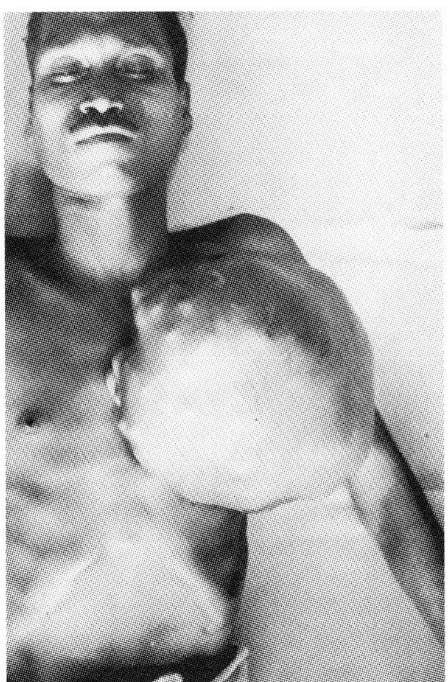

Fig. 17.3A: A giant osteochondroma from left second rib

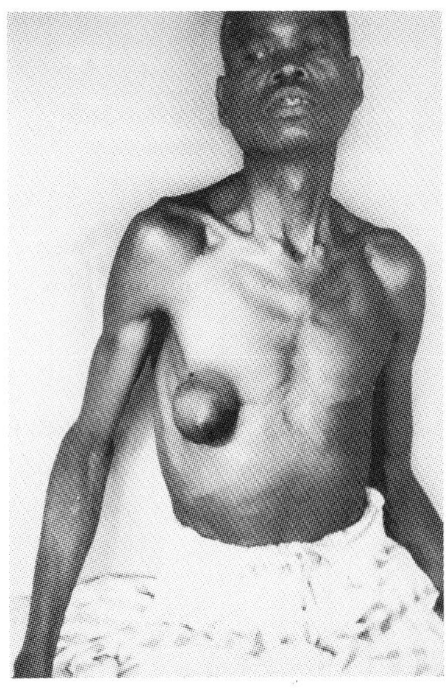

Fig. 17.3C: Ball like osteochondroma from right ninth rib

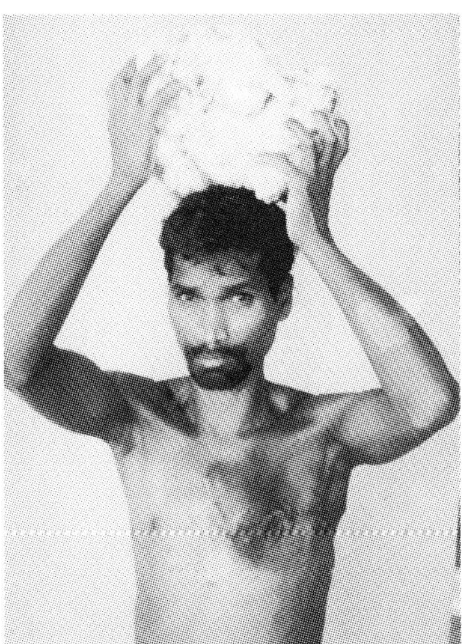

Fig. 17.3B: Same patient with the growth on his head after its removal (9.5 kg). Note the cut end of rib pointed by the patient s left ring finger

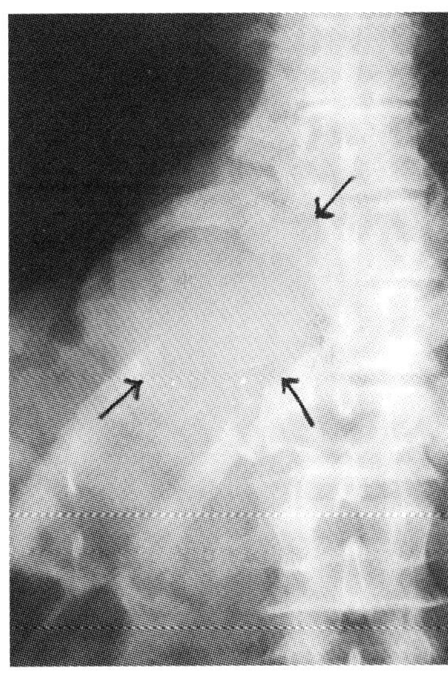

Fig. 17.4: Haemangioma of vertebrae extending into the ribs

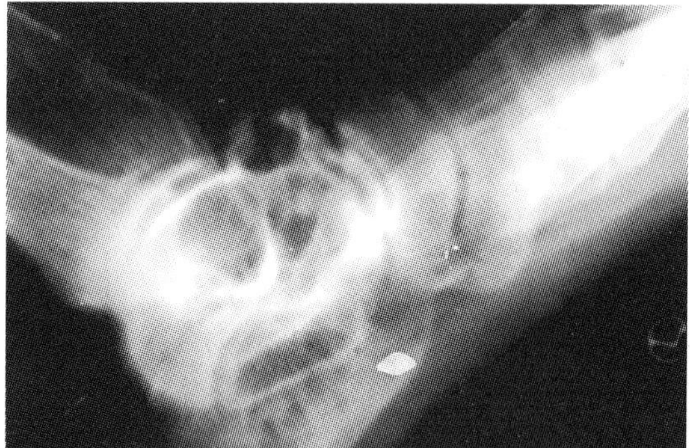

Fig. 17.5A: Giant cell tumour in talus

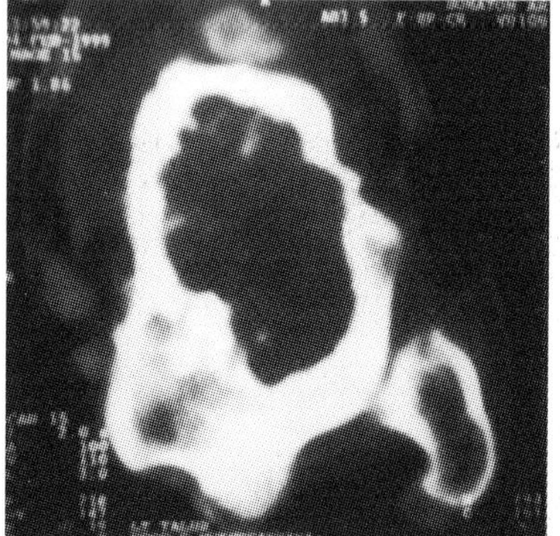

Fig. 17.5B: CT scan of the same patient with giant cell tumour of the talus

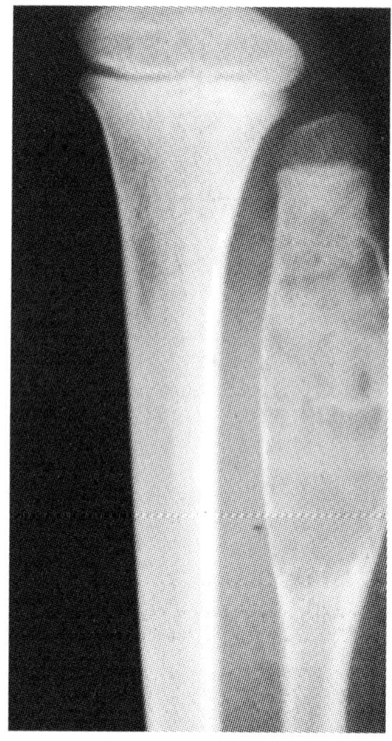

Fig. 17.5D: Fibrous dysplasia from upper end of fibula

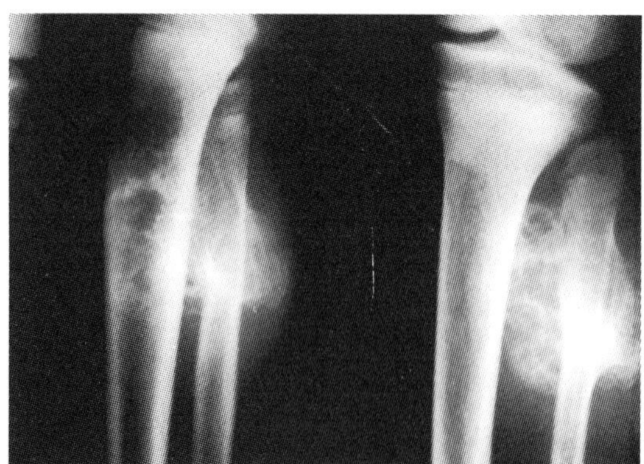

Fig. 17.5C: Solitary exostosis (osteochondroma) from upper end of fibula producing mechanical pressure leading to paralysis of lateral popliteal nerve

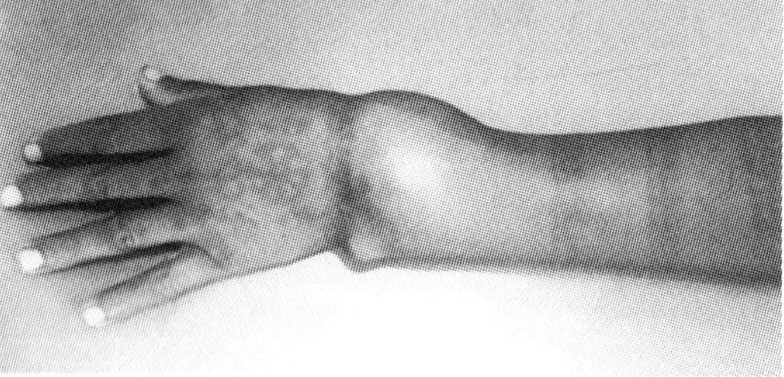

Fig. 17.6: Typical giant cell tumour of lower end of radius—eccentric growth

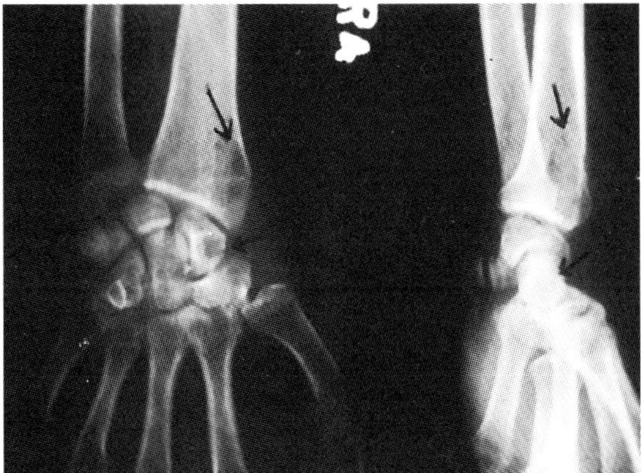

Fig. 17.7: X-ray of wrist region showing early giant cell tumour of lower end of radius

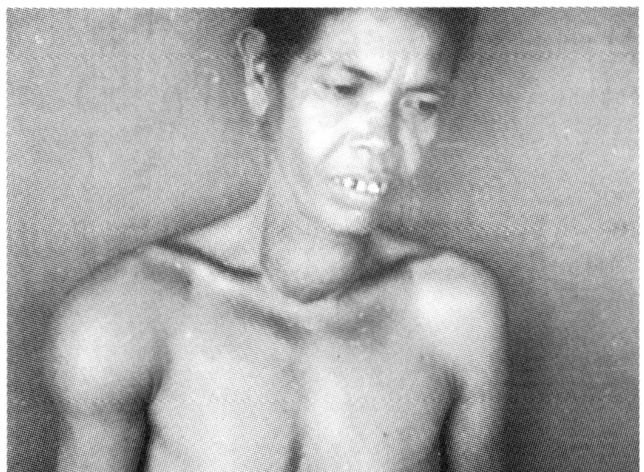

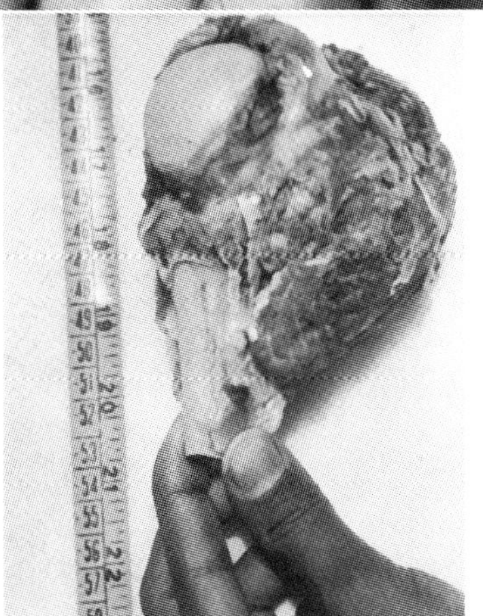

Figs 17.8A and B

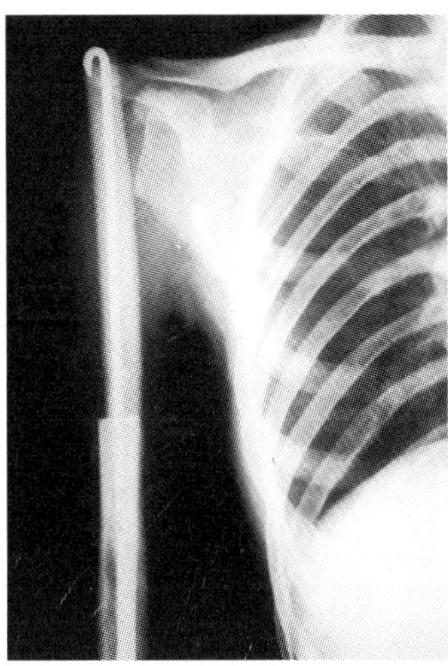

Figs 17.8A to C: (A) Malignant giant cell tumour from upper end of humerus (B) The growth was totally excised with the upper 2/5th of humerus and the deficiency of the humerus was reconstructed by the ipsilateral fibula (Fig. 17.8C)

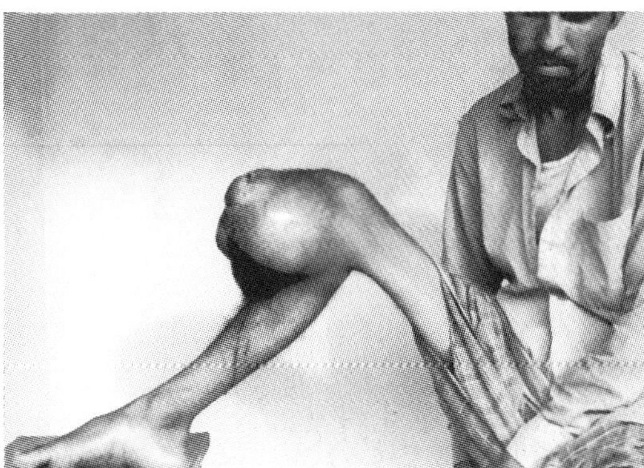

Fig. 17.9A: Huge giant cell tumour from upper end of tibia producing triple deformity of knee joint. Indigenous cauterisation produced ulcers over the growth

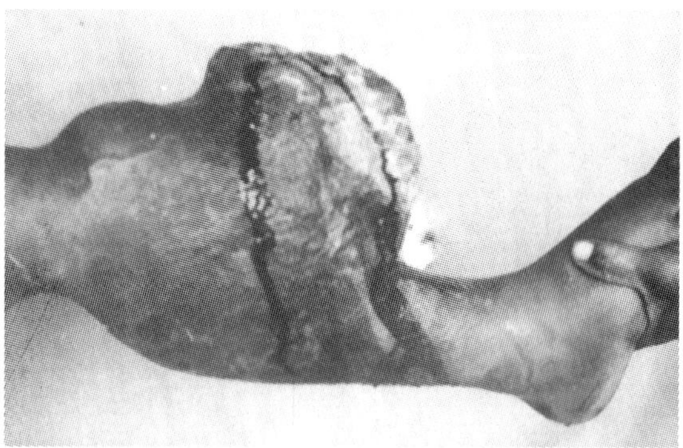

Fig. 17.9B: Fungating huge osteosarcoma giant cell tumour from upper end of tibia history of some local chemical application

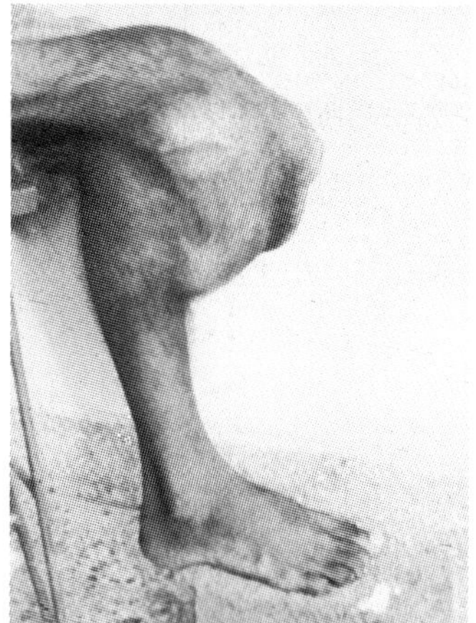

Fig. 17.9C: Chondrosarcoma arising from solitary exostosis from upper end of tibia

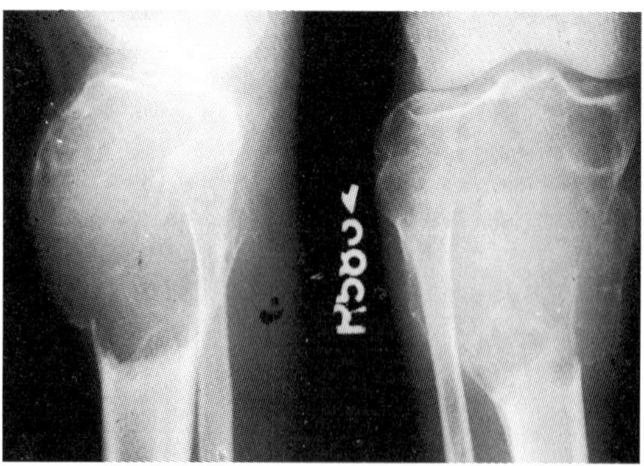

Fig. 17.10: Invasive giant cell tumour from upper end of tibia with pathological fracture

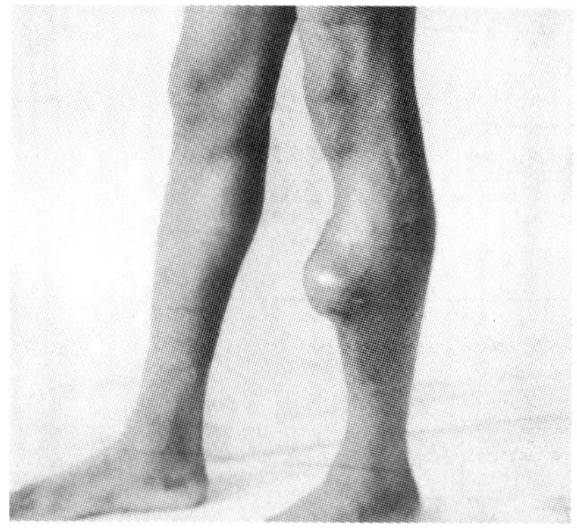

Fig. 17.11: Adamantinoma of tibia, a rare tumour from inclusion tissues

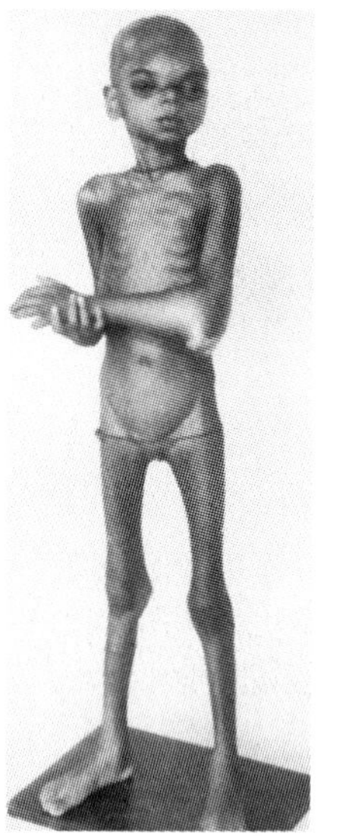

Figs 17.12A and B: Multifocal lymphoma affecting skull, clavicle, elbow region, right ankle. One at elbow ulcerated due to indigenous application

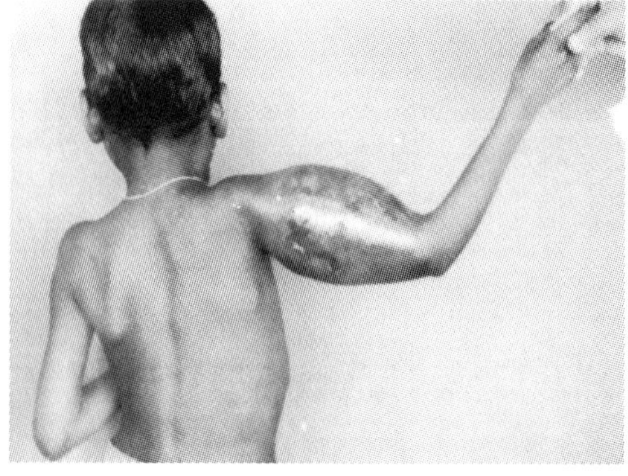

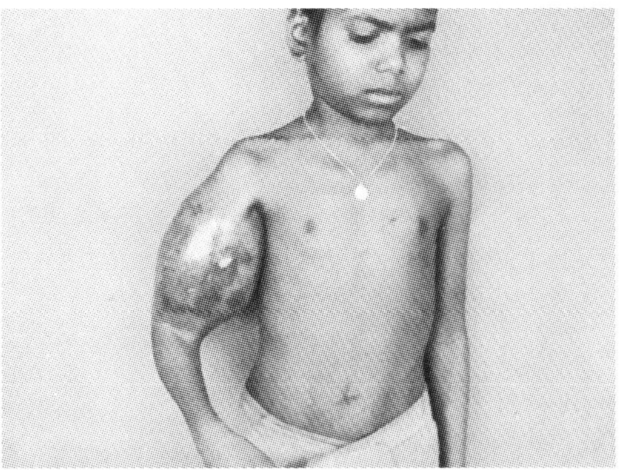

Fig. 17.13B: Haemangio-endothelioma of humerus (front view)

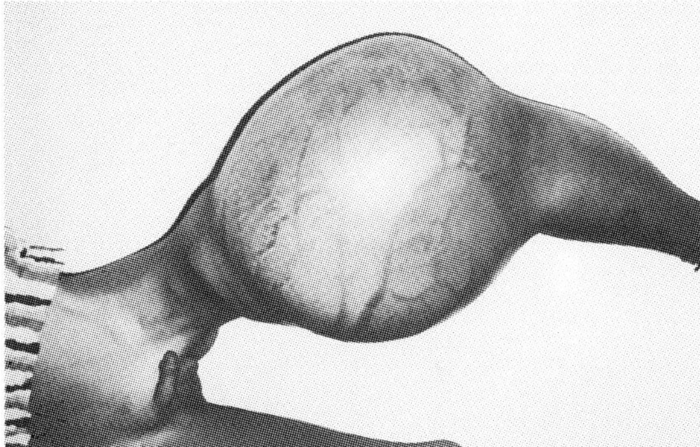

Fig. 17.14: Osteosarcoma from lower end of femur in a boy aged 5 years. Note size of growth and vascular prominence

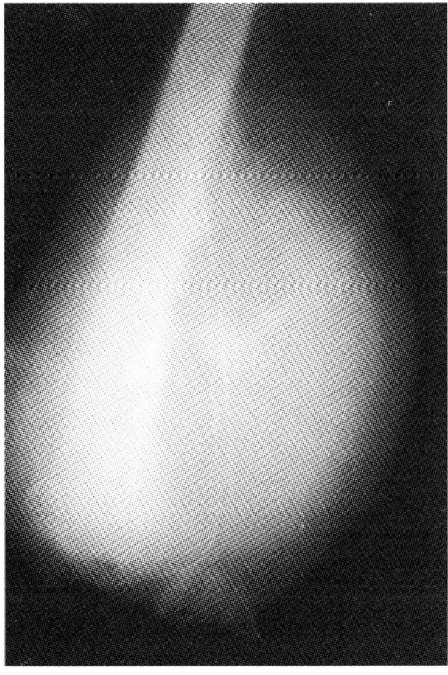

Fig. 17.15: Osteosarcoma of lower end of femur

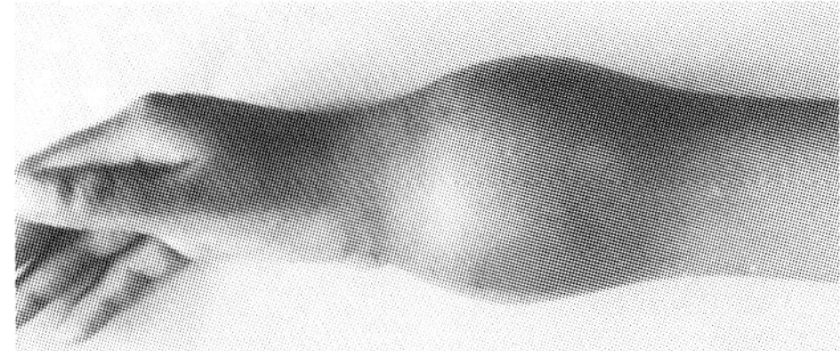

Fig. 17.16: Osteosarcoma of lower end of radius fusiform growth (cf. giant cell tumour with eccentric growth)

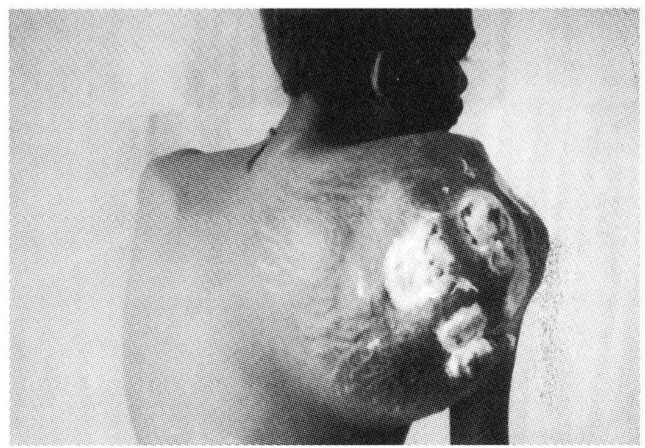

Fig. 17.17: Osteosarcoma from scapula with fungations due to some indigenous applications

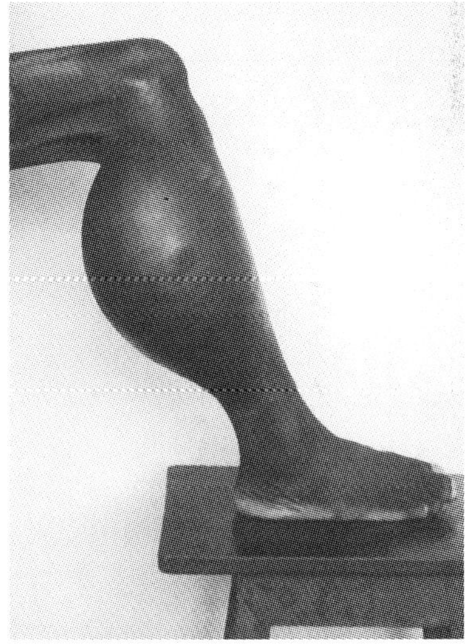

Fig. 17.18: Huge soft tissue growth from upper calf (rhabdomyosarcoma) mimicking osteosarcoma of fibula

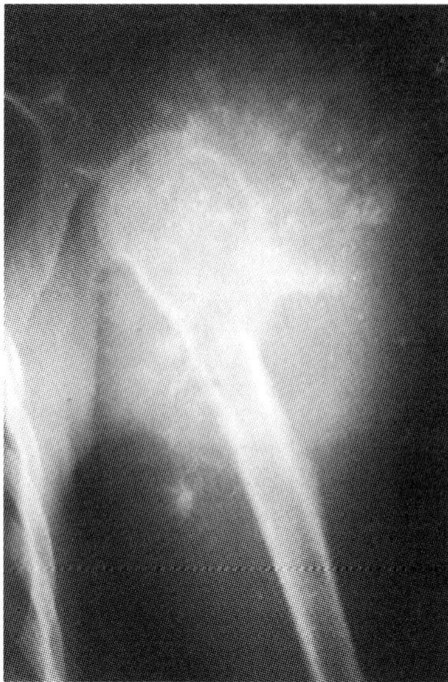

Fig. 17.19: Chondrosarcoma from upper end of humerus

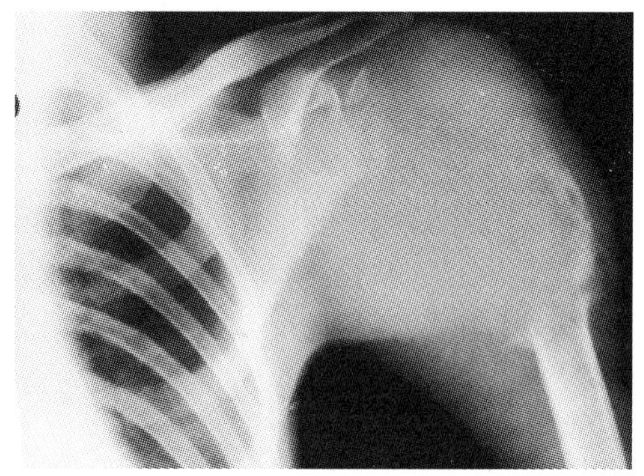

Fig. 17.20: Osteosarcoma from upper end of humerus

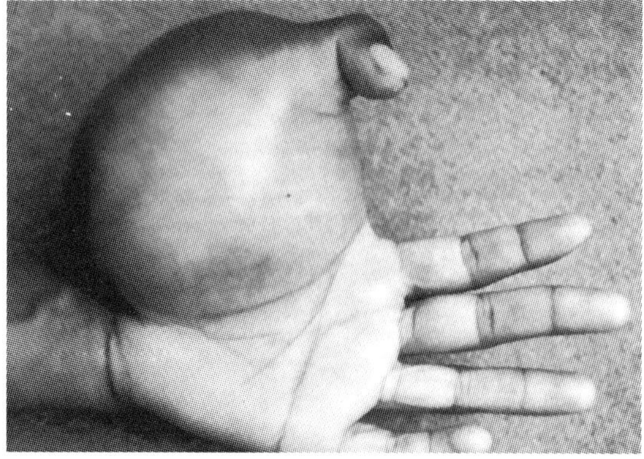

Fig. 17.21: Clinical photogaph (palmar aspect)—Osteosarcoma from first metacarpal

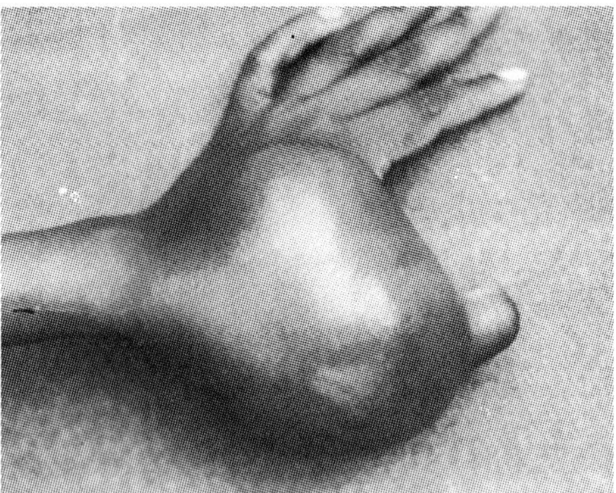

Fig. 17.22: Clinical photograph (dorsal aspect)—Osteosarcoma from first metacarpal

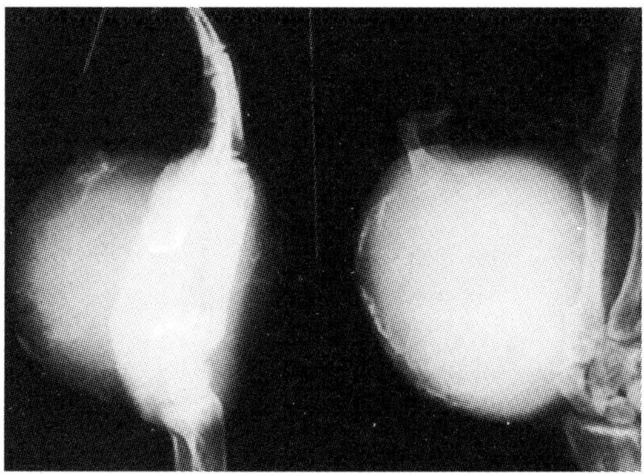

Fig. 17.23: X-ray of same patient (Figs 17.21 and 17.22)

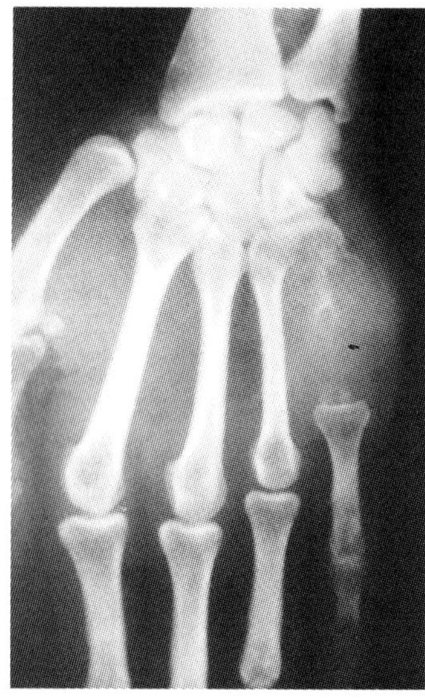

Fig. 17.24: Ewing's sarcoma from fifth metacarpal

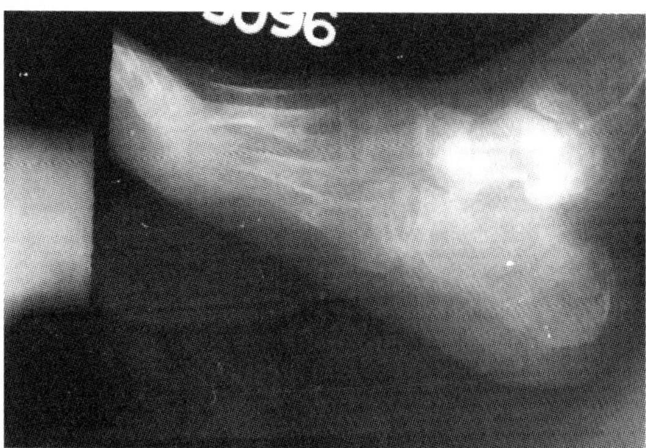

Fig. 17.25A: Ewing's sarcoma of talus

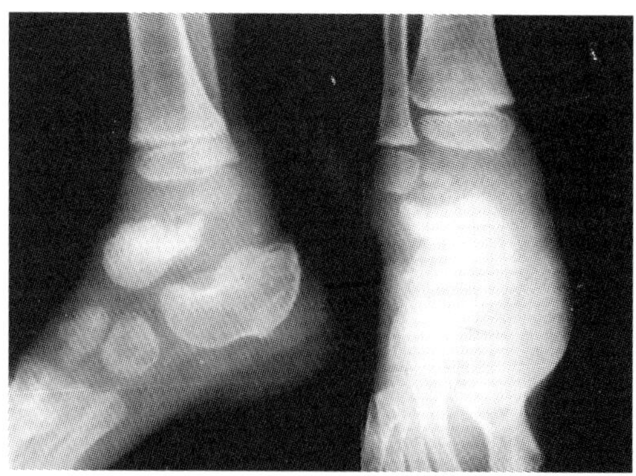

Fig. 17.25B: Pyogenic arthritis of ankle with osteomyelitis of talus

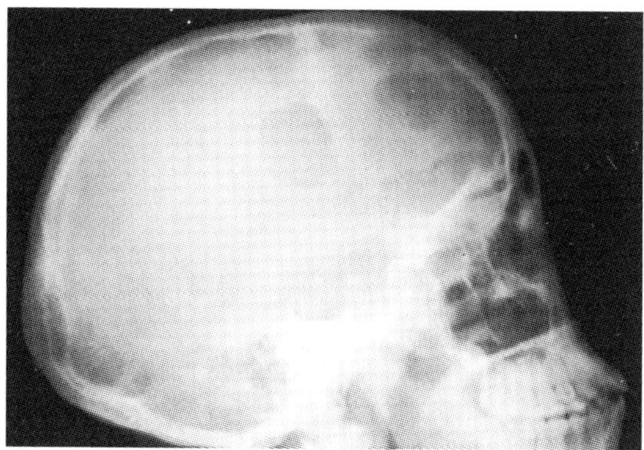

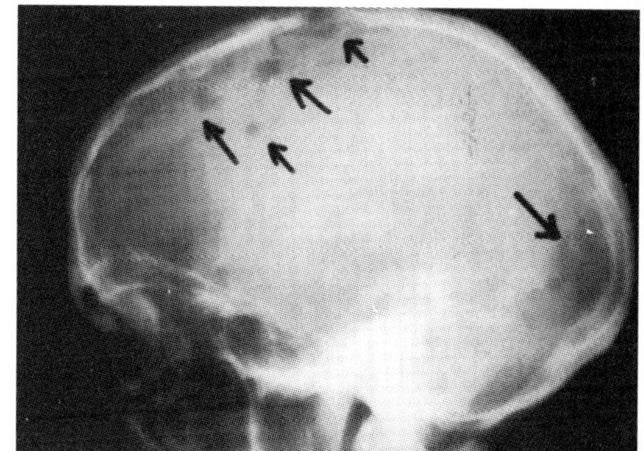

Figs 17.26A and B: Multiple myeloma

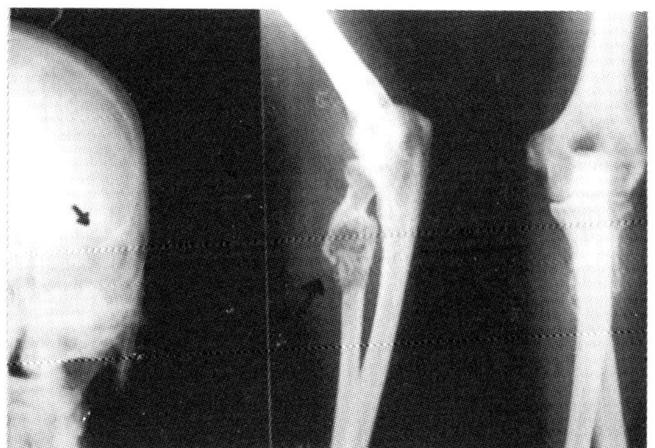

Fig. 17.27: Multiple myeloma in upper end of radial shaft with pathologial fracture and lesions also in skull

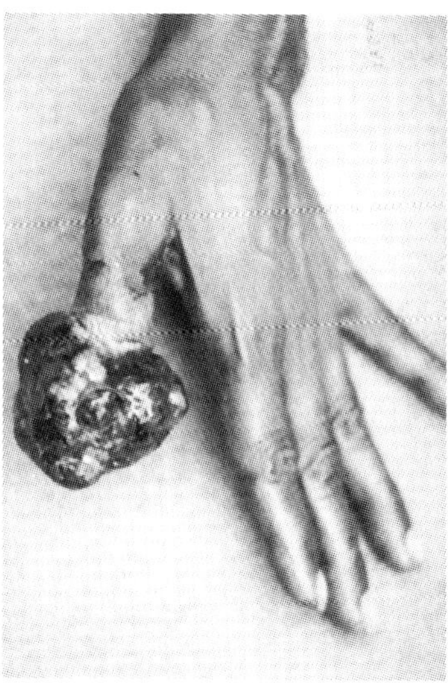

Fig. 17.28: Melanoma from thumb

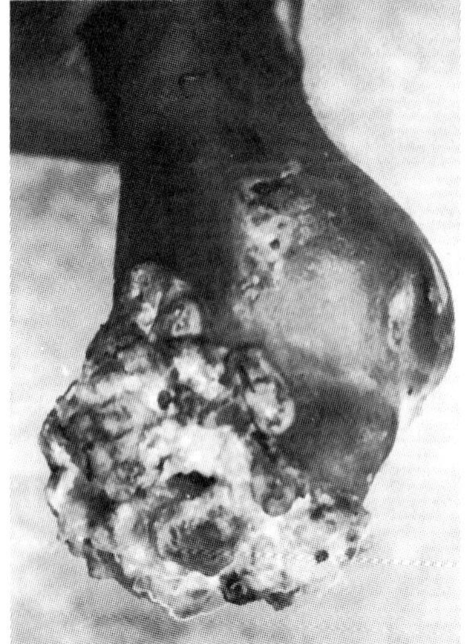

Fig. 17.29: Melanoma from foot

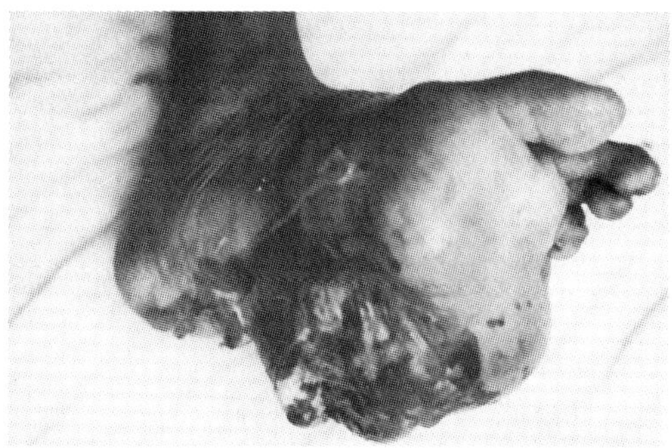

Fig. 17.30: Melanoma from sole

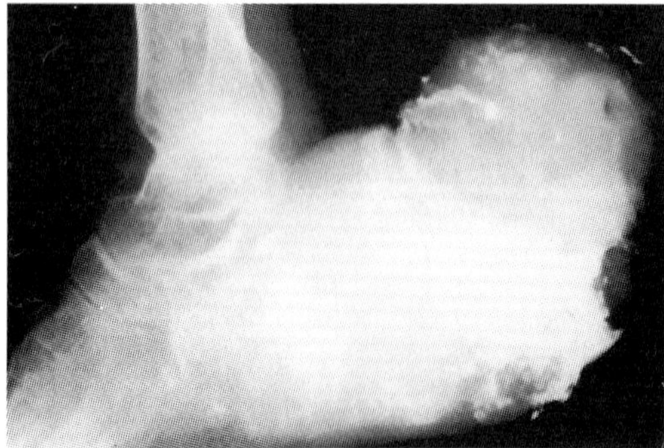

Fig. 17.30A: Melanoma of heel (calcaneum)

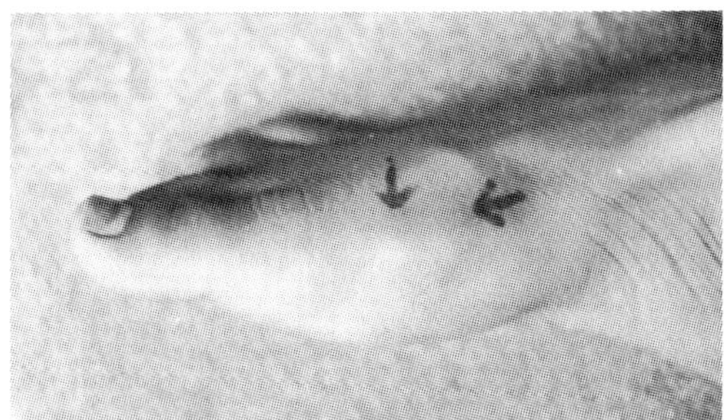

Fig. 17.31: Synovioma from tibialis anterior tendon sheath

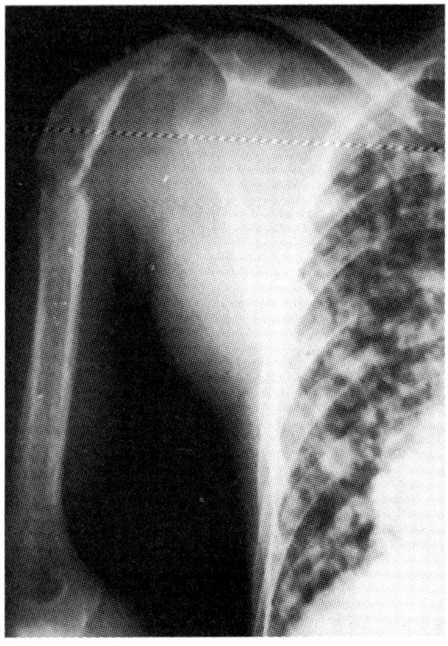

Fig. 17.32A: Metastatic carcinoma in upper end of humerus (with pathological fracture) and carcinomatosis lung

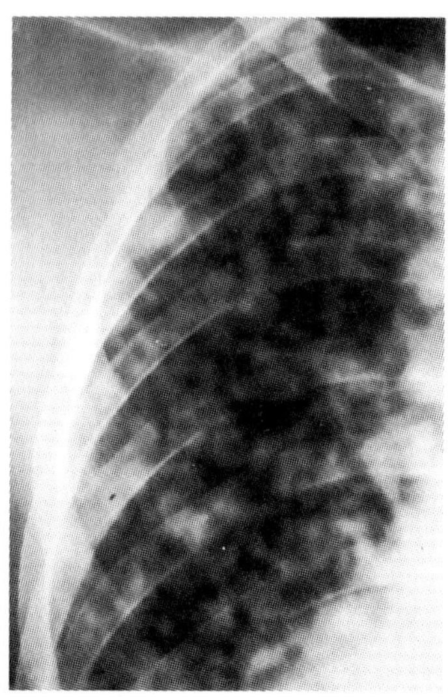

Fig. 17.32B: Carcinomatous lung

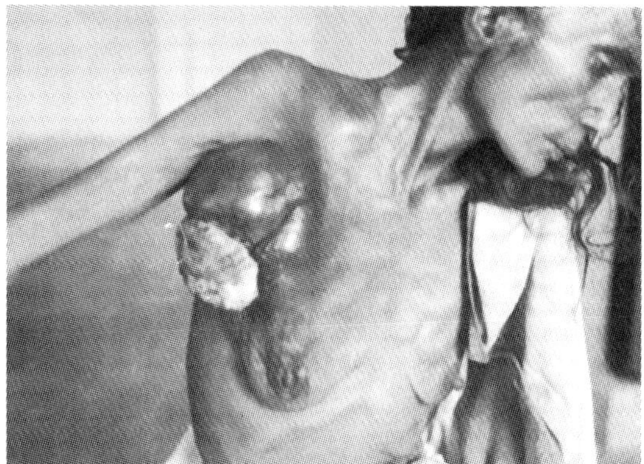

Fig. 17.33: Fungating carcinoma from axillary gland

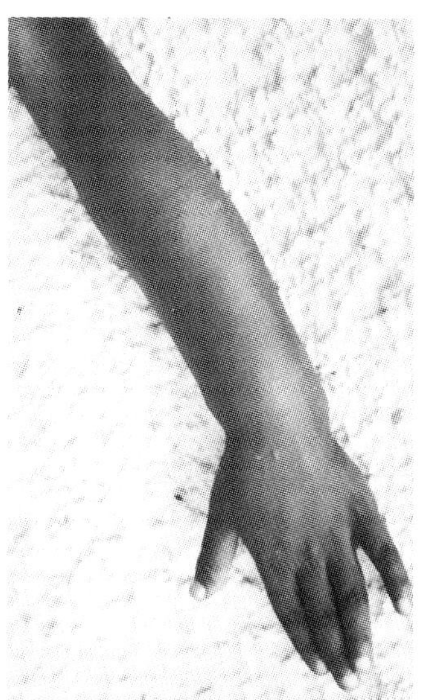

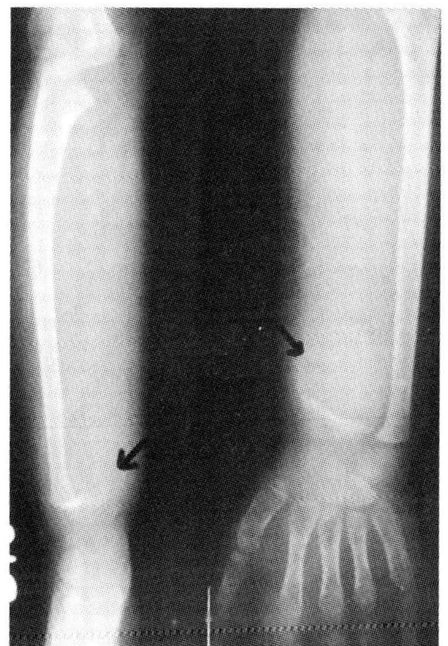

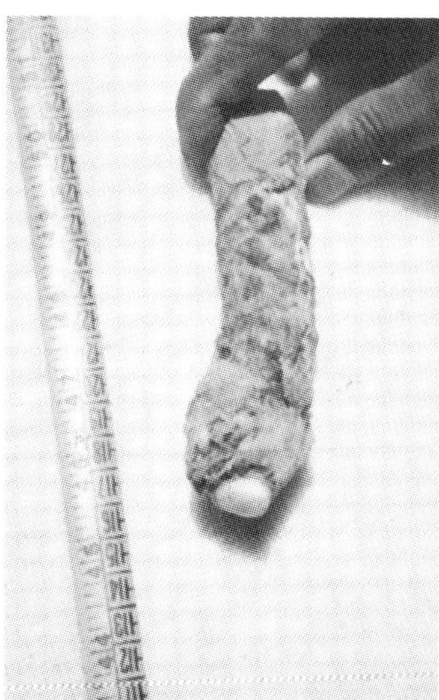

Bone dissolving disease in a boy aged 6 years (Gorham-Stout syndrome

Fig. 17.34A: Note the swelling of the forearm

Fig. 17.34B: X-ray of same patient. Note almost complete dissolution of radius, except little bone at the lower end

Fig. 17.34C: Specimen; of the totally removed radius (and reconstructed with fibula) which histologically showed markedly vascularised fibrous tissue

BIBLIOGRAPHY

1. American Joint Committee on Cancer Bone. In ID Feming, J Copper, DE Henson *et al* (Eds). *AJCC Cancer Staging Manual* (5 edn) Philadelphia: Lippincott-Raven, 143-47, 1997.
2. Enneking WF, Spanier SS, Goodman MA: A system for the surgical staging of musculoskeletal sarcoma. *Clin Orthop* **153**: 106, 1980.
3. Enneking WF: Staging musculoskeletal tumors. In WF Enneking (Ed): *Musculoskeletal Tumor Surg* New York: Churchill Livingston, 87-88, 1983.
4. Pandey S, Pandey AK: Osseous haemangiomas. *Arch Orthop Traumat Surg* **99**: 23-28, 1981.
5. Pandey S: Ewing's sarcoma of the third metacarpal. *Int Surg* **57**: 984-85, 1972.
6. Pandey S: Ewing's tumour of talus. *J Bone Joint Surg* **52-A**: 1672-73, 1970.
7. Pandey S: Giant cell tumour of talus. *Int Surg* **55-3**: 179-82, 1971.
8. Pandey S: Giant chondromas arising from the ribs. *J Bone Joint Surg* **57B**: 519-25, 1975.
9. Pandey S: *Intraosseous haemangioma.* Abst Book SICOT, Japan: Kyoto, 1978.
10. Pandey S: Pulsatile skeletal metastasis from thyroid carcinoma. *Int Surg* **53-1**: 62-64, 1970.
11. Pandey S: Voluminous osteochondroma of the second rib. *Int Surg* **56-6**: 419-21, 1971.

18

Mandible and Temporomandibular Joint

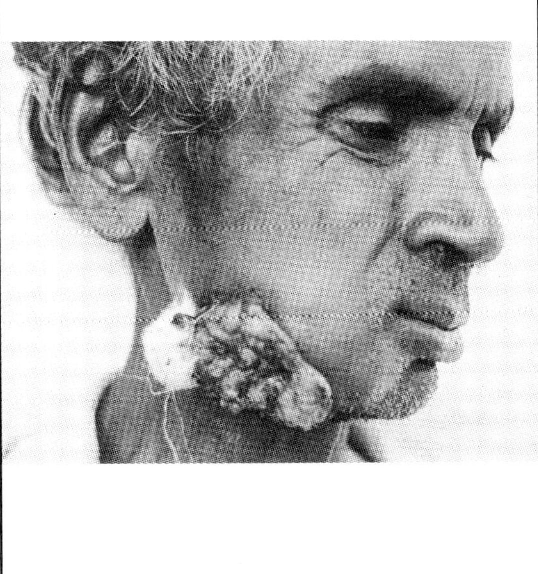

INTRODUCTION

Ideally, the temporomandibular joint should fall in the domain of an orthopaedic and facio-maxillary surgeons. However, an orthopaedic surgeon primarily comes in the picture for managing traumatic, congenital, and other acquired pathologies of the temporomandibular joint.

ANATOMICAL CONSIDERATIONS

i. The temporomandibular joint is the articulation between the articular tubercle and the anterior portion of the mandibular fossa of the temporal bone above and the condyle of the mandible below. A fibrous articular disc divides the joint into an upper and a lower part. As such the condyle and disc move together during retraction and protraction of the mandible. Derangement of this articular disc may result in clicking and pain on jaw movements (e.g. in various trauma, over-grinding).
ii. The disposition of the temporomandibular joint (a condylar joint) is such that the condyloid process of the mandible is at a disadvantageous position. In fact, when the mouth is open, the mandibular condyles sit almost on the watershed, i.e. articular eminences. In this mechanically disadvantageous position any sudden violence (even muscular spasm or yawning) may thrust one or both condyles into the infra-temporal fossa.
iii. The mandible at the temporomandibular joint remains almost suspended through muscular and facial attachments. Though the joints are quite small, the joint space more or less, always remains maintained due to the passive distractive force of gravity. Still, ankylosis is perhaps the most common pathology, which involves this joint. Of course, in most of the cases, the causes are in the soft tissues in and around the joint.
iv. Both temporomandibular joints act in harmony, forming together a bicondylar arrangement. Therefore, affection of one

joint is bound to affect the function of the other.

v. The main function of the temporomandibular joint is for mastication. Secondarily, they help in articulation, phonation, and certain facial expressions.

Muscles of mastication—Main muscles are (i) Temporalis, (ii) Masseter, (iii) Lateral pterygoids, (iv) Medial pterygoids. Assisted by: (i) Digastric, (ii) Mylohyoid, (iii) Omohyoid, (iv) Stylohyoid, (v) Sternohyoid, (vi) Thyrohyoid.

OSSIFICATION OF MANDIBLE

Mandible is ossified in dense membranous tissue. Each half develops from one centre appearing at the sixth week of intrauterine life. The mandible is the second bone to ossify in the body, first being clavicle.

ANATOMICAL LANDMARK OF TEMPOROMANDIBULAR JOINT

Just in front of and slightly above the tragus, the transverse slit of the temporomandibular joint can be felt. Put your index finger tip over this slit and ask the patient to open and close the mouth repeatedly. Movements of the condyloid process of mandible can be felt under the finger tip.

METHODOLOGY

History

Besides taking history in the usual way, few important points to be enquired about are—(i) Biting any hard/tough stuff, (ii) Malocclusion, (iii) Any history of discharge (blood tinged, serous, black grain and/or pus) from gums or buccal region, (iv) Any discharge from ear, (v) History of infection (intra/periarticular) in that region, (vi) Past history of tetanus with prolonged illness.

General and systemic examinations: As in the chapter on Introduction (special reference to speech, swallowing, dribbling of saliva).

Regional examination: It includes examination of cranial nerves, cervical spine, different groups of cervical lymph nodes, examination of the throat (naso-oropharynx) and examination of the ear (external auditory meatus may be fractured in temporomandibular injury; middle ear infection can cause pain and ankylosis of the joint).

Local Examination

Attitude: Certain peculiar attitudes of the lower jaw can indicate certain pathologies at the temporomandibular joint.

Certain Fixed Attitudes

i. A retracted or small chin with shrunken lower cheeks, assuming more or less a triangular shape with an imaginary line joining temporomandibular joints, indicates *micrognathia* (hypoplasia); congenital bilateral ankylosis of temporomandibular joint; symmetrically underdeveloped chin can be associated with cleft palate and breathing problems (Pierre Robin Syndrome); *Agnathia* (absence of mandible); *Prognathism* (hyperplasia of mandible)—commonly symmetrical and manifests in late childhood—chin and lip protruded with dental malocclusion.

ii. Asymmetric shape of mandible, more or less in one half, with chin deviated to one side indicates unilateral temporomandibular ankylosis (a very rare congenital condition).

iii. Protracted chin with massive body of mandible, thick and extruded lower lip, broad lower jaw, wider lower face, more or less quadrangular shape of lower jaw (lantern jaw)—indicates *acromegalic jaw* (hyperpituitarism).

iv. Partially opened up mouth, protracted chin, lower lip at a level distal to that of the upper, patient unable to close the mouth, difficulty in speaking clearly, any passive attempt of closing mouth causing marked pain at temporomandibular joints—indicates bilateral dislocation of temporomandibular joints.

v. Mouth partially opened up, more on the opposite side, chin deviated to the opposite side, angle of mandible at a higher level on the side of affection; difficulty in articulation, passive attempts at closure causing pain in the affected temporomandibular joint indicates unilateral dislocation of the temporomandibular joint.

vi. Post-burn contractures at the neck cause pulling down of the lower jaw with or without subluxation at the temporomandibular joints. Facial burn contractures affect the facial symmetry and may lead to ankylosis of the temporomandibular joint. The attitude of the chin, rather the lower jaw, will vary as a whole according to the contracture.

Inspection

Look for the symmetry of the zygomatic processes. At the posteroinferior end of the zygomatic process, a shallow depression in seen. This should be symmetrical on both sides. Any fullness in this area may be due to some pathology of the temporomandibular joint or overlying tissues. Fullness below this region is due to parotid affection. The parotid swellings may also encroach below and behind the lobules of the ears.

Any abnormality in the skin condition, shape and size of mandible and any swelling in its relations should be noted. Certain peculiar attitudes of the lower jaw (as described earlier) usually indicates some pathology at the temporomandibular joint.

Large glandular enlargements in posterior digastric fossa or behind the ear, if present, may be obvious on inspection.

Inspection through Buccal Cavity

i. Look for the number and inter-dental relations of the teeth on the lower jaw and their interrelations with their counterparts on the upper jaw. In case of fracture—displacement of the jaw bones, the disturbed relation in the level of the teeth is an important finding.

ii. Ask the patient to clench the teeth—normally the teeth should sit on their counterparts. Note any asymmetry in the relations of the teeth.

iii. Look at the relations of the teeth and gums. Any obvious space occupying lesion in gingivolabial fold should be clearly noted. Alongwith, also note its surface, vascularity, size, shape, relation to the corresponding tooth (present or missing).

iv. Any obvious infection in any tooth should be noted.

v. Look at the buccal mucosa. Normally it should look pink with a slight bluish tinge here and there due to venous channels. In the posterior part of the oral cavity the mucosa gives an impression of its more firm adherent relation as mucoperiosteum. Note for any change in colour and texture of the mucosa and periosteum.

In a very rare condition which may be called *'pale mucosal fibrosis'*, the mucosa becomes pale and tightly adherent to the underlying surface. The same pathology also spreads over the tonsillar pillars. Consequently, there is gradual extra-articular ankylosis of the temporomandibular joint. We have seen only four cases and all were females in their twenties/thirties.

Look for the symmetry of the tonsillar folds, tonsils, oropharynx, tongue, salivary ducts and sublingual surfaces and note any abnormality in the form of swelling, adhesions, puckering, discolouration, sinuses and abnormal discharge.

All fractures involving the teeth are compound within the mouth due to rupture of firmly attached mucoperiosteum. Subperiosteal haematoma, due to fracture of body of mandible, may present as a soft or cystic swelling in the floor of the mouth.

Palpation

Superficial palpation: Feel for texture, temperature and sensation of skin (affection of inferior dental nerve, usually in fracture of mandible, disturbs the sensation of lower lip).

Deep palpation: Temporomandibular joint can be palpated easily from outside than from inside. Both joints must be palpated simultaneously.

Method (Fig. 18.1): Stand behind the patient who is sitting on a stool, keeping her head erect as far as possible. With both thumbs, support the back of the head while both ring fingers gently rest at the angle of the mandibles to appreciate movements of the lower jaw, the tips of index fingers being kept in front of the tragus. The patient is asked to gently open and close the mouth. Your index fingers will appreciate the movements of the condyloid processes of the mandible with each movement of the jaw. Note the excursion of the movements by:

i. Appreciation of going down of jaw on your ring finger.
ii. Looking from the front, see the approximate gap created at the angles of the mouth. In the mid line note the maximum extent of opening up of the mouth by fingers-width assessment. Accurate measurement for prognostic value should be done by a graduated scale or graduated mouth blocks.

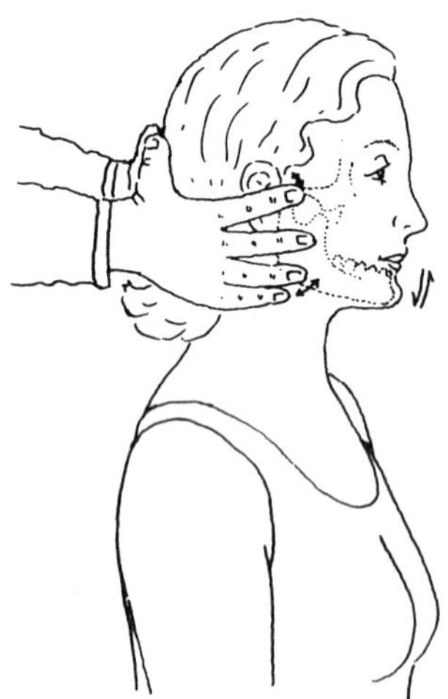

Fig. 18.1: Method of palpation of temporomandibular joint

The joint is felt as a transverse slit running anteroposteriorly below the posterior end of the zygomatic process. Note shape, size, regularity and any abnormal swelling or tenderness of the condyloid process.

Palpating the joint from the buccal cavity is neither easy nor much informative. However, putting one index finger through the mouth cavity along the line joining the angle of mouth to the tragus, and the other outside in front of the tragus, one can appreciate movements at the joint (only limited assessment is possible since the patient cannot close the mouth fully).

From inside, also palpate the gum, gingiolabial fold, palate, mucosa, sublingual region, salivary ducts and floor of the mouth, and note any abnormality.

Note pliability of the mucosa, any tenderness, any firm to hard structure in the salivary ducts (stone) and enlargement of salivary glands (usually sub-mandibular). Count the teeth and note any distortion, infection, or impaction of the tooth, specially in the molar region.

In case of trauma, palpate the mandible through the submandibular region for its contour, shape, size, any tenderness, crepitus, swelling, irregularity, and displacement of the fracture.

In case of any scar or sinus, palpate as in the chapter on Introduction.

MOVEMENTS (Table 18.1)

Anatomically, movements of the temporomandibular joint may be described as depression, elevation, protrusion, retraction and lateral rotating movements. The actual physio-mechanics, though, is not that simple, functional mandibular movements are actually the resultant of complex rhythmic movements of the aforesaid types. However, clinical assessment must be for individual anatomical movements.

Investigations

1. X-ray is the main investigation. For mandible posteroanterior, lateral, oblique and inferosuperior views are helpful. For

Table 18.1: Movements of temporomandibular joint

Movement	*Physiomechanics*	*Muscles involved in movement*	*Nerve supply*
Depression	When the mouth is open, head of mandible first rotates, then glides downwards and forwards with the lower surface of the articular disc	1. Lateral pterygoids assisted by Digastric 2. Omohyoids 3. Mylohyoids	Mandibular division of trigeminal nerve Trigeminal and facial nerve Hypoglossal nerve Trigeminal nerve
Elevation	In closure of the mouth, the head of the mandible glides upwards and backwards along with the articular disc back into the temporal fossa	1. Temporalis 2. Masseter 3. Medial pterygoids of both sides	Mandibular division of trigeminal nerve
Protrusion	Jaw remaining occluded, the lower teeth are drawn forward over the upper	Lateral and medial pterygoids	Mandibular division of trigeminal nerve
Retraction	Mandible is drawn backwards from protrusion to the position of rest	1. Temporalis assisted by middle and deep parts of Masseter, 2. Digastric 3. Geniohyoids	Mandibular division of trigeminal nerve Trigeminal and facial nerve. Hypoglossal nerve
Rotatory movements	In grinding or chewing the head of one side along with the corresponding disc glides forwards, rotates around a vertical axis and then glides backwards rotating in an opposite direction as the head of the opposite side comes forwards in its turn	Medial and lateral pterygoids of each side acting alternately	Mandibular division of trigeminal nerve

temporomandibular joints lateral, oblique and 35° fronto-occipital views are useful. However tomography may be very useful.

2. Aspiration from the distended temporomandibular joint may be useful to know and examine the nature of collection.

Key Diagnostic Points of Common Pathologies of the Mandible, Temporomandibular Joints, and Swellings of the Jaw

I. Disease

1. *Congenital*

Absence of lower jaw (agnathia).

— Hypoplasia or deficient development of lower jaw (micrognathia).

— Hyperplasia or over development of lower jaw (prognathism).

— Asymmetric development of lower jaw.

— Congenital ankylosis of temporomandibular joint (ankylosis develops during ossification of Schmidts parietal bone and is a rather rare condition).

2. *Ankylosis of Jaw* (Fig. 18.2)
   a. Congenital ankylosis—leads to deficient development of lower jaw.
   b. Acquired ankylosis—Usually follows:
      i. inflammatory lesions, e.g. septic arthritis, osteomyelitis, mumps, measles, scarlet fever, enteric fever, tetanus, rheumatic fever, otitis media, mastoiditis, parotitis, caries teeth, parotid stones, cancrum oris.
      ii. Collagen arthropathy—e.g. rheumatoid arthritis, ankylosing spondylitis.

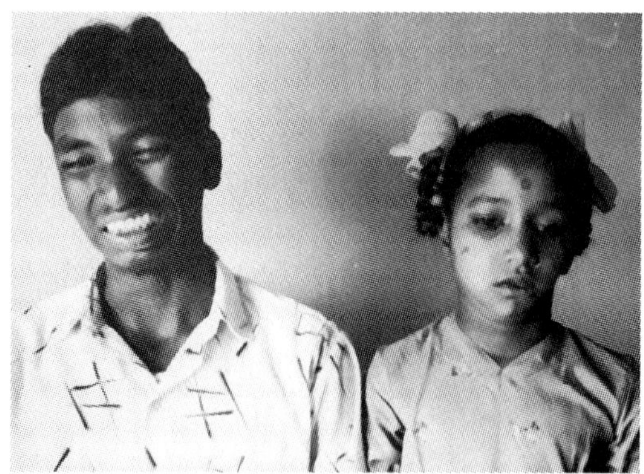

Fig. 18.2: Ankylosis of jaw: On the left acquired type; on the right congenital

iii. Traumatic—fractures of condyles, neck, ramus of mandible; subluxation, dislocation; fracture-dislocation; even strains and sprains have been seen to cause ankylosis to some extent.
iv. Neoplastic—malignant neoplasm of parotid gland, gums, jaw and ear may lead to ankylosis of jaw.
v. Miscellaneous—pale mucosal fibrosis, hysterical.

Ankylosis can otherwise be classified as:

i. Unilateral (often marked by asymmetry of face with the chin deviated to the side of ankylosis).
ii. Bilateral—congenital or acquired ankylosis in childhood leads to symmetrically retarded growth of the jaw. Inability to open the mouth results in bad oral hygiene and foul smell.

3. *Diseases Affecting the Temporomandibular Joint*

A. *Infective:*
  a. Following open injuries.
  b. Through haematogenous route (e.g. in rheumatic fever, tonsillitis, influenza).
  c. Spread from surrounding tissues (e.g. otitis media, osteomyelitis of mandibular process, parotid abscess).

B. *Arthrosis*—following:
  a. Involution.
  b. Developmental defects of jaws.
  c. Malocclusion of the teeth.
  d. Reduced occlusion of teeth.
  e. Improper prosthetic management following excisional surgery.
  f. Collagen arthropathy.

In arthrosis, symptoms are—

i. Articular—pain, crackling and clicking in the joint.
ii. Regional—pain, feeling of obstruction in nose and ears, tinnitus, glossalgia, pain in face and eyes, dryness of mouth, hearing defects, headache, etc.

II. Traumatic Conditions

i *Dislocation*

a. Most commonly anterior dislocation (mouth remains open and cannot be closed) (Fig. 18.3).

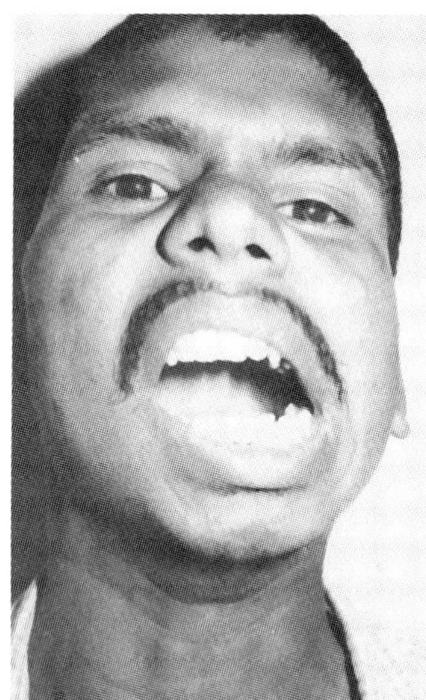

Fig. 18.3: Anterior dislocation of left temporomandibular joint

b. Very rarely posterior dislocation. Here, following a direct blow on the lower jaw, the condyles rest against the mastoid process after fracturing the auditory meatus or slipping underneath it. In this condition, it becomes impossible to open the mouth.

c. Lateral dislocation—The condyle is displaced lateral to the zygomatic process. This is encountered in fracture of the mandible. The chin is displaced in the direction of the fracture. The mouth is easily opened.

d. Habitual mandibular dislocation—Patients, usually ladies in late teens and twenties, complain of click and slipping of the temporomandibular joints; they can voluntarily repeatedly reproduce and reduce subluxation/dislocation of the joints.

ii. *Subluxation of the Temporomandibular Joint*

a. Traumatic

b. Habitual subluxation is more common—The patient manages herself to produce and reduce the subluxation. The symptoms are—annoying discomfort in temporomandibular joint, with or without clicking of the joint.

iii. *Fracture of the Mandible*

For all practical purposes, fractures of the jaw are potentially infected open fractures, having communication with the (dirty) oral cavity.

Any part of the body, angle, ramus or neck may sustain a fracture. Fractures up to the body and angle are usually displaced, which becomes obvious by the displacement in the teeth level (Fig. 18.3). Patient articulates with difficulty and there is swelling of the jaw. Gentle and cautious palpation through the submandibular region can provide the clue regarding the site of fracture. Bilateral fractures may lead to serious complication, like—drooping of the jaw, swelling of the tongue, oedema of the glottis or even endanger the patency of the air way. There will also be disruption in the teeth level.

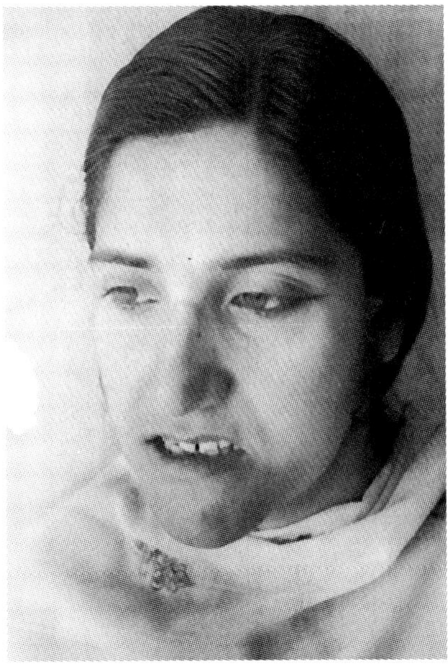

Fig. 18.4: Subacute osteomyelitis or Jaw due to periapical abscess

Swellings of the Jaw (Table 18.2)

As such, any osseous or soft tissue swelling, right from inflammatory to neoplastic, may arise in the jaws. However, there are a few swellings which are peculiarly localised only to the jaw and deserve separate consideration.

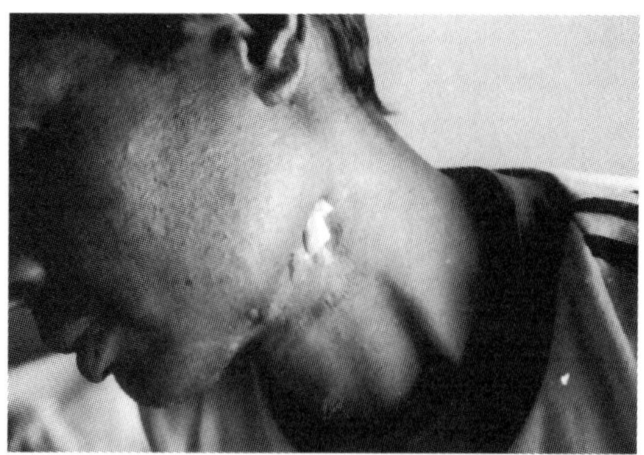

Fig. 18.5: Chronic osteomyelitis of mandible with a sequestrum ejecting through the sinus

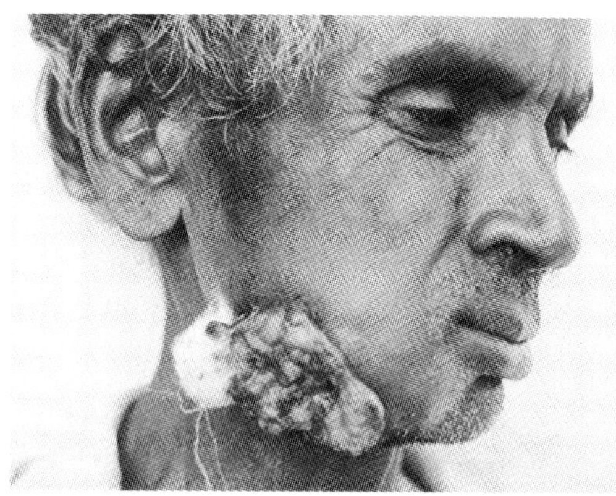

Fig. 18.6: Carcinomatous epulis fungated out after biopsy

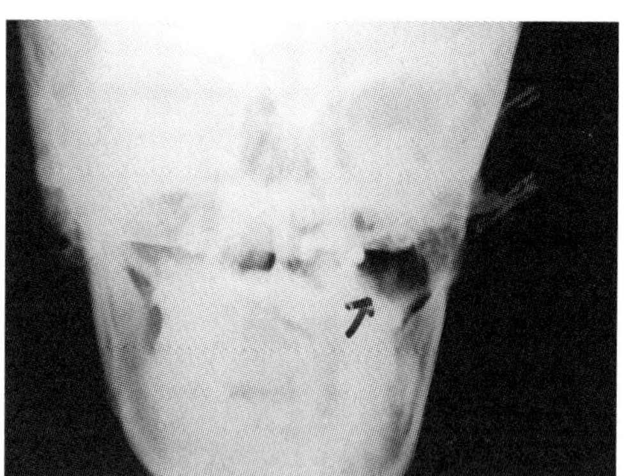

Fig. 18.7: Dental cyst

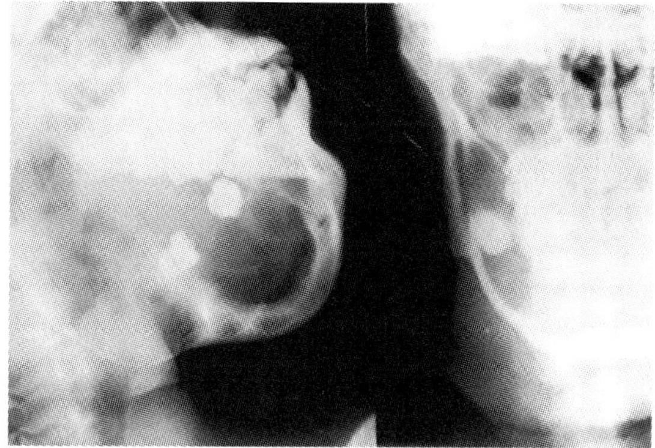

Fig. 18.8: Dentigerous cyst in the mandible

Table 18.2: Swelling of the jaw

Type of swelling 1	*Site* 2	*Presenting features* 3	*X-ray findings* 4
1. Inflammatory swellings (Fig. 18.4)	Any where, but common are alveolar abscess, gum abscess, tooth-gum infection, osteomyelitis, tuberculosis, actinomycosis, submandibular salivary gland infection with or without stone in duct. Acute osteomyelitis is rare, seen mostly in infants as a complication of scarlet fever and measles Subacute osteomyelitis is common and occurs due to infections in and around the tooth and open fractures. Chronic osteomyelitis affects mandible (Fig.18.5) following infections of tooth, open fractures, irradiation and chemical necrosis (phosphorus poisoning)	— Varying constitutional features. — Local tenderness, pain, swelling, with or without fluctuation. — Thickening of the bone. — Sinuses. — Earlier difficulty in opening mouth due to spasm, later on ankylosis of jaw (if neglected)	If bone is involved, areas of destruction, may be new bone formation, bone abscess shadow, sequestrum (Fig. 18.5).
2. Epulis word is derived from the Greek eπ (on top of) and (gum) Epulis (Swelling arising from gum) classified as:	Mucoperiosteum of gum		Soft tissue shadow; if bone is involved, areas of rarefaction or destruction
i. Congenital	Like fibrous epulis of older people, it occurs as a pink swelling on the gums in relation to unerupted incisor teeth		
ii. Fibrous	Slow growing regular fibrous growth.		
Pregnancy epulis or pregnancy tumours	Arise at sites of local irritation, usually as an enlargement of an interdental papilla. In pregnant women, insignificant deposit of calcium causes irritation and hormonal changes in pregnancy	Soft, pink, vascular, rapidly enlarging lumps appear on the gums	
iii. Myelomatous	Purple looking swelling, osteoclastomatous feel, expansile nature.	Foul smell, salivation	
iv. Granulomatous	Granular mass around an infected tooth.	Caries tooth, foul smell, salivation.	
v. Carcinomatous (Fig. 18.6)	Epithelioma, fungating margin	Arising from the gum, having firm ulcer, irregular surfaces, everted margin, bleeding, tenderness	
vi. Sarcomatous	Rapidly growing, firm, vascular, tender swelling from the gum		

Contd.

Table 18.2: Contd.

Type of swelling 1	*Site* 2	*Presenting features* 3	*X-ray findings* 4
3. Odontomes: (Swelling usually arising from tooth germs. The epithelial debris left out in the process of development of enamel of tooth are supposed to be the site of origin of odontomes)	A tumour arising from any tissue taking part in the development of a tooth		
Classification of odontomes:			
I. Epithelial odontomes:	Cysts of eruption—bluish swellings of the gum, occurring where deciduous or permanent teeth are to erupt		
i. Dental cyst (Fig. 18.7)	Usually upper jaw, arises from the root of normally erupted but chronically infected tooth	Expansion of bony cortex, leading to thinness or even pathological fractures. It contains clear watery fluid with sparkling cholesterol crystals. Under finger pressure yielding tendency of cystic wall—may even be fluctuant	Expansion of the cortex with a clear cavity in relation to the root of a tooth
ii. Dentigerous cyst (Follicular odontomes) (Fig. 18.8)	More common in mandible. Associated with unerupted permanent tooth. No relation with infected caries tooth	Any age but common in teens Expanded cystic wall occupies floor of the mouth	Evidence of tooth in the cyst.
iii. Adamantinoma—(Cusaic 1827) (Akin to osteoclastomatous lesion).	Lower jaw mostly affected near about angle of mandible, rarely in maxilla	Most common in the age of 40 or more in females, slow growing. Can occur 11 years upwards	Expansion of cortex, multiple septae, soap bubble appearance
Synonyms: Carcinoma of tooth-germ residue	Multilocular hard to firm swelling (may even burst in the mouth and get infected)	Swelling more obvious from cheek side than from mouth, egg shell crackling may be elicited	
Ameloblastoma (formerly known as adamantinoma and clinical features are same	Difficult to differentiate from osteoclastoma clinically or even histopathologically	Has been known to metastasise to bones, lung. Locally invasive within medullary bone and soft tissues; not radiosensitive Excision with 1 cm margin and substitution by iliac crest graft	Cluster of small cysts in the centre of the lesion.

Contd.

Table 18.2: Contd.

Type of swelling 1	*Site* 2	*Presenting features* 3	*X-ray findings* 4
Eve's disease			
II. Connective tissue odontomes—			
i. Fibrous odontomes—	Usually in rachitic children, more or less features of dentigerous cyst, but here the cyst is small and with a dense fibrous wall.		
ii. Cementoma—	Occurs as a mass of cement in nodular form in relation to the root of an erupted tooth.		
iii. Osseous odontomes—	Bone deposition in the wall of a fibrous odontomes.		
III. Composite odontomes—			
i. Radicular odontomes—	A very rare tumour, developing in connection with tooth fang.		
ii. Compound follicular odontome—	A number of ill-formed teeth are produced due to disordered activity in the cells of dental papilla. Other conditions like—extra cups and roots, dichotomy (two or more teeth developing as one), enamel nodule and extra-denticle have also been described as composite odontomes.		
4. Neoplastic conditions—			
I. Benign—(i) solitary cyst (ii) fibroma (iii) chondroma (iv) osteoma—may occur in the jaw.			
II. Locally malignant—			
Osteoclastoma (GCT)	Difficult to differentiate from adamantinoma, may develop centrally in the jaw. Jaw may be affected by xanthomatosis, osteitis fibrosa cystica, Paget's disease.		
III. Malignant—			
i. Sarcoma			
ii. Carcinoma	Usually from the antrum.		
iii. Melanoma	Maxilla is usually involved secondarily from the palate.		
iv. Metastatic carcinoma	Mandible is commonly involved in advanced carcinoma of tongue or the floor of mouth or from secondarily involved cervical/submandibular lymph glands.		

BIBLIOGRAPHY

1. Cusaic: Dublin Hosp Rep **4**: 1, 1827.

19 Gross Examination of Head Injury

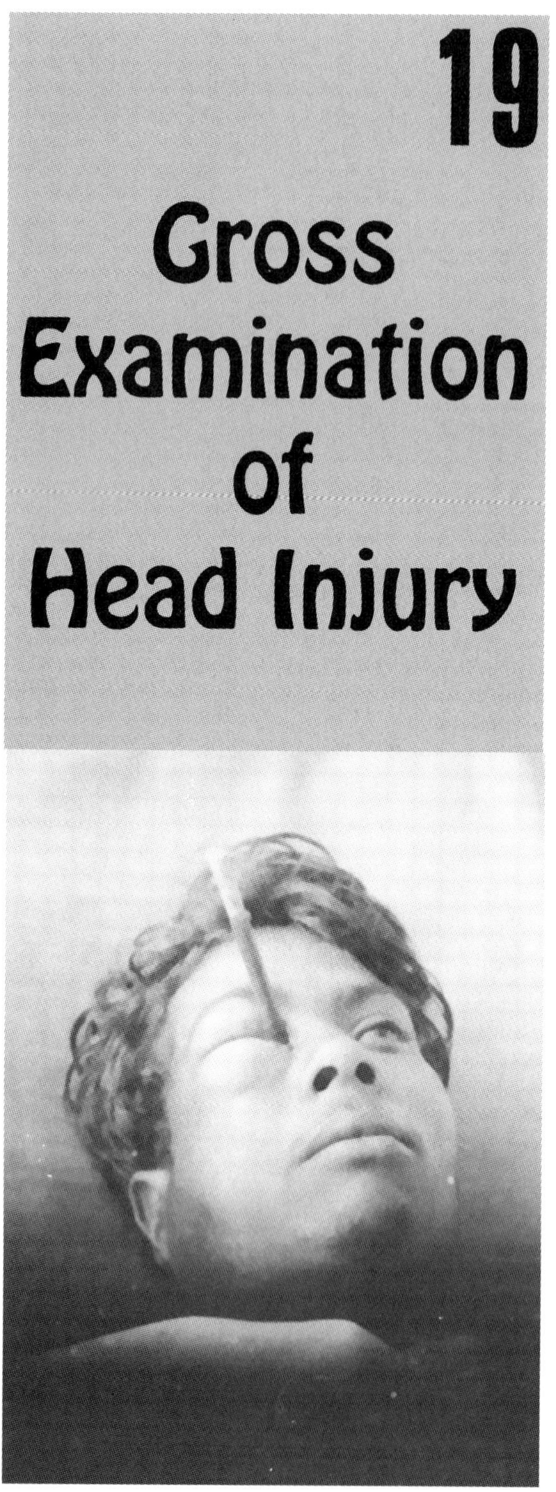

Head injury is one of the most common injury in accidents especially the road traffic accidents by motorcyclists. However, the use of crash helmet and legislation concerning head protection and body constraint for traffic and sporting events have definite effect in reducing the incidence.

With the highly advanced diagnostic and therapeutic aids (angiography, ultrasonography, CAT scanning, stereoscopic examination, MRI, 3-D and 4-D NMR with isotopic labelling) being used in managing head injuries, it has become further imperative to suspect and diagnose head injuries at the earliest. The aphorism of Hippocrate's—"No head injury is so slight that it should be neglected, or so severe that life should be despaired of" is a moral and duty bound incentive for any clinician confronted with this injury.

Head injury is often an accompaniment of multiple injuries—as occurs commonly in road traffic accidents, fall from height, industrial accidents, sports injuries, etc. Here again, the orthopaedic surgeon, being the team leader of the 'accident services', owes the responsibility of seeking the help of a neurosurgeon at the earliest in managing this injury.

In any head injury, the first assessment is of A, B, C (A = Airway, B = Breathing, C = Circulation). The real assessment (Tables 19.2 to 19.4) must begin only after the above are attended to. Following that, a quick general assessment of the patient should be made regarding level of consciousness (comatose, semiconscious, stuporose, delirious, irritable, confused) however, he may not be unconscious initially; patency of air way; any other obvious vital injury (severe chest injury, severe abdominal injury; injury to neck or groin (especially penetrating injury); pulse; respiration; blood pressure; pupillary condition; temperature (on both halves of the body); bladder condition (wetting of bed), if bladder is full, catheterise and collect sample of urine for examination; smell coming from mouth (alcoholic, uraemic, diabetic); scalp (any obvious bruising, haematoma, cut lacerations; bony depression, deformity, etc), bleeding (or CSF or very rarely brain matter) through—nose, ear and mouth, CSF leak through nostrils (rhinorrhoea) or through external auditory meatus (otorrhoea) is usually mixed with blood. If a drop of it is dropped on a sheet it produces the double ring of blood and CSF. Further the clotting of this blood is delayed due to the presence of CSF. Note for any neck rigidity (may be due to meningeal irritation in subarachnoid haemorrhage) and also look for evidence of Jacksonian fits. Then neurological examination should be done in detail if the condition of the patient permits. Following this a quick but thorough systemic examination, should be done.

Make a note of each finding. Frequent repeated and thorough examinations at short regular intervals (half to two hourly) is mandatory.

Patient is usually brought unconscious. Whenever possible, take a detailed history from the attendants and/or the patient (if conscious) regarding:

i. Mode of injury, circumstances and time of accident, use of a crash helmet.
ii. Immediate status after injury (transient unconsciousness, vomiting, continued unconsciousness). Transient unconsciousness should be differentiated from 'syncope'[(Gr synkopi, fainting) i.e. a transient loss of consciouness due to inadequate blood flow to the brain].
iii. Intake of alcohol.
iv. Known history of diabetes, epilepsy, renal failure, any addiction (i.e. opium or any drug, etc).
v. If patient can respond, the initial history should be taken for the followings: A-allergies (e.g. to drugs, etc like penicillin); Medicine taken regularly (e.g. steroids, hypotensives, antidiabetics, anticoagulents, etc); Past-illness; Last meal taken, Events of accident (AMPLE).

Certain attitudes and postures provide clues in the assessment of head injuries, e.g.—Lying flaccid with the mouth relaxed and angle of mouth sagging denotes a serious condition. Decereberate posturing, whether unilateral or bilateral, is of grave prognostic significance, since it usually signifies severe and most likely, irreversible mid brain damage. If patient is curled up on his side and resents interference, it indicates cerebral irritation, which is a favourable sign in head injury.

Besides examinations on general principles, certain factors deserve special mention.

- *Pupil*: Size and equality of the pupils are of more importance than the reaction to light. The pupil can be fixed and dilated immediately after injury due to direct involvement of the oculomotor nerve in case of fracture of the anterior cranial fossa. It is of particular importance when the patient is not in deep coma.
- *Ciliospinal reflex:* This reflex (minor pupillary dilatation of both eyes on painful stimuli) signifies integrity of the sympathetic pathway and thus the mid brain. This reflex is usually more marked in comatose state.
- *Oculocephalic reflex* (Doll's eye phenomenon): On rapid rotation of the patient's head, the eyeball moves away from the direction in which the head is turned. Proprioceptive impulses transmitted from the neck muscles to the longitudinal fascicle are responsible for this reflex, which denotes severe brain damage.
- *Oculovestibular* (Caloric) *reflex*: Integrity of the brainstem function can be finally assessed by this reflex. If the brain stem is functionally intact, injection of cold water into the ear, while head is supported in 30° elevation, stimulates movements of the eyeball. No response of the eyeballs to this denotes a very grave sign, and if it persists for more than an hour, death is certain.
- *Analysis of motor response to command and stimuli*: Obeying commands is a good prognostic sign. Flexion response, and attempt at avoiding painful stimuli indicate good prognosis. On the other hand, extensor responses and/or assumption of decereberate posture have a grave prognosis.

Even in noncomatose patients, the motor responses are more informative than sensory charting.

In subarachnoid haemorrhage, the meningeal irritation leads to neck rigidity.

- *Post-traumatic amnesia* (Return of continuous memory after head injury): It is the best guide for assessing the ultimate prognosis. If it exists less than twenty four hours, the prognosis is good. Its extension beyond twenty four hours is not a good prognostic sign.
- Due to loose attachment and pliability of the epicraneal aponeurosis, the external wound may not overlie the underlying fracture in a compound injury.
- *Cardiac arrhythmias* (atrioventricular nodal and ventricular arrhythmias) are frequently associated with severe brain injuries.
- *Assessment of level of consciousness:* Though not universally accepted, Glasgow Coma Scale has been observed to be reliable, and on the whole satisfactory in prognostising the ultimate outcome of a head injury. Though it is fallacious when there are associated orbital injuries, diseases, speech problems, and pre-existing mental conditions, these can be out-weighed by its overall simplicity and practicability, since it gives an actual description of the patient's condition, rather than expressing in terms of coma, semicoma, and stupor.

Three parameters (E, M, V) are mainly observed to assess the depth of the coma.

By adding the scores of each component, the total Glasgow Coma Scale (Table 19.1) is determined. If the total score is 15 (E 4 + M 6 + V 5), the patient's level of consciousness is completely normal. A patient in deep coma will score only three. The higher the score, better is the prognosis.

Investigations

1. In any patient of head injury (specially unconscious ones);
   - Examination of vomitus—if it is there.
   - Routine examination of urine—specially for sugar.
   - Breath—analysis for alcohol, etc.
   - Blood urea and serum creatinine.
2. X-ray (in addition to the skull, the neck should be included) whenever possible, but not at the cost of management of the head injury. Two real indications for an emergency X-ray are, depressed fracture and intracranial foreign body. This is also important from medicolegal point of view.
3. Lumbar puncture—(Usually not to be done in acute head injury), very cautiously (to avoid formation of pressure cone—which may be fatal) to see tension of CSF, any blood in CSF.
4. Cerebral/carotid angiography.
5. EEG—Not of much significance in acute head injury, but may be useful later on.
6. CAT scanning.
7. Stereoscopic studies.
8. NMR (MRI)
9. Ultrasonogram.
10. Inspection burr holes in the skull.

Table 19.1: Glasgow Coma Scale

E = Eye opening		*M = Best motor response*		*V = Verbal response*	
Spontaneous	—4	Obeys	—6	Oriented	—5
To speech	—3	Localises	—5	Confused conversation	—4
To pain	—2	Withdraws	—4	Inappropriate words	—3
Nil	—1	Abnormal flexion	—3	Incomprehensible sound	—2
		Nil	—1	Nil	—1

Table 19.2: Features of fracture of base of the skull*

Anterior cranial fossa		*Middle cranial fossa*	*Posterior cranial fossa*
Compounding through paranasal sinuses, bleeding and/or CSF or brain matter leak through nose; may be damage of 1, 2, 3, 4, 5, 6 cranial nerves; subconjunctival haemorrhage. Clinical difference between subconjunctival haemorrhage following fracture of anterior cranial fossa and black eye (direct injury over face/eye)		May be internal compounding through auditory meatus, blood and/or CSF through nose or mouth; may vomit swallowed blood; may be affection of 7th and 8th cranial nerves. By 48 hours following injury, bruising appearing at the mastoid process almost confirms fracture of middle cranial fossa (Battle's sign)	May cause serious haemorrhage due to rupture of the venous sinuses; may produce lesion of brain stem which may prove fatal; blood extravasates posterior to mastoid process; may be nystagmus and ataxia; 9th, 10th and 11th cranial nerves may be affected
Subconjunctival haemorrhage	*Black eye*		
— Ecchymosis develops gradually (usually after 24 hours)	— Ecchymosis develops soon after injury		
— Ecchymosis is circular, limited by attachment of orbital fascia to orbital margin	— Ecchymosis spreads even to the cheek and forehead		
— Colour is usually purple-blue	— Reddish-purple colour		
— Haemorrhage is subconjunctival and can not be moved with conjunctiva, and its posterior limit cannot be seen	— Haemorrhage is conjunctival and moves along with conjunctiva, also posterior limit can be seen		
— Eyeball may protrude due to retrobulbar collection	— Eyeball not protruded		
— Conjunctiva may be swollen	— Eye lid swollen		
Bilateral symmetrical black eye is suggestive of fracture of the anterior cranial fossa			

*NB. An unusual arrow injury caused the crack fracture of base of skull, and the arrow tip was almost to pierce the medulla oblongata region. Very cautious removal of the arrow left behind no legacy, except the scar (Figs 19.1 to 19.3).

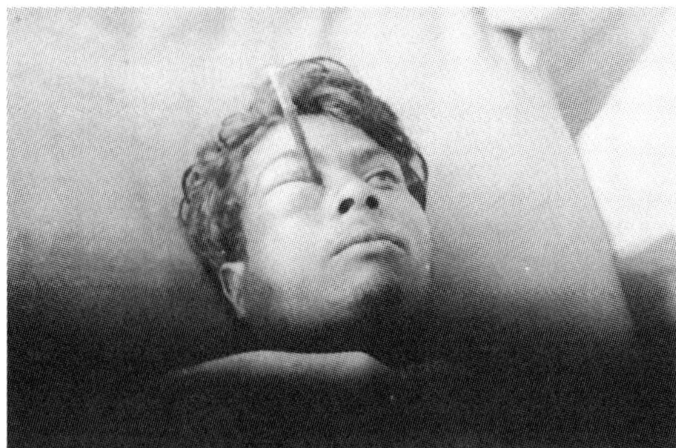

Fig. 19.1: An unusual arrow injury piercing through the inner canthus of right eye

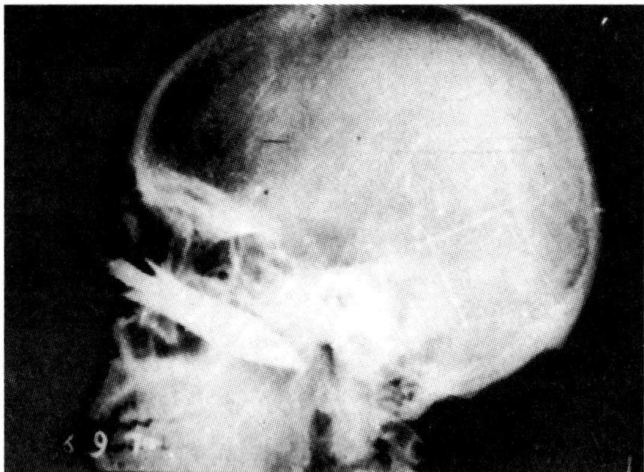

Fig. 19.2: The arrow tip almost to pierce the medulla oblongata region

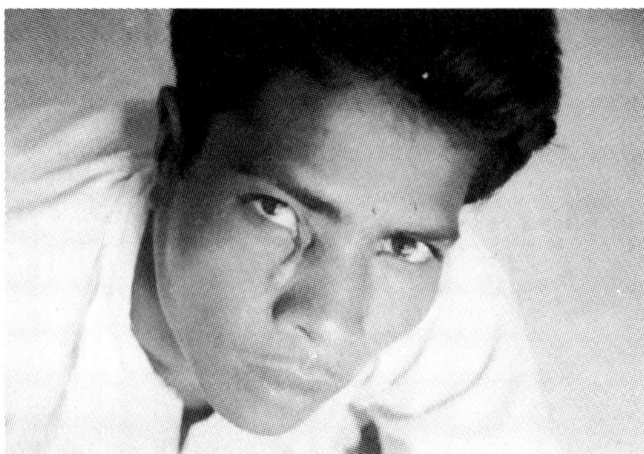

Fig. 19.3: After cautious removal of the arrow, the patient recovered fully

Table 19.3: Brain injuries

		Cerebral concussion	Cerebral irritation	Cerebral compression
1.	Effect of head injury	Mild	Mild to moderate	Severe
2.	Onset	Immediate	Delayed	Immediate or delayed
3.	Cause	Shock of brain	Irritation due to cerebral oedema, contusion of brain	Usually due to cerebral haemorrhage (clot), bony fragment, foreign body or laceration of brain
4.	Consciousness	Initial unconsciousness for a short period	May be history of initial unconsciousness, remains drowsy and irritable, avoids light and keeps eyes closed, preferring darkness.	Concussion may continue in deep unconsciousness — Initial restlessness, ending in deep unconsciousness — Concussion—lucid interval—deep unconsciousness
5.	Attitude	While unconscious, the patient may be completely flaccid but recovers soon	Assumes attitude of flexion and lies curled up on the side	— May be flaccid in the beginning — One side may be paralysed, while the other shows incoordinated contractions and may later on become paralysed
6.	Pulse	Rapid with low volume	Initially rapid, gradually settles	— Initially rapid, gradually becomes slow and bounding, may again become rapid in terminal stage
7.	Blood pressure	Falls	Initially falls, later on maintained.	Falls initially, then gradually rises to maintain the cerebral circulation and again falls in the terminal stage
8.	Respiration	Slow, shallow and rapid	Almost normal	— Initially slow, shallow and rapid; gradually becomes slow and deep suggestive of Cheyene-stokes breathing. Stertorous breathing may develop (Cheeks puffing in and out with snoring noise) indicating onset of bulbar compression.
9.	Temperature	Subnormal	May be slightly higher	— Initially subnormal, then moderate pyrexia. Intracranial haematoma/secondary infections may lead to higher temperature. Extremely high temperature (40°-42° C) indicates pontine haemorrhage.
10.	Eye (pupil)	Slightly dilated, equal and reactive	Equal, reactive, remains slightly dilated but instantaneously constricts on testing	Hutchinson's pupil— *Normal side* / *Affected side* Initially normal reactive / — Contracted reactive Later on contracted / — Dilated, may be fixed Last stage dilated and fixed / — Dilated and fixed In pontine haemorrhage pin point fixed pupils
11.	Reflexes	Absent, but recover	Irritable jerks	Paralysed side flaccid (jerks absent)
12.	Residual effects	— May recover fully — May be followed by stage of irritation — May be followed by compression features either in continuity or with lucid interval	— May recover completely — May be residual headache, irritability, forgetfullness, lack of concentration, abnormal psychic behaviour	— May end fatally If recovery—usually incomplete. Residual paresis, speech defects. Abnormal psychic behaviour. Lack of concentration, insomnia. Intracranial abscess Jacksonian fits

Table 19.4: Injuries of intracranial blood vessels

	Extradural (middle meningeal haemorrhage)	*Subdural haemorrhage*	*Intracerebral haemorrhage*	*Subarachnoid haemorrhage*
Incidence	Not common	Common	Common	Not common
Onset	Delayed manifestation (1-2 days)	Quite early manifestation	Early manifestation	Early manifestation
Site of injury on skull	— Temporal injuries—fracture skull with rupture of branches of middle meningeal artery. (rarely anterior meningeal) — Haematoma on temporal region	Injury anywhere on the skull, even without fracture. Usually rupture of large cortical veins and/or laceration of the cortex	—Injury anywhere on the skull —With any type of brain injury	—
Stages of manifestation	— Initially in a state of confusion or irritation, or concussion features—recovers—after a variable period (few hours to days—lucid interval) again gradually becomes drowsy, and comatose — Gradually accumulating haematoma/clot presses the cerebral cortex from below upwards—producing facial, then upper limb, then lower limb paralysis	—No lucid interval. Patient remains unconscious Develops paralysis from the beginning (not in an orderly fashion) Rapid deterioration	—No lucid interval Patient unconscious. Develops paralysis from the beginning (not in an orderly fashion)	—Soon after injury rapid pulse, pyrexia, neck rigidity, severe headache, restlessness, positive Kernig's sign. After few hours lumbar discomfort with bilateral plantar response upgoing
Lumbar puncture	No blood in CSF	Blood in CSF	Blood in CSF	Blood in CSF

Lateralisation of the lesion in extradural haemorrhage: (i) Swelling and bruises in the temporal region—usually opposite to the side of paralysis (except in countre-coupe injury), (ii) Observation of Hutchinson's pupils, (iii) Temperature is higher on the paralysed side, (iv) Babinski positive on the side opposite to the haematoma pressing side, (v) Speech will be affected in case of left sided injury of a right handed person, (vi) Fracture of the skull usually denotes the underlying brain tissue damage—paralysis on the opposite side.

BIBLIOGRAPHY

1. Iversen LD, Swiontkowski MF. The diagnosis and management of musculoskeletal trauma. In Iversen LD, Swiontkowski MF (Eds): *Manual of Acute Orthopaedic Therapeutics* (4th ed), Boston: Little Brown and Company, 1-19, 1995.
2. Pandey S, Sinha SN, Jha B *et al*. An unusual arrow injury. *Int Surg* 57-589, 1972.

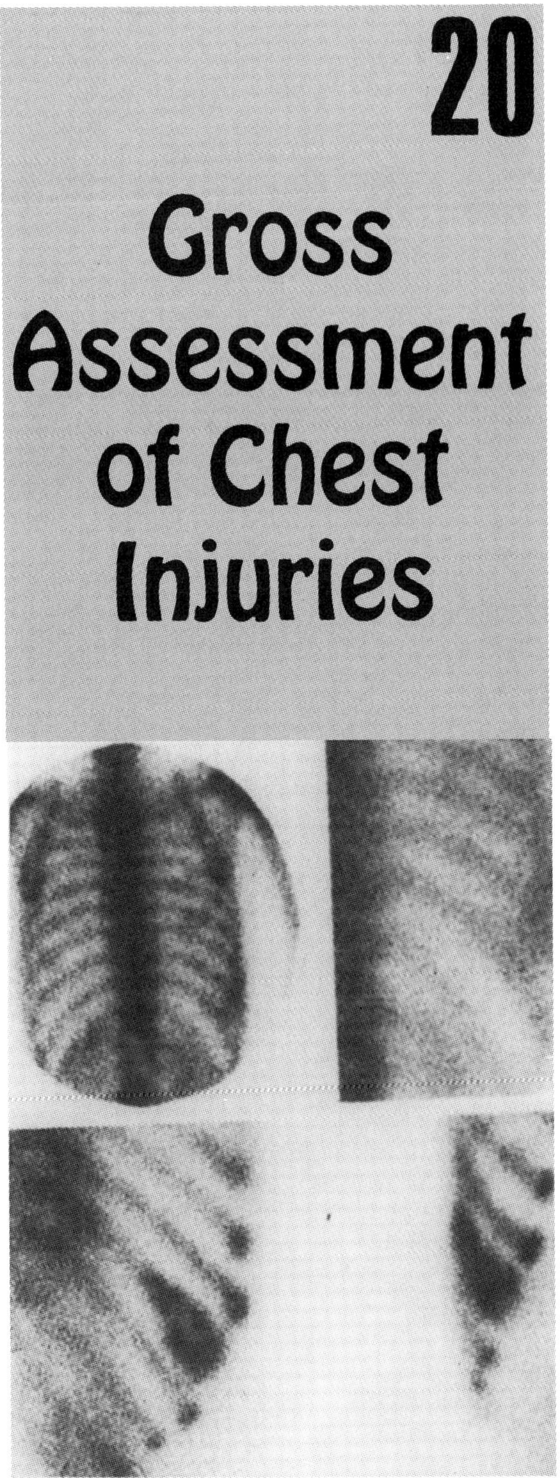

20 Gross Assessment of Chest Injuries

Chest injuries cause approximately 25% of the deaths occurring due to war and allied injuries. Hence, their accurate diagnosis and prompt treatment is of great importance. In civil practice, causes of chest injuries include road traffic accidents; increasing criminal violence, (stab injuries, gunshot/missile injuries) and sports injuries. The main importance of chest injuries is in their effects on the vital organs of the chest, like lungs, heart and major blood vessels, giving rise to traumatic pneumothorax, haemothorax, mediastinal flutter, stove-in-chest, rupture of aorta and other catastrophies.

According to mode of violence chest injuries can be: (i) non-penetrating (blunt trauma to thoracic cage), which usually produce contusion to lung, haemorrhage and oedema in alveoli and interstitial tissue, but rarely, even transection of trachea and/or bronchus leading to emphysema, pneumothorax and respiratory distress, (ii) penetrating injuries (minor pleural puncture to catastrophic heart, aortic and lung injuries).

Chest injuries may be classified as follows:

Group I Those peculiar to the chest wall:

a. Subcutaneous emphysema.
b. Flail chest (paradoxical respiration).
c. Open pneumothorax.

Group II Those peculiar to the inner region of the chest:

a. Closed pneumothorax.
b. Haemothorax.
c. Obstruction of lower air ways due to secretions, leading to "wet lung" and aspiration pneumonitis.

Group III Those peculiar to the inner most region of chest:

a. Mediastinal emphysema and injury.
b. Cardiac tamponade.
c. Traumatic diaphragmatic hernia.

The mortality rate due to injuries of heart and great vessels and pulmonary insufficiency is still high.

Regardless of the classification, it is important to detect whether the thoracic cage was penetrated by a pointed object.

Chest Wall

Fracture of single or multiple ribs is not alarming, if the lung parenchyma or pleura has not been pierced. However, the patient feels pain even in regular breathing. The fracture can be best localised by asking the patient to point out the site of 'catch' due to pain while taking a deep breath. Palpation with the finger tip along the suspected rib will elicit maximum tenderness at the fracture site. One may feel crepitus as well.

Chest compression test should be avoided as far as possible, except in doubtful cases.

Compression Test

While sitting on a stool, the patient elevates his arms over the head. The base of one hand is placed over the sternum and the base of the other over the spine at the same level. The thorax is then gently compressed anteroposteriorly. When a rib has been fractured, this manoeuvre causes pain at the site of lesion.

Side to side compression may also be done if the fracture is located more anteriorly or in the sternum.

In multiple fracture of the ribs, though there may not be immediate complications, injury to the underlying pleura and lungs, later on, is a possibility. The pain in such case is of greater magnitude with limited excursion of that side of the chest, leading to post-traumatic atelectasis of the lung.

Injury of Lungs

There are two early features:

a. Haemoptysis—In every case of chest injury, an early enquiry about coughing out of blood should be made.
b. Surgical emphysema—Due to traumatic rupture of pulmonary tissue, air percolates from beneath the visceral pleura to enter the hilum of the lung and via the mediastinum it appears in the neck. However, air may directly enter the subcutaneous tissue after rupture of both the layers of pleura.

EXAMINATION OF INJURIES OF THE CHEST (Table 20.1)

Usual complaints are: Swelling, pain, fever, difficulty in breathing, cough, haemoptysis. Enquire about the nature of violence and history of any previous chest disease.

General and systemic examinations: See whether the patient is in shock, restless, cyanosed, dyspnoeic or gasping. Pulse, temperature and blood pressure should be recorded. Also, look for any associated injury.

Attitude of the Patient

Fracture of sternum: The attitude of characteristic. The body is bent forwards with the shoulders rotated inwards, the head is held downwards and forward.

Respiration: Note the type of the breathing patterns. The respiration may be:

— Abdomino-thoracic or abdominal or thoraco-abdominal or only thoracic.
— Paradoxical breathing, i.e. indrawing of chest wall during inspiration and expansion during expiration.

Also note whether respiration is easy or laboured.

Local Examination

Inspection

Inspect the chest wall from all around (the clothes must be removed or cut open to see clearly) for any wound especially penetrating (whether it has penetrated the pleura) or sucking chest wound or for a paradoxical movement of a flail chest wall.

In case of penetrating wound, air and blood passes in and out of the wound with a loud sucking noise.

Look for any swelling on the chest. Surgical emphysema gives rise to a diffuse swelling.

Table 20.1: Acute traumatic conditions of chest

	Type of injury 1	History 2	Clinical feature 3	Radiology 4	Investigation 5	Complication 6	Treatment 7	Prognosis 8
1.	Single rib fracture	—Injury —Heavy coughing	Pain at the site of fracture (aggravated by deep breathing and coughing). Local tenderness; may be crepitus; compression test indicates sight of fracture Fractures of lower ribs may involve underlying abdominal viscera.	Fracture may not be shown in X-ray		Surgical emphysema —felt as crepitus on gentle palpation	—May be ignored —Analgesics —Prophylactic antibiotics —Local infiltration of long acting local anaesthetic agent —Encourage normal respiratory pattern —Effective coughing after pressing the injured portion of chest —Ambulation (not bed rest) —Strapping of chest (not being preferred as regular procedure) —In case of massive surgical emphysema putting a wide bore needle or tube in subcutaneous tissue is needed	Good
2.	Multiple rib fractures (on one side)	—Severe injury —Chest compression against hard object	Marked pain at the site of fracture even on normal breathing; breathing is shallow. Local tenderness ++, crepitus, (compression test should be avoided lest it may produce complications)	Fractures visible usually with overlap	— — — —	Surgical emphysema Pneumothorax Haemopneumothorax Contusion of lungs	—Hospitalise the patient (some may require positive pressure ventilation) —Strapping of chest —Long-acting local anaesthetic infiltration —Analgesics —Chest binder (Elastic corset) with pressure pads. In certain conditions, fixation of fractures by stainless steel wire, intramedullary rush pin, Judet clips, may be required	Fairly good
3.	Fracture sternum	Severe direct injury from the front, e.g. impact of steering wheel (getting less); deceleration on to seat belts, closed cardiac massage	Pain in the sternal zone, tenderness at the fracture site, irregularity usually in a transverse line due to slight overlapping tendency of the fragments	Lateral and oblique views must be taken to exactly localise the site of fracture and displacement	ECG (for any concomitant myocardial injury). X-ray of dorsal spine (for any concomitant vertebral fracture	Myocardial injury, Vertebral injury, Mediastinal emphysema may be due to ruptured bronchus. Air may enter peribronchial space. Emphysema first appearing over suprasternal notch spreads, to neck, face, chest, abdomen and scrotum. (Some are associated with multiple segmental rib fractures leading to flail chest and severe pulmonary insufficiency) rupture of aorta	—May be ignored —Analgesics —Rarely reduction by hooking the fragment, if markedly displaced —Management of associated serious injuries (e.g. myocardial injury, unstable chest injury, paradoxical movement of flail chest, etc)	Fairly good

NB. The fracture of first rib is potentially serious chest injury, since it is well protected and requires a severe force to fracture, which may also lead to injuries to big vessels, head, neck, and abdomen. Mortality rate with fracture of first rib may be about 30%

Contd.

Table 20.1: Contd.

	Type of injury 1	History 2	Clinical feature 3	Radiology 4	Investigation 5	Complication 6	Treatment 7	Prognosis 8
4.	Multiple rib fractures at two sites (flail chest, stove-in chest) Flail—when ribs are fractured at two sites, usually anteriorly and posteriorly)	Severe injury usually traffic accidents	Severe pain, respiratory distress. Cyanosis, features of shock, paradoxical breathing (the portions of the ribs intervening the fracture sites forms a flail segment). With every inspiration, due to negative pressure in pleural cavity, this flail segment is sucked in and in expiration the flail segment is blown out and air comes from the opposite lung along the carina	Affected lung space is collapsed to varying extent. Fractured fragment obvious—usually with overlap	Screening to confirm the paradoxical breathing	Shock, cyanosis Traumatic wet lung (lung secretions fill in bronchi) May be lethal	First aid is by padded pressure over the flail segment —Endotracheal intubation and suction and cleaning of trachea and bronchial tree —Positive pressure ventilation —Towel clip traction of the flail fragment and stabilisation with a crammer wire circular frame —Internal fixation of the fractured ribs	If managed well —fairly good —may be lethal
5.	Haemothorax (Blood in pleural cavity)	Laceration of lung parenchyma. Rupture of intercostal or internal mammary vessel	Pain chest. Respiratory distress. Cyanosis in severe cases. Tendency of silent chest. Dullness on percussion from below upwards. Muffled or absent breath sounds. Impaired vocal resonance	Radiopaque shadow filling the costophrenic and cardiophrenic angles and proceeding upwards	Aspiration (frank blood in pleural cavity)	May lead to clotting (clotting is rare due to churning), Pyothorax or Empyema	—Aspiration —Antibiotics —Respiratory exercises —Catheter drainage through 8th intercostal space in mid axillary line connected to water seal drainage	Fairly good
6.	Haemopneumothorax	Rupture of lung parenchyma or entry of air from outside	As above, hyperresonance and vocal fremitus, above the level of dullness. The line of dullness is horizontal when examined in the sitting position	Radiopaque shadow at the bottom of the lung field having a horizontal level, over which there is air in the pleural cavity.	Aspiration (frank blood in pleural cavity)	May lead to clotting (clotting rare due to churning). Pyothorax or Empyema, Respiratory distress may increase, pyopneumothorax	—Aspiration —Antibiotics —Respiratory exercises —Catheter drainage through 8th intercostal space —If needed, a 2nd catheter drainage in 2nd intercostal space anteriorly and connected to water seal drainage	Fair
7.	Pyothorax (Empyema) —pus in the pleural cavity.	Rupture of lung abscess in pleural cavity. Infection of haemothorax Penetrating injury of chest	Constitutional features of infection (febrile attacks and feature of toxaemia) Findings of haemothorax exaggerated.	Findings of haemothorax exaggerated	Aspiration of pleural cavity—pus	—Fever —Toxaemia, may even lead to lethal stage —Secondary lung abscess —May end in bronchopleural fistula or break subcutaneously (Empyema necessitence —Impulse on coughing) or may even lead to sinus to exterior	—Repeated aspiration —Catheter drainage through 8th intercostal space in mid axillary line connected to water seal system —Antibiotics —General restorative measures —Surgery—Evacuation of pus. Excision and/or decortication	Fair

NB. The **major life threatening problems** are tension pneumothorax, massive haemothorax, flail chest, thoracic major blood vessels injuries, open cardiac injury and traumatic asphyxia.
A tension pneumothorax is diagnosed by the signs of massive pneumothorax alongwith positive pressure in the intrapleural hemispace, causing mediastinal shift and decreasing venous return—which leads to a rapidly deteriorating respiratory and cardiovascular condition. Urgent aspiration of air relieve symptoms.
In **flail chest** patient can ventilate, but dyspnoea and cynosis persist. There is dissociated (discordinated) movements of the chest wall.
Besides definitive management, patient should be given immediate oxygen and put on ventilator

Contd.

Table 20.1: Contd.

	Type of injury 1	History 2	Clinical features 3	Radiology 4	Investigations 5	Complications 6	Treatments 7	Prognosis 8
8.	Traumatic asphyxia	—Sudden compression of chest (crush injury) —Sudden retropulsion of blood into the bigger veins of chest, neck and head—leads to extravasation of blood into loose subconjunctival and subcutaneous tissues of face	—Marked subconjunctival congestion —Bleeding from nose and ears —Congested skin at face and neck —Petechial haemorrhage	Shock	— —	May be lethal unless and until atteneded very promptly.	—Management of shock —Hyperbaric oxygen	Poor
9.	Injury to lung parenchyma (contusion or laceration)	Closed or open chest injury	Haemoptysis, pain chest, surgical emphysema, respiratory distress, restricted chest movement, weak breath sounds.	Features of localised consolidation of lung	—	Pneumonia Lung abscess	—Symptomatic —Antibiotics —Other expectant line of treatment	Fair
10.	Cardiac injury (usually haemopericardium)	Closed or open chest injury	—Typical *triad of cardiac tamponade*—increased area of cardiac dullness, muffled/inaudible heart sounds, gradual increasing of venous, and falling of arterial blood pressure. (rise in diastolic and fall in systolic blood pressure) —Features of shock	Increased cardiac shadow	Aspiration through left anterior 4th intercostal space—diagnostic (as blood comes out) and therapeutic, (as symptoms and signs improve)	Respiratory distress, cardiac shock—may be lethal.	—Aspiration (may be repeated) through 4th intercostal space —Antibiotics —Specialised treatment	Fair
11.	Thoracic major vessels injury (specially aorta)	Severe chest injury (specially penetrating injury) rapid deceleration, e.g. in car crash or fall from a great height	Fever Shock Features of cardiopulmonary failure	In presence of minor leaks —Widening of mediastinum	—	Usually lethal	—Prompt treatment by specialised cardiothoracic team may save the patient	Poor
12.	Injury to diaphragm (rupture of diaphragm) occurs in about 4 to 5% of chest injuries	Close crush injuries —Penetrating abdominothoracic/thoraco abdominal injuries	Features of shock Features of peritonitis Respiratory distress Basal dullness Muffled/inaudible breath sound	Radiopaque shadow in continuity with diaphragm (as if raised diaphragm) akin to haemothorax. —On left side—herniated stomach may show gas. (cf. haemothorax)	Barium meal reveals position of stomach inside the chest Aspiration at lower chest does not reveal blood	Cardiopulmonary compression features, profound shock (haemorrhagic), Peritonitis	Thorough repair of rupture through thoracoabdominal approach	Poor to fair

Contd.

— Presence of ecchymosis on the chest wall.
— Presence of petechial haemorrhage in supraclavicular region at the side of the neck (traumatic asphyxia).

Examination of sputum: If sputum is blood stained, it indicates injury to the lung.

Palpation

Palpate the ribs, besides the tenderness, which will be present in all injuries, crepitus [if present, indicates rib fractures (cf. crepitus in subcutaneous emphysema)], sternum, thoracic vertebrae, and any swelling if present. Ascertain the position of apex beat of heart. Feel for the vocal fremitus.

In the fractures of lower ribs, there is possibility of injury to abdominal organs, e.g. liver, spleen, etc.

Percussion: Undue resonance over the chest is suggestive of pneumothorax; normal cardiac dullness may be obliterated. Haemothorax and haemopericardium will be dull on percussion.

Auscultation: Auscultate for any crepitus.
— Diminution or absence of breath sounds indicates haemo/pneumothorax.

Heart: Muffled heart sounds with low pulse pressure and high diastolic pressure occur in haemopericardium.

A rapid thready pulse, falling blood pressure, distended neck veins, and distant muffled heart sounds indicate the development of cardiac tamponade.

If on inspection the patient appears to be in great respiratory distress, immediate management must be started.

21 Gross Examination of Abdomen

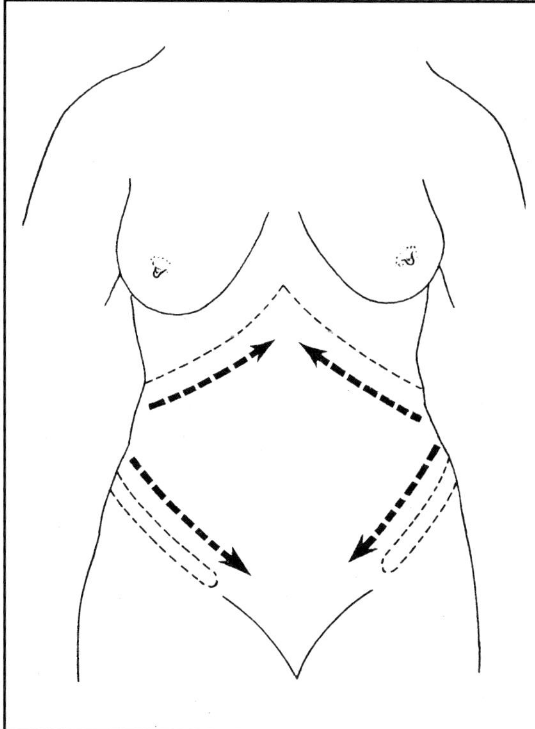

No branch of medicine is independent, and interdisciplinary basic knowledge is essential for examination of any patient. After all we are examining a patient, not just a system.

In orthopaedic practice, examination of the abdomen is *required mainly after an accident*, since it is the third most commonly injured region of the body. In an accident service, the orthopaedic surgeon, being the chief of the team, has an obligation to ensure that the patient has no other vital injuries. In severe accidents, the abdomen may be involved both as closed or as open injuries.

Open injuries are usually obvious and they must get the attention of an abdominal surgeon at the earliest, because though it may look small on the surface, it may be grievously damaged in the deep. In closed injuries, one must be on the lookout to detect any visceral damage or internal haemorrhage. In managing abdominal injury one should never forget the dictum that 'it is always better to open and see the abdomen than to wait and repent'.

HISTORY

In case of injury, enquire in detail regarding the nature of blow/hurt/or crush over the lower chest or abdomen. Note the site, character, progression and reference of pain; distention, *borborgymi*; and passing of urine, flatus, and stool. Enquire about the colour of urine, stool and vomitus.

Pain in the shoulder region during inspiration usually suggest subdiaphragmatic irritation due to blood or leaked gastrointestinal content [(in case of penetrating injury or rupture) of abdominal organ or viscera] or inflammatory lesion in that region.

Blunt abdominal trauma (e.g. severe blow, hurt by or fall on blunt hard object) may produce severe intra or retroperitoneal injuries with relatively few clinical signs.

Repeated examination is essential regarding:

I. General condition of the patient.

II. Local condition of the abdomen.

I. General Condition of the Patient

Look for facial expression, pulse—rate and volume, respiration (type of respiration), blood pressure, temperature, features of internal haemorrhage, i.e. increasing restlessness, increasing pallor, feeble to imperceptible pulse, gradual fall of blood pressure, sweating, air hunger, drowsiness, collapse.

In case of injury, a rising pulse rate combined with falling blood pressure is highly suggestive of *intra-abdominal injury.*

A quick systemic examination should be done to rule out any other vital injury.

II. Local Condition of the Abdomen

Certain helpful criteria while examining the abdomen:

i. Patient should lie supine on a flat bed, *preferably* with flexed lower limbs.
ii. Ask him to breath through the mouth, to relax the abdomen.
iii. Now proceed by gently starting from the non-affected side to overcome the possible resistance offered by an apprehensive patient.
iv. Always examine in supine position for abdominal complaints.

Inspection

Inspect from all sides, including the back. Look for skin condition, any prominence of veins, umbilicus, protuberance of abdomen, tattoo marks and any localised bulging on straining. In case of injury—look for bruising, abrasion, wound (site, number, entry/exit, protruding structure, discharge), abdominal distention, localised discolouration of skin.

Any lacerated wound or eviscerated bowel is covered with a large sterile pack soaked in warm saline.

Palpation

Palpate from all sides. Be very gentle in abdominal palpation.

a. *Abdominal wall*: For guarding, tenderness, herniation, and crepitus (surgical emphysema due to colonic injury, sternal fracture).
b. *Abdominal cavity*: For viscera (liver, spleen, gallbladder, kidney, urinary bladder) any distention, and evidence of fluid in the abdomen, any palpable lump (note its characters in detail).

Percussion

Obliteration of liver dullness indicates *perforation of hollow viscus*. Shifting dullness indicates fluid in the peritoneal cavity. Suprapubic dullness signifies distension of urinary bladder. *With dullness in iliac fossa, suspect iliac abscess.*

Auscultation

Auscultation of all quadrants is mandatory. The continuous presence of normal bowel sounds in all quadrants is against the diagnosis of intra-abdominal injury (complete absence of bowel sounds indicates paralytic ileus or serious abdominal injury). Muffled and interrupted bowel sounds may be heard in mild intra-abdominal injury, paralytic ileus or early intra-abdominal bleeding. Increased bowel sounds indicate early intestinal obstruction (which may later turn into paralytic ileus). Note for any adventitious sound (arterial bruit).

Measurements

Repeated measurement of the girth of abdomen at the umbilicus should be done in cases of injury. Gradual increase, coupled with clinical deterioration, is an important evidence of intraperitoneal bleeding.

Per Rectal/Per Vaginal Examination

Tenderness and soft swelling in the rectovesical pouch, may indicate intraperitoneal haemorrhage or rupture of bladder.

INVESTIGATION

i. *X-ray*: In plain X-ray of abdomen in sitting posture, air (gas) shadow under diaphragm, indicates perforation of hollow viscus. Distended intestinal loop shadows signify distention (obstruction). Multiple horizontal fluid levels, indicate paralytic ileus/obstruction.

ii. *Paracentasis and peritoneal lavage*: Aspiration of blood from sub-umbilical midline region helps in establishing the diagnosis of abdominal injuries.

Diagnostic peritoneal lavage is particularly useful in comatose or semicomatose patients due to associated head injuries, alcoholic intoxication or drug ingestion.

iii. *Ultrasound*: In case of injury, increase in visceral shadow indicates perivisceral haematoma. Repeated ultrasonography, may be prognostic regarding increasing or regressing perivisceral haematoma.

iv. *CT scan*: It may help in diagnosing and localising the retroperitoneal haematoma.

v. *Magnetic resonance imaging (MRI)*: It helps in localisation of the pathology/injury more clearly.

vi. *Exploratory laparotomy*: Even diagnostic laparotomy may prove more rewarding, especially in case of unresolved suspicion, and may provide a chance of therapeutic surgical measures.

Key Diagnostic Points

Rupture Liver

Due to direct injury on right lower thorax and right upper abdomen (e.g. steering wheel injury).

— General features of extreme shock.

— Tenderness and rigidity, more in right hypochondrium and lower right intercostal spaces.

— Increased area of liver dullness.

— Shifting dullness.

— May be associated with fracture of right lower ribs.

Splenic Rupture

— Due to crush injury over left lower chest/left upper abdomen.

— Usually with overlying fracture of left lower ribs.

— Local tenderness and rigidity, more in left hypochondrium.

— Hyperaesthesia and pain in left shoulder, referred from the left sub-diaphragmatic area (Kehr's sign).

— Persistent dullness mainly in left upper abdomen, and left flank, but shifting dullness in the right flank (Ballance's sign).

— Pointed finger tip pressure in between sternomastoid and scalenus medius in supraclavicular region initiates severe pain (Saegessar's splenic point).

Renal Injury

— Usually due to injuries in lumbar region (blow or fall or runover).

— Tenderness in and around the renal angle.

— Varying swelling and dullness over the renal angle.

— Passing of blood in urine.

— All the samples of urine should be preserved to look for presence of blood in the urine. (Haematuria may occur even after three weeks due to dislodgement of clot).

— Abdominal distention may develop due to irritation of splanchnic nerves by retroperitoneal haematoma.

Urinary Bladder Injury

— Intraperitoneal rupture of bladder (20%)—follows injury while bladder is full and leads to peritonitis.

— Extraperitoneal rupture (80%)—follows pelvic injuries (see chapter on Pelvic Injury)—suprapubic tenderness, little dullness in hypogastrium, blood/clot in urine.

- Severe injuries of most of the abdominal viscera produce profound shock.
- Rupture of hollow abdominal viscera leads to severe peritonitis (abdominal pain, features of shock, rigid abdomen, muffled or absent bowel sounds).
- Rupture of major blood vessels is usually fatal.

In spinal injuries or following surgery on the spine, or a peritoneal lavage, the features of paralytic ileus commonly develop (distended abdomen and with tinkling bowel sounds). In these cases, or even after applying plaster jacket/spica a very severe complication—acute dilatation of the stomach—may occur (acute distention of upper abdomen, very weak/absent bowel sounds, left diaphragm pushed up in chest which develops increased resonance, persistent vomitting, profound shock, unless managed very promptly, this condition is fatal).

Among nontraumatic conditions, the abdomen and allied zones requires examination for:

i. Any referred pain (e.g. caries spine, spinal injury).
ii. Search for a cold/hot abscess (e.g. in abdominal wall; in pelvis—psoas abscess, iliac abscess).
iii. Palpating lower abdomen for vertebral prominence (e.g. spondylolisthesis).

Iliac Abscess

— It is commonly confused with hip pathology.
— Patient can be of any age—from a young child to an adult.
— Constitutional features—fever rangingp up to 38.5°C or even more. Patient toxic.
— Keeps the hip flexed and slightly externally rotated.
— Resistant, firm tender mass felt in iliac fossa (which should be normally empty).
(cf.) In *psoas abscess* resistant firm tender mass is felt by the side of the vertebrae. While palpating psoas abscess support the flank from behind by one hand and palpate by tips of four fingers of opposite hand against the sides of the lumbar vertebrae.
— Iliac fossa dull on percussion (compare with the other side).
- Take the patient in confidence, further flex the hip and demonstrate the free rotational movements of the hip (this rules out any hip pathology).
— Aspiration of pus is confirmatory.

22 How to Read an X-ray Plate

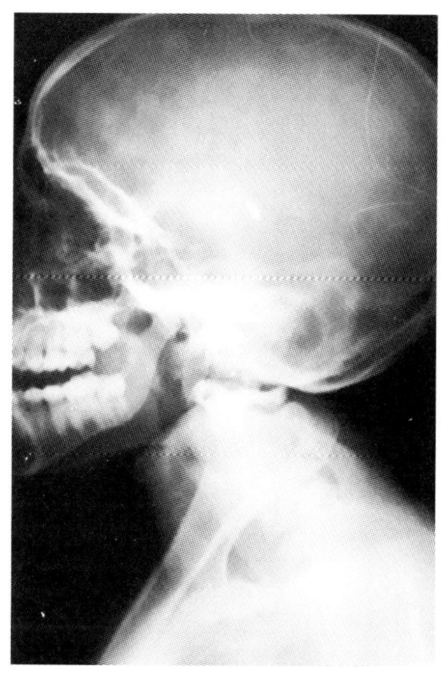

For proper diagnosis the quality of X-ray must be of good standard, i.e. adequately positioned, exposed, developed (so as to show all gradations of the gray scale by which fine differences of skin, subcutaneous tissues, muscle mass, intervening fascial planes, bone and joint details can be delineated), properly washed, nicely dried up and should be free from artifact.

While exposing for the bone and joint pathologies following general principles should be observed:

- Full length of the limb bone should be exposed if possible.
- X-ray plate should be long enough to include the zones beyond the suspected length, and should include at least one joint nearer to the pathology.

In case of a joint, at least 1/3rd to 1/2 of the adjoining bones on either side must be included.

- All soft tissues from all around the bone/joint should be included.
- X-ray must be taken in at least two planes—anteroposterior and lateral—and preferably the oblique view should also be always taken.
- Special views are required for special visualisation whenever needed.
- Stress views are required in suspected instability of any joint or suspected nonunion of a fracture.

Inspect a plate against a bright light. Proceed in the following order—Confirm the name of the patient; type of X-ray (plain, contrast, tomogram, etc.) view taken, part exposed, extent of inclusion and side of the limb or part. Then read systematically:

A. *Soft Tissue Shadow*

Increased (generalised or localised), normal, decreased; texture, i.e., clear delineation of different layers; ground glass appearance (homogenous), etc. Any abnormal content, e.g. shadow in soft tissue zone, e.g.

a. radiopaque shadow, e.g. metallic foreign body, bony piece (e.g. sequestrum, calcified parasites, cysticerci, guinea worm, new bone forming tumours, calcified blood vessel wall, phleboliths, calcification in ligaments, faecolith (in case of pelvis and lumbar and sacral and coccygeal region of spine), myositic mass.

b. entrapped transluscent area—e.g. air in sinus tract, gas in muscle plàines (gas gangrene), surgical emphysema.

B. *Joint*

Joint space—(Radiological space = anatomical joint space + area occupied by articular cartilage)

- Periarticular tissues
- Clear, fuzzy
- Increased, normal, decreased
- Regular, uniform
- Any radiopaque shadow in the joint space
- Any bony trabeculation across the joint.

C. *Articulating Bones*

- Interrelation between the articulating bones (always compare with opposite side if possible) for congruity—normal, subluxated (partial dissociation), dislocated (complete dissociation)
- Margins—uniform, erosion, destruction, osteophytes, collapse
- Subchondral area—condensations, rarefaction, cysts/cyst like spaces, destruction, sequestrum

D. *In a Long Bone Shadow Look for*

- Overall alignment
- Average bone age, and sex (if possible)
- Different areas—articular ends, metaphyseal areas, diaphyseal area.
- Cortical shadow—texture—normal, thickened, thinned, destruction, breach in the continuity—pseudo or real fractures, reactionary bone laying—its type, pattern, extent, any associated lesions (subperiosteal longitudinal or sunburst).
- Medullary shadow—mainly in the diaphyseal area—any cystic area, texture, any abnormal content, expansion of medulla, trabecular pattern.
- Corticomedullary delineation.
- Condition of growth plate shadow (in case of infants, children and adolescents)—uniformity, widening, destruction, premature fusion, irregular fusion.

23 Advanced Diagnostic Imaging

Technology has become the symbol of today's life and so also of the modern medicine. After the discovery of X-rays by physicist Wilhelm Conrad Röentgen (1845-1922), this has become the most useful method of diagnostic imaging. The advanced techniques of imaging are more or less 'developed and modified' forms of X-ray technology. The goal of any imaging study is to define accurately the pathomorphological changes in any specific tissue, organ or part of body.

Earlier radiographic imaging studies, e.g. plain radiography, computed tomography and radionuclide studies played major role in evaluation of musculoskeletal disorders. However, they focussed mainly on detection of osseous abnormalities. With the development of MRI, it is now possible to evaluate non-invasively the soft tissue structures as well.

Contrast media (air, gas, or iodine based liquids) is used with X-rays for delineating the tract, cavities or spaces for knowing their size, patency, direction and occupancy. The contrast material is introduced (injected) into blood vessels, body fluids, cavities, tracts, and organs. This leads to a marked differences in the coefficient of absorption of the X-rays by the adjacent structures which provides diagnostic contrast between the tissues.

Usually contrast media are of following types (Table 23.1).

Iodine based liquids can be ionic, water soluble, or oily. The former two are less irritant, less toxic, miscible, and get rapidly absorbed and excreted. The latter is more irritant, more toxic, non-miscible and very slowly absorbable. Of the iodides, metrizamide—a non-ionic and least toxic and least irritant—is most commonly used. Contrast media is usually used for following investigations (Table 23.2).

MRI—Paramagnetic contrast agents are used to delineate the lesion in better way. They decrease the T_1 and T_2 of adjacent protons and act as proton relaxation enhancers. The contrast media dimeglumine gadopentate (Magnevist) is commonly used.

Table 23.1: Contrast media

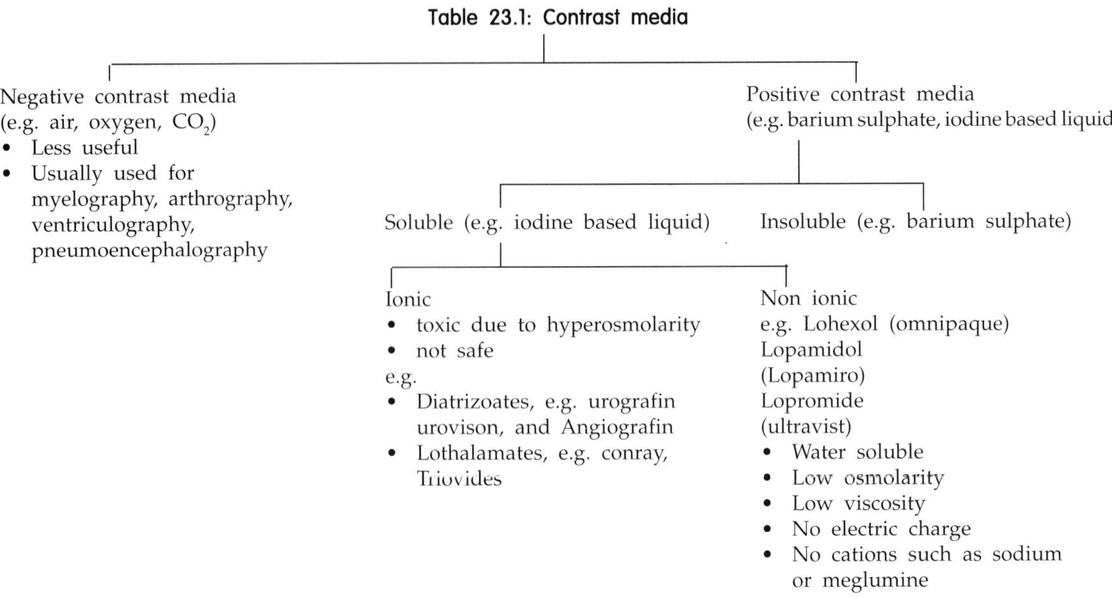

Table 23.2: Investigations where contrast media is usually used

Name of investigation		*Place where dye is injected*	*Indications*
Sinography or fistulography	Ionic contrast media is used.	Contrast liquid is injected into the sinus through its mouth	To know the direction, extent, source, and cause of sinus
Arthrography	6 to 10 ml of conray 280 or urografin 60% or non-ionic Omnipaque or Lopamidol	Contrast liquid is injected into the joint	To know the damage of intra-articular structures, e.g. ACL, meniscal tears in knee; to outline the intra-articular cartilaginous structures, e.g. femoral head in CDH To confirm the loosening of the prosthesis where the dye will percolate around the loosened stem, i.e. bone-cement interface; to confirm the capsular tear, etc.
Discography		Contrast liquid is injected in the intervertebral disc	To diagnose the disc degeneration and prolapse
Facetography		Contrast liquid is injected into the facet joints	To delineate the abnormalities of the facet joints; rupture of the facet joint capsule
Myelography and Radiculography. Nowadays, it is usually combined with CT (postmyelogram CT or myelo CT or even MRI. 100 ml of contrast media is used to obtain optimal scans.	10 ml of iohexol (omnipaque 180 to 240 mgm/ml) or 10 ml of iopamidol 200 to 250 mgm/ml	Contrast liquid is injected into the subarachnoid space	To delineate any pressure on the spinal cord and roots, e.g. extramedullary spinal tumours; intervertebral disc herniation; to know the dimensions of the vertebral canal (e.g. canal stenosis)

Non-invasive diagnostic aids, such as tomography, xeroradiography, ultrasonography scintigraphy, computed axial tomography, and magnetic resonance imaging have definitely improved the accuracy of diagnosis without many of the attendant risks. However, certain disadvantages of these diagnostic aids, as noted below, prevent them from being ordered as a routine procedure.

Disadvantages

- Most of them are too expensive.
- The findings are too difficult for interpretation by average clinicians, except in too obvious pathologies, most of which can be fairly and accurately diagnosed by much less cheap good quality X-rays.
- One has to mostly rely on the radiologist's report which is usually written without interaction with the clinicians and the patients. Hence at times, the reports confuse the clinical diagnosis.
- Unless two or more of the above aids are combined, there is lack of specificity and accuracy in diagnosis.

TOMOGRAPHY

Tomography is the X-ray image focused on a desired plane. The word tomogram is derived from the word 'tomos' (= cut or section). By rotating the tube and the X-ray film in opposite directions on any imaginary pivot, the pictures produced on either side of the pivotal plane are blurred out. The object under study is demonstrated in a succession of different layers of the object cut into a number of sections or slices. Pictures obtained on different plane-cuts, reveal the lesions which are obscured on plane X-rays.

Its disadvantage is relatively high dose of radiation to the patient. Advent of CT and MRI are outdating the tomography.

Uses of Tomography

- Tomography can be helpful in clarifying the vague and obscured findings of plane X-rays, and occult injuries. It can assist in further assessment of a known fracture or fracture-dislocation.
- It reveals the deep seated lesions, e.g. osteoid osteoma, brodies abscess, infective focus, etc.
- It may help identify a less obvious sequestrum or subchondral bony plate destruction in septic arthritis and thus distinguish it from periarticular osteoporosis, where the subchondral plate remains intact.
- In spinal region, tomography is very useful for identifying the facet fractures and the obscured defects in the pars interarticularis.
- It was earlier used to demonstrate the tuberculous infilterations and cavities in the lung.

XERORADIOGRAPHY

'Xero' means 'dry'. The xeroradiography is dry procedure in which the wet process of developing and fixing the films are not used.

Routine X-ray exposures are also used in Xeroradiography. An aluminium plate is coated with the thin layer of selenium and charged electrically. Selenium plate has photoconductive behaviour. The X-ray beam is passed through the part of body, to be studied, to reach the plate. Here the response is registered as an electrically charged density pattern on the recording plate as the latent image, which is developed by blowing a thin powder (Toner) over selenium coated plate on which the powder adheres in the proportion of the charge present over there. Then it is reproduced in the form of positive images on a plastic coated paper which becomes the permanent record. The photoelectrical process involved here, is mainly sensitive to variations in the tissue density.

Uses of Xeroradiography

Xeroradiography produces a very high grade of soft tissue contrast, which is not obtained on routine radiography.

Vague, obscured and fuzzy lesions, e.g. subperiosteal erosions (e.g. in early osteomyelitis), early soft tissue calcification (e.g. in myositis ossificans), early cartilaginous calcification (e.g. in chondrocalcinosis, foreign bodies of low density), etc. can be displayed not only more easily but also earlier than by the use of plane X-rays. It is widely used for mammography.

Disadvantage of xeroradiography is that, for exposing the deeper and thicker part, a high dose of radiation is required.

ULTRASONOGRAPHY

Sounds of frequency higher than 20,000 Hz are called 'ultrasonics'. Sounds of frequency lower than 20 Hz are called infrasonics or subsonics. We cannot hear the ultrasonic and infrasonic sounds. They travel with same speed as the audible sound.

Ultrasonography can be utilised for diagnostic (ultrasonography) and therapeutic purposes. The principle of ultrasonography is based on the recording of reflection of sound waves from the resistances of different densities. High frequency sound waves produced by a transducer can penetrate several centimetres through the soft tissues. While passing through the tissue-interfaces, few of these sound waves are reflected back as echoes to the transducer. As the echoes are received as electrical signals, these can be registered as images on a screen or a plate with the help of various equipments. The tissues of different densities can be reproduced as images in gradations of grey, which can reasonably delineate the anatomical outline.

According to the structural character of the tissues, their echogenisity vary. They can be highly echogenic (mostly solid, e.g. fat), mildly echogenic (e.g. semisolids) or echofree (e.g. fluid filled cysts).

Uses of Ultrasonography

- Due to contrast echogenisity of solid and cystic masses, ultrasonography is mainly useful in diagnosing the deep seated cystic lesions, e.g. abscesses, haematomas, cysts, aneurysms, intra-articular fluids, etc. in differentiating between cellulitis, abscess, osteomyelitis.
- It is almost routinely used to screen the neonates for the dysplasia (CDH) of hip. Ultrasonography can well demarcate the relation between acetabular labrum and cartilaginous femoral head epiphysis.
- Ultrasonography can be helpful in diagnosing the rotator cuff injuries of the shoulder; internal derangements of the knee; in Perthes' disease of hip-growth and development in bony and cartilaginous portions of the femoral head, early changes like irregularity and fissuring and late changes like flattening and fragmentation. However, the interpretation may be difficult and even inaccurate.
- Study of extent and nature of soft tissue masses; muscle pathologies (e.g. rupture, inflammation, haematoma, myositis ossifans); tendon pathologies (e.g. tendinitis, tears, tumours); bursal pathologies (bursitis, chronic degenerative changes, etc.).

SCINTIGRAPHY (Radioactive Isotope or Radionuclides Studies)

Different tissues take up radioactive isotopes (radionuclides) according to their activities, and emit photons, which can be recorded by simple rectilinear scanner or a gamma camera to produce an image. Radiotracers are injected intravenously and their passage through organs and parts being studied, is seen with gamma camera.

In orthopaedic practice, radioactive isotopes commonly used are technetium 99 m phosphate (99mTc to study vascularity and osteoblastic activity), gallium 67 citrate (67 Ga to study macrophage uptake for diagnosing inflammation and infection), technetium-labelled sulphur colloid (99 m Tc-Sc), and indium-111-labelled leucocytes to assess leucocyte concentration, e.g. in infections; Indium chloride is used to diagnose loosening of prosthesis. Of these isotopes, technetium 99m has been found to be ideal for radionuclide imaging and it emits gamma rays. It has a short half-life (6 hours) and appropriate energy characters for recording by gamma camera. It is excreted rapidly by the kidney into the urine. Combined with bone seeking phosphate compound, it is selectively concentrated in bony structures. The low background activity indicates clear visibility of any increased uptake.

Of recently, the radioactive technetium-labelled hydroxymethlene diphosphonate (99 mTc-HDP) is being used intravenously and the uptake activities are recorded in three phases.

i. The 'flow phase': It is akin to radionuclide angiogram demonstrating the blood flow.
ii. 'Immediate' or 'perfusion' or 'equilibrium' or 'blood-pool' phase: immediately after the injection, the image shows relative vascular flow and distribution of radioisotope in the perivascular and extracellular space.
iii. Delayed or bone phase: Two to four hours after the injection, when most of the isotope has been excreted, except that taken up in the bone by its osteoblastic activities.

Normally in the equilibrium phase, the periarticular vascular tissues take up the isotope most actively and produce darkest images, which gradually fade away.

Two to four hours later in the 'delayed phase', the uptake is more in the metaphyseal cancellous area showing more activity, and the outlines of bones are shown more clearly.

Abnormal recordings of the uptake are significant when it is sharply localised or obviously asymmetrical. Broadly the abnormal recordings can be of four types:

i. Increased uptake (activity) in the 'equilibrium' or 'perfusion' phase: It indicates increased vascularity of the soft tissues, e.g. in acute (or even chronic) inflammatory changes.
ii. Decreased uptake (activity) in 'equilibrium' phase: It indicates decreased vascularity of the soft tissues. It is an unusual finding.
iii. Increased uptake (activity) in 'delayed' phase: It indicates increased activities in the extracellular fluid or more enthusiastic cellular activities in the process of new bone formation in fracture healing, inflammation of bone, bone tumours (Fig. 23.1), revascularisation in osteonecrosis, myositic activities and hetrotropic bone formation.

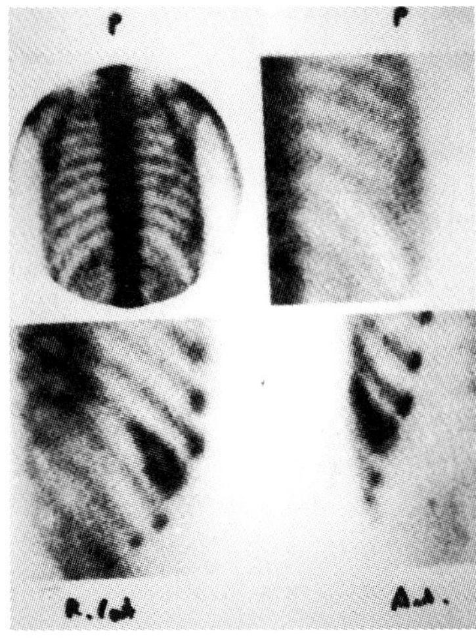

Fig. 23.1: Bone scintigraphy using technetium, showing increased uptake in right 8th rib (neoplasm) against the normal low background activity in rest of bones

Osteomyelitis focus usually presents as an area of increased tracer uptake (hot area), but in infants, due to oedematous occlusion of the intramedullary vessels, there decreased delivery of the isotope leading to decreased tracer uptake (cold area).

The tracer (technetium 99 m) uptake will be more in the active bone tumours, bone involvements in malignant soft tissue tumours and occult bone metastasis.

iv. Decreased uptake (activity) in 'delayed' phase: It indicates decreased vascularity of the bone, e.g. in avascular necrosis of femoral head, fibrotic replacement of bony tissues, etc.

Uses of Scintigraphy

- Enthesopathy (disease activities at the sites of tendon and ligament attachment to the bone), e.g. inflammatory, degenerative, metabolic, traumatic disorders affecting the pelvis, trochanter, humeral tuberosity, patella, osteitis pubis, etc.

- Early detection and localisation of inflammatory changes, e.g. acute osteomyelitis focus, bone abscess.
- Early detection of bony metastasis.
- Detection and localisation of avascular necrosis of bone (e.g. in Perthes' disease, idiopathic osteonecrosis, avascular necrosis following fractures, etc.). In Perthes' disease it can be used to evaluate early stages of pathological process. In the very early stage, uptake of technetium 99 m is decreased, and it remains variable or is increased when the symptoms appear.
- Detection of infection in prosthetic replacement.
- Early detection of stress fracture.
- Detection of degenerative joint diseases.
- Studies of joint pathologies, e.g. activity in rheumatoid arthritis, ankylosing spondylitis, osteoarthritis.
- Bone graft viability, uptake, etc.

Coregistration Imaging

To localise the pathology more accurately selective use of coregistration scanning can be a useful technique (e.g. for investigating patients with pain in foot, ankle or wrist, etc).

Coregistration Processing

The X-ray is processed and digitised on a UMAX vist 58 flat bed scanner at 75 dpi. The co-ordinates of the position of the equivalent markers in the two images are identified. From the sets of pairs of markers a transformation matrix is devised, which coregisters the radiograph and isotope scan so that these images can be superimposed on each other (Robinson *et al* 1998).

IMMUNOSCINTIGRAPHY

Whereas X-ray, including CT, sonography, and MRI all visualise tumours by reason of the morphologic differences between the neoplasm and the surrounding healthy tissue, the nuclear medicine (scintigraphy) makes use of specific actions or reactions or special surface structure of tumour cells to demonstrate neoplastic tissue. In immunoscintigraphy, the radioactive labelled antibodies, directed against tumour-associated-surface antigens, are injected intravenously and the site of the antigen-antibody reaction is located and imaged by recording the emitted gamma rays with a gama camera. The development of monoclonal antibodies and the possibilities of labelling them with short-lived technetium has significantly increased the use of immunoscintigraphy in clinical practice.

Attempts are being made to use the antibodies for therapeutic purposes after labelling them with the substances, which emit alpha and beta rays rather than the gamma rays.

Presently, immunoscintigraphy is being utilised for making specific diagnosis of recurrence and metastasis in colorectal cancer and other tumours producing carcinoembryonic antigen (CEA), ovarian carcinomas, lymphomas and melanomas. This technique is rarely a meaningful method for primary tumour diagnosis. (Weib, ML 1993).

CAT SCAN

In 1974, Douglas Hounsfeld discovered the CAT scan machine, which opened the vistas of human anatomy with great precision and most of the time help patients get rid of an eager scalpel.

CT (computed tomography) produces transaxial cutting images through selected tissue planes, by which the anatomical planes, not delineable by plane X-rays, can be visualised. In CT scanning also the X-ray is utilised. The X-ray emits from a X-ray tube installed inside a machine known as 'gantry'. The part to be CT scanned is kept in the round portion of the 'gantry'.

At first a 'survey view' of the region should be taken in which the affected area is selected and through it a series of cross-sectional images are obtained. Cutting slices are usually 5-10 mm apart, when done through the bigger joints or the tissues. However much thinner slices are cut in case of small joints, intervertebral disc or smaller tissues.

The value of CT is further increased when with the help of special equipment, different transaxial cut images are reconstructed in coronal or sagittal or even three dimensional (3D) images of bones with complicated shape, e.g. vertebrae.

CT displays the bony structures clearly but does not define accurately the soft tissues.

Advantages of CT Scan

- Cross-sectional images
- No hinderances by overlying soft tissues
- Superior contrast resolution
- Detection of even early calcification
- Detection of soft tissue involvement in neoplasms
- Visualisation of joint details—cartilages and ligaments are better visualised
- Various tissue characteristics can be delineated by measuring the Housefield units, especially in differentiating fat from other soft tissue and bones.
- Contrast enhancement is possible by intravenous injection of iodine based contrast medium.

The *main recent advances* in CT Scanning are:

- (3D) Three dimensional CT
- Real time Multiplaner Reconstructions
- High resolution CT
- Dynamic CT
- Dental CT.

Uses of CT

CT has proved to be a very useful diagnostic aid in assessing the anatomical dimension of spinal canal, spinal trauma and diseases.

Canal Stenosis

Standard CT in cross-sectional mode can suggest foraminal narrowing. CT is useful in defining the lateral recess stenosis and foraminal stenosis, which is hardly possible in myelography.

CT is helpful in assessing the degree of encroachment of spinal canal by a fractured fragment, herniated intervertebral disc or any other space occupying lesion. The best way of confirming the diagnosis is by metrizamide or iohexol myelography combined with a reformatted computed tomography scan of the suspected segment. Combined with MRI, postmyelogram contrast CT can suggest 96-97 per cent accurate diagnosis.

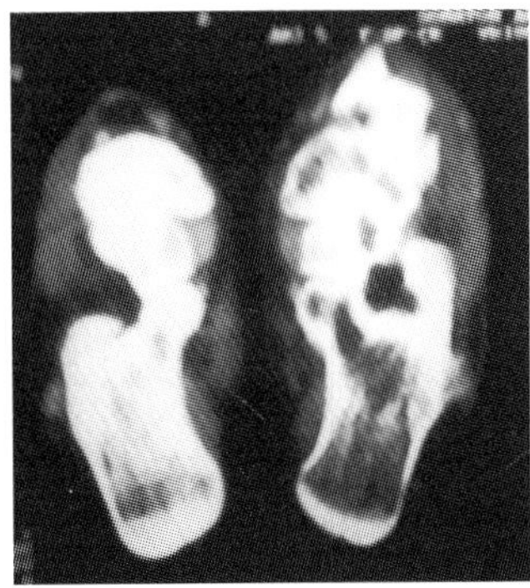

Fig. 23.2A: CT of both hind feet showing a cystic destruction in right talus (giant cell tumour)

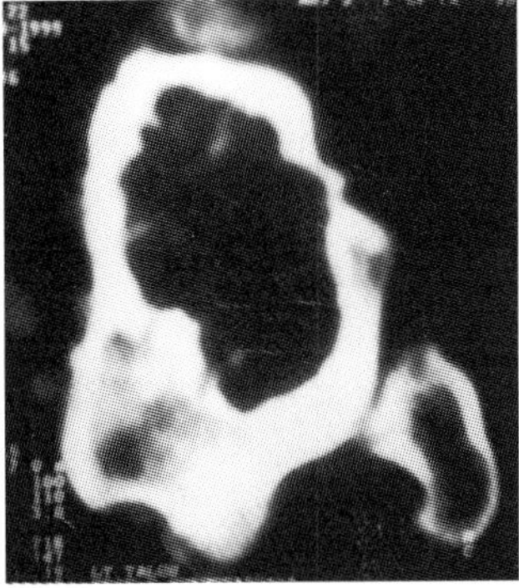

Fig. 23.2B: Enlarged view of right talus showing large areas of destruction in the neck, head and part of body of talus

Radiation exposure of 4.8 to 7 rads, and the need for an invasive procedure for injecting the dye are disadvantages of contrast CT.

Spinal Trauma

Fractures of cervicothoracic and thoracic or thoracolumbar regions may be missed on plane X-rays. Injuries to osseous, ligamentous, and neurological structures can be evaluated with a high degree of accuracy through the sophisticated imaging technique like tomography, contrast myelography, postmyelogram CT with sagittal reconstruction, and MRI.

CT is helpful in assessing the degree of compromise of the spinal canal.

Reformatted CT scans of the cervical spine usually present less distinct picture than in the lumbar spine.

Infections of Spine

Broad findings of the CT scan are more or less similar to those of plane X-rays including the lytic lesions in the subchondral zones, destruction of the end plate, sclecrosed margin of the lytic lesions, lesser density and flattening of the disc, disruption of bone in the paradiscal and peridiscal regions, soft tissue shadows in epidural, paravertebral and paraspinal areas, and abscesses.

Postmyelogram CT clearly defines the compression of the spinal cord and other neural elements by abscess or sequestrum or bone or other materials.

Spinal Tumours

CT is of much use in assessment of the size, shape and infiltration of the tumours. Postmyelogram CT (myelo. CT) clearly defines the space, occupying growths in vertebral canal.

CT cannot demonstrate intra-spinal tumours (unlike MRI) and archnoiditis. It also cannot differentiate between old scars and new disc herniation.

CT is a very sensitive investigation for detecting pulmonary metastases in malignant tumours.

Myelography combined with multiplanar CT scans can be of much use in assessing the intraspinal and extraspinal effects of spondylolisthesis including the evaluation of disc degeneration.

Other Places, beside Spine, where CT can be Helpful

Fractures not clearly delineable in plane X-ray, can be displayed by CT, e.g. carpal, tarsal (mainly calcaneal fractures and osteochondral fractures of talus), tibial condylar, and pelvic fractures (including the injuries and pathologies of sacroiliac joints); hairline fractures.

High resolution computed tomography has been found to be very useful in studying the meniscal tears, cruciate ligament tears, disorders of complicated joints, e.g. sacroiliac, sternoclavicular, etc.

CT can be useful in assessing the patellofemoral joint, synovial cysts and soft tissue tumours in and around the knee.

MAGNETIC RESONANCE IMAGING (MRI)

The Nobel laureate Felix Bloch and EM Purcell discovered the physical phenomenon of Magnetic Resonance Imaging (MRI) in 1946, based upon assessment of radiofrequency emissions from atoms and molecules in tissues, exposed to an external magnetic field.

The medical application of NMR (Nuclear Magnetic Resonance) was pioneered by Odebald and Lindstorm in 1955, while Damadian and Hinslow were the first to produce the NMR images on 3rd June, 1977.

The images recorded in MRI are more or less similar to those of CT scans, but have more clarity and tissue contrast. It gives detailed images of both bones and different soft tissues. The sectional images can be produced in any plane, and reconstituted to project three dimensional (3D) pictures. MRI is a noninvasive procedure and allows to visualise the structures directly in all orthogonal planes.

In this technique there is interaction of nuclei of a selected atom with an external oscillating electromagnetic field, which is changing as a function of time at a particular frequency. Even though all atoms with odd number of protons have property of magnetic resonance, the hydrogen nucleus, because of its abundance in tissues and easy detectability, is used in the current technique of MRI.

The intensity of MR signals depends upon the concentration of hydrogen nuclei in the tissues underscanning and their spinning character and relaxation rates following proton excitation. The physical phenomenon of relaxation is expressed by two independent tissue constants T1 and T2, producing two signals simultaneously. While the images are produced the tissue character can be 'weighted' or enchanced to provide complementary informations. The T1 weighted images are sharp, well defined and almost anatomical in appearance. The T2 weighted images project more of the pathological characters of the tissues.

Tissues with maximum concentration of hydrogen nuclei emit high intensity signals producing the brightest images (e.g. fat, bone marrow, cancellous bone, etc.); those with little concentration of hydrogen emit low intensity signals projected as black (e.g. ligaments, bony cortex, tendons, air, etc.); and those with intermediate concentration are produced in the grey scale (e.g. cartilage, muscle, spinal canal, etc.).

Other frequently used pulse sequences are proton density and short tau inversion recovery (STIR), which has the property to suppress the signals from fat and increase the contrast for water containing tissues.

Various tissues and organs can be imaged clearly by properly adjusting the anatomical plane, type of coil, thickness of cut slice, and sequence of pulse and magnification.

Uses of MRI

MRI is marginally superior to spine myelo-CT in identifying the spinal lesions. It can suitably examine the entire spine, identify the degenerated disc, delineate the cord and root impingement (Figs 23.3A and 23.9), demonstrate the intra-spinal tumours (Figs 23.4A1, A2, 23.4B and 23.5A), and evaluate the thecal spaces and tissues in the foramen (Fig. 23.6). If combined with post-myelogram CT, the accuracy of diagnosis may be up to 95 per cent, and even non-symptomatic lesions can be identified (Fig. 23.7).

- Spinal infections (Figs 23.3B, 23.4B, 23.8A and B, 23.13) can be identified quickly and more or less accurately, and the extent of normal and infected tissues can be delineated in high quality MRI. To detect infection, T1-intermediate and T2-weighted views should be obtained in sagittal plane.

The MRI sequences typically used to evaluate the musculoskeletal system are the spin-echo, gradient echo, and short tau inversion recovery (STIR) sequences. They provide excellent contrast and spatial resolution for the evaluation of normal anatomical structures and pathological changes within the body. Spin-echo T1 weighted sequences (a short relaxation time and a short echo time) are optimum to delineate tissues containing fat or blood and provide excellent anatomical detail. Spin-echo proton-density-weighted sequences (a long relaxation time and a short echo time) are also used to assess soft tissue and bone anatomy. Spin-echo-T2 weighted sequences (a long relaxation time and a long echo time) are used to delineate tissue containing fluid or oedema. Short tau inversion recovery (STIR) and spin-echo-fat-saturated T2-weighted sequences are particularly sensitive to fluid or oedema in soft tissues and osseous structures.

The high signal intensity in cancellous bone on T1 weighted sequence. If the abnormal process contains increased free water (as with an inflammatory lesion or malignant cells), there is increased signal intensity in the cancellous bone on spin-echo T2 weighted and short tau inversion recovery sequences. If the pathology replacing the marrow fat contains fibrous tissue or additional mineralization there is low signal intensity on all of the magnetic resonance images.

With MRI it is now possible to follow non-invasively the evolution of injury, repair and remodelling of tissue and the changes of tissue-aging.

Recent advances in MRI, including faster imaging sequences and improved surface coil design have markedly increased the amount of informations provided by these images.

MRI cannot differentiate between the pyogenic and non-pyogenic infections. The calcified areas of tuberculous abscesses, so well demonstrable in plane X-ray are not identified in MRI.

In infections the patients usually remain in pain and agony, due to which they face a lot of difficulty in remaining still in a particular position for long periods. Hence motion-induced

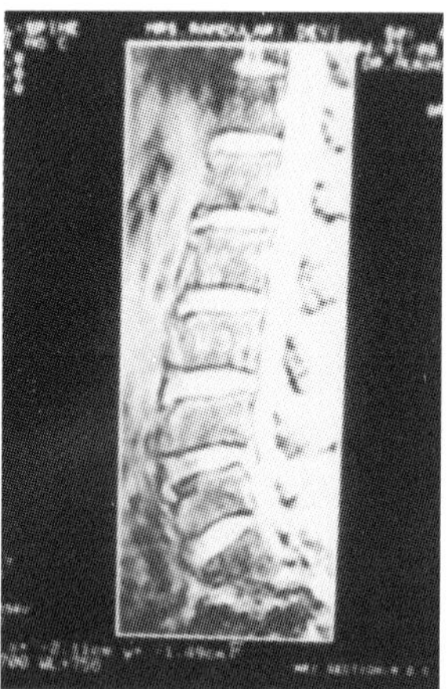

Fig. 23.3A: MRI of lumbosacral spine showing lumbar canal stenosis and posterior herniation of degenerated discs seen in mid-sagittal T1 and T2 weighted images

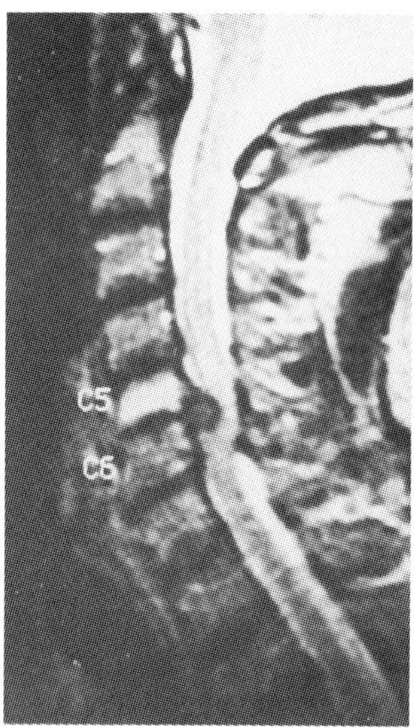

Fig. 23.3B: T1 weighted mid sagittal image showing compression at C5-6 levels due to tuberculous abscess

degradation of the findings and artefact are common and misleading.

To increase the accuracy of early detection of infection and to monitor its various pathological processes, the contrast material gadolinium-labelled diethylenetriamine pentacetic acid (Gd-DT PA) is being used in MRI. Though it is useful in detection of even doubtful infection and also

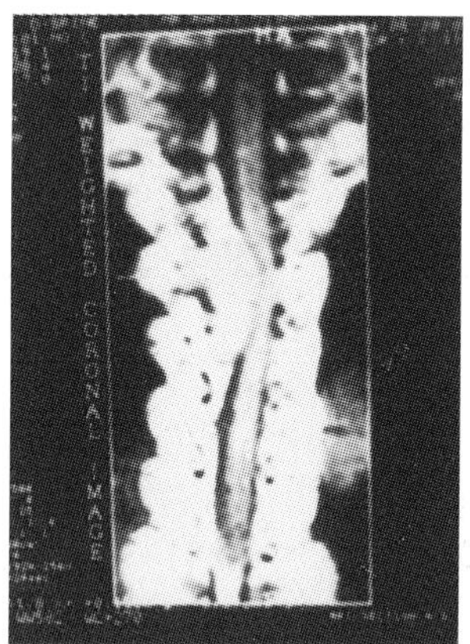

Fig. 23.4A1: MRI of dorsal spine T1 weighted image showing isointense extramedullary dumb-bell shaped spinal tumour, which looks hyperintense on. T2 weighted image. The possibility is of neurofibroma

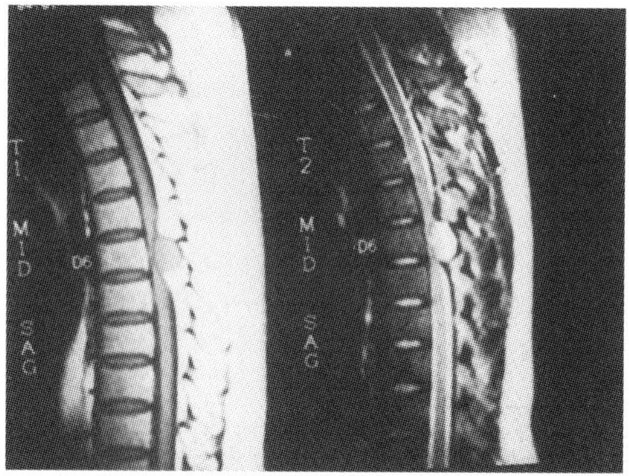

Fig. 23.4A2: MRI showing compression of the spinal cord by an oval extradural mass (neurofibroma)

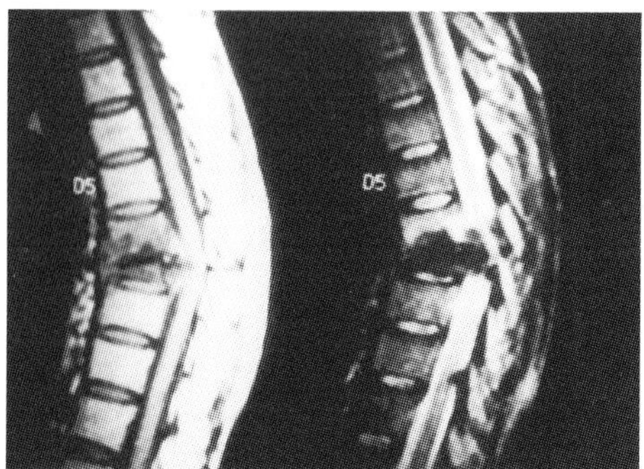

Fig. 23.4B: T1 and T2 weighted mid sagittal images showing extra-dural compression by a space occupying lesion (neoplasm or abscess)

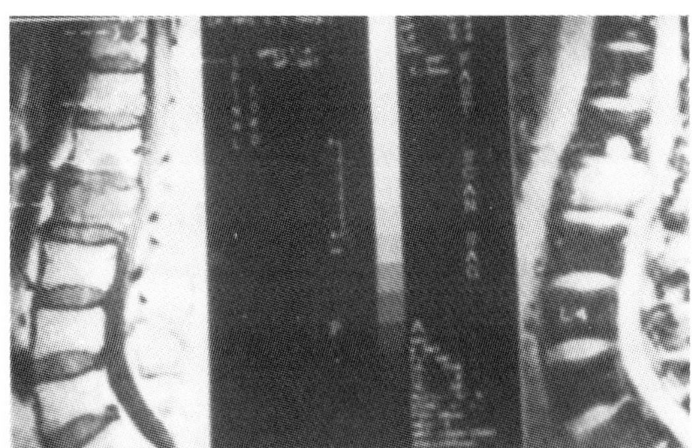

Fig. 23.5A: MRI of lumbar and lumbosacral sagittal section showing multifocal hypointense areas L2 vertebral body on T1 weighted image. Wedging of L2 vertebra, and impingement of the spinal cord by the posteriorly displaced portion of vertebral body (due to secondary metastasis)

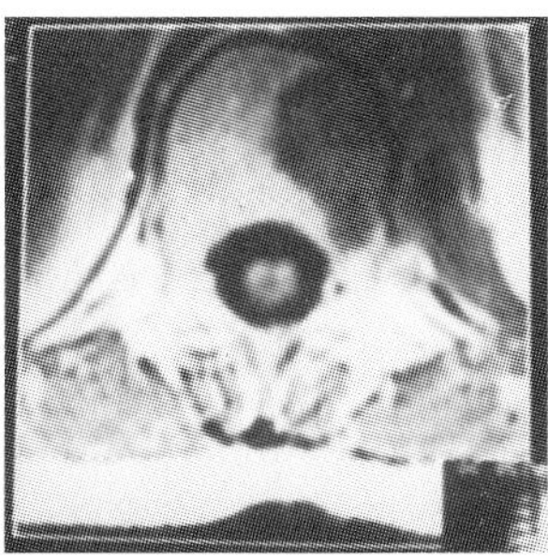

Fig. 23.5B: Coronal weighted image of the same patient (Fig. 23.5a) reveals involvement of large area of soft tissues and destruction of right pedicle of L3 level

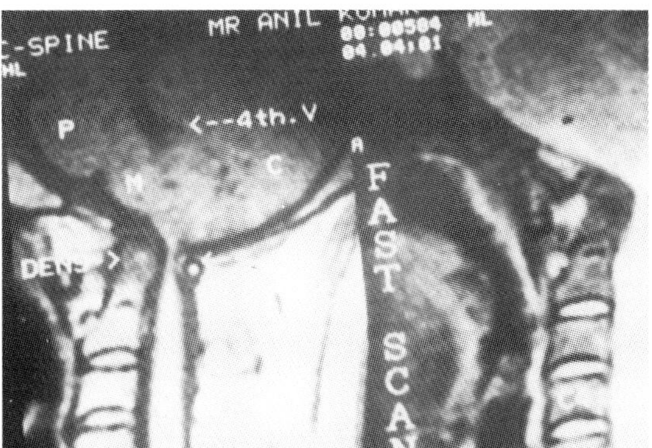

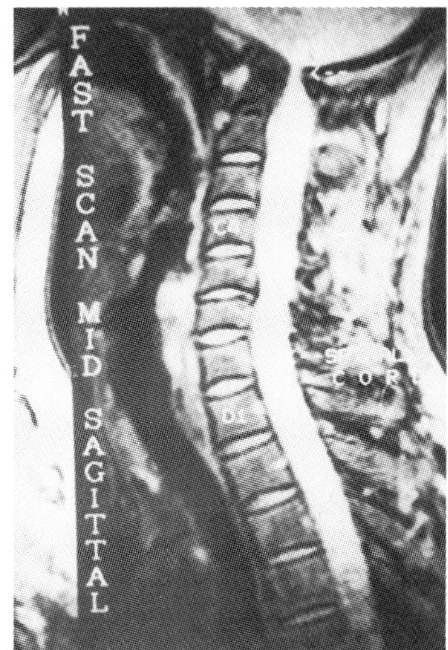

Figs 23.6A and B: MRI of craniovertebral region. Mid-sagittal T1 weighted image shows the odontoid process lying above the plane of foramen magnum, causing marked reduction in the space and pressure over the spinal cord platybasia with basillar impression in craniovertebral junctional congenital anomaly

enhances the sharp appearances of epidural and spinal infections, the added risk, expenses, and time have put reservations on its regular use.

Spinal Injuries

The role of MRI in spinal trauma is still evolving. It presents superior images of the lesions in the craniocervical and cervicothoracic regions. Its role in determining the prognosis for neurological recovery in traumatic quadriplegia or paraplegia, is being favourably reported.

In investigating the low back pain MRI must be better related to the clinical features. The recent development of MRI scanning in the erect posture may well reveal biomechanical defects and spinal pathology, which are unrecognisable when the patient is supine.

In general bone and joint infections, MRI is not much helpful. In osteomyelitis the marrow fat is replaced by oedematous fluid and cellular infiltrates. Hence in MRI there is a decrease in normally present high marrow signals on T1 weighted images and a normal or increased signal on T2 weighted images.

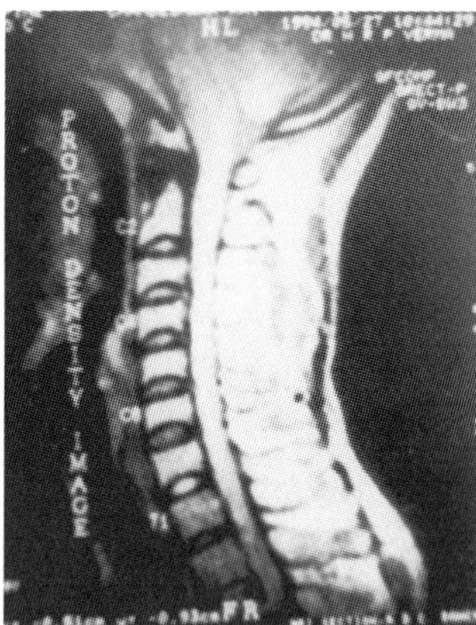

Fig. 23.7: MRI of cervical spine: Proton density and T2 weighted image shows a focal hyperintense area within the spinal cord at C3-C4 level suggestive of traumatic cord contusion

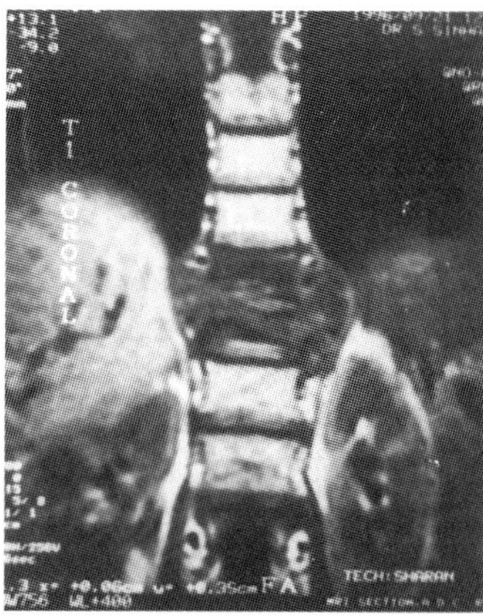

Fig. 23.8B: Coronal section showing paravertebral abscess due to tuberculous infection

MRI has a definite role (about 75 per cent positive) in early detection of the avascular necrosis of femoral head, but its regular use for clinical decision making is still being developed. Accurate estimation of the extent of osteonecrosis of the femoral head and to calculate the volume and surface area of the osteonecrosis MR images can be used but at the present time this method is too complicated for clinical application.

In carpal tunnel syndrome, the synovial diseases, narrowing of the tunnel, and median nerve compression can be well delineated in MRI.

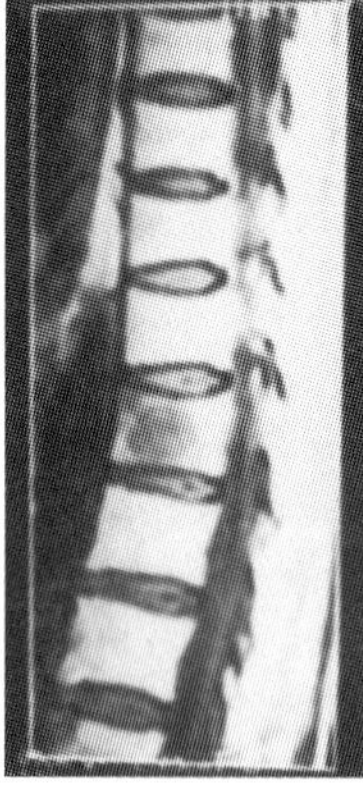

Fig. 23.8A: MRI of dorsal spine showing focal hypointense area on T1 weighted image (which appears as hyperintense area on T2 weighted image) in D12 vertebral body suggestive of tuberculous focus

MRI appears to be a very accurate investigation for assessing the extent of bone and soft tissue involvement by the tumour. There is also possibility of assessing the actual nature of the tissues which can help in the pathological diagnosis besides anatomical delineation.

The Obvious Advantages of MRI are

1. It is a non-invasive, versatile, and sensitive technique with fairly high degree of specificity and accuracy, and with no risk of ionizing radiation.
2. It does not require frequent repositioning as in myelography.

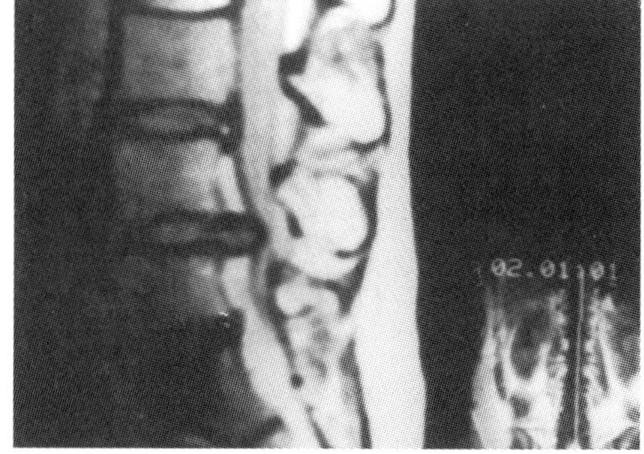

Fig. 23.9: MRI of lumbar region showing compression by L4-5 disc herniation

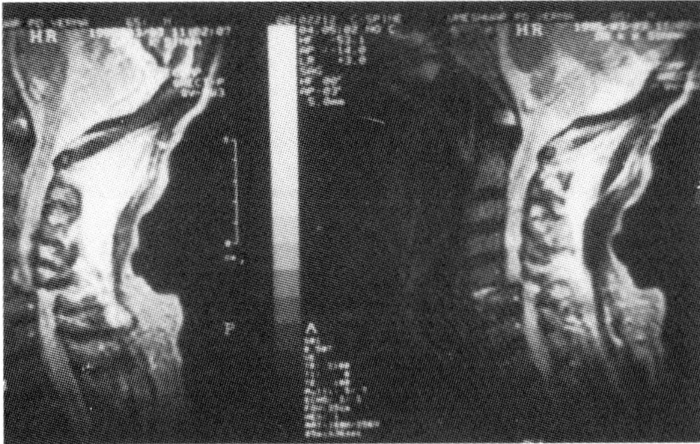

Fig. 23.10: T2 weighted image showing complete transection of cord at C6-7 levels

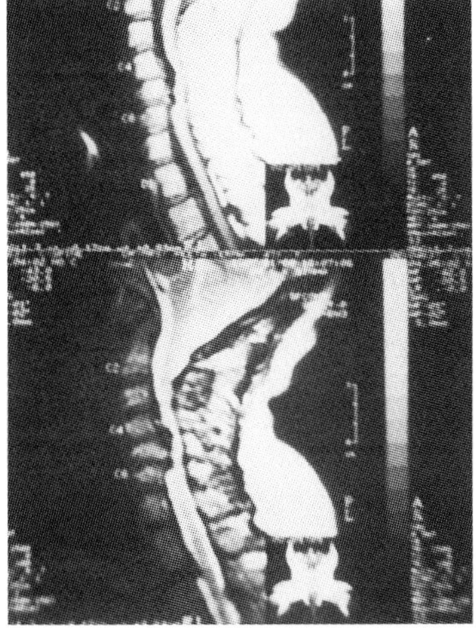

Fig. 23.11: T2 weighted image in mid-sagittal section showing epidural compression at C4-5 level probably due to calcification of posterior longitudinal ligament or thickened ligamentum level

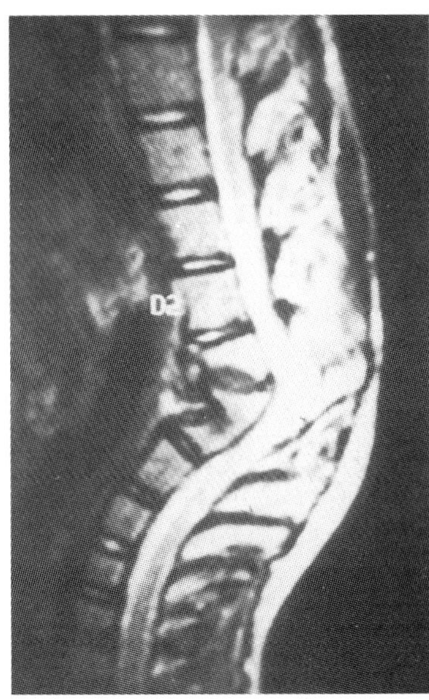

Fig. 23.12: T2 weighted mid-sagittal section showing destruction at D3-4 with compression of cord due to internal gibbus

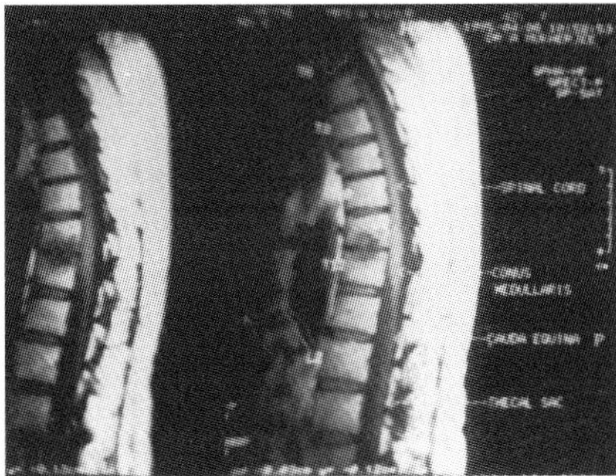

Fig. 23.13: T1 weighted mid-sagittal image showing almost kissing lesions of D10-11 and destruction of the intervertebral disc due to tuberculous infection

3. It produces clear and high soft tissue contrast differentiating the bone and soft tissues.

Disadvantages of MRI

Besides those enumerated in the beginning of the chapter, other noticeable disadvantages of MRI are:

1. It is a costly investigation.
2. It requires the patient to lie still in a particular position, which can become painful and annoying.
3. The fear of remaining in a closed container for a long period (claustrophobia) may create a problem, affecting the final result of MRI.
4. MRI is absolutely contraindicated in the persons with pace-makers, replaced joints or implants, a metallic foreign body in the eye or spine, a cerebral aneurysmal clip, some types of infusion pumps, bone or nerve stimulators and an ocular or cochlear implant. Hence the patient must

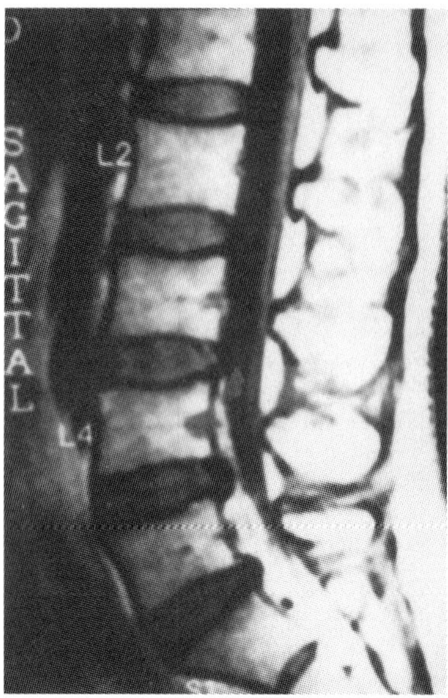

Fig. 23.14: T1 weighted mid-sagittal images showing intervertebral disc herniation pressing on cauda equina. CT myelography revealing paracentral herniation of L5-S1 compression of the nerve roots

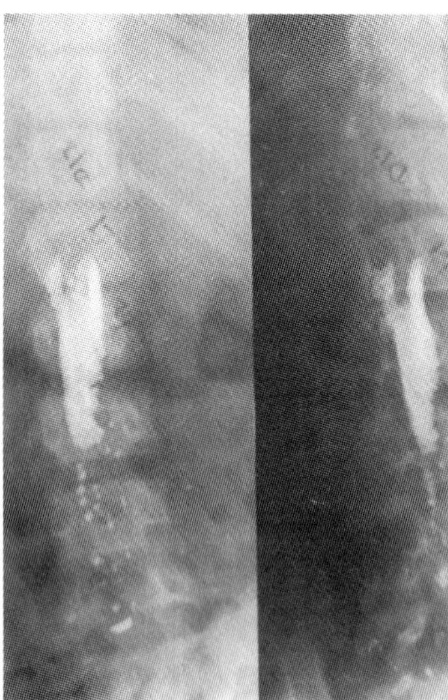

Fig. 23.15: Descending myelogram showing complete block at lower border of L4 cauda equina lesion due to massive intervertebral disc herniation

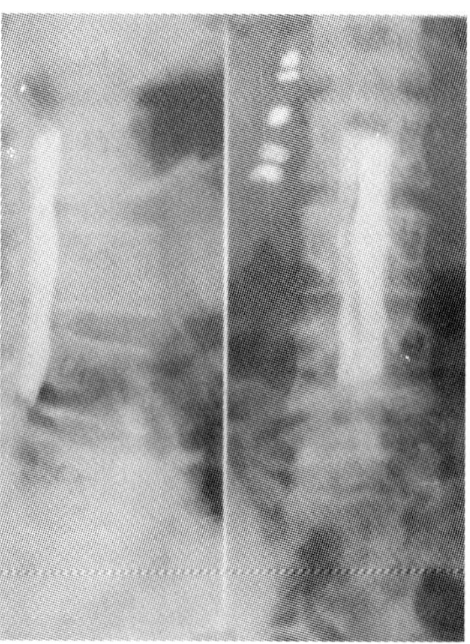

Fig. 23.16: Ascending myelograph showing block at L1 level due to meningioma

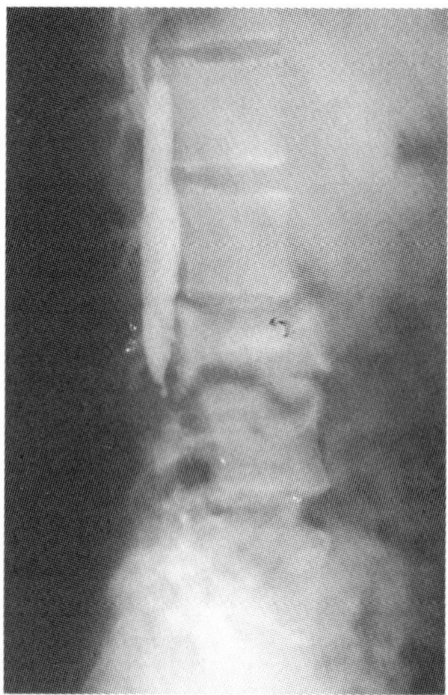

Fig. 23.17: Descending myelogram showing tapering block at the lower border of L3 vertebra due to unusual tuberculous concentrina collapse of L3

be thoroughly screened before ordering for MRI.

Redundant and unnecessary MRI must be eliminated to control the spiraling costs of health care.

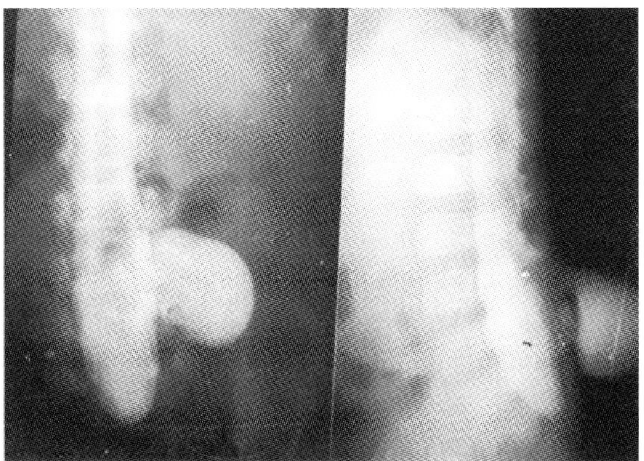

Fig. 23.18: Myelogram showing dye in pouch of meningocele

BIBLIOGRAPHY

1. Armstrong P, Keevil SF: Magnetic resonance imaging-1: basic principles of image production. *BMJ* **303**:35-40,1991.
2. Bloch F, Hanson W, Packard ME: Nuclear induction. *Physical Review* **69**: 127, 1946.
3. Damadian R: Tumour detection by nuclear magnetic resonance. *Science* **171**: 1151-53, 1971.
4. Herzog RJ: Magnetic resonance imaging of the shoulder. An instructional course lecture. *J Bone Joint Surg* **79-A**: 934-51, 1997.
5. Mansfield P. Multiplanner image formation using NMR spin echoes. *J Physical Chem* **10**: 55-58, 1977.
6. Purcell EM, Torrey HC, Pound RV. Resonance absorption by nuclear magnetic moments in a solid. *Physical Review* **69**: 37-38, 1946.
7. Robinson Ahn, Bird N, Screaton N, *et al*: Coregistration imaging of the foot. *J Bone Joint Surg* **80-B**:777-80, 1998.
8. Ullrich Sprect (Ed). X-ray Contras Media. Berlin: Springer Verlag, 1989.
9. Weib ML: Nuclear medicine methods in oncology. *Medical Focus International* **XI.5**: 16, 1993.
10. Young-Min Kim, Ahn JH, Kang HS, *et al*. Estimation of the extent of osteonecrosis of the femoral head using MRI. *J Bone Joint Surg* **80-B**: 954-58, 1998.

Appendices

Appendix 1
Syndromes related to Orthopaedics and Traumatology

ADULT RESPIRATORY DISTRESS SYNDROME (ARDS)

ARDS is a clinical syndrome which *commonly develop after severe trauma, multiple fractures, lung contusion, and fat embolism.* It can also occur after septicaemia, prolonged hypotension, gastric aspiration, massive blood transfusion, overdoses of certain drugs.

It manifests as:

- *Severe hypoxaemia,* resistant to supplemented oxygen therapy. The partial pressure of oxygen (PO2) is less than 75 in patient receiving more than 50% oxygen.
- *Diffuse fluffy pulmonary infilterates* which involve both the lungs.
- *Absence of increased pulmonary capillary hydrostatic pressure* probably due to cardiogenic cause. The pulmonary wedge pressure is less than 18.
- No other explanation for the above findings. Lungs develop diffuse alveolar damage and become stiff.

Management of ARDS is primarily the treatment of its cause. Acute cases may need mechanical ventilation. Complication should be apprehended and prevented as far as possible.

ANTERIOR CORD SYNDROME

In this syndrome there is *loss of neural functions* of the *anterior two-thirds of the spinal cord* (e.g. in spinal injury, space occupying lesions, etc.). Patient has *complete loss of motor functions below the level* of lesion (cortico-spinal tracts) and *pain, touch and temperature* sensations (spino-thalamic tracts), but has sensations of vibration, proprioception, position and light touch due to intact posterior column. These preserved sensations help in improving the rehabilitation processes and overall prognosis.

ANTERIOR IMPINGEMENT SYNDROME

It is an inflammatory process in which the *anterior capsule of the ankle joint is repeatedly impinged* with dorsiflexion in running and jumping sports. It leads to the formation of a bony spur at the anterior distal tibia and chronic pain in the ankle. It should be managed by ice *fomentation, NSAID* and *heel raise* in the footwear. The persistant problems can be relieved by athroscopic debridement and removal of bony spur.

ANTERIOR INTEROSSEOUS SYNDROME

It is the *compression neuropathy of anterior interosseous nerve* (a branch of median nerve emerging at about 5 cm below the elbow and it contains only the motor fibres for supplying the flexor pollicis longus, flexor digitorum profundus (to the index and middle fingers) and pronator quadratus muscles. Though this nerve contains only motor fibres, *pain in the forearm is the common complain* in this syndrome, which is *exacerbated by exercises and relieved by rest.* There is no significant sensory problems, except unexplained pain.

The Kilon-Neven sign is positive.

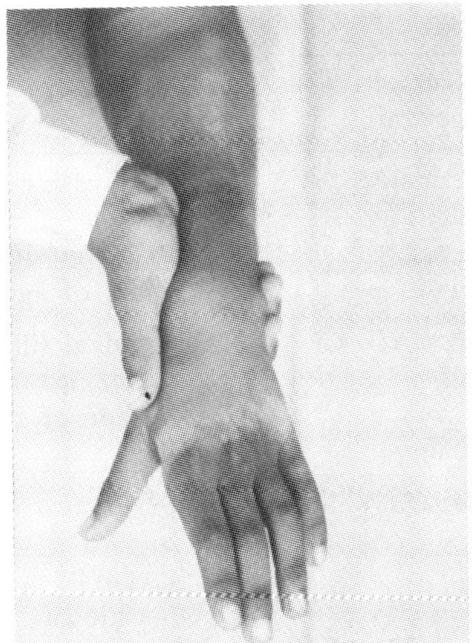

Fig. A1.6: Aquired constricting flat fibrous band following trauma (devitalised skin and subcutaneous tissue in a fan-belt injury, sloughed out and healed by second intention

or its branches (the calcaneal branch, lateral and medial plantar nerve) *in the tarsal tunnel* (a fibroosseous tunnel formed by the medial wall of calcaneum and talus and medial malleolus, and roofed by the flexor retinaculum or laciniate ligament. It contains the posterior tibial nerve and its branches, posterior tibial artery and vein, tendons of tibialis posterior, flexor digitorum longus, and flexor hallucis longus). Compression may be due to engorged veins, growths (like lipoma), fracture callus, ganglion from tendon sheath, exostosis, excessive valgus deformity, etc.

Patients complain of burning, tingling, numbness and/or pain in the sole, which increases with activities and overuse and gets relieved with rest. Occasionally the pain may radiate along the posterior tibial nerve and/or its branches.

Diagnosis is based on clinical findings, positive Tinel's sign, and EMG studies.

Management consists of NSAID, shoe-modifications, treatment of identified cause, corticosteroid injection, and surgical decompression especially in resistant cases.

THIGH COMPARTMENT SYNDROME

As in the leg, compartment syndrome can occur in thigh as well due to blunt injury to thigh with prolonged compression by any heavy object or even body weight, with or without fracture of femur. It can occur *in any of the three compartments* of thigh (i.e. quadriceps, hamstring, adductor) but *quadriceps compartment* is *mostly involved.*

THORACIC INLET SYNDROME

See page 173 in the chapter on Spine.

THORACIC OUTLET SYNDROME (Adson's Sign)

In a vice lake action, the axillary artery and brachial *plexus coursing over the first rib, may be compressed by the cervical rib* (rib, or rudimentry rib with fibrous band originating from the seventh cervical vertebra and insering onto the first rib) producing various symptoms, e.g. burning, tingling, numbness in palm and/or finger tips. The lower trunk of the brachial plexus (mainly T1) is usually compressed leading to wasting of the interossei. Axillary artery compression may gradually lead to the post-stenotic dilatation with thrombus formation and embolism. Persistant symptoms can be only relieved by decompression (removal of cervical rib and/or fibrous band).

TIETZE'S SYNDROME

It is idiopathic self-limiting *costchondritis* occurring at the *costo-sternal junctional regions* usually in the age group 25 to 50 years characterised by painful tendor enlargement of one or *more ribs (4th to 7th).* The pain increases on deep breathing, coughing, sneezing, local deep pressure and chest compression. Reassurance and NSAID usually help. In resistant cases local infiltration of corticosteroids is indicated.

TITHERED CORD SYNDROME

The filum terminale and lower end of spinal cord/or roots may get tethered to the vestigial remnants of spina bifida, which in due course may lead to various neurogenic disorders and deformities especially in ankle and foot region.